Tumors of the Testis and Adjacent Structures

AFIP Atlas
of
Tumor Pathology

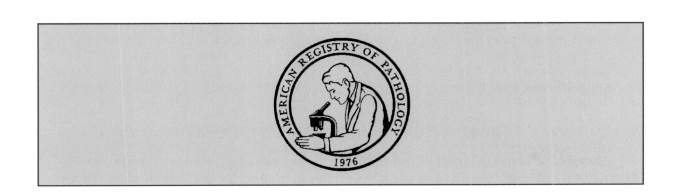

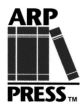

ARP PRESS

Silver Spring, Maryland

Editorial Director: Mirlinda Q. Caton
Production Editor: Dian S. Thomas
Editorial Assistant: Magdalena C. Silva
Editorial Assistant: Alana N. Black
Copyeditor: Audrey Kahn

Available from the American Registry of Pathology
Silver Spring, Maryland 20910
www.arppress.org
ISBN 1-933477-21-0
978-1-933477-21-3

AFIP ATLAS OF TUMOR PATHOLOGY

Fourth Series
Fascicle 18

TUMORS OF
THE TESTIS AND
ADJACENT STRUCTURES

by

Thomas M. Ulbright, MD
Lawrence M. Roth Professor of Pathology & Laboratory Medicine
Indiana University School of Medicine
Indiana University Health Pathology Laboratory
Indianapolis, Indiana

Robert H. Young, MD, FRCPath
Robert E. Scully Professor of Pathology
Department of Pathology
Harvard Medical School
Pathologist, James Homer Wright Pathology Laboratories
Massachusetts General Hospital
Boston, Massachusetts

Published by the
American Registry of Pathology
Silver Spring, Maryland
2013

AFIP ATLAS OF TUMOR PATHOLOGY

EDITOR
Steven G. Silverberg, MD
Department of Pathology
University of Maryland School of Medicine
Baltimore, Maryland

Manuscript reviewed by:
Ronald A. DeLellis, MD
Alberto G. Ayala, MD

EDITORS' NOTE

The Atlas of Tumor Pathology has a long and distinguished history. It was first conceived at a cancer research meeting held in St. Louis in September 1947 as an attempt to standardize the nomenclature of neoplastic diseases. The first series was sponsored by the National Academy of Sciences-National Research Council. The organization of this Sisyphean effort was entrusted to the Subcommittee on Oncology of the Committee on Pathology, and Dr. Arthur Purdy Stout was the first editor-in-chief. Many of the illustrations were provided by the Medical Illustration Service of the Armed Forces Institute of Pathology (AFIP), the type was set by the Government Printing Office, and the final printing was done at the Armed Forces Institute of Pathology (hence the colloquial appellation "AFIP Fascicles"). The American Registry of Pathology (ARP) purchased the Fascicles from the Government Printing Office and sold them virtually at cost. Over a period of 20 years, approximately 15,000 copies each of nearly 40 Fascicles were produced. The worldwide impact of these publications over the years has largely surpassed the original goal. They quickly became among the most influential publications on tumor pathology, primarily because of their overall high quality, but also because their low cost made them easily accessible the world over to pathologists and other students of oncology.

Upon completion of the first series, the National Academy of Sciences-National Research Council handed further pursuit of the project over to the newly created Universities Associated for Research and Education in Pathology (UAREP). A second series was started, generously supported by grants from the AFIP, the National Cancer Institute, and the American Cancer Society. Dr. Harlan I. Firminger became the editor-in-chief and was succeeded by Dr. William H. Hartmann. The second series' Fascicles were produced as bound volumes instead of loose leaflets. They featured a more comprehensive coverage of the subjects, to the extent that the Fascicles could no longer be regarded as "atlases" but rather as monographs describing and illustrating in detail the tumors and tumor-like conditions of the various organs and systems.

Once the second series was completed, with a success that matched that of the first, ARP, UAREP, and AFIP decided to embark on a third series. Dr. Juan Rosai was appointed as editor-in-chief, and Dr. Leslie Sobin became associate editor. A distinguished Editorial Advisory Board was also convened, and these outstanding pathologists and educators played a major role in the success of this series, the first publication of which appeared in 1991 and the last (number 32) in 2003.

The same organizational framework applies to the current fourth series, but with UAREP and AFIP no longer functiong, ARP is now the responsible organization. New features include a hardbound cover and illustrations almost exclusively in color. There is also an increased emphasis on the cytopathologic (intraoperative, exfoliative, and/or fine needle aspiration) and molecular features that are important in diagnosis and prognosis. What does not change from the three previous series, however, is the goal of providing the practicing pathologist with thorough, concise, and up-to-date information on the nomenclature and classification; epidemiologic, clinical, and pathogenetic features; and, most importantly, guidance in the diagnosis of the tumors and tumorlike lesions of all major organ systems and body sites.

As in the third series, a continuous attempt is made to correlate, whenever possible, the nomenclature used in the Fascicles with that proposed by the World Health Organization's Classification of Tumors, as well as to ensure a consistency of style. Close cooperation between the various authors and their respective liaisons from the Editorial Board will continue to be emphasized in order to minimize unnecessary repetition and discrepancies in the text and illustrations.

Particular thanks are due to the members of the Editorial Advisory Board, the reviewers (at least two for each Fascicle), the editorial and production staff, and the individual Fascicle authors for their ongoing efforts to ensure that this series is a worthy successor to the previous three.

Steven G. Silverberg, MD
Ronald A. DeLellis, MD
William A. Gardner, MD
Leslie H. Sobin, MD

PREFACE AND ACKNOWLEDGMENTS

We are honored again for the opportunity to work on the male gonad for what has become, since the inauguration of the first series in 1949, one of the prime resources for diagnostic pathologists concerning neoplasms and their mimics. Our goal has been to cover not only the common lesions but also the unusual. If we have been successful, it is in no small part due to the help of the pathology community as a whole, as many of the illustrated cases were received in consultation. We thank the many who have sent us interesting cases and who have been generous in numerous instances when we requested gross photographs. We have also continued to use material from the consultation files of Dr. Robert E. Scully, one of the true masters of gonadal pathology, and we remain grateful for having this remarkable resource to draw upon. Sadly, Dr. Scully died late in 2012 when these remarks were being prepared, so they are tinged with great sadness. One of us, Dr. Young, had the privilege of a close professional and personal association with Dr. Scully for over 30 years, an experience second to none because of Dr. Scully's remarkable skills and his wonderful personal qualities. The senior author, Dr. Ulbright, did not personally work with Dr. Scully, but got to know him well over the years and was equally aware of his kind, gentle nature and remarkable contributions to the field of pathology, including testicular pathology.

A large proportion of the material also derives from the urology services at the Indiana University Health Hospitals (IU) and the Massachusetts General Hospital (MGH). The long tradition of excellence in urologic services at these institutions, initiated by the late Dr. John P. Donohue at IU and for three decades under the stewardship of Dr. W. Scott McDougal at the MGH, has provided us with a wealth of material and insight into the clinical significance of our interpretations, something of utmost importance to practicing pathologists. It has also been a privilege for one of us, Dr. Ulbright, to collaborate over the years with Dr. Lawrence H. Einhorn, a consummate clinician who headed the Division of Oncology at IU for many years and developed the chemotherapy protocols that have made many testicular cancers curable.

As mentioned in our preface to the Third Series edition, we stand on the shoulders of giants in the field of genitourinary pathology. The homage made at that time remains. We have reached our current state of knowledge thanks to the work of these investigators, and those who have made the most seminal contributions have been paid tribute in Dr. Young's 2005 *Modern Pathology* article, "A brief history of the pathology of the gonads."

This edition represents a significant expansion of both the textual and illustrative material of the Third Series Fascicle. The numerous images reflect our belief that the "atlas" role that was the intent of the original Fascicles of the Armed Forces Institute of Pathology is of paramount importance in these works. At the same time, the current scope is no longer primarily a visual resource, but also a comprehensive description of clinical, pathologic, immunohistochemical, molecular biologic, prognostic, and to a limited extent, therapeutic aspects of the various entities. For this reason, we have greatly expanded our coverage of the immunohistochemical and molecular features of the various lesions, recognizing that such information is quickly supplemented by new observations. Nonetheless, we continue to believe that careful gross examination and routine light microscopic observations are the foundations for diagnosis of these neoplasms and neoplastic-like processes. The reader will notice that scrotal pathology, which had been ably discussed by Dr. Mahul Amin in the Third Series Fascicle, is no longer represented in this Fascicle. It is covered in the now published Fourth Series Fascicle, *Tumors of the Prostate Gland, Seminal Vesicles, Penis, and Scrotum.*

We are greatly indebted to Dr. Judith Ferry, who helped us avoid errors in the sections dealing with lymphoma and hematopoietic neoplasms in chapter 7 by generously reviewing our drafts and providing editorial suggestions. Dr. G. Petur Nielsen also helped us update the section dealing with soft tissue neoplasms in chapter 7 by playing a similar role. Needless to say, the authors are solely responsible for any persistent deficiencies. Ms. Tracey Bender did an outstanding job with the clerical work, including numerous revisions. The staff at the American Registry of Pathology, and especially Ms. Mirlinda Caton, provided us with excellent editorial support.

Thomas M. Ulbright, MD
Robert H. Young, MD, FRCPath

Permission to use copyrighted illustrations has been granted by:

American Association for Cancer Research
Cancer Epidemiol Biomarkers Prev 2004; 13: 2160. For figure 1-25.

American Society for Clinical Pathology
Am J Clin Pathol 1956;26:1305. For figure 8-94.
Testicular Tumors. Chicago: ASCP Press; 1990. For figures 3-4, 3-6, 3-36, 3-42, 3-73, 3-90, 4-4, 4-66, 4-121, 4-160, 5-14, 5-30, 5-31, 6-68, 6-71, 6-100, 6-108, 7-26A, 7-38, 7-70, 7-106, 8-11, 8-17, 8-27, 8-37, 8-38, 8-40, 8-41, 8-43, 8-44, 8-51 left, and 8-102.

Elsevier
Atlas of Surgical Pathology of the Male Reproductive Tract. Philadelphia: W.B. Saunders; 1997. For figures 7-37 and 7-95.
J Urol 1963; 90: 25. For figure 8-5.
Semin Urol 1984; 2: 220, 222. For figures 1-22 and 1-23.
Urol Oncol 2007; 25: 34. For figure 1-26.
Urologic Surgical Pathology. St. Louis: Mosby; 1997. For figures 1-5, 2-2, and 8-97.
Uropathology. New York: Churchill Livingstone; 1989. For figure 1-8.

Lippincott
Diagnostic Surgical Pathology. New York: Raven Press; 1994. For figures 3-7 and 4-36.
Medical Embryology: Human Development—Normal and Abnormal. Baltimore: Williams & Wilkins; 1969. For figures 1-1 to 1-4.
Sternberg's Diagnostic Surgical Pathology. New York: Lippincott Williams & Wilkins; 2010. For figure 2-1.

Massachusetts Medical Society
N Engl J Med 1966: 274: 928-929. For figure 8-55.

Oxford University Press
Cunningham's Textbook of Anatomy. Oxford. For figure 1-6.
Int J Epidemiol 1986; 15: 165. For figure 1-24.

Pulso Ediciones
Algaba F. Atlas de Patología de los Tumores Urogenitales. Barcelona: Fundación Puigvert; 1991. For figure 8-28.

Wiley
Am J Anat 1963; 112: 39. For figure 1-11.

CONTENTS

1 TESTICULAR TUMORS: GENERAL CONSIDERATIONS

Since the last quarter of the 20th century, great advances have been made in the field of testicular oncology. There is now effective treatment for almost all testicular germ cell tumors (which constitute the great majority of testicular neoplasms); prior to this era, seminoma was the only histologic type of testicular tumor that could be effectively treated after metastases had developed. The studies of Skakkebaek and his associates (1–9) established that most germ cell tumors arise from morphologically distinctive, intratubular malignant germ cells. These works support a common pathway for the different types of germ cell tumors and reaffirms the approach to nomenclature of the World Health Organization (WHO) (10). We advocate the use of a modified version of the WHO classification of testicular germ cell tumors so that meaningful comparisons of clinical investigations can be made between different institutions.

Cytogenetic and molecular studies have provided new insights into possible relationships between different morphologic types of germ cell tumors (11–21) but, from a practical viewpoint, careful gross evaluation and, even more so, sound light microscopic evaluation remain the bedrocks for the assessment of these tumors, although immunohistochemistry plays a significant role in specific situations. Advances in the field of sex cord-stromal tumors have allowed recognition of several new variants within that group of tumors (see chapter 6), and a number of large clinicopathologic studies have significantly increased the knowledge of a variety of miscellaneous primary neoplasms (see chapter 7), as well as of metastatic tumors and hematopoietic neoplasms. There is also a better understanding of the diverse spectrum of neoplasms and tumor-like lesions that affect the paratestis, including morphologic variants that may lead to misinterpretations.

EMBRYOLOGY, ANATOMY, HISTOLOGY, AND PHYSIOLOGY

Several thorough reviews of the embryology (22–31), anatomy (22,25,32,33), and histology (34–36) of the testis may be consulted for more detailed information about these topics.

Embryology

The primordial and undifferentiated gonad is first detectable at about 4 weeks of gestational age when paired thickenings are identified at either side of the midline, between the mesenteric root and the mesonephros (fig. 1-1, left). Genes that promote cellular proliferation or impede apoptosis play a role in the initial development of these gonadal ridges, including *NR5A1 (SF-1)*, *WT1*, *LHX1*, *IGFLR1*, *LHX9*, *CBX2*, and *EMX2* (31). At the maximum point of their development, the gonadal, or genital, ridges extend from the sixth thoracic to the second sacral segments of the embryo. They are covered by layers of proliferated coelomic epithelium (fig. 1-1, right).

By 6 weeks of development, germ cells have migrated into the developing gonad, following a pathway from their initial site of formation in the caudal portion of the wall of the yolk sac, close to the allantois, along the wall of the hindgut and the dorsal root of the mesentery, and from there to the adjacent gonads (fig. 1-2). Such cells are distinctive and recognizable by their high content of placental-like alkaline phosphatase (PLAP), expression of nuclear transcription factor OCT3/4 (POU5F1) and stage-specific antigen 1, and abundant cytoplasmic glycogen. This migration is accomplished by amoeboid movement of the germ cells, and depends, at least in part, on transforming growth factor-beta and the *FOXC1* gene (37,38). It is hypothesized that the occurrence of extragonadal germ cell tumors is explained by the

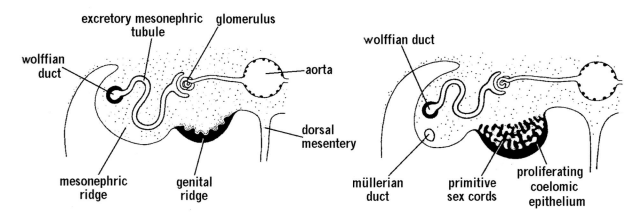

Figure 1-1

EMBRYOLOGY OF TESTIS

Left: At 4 weeks of gestation, the genital ridges are apparent as mesenchymal condensations covered by coelomic epithelium that has proliferated.

Right: At 6 weeks, there is ingrowth of the coelomic epithelium with extension into the mesenchyme to form the primitive sex cords. (Fig. 11-13 from Langman J. Medical embryology and human development—normal and abnormal, 2nd ed., Baltimore: Williams & Wilkins, 1969:164.)

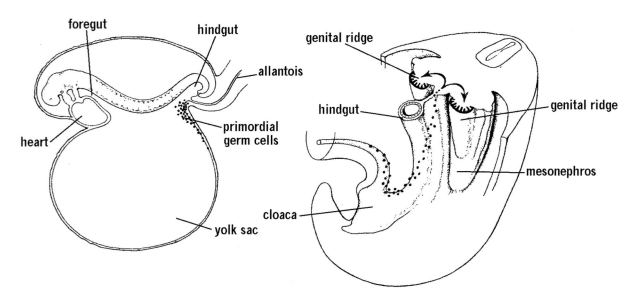

Figure 1-2

EMBRYOLOGY OF TESTIS

Left: At 3 weeks of gestation, the primordial germ cells form in the wall of the yolk sac.

Right: At 6 weeks, the primordial germ cells migrate to the wall of the hindgut, along the dorsal mesenteric root, and into the genital ridges. (Fig. 11-14 from Langman J. Medical embryology and human development—normal and abnormal, 2nd ed., Baltimore: Williams & Wilkins, 1969:165.)

aberrant midline migration of some germ cells to involve such sites as the pineal region, the anterior mediastinum, the sacrococcygeal area, and possibly, the retroperitoneum.

At 6 to 7 weeks of gestation, the proliferated coelomic epithelium on the surface of the gonadal ridge migrates into the underlying mesenchyme to develop into the primitive sex

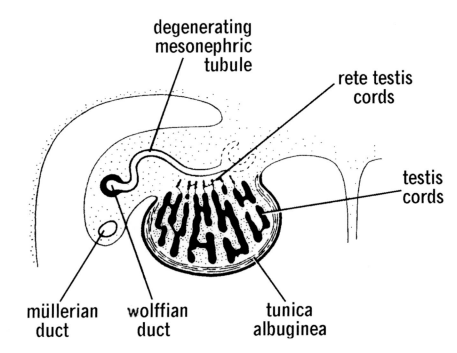

degenerating
mesonephric
tubule

rete testis
cords

testis
cords

müllerian
duct

wolffian
duct

tunica
albuginea

Figure 1-3

EMBRYOLOGY OF TESTIS

At 8 weeks of gestation, the tunica albuginea surrounds the developing testis and the rete testis cords intermingle with mesonephric tubules at the hilum. (Fig. 11-15A from Langman J. Medical embryology and human development—normal and abnormal, 2nd ed. Baltimore: Williams & Wilkins, 1969:165.)

cords (fig. 1-1, right). The molecular signals for this process appear to involve several genes, including *GATA4*, *ZFPM2*, and *WT1+KTS*, which, in turn, activate the *SRY* gene on the Y chromosome, a key event for the formation of Sertoli cells and the initial molecular difference in the development of a testis as opposed to an ovary. Subsequently, a longitudinal groove forms between the gonadal ridge and the more lateral mesonephric body, resulting in a separation of these structures. At this point (approximately day 42), the developing testis becomes morphologically distinct from a developing ovary.

SRY, also known as *TDF* (testis-determining factor), gene activation causes downstream activation of *SOX9*, *FGF9*, and *DAX1*, which appear to play roles in the differentiation of Sertoli cells and their migration. This gene is also important in the induction of the *AMH* (anti-müllerian hormone, also known as müllerian-inhibiting substance) gene in Sertoli cells, which produces the hormone that causes regression of the müllerian ductal system. The Sertoli cells aggregate around the primitive germ cells, incorporating them into solid tubular structures. Activation of several genes, including *PDGFRA*, *DHH*, and *ARX*, contribute to this process and to the formation of Leydig cells. With continued proliferation, the sex cords penetrate deep into

the medulla of the testis, forming the testis, or medullary, cords. The testis cords are, therefore, composed of a dual population of cells: one derived from the primitive sex cords and destined to form the Sertoli cells of the seminiferous tubules, and the second representing the migrated germ cells that become the spermatogonia of the testis. At this stage (day 42), the anlage of the tunica albuginea is apparent at the periphery of the embryonic testis as a layer of flattened cells. With further development, the testis cords lose their original connection with the surface epithelium and the tunica albuginea becomes better defined (fig. 1-3).

With the formation of distinct testis cords, a third cellular element of the developing testis becomes apparent as the interstitial component occupying the area between the cords. The origin of these interstitial (Leydig) cells is not entirely clear, although a steroidogenic population of cells appears to form along the anterior aspect of the mesonephros to supply both the gonad and adrenal gland, with segregation between the two organs perhaps mediated in part by the *WNT4* gene (31). Leydig cells become morphologically distinct at about 8 weeks of development. They are particularly prominent between the 4th and 6th months of gestation, only to regress following birth and to reappear at puberty.

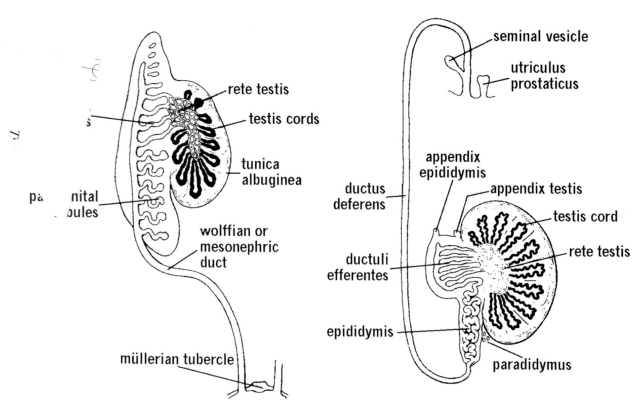

Figure 1-4

EMBRYOLOGY OF TESTIS

Left: By 4 months of gestation, the rete testis cords have merged with the epigenital tubules of the mesonephros.
Right: Diagram of the mature testis after descent showing the relationship of various structures. (Fig. 11-18 from Langman J. Medical embryology and human development - normal and abnormal, 2nd ed. Baltimore: Williams & Wilkins, 1969:169.)

Near the hilum of the developing testis, the testis cords break up into a network of very small strands of cells that intermingle with mesonephric cells. The rete testis forms out of these components, although the contribution of the sex cords and mesonephros to its structure remains controversial (39). During subsequent development, the rete testis cords merge with portions of the regressing mesonephric tubules, establishing the basis for the subsequent continuity between the seminiferous tubules and the excretory duct of the mesonephros (wolffian duct) (fig. 1-4). Continued growth of the testis cords, now designated seminiferous cords, results in a looped configuration, with the ends of the loops developing into the narrow tubuli recti. The seminiferous cords remain solid until spermatogenesis begins at puberty at which time lumens develop within the cords to pro-

duce seminiferous tubules. These structures are, in turn, invested by peritubular myoid cells. At this time, continuity is established between the tubuli recti and the tubules of the rete testis.

The initially elongated configuration of the developing testis becomes contracted to a more adult-like ovoid form by about 8 weeks of gestation; at this time, the testis extends from the diaphragm to the site of the abdominal inguinal ring. During subsequent development, the testis attains a position in the iliac fossa near the internal inguinal ring until descent, which normally begins at the 7th month. The excretory ducts of the testis develop as some of the mesonephric tubules (epigenital tubules) establish continuity with the cords of the rete testis to become the efferent ductules (fig. 1-4). Just caudal to the efferent ductules, the mesonephric, or wolffian, duct, under the trophic influence of testosterone

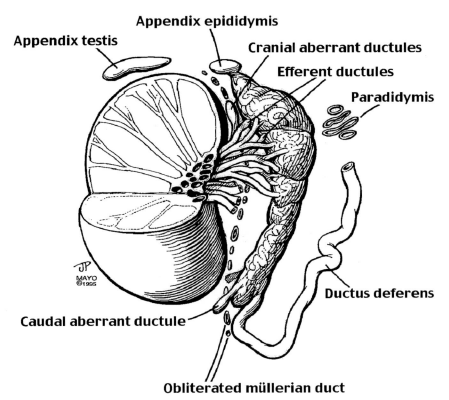

Appendix testis

Appendix epididymis

Cranial aberrant ductules

Efferent ductules

Paradidymis

Ductus deferens

Caudal aberrant ductule

Obliterated müllerian duct

Figure 1-5

ANATOMY OF TESTIS

Diagram of testicular anatomy, with vestigial embryonic remnants. The appendix testis, the appendix epididymis, the aberrant ductules, and the paradidymis are seen. The efferent ductules of the epididymis bridge to the testis at the hilum. (Fig. 12-1 from Bostwick DG. Spermatic cord and testicular adnexa. In: Bostwick DG, Eble JN, eds. Urologic surgical pathology. St. Louis: Mosby, 1997:648.)

produced by the fetal Leydig cells of the ipsilateral testis, becomes briefly elongated and convoluted, forming thereby the body and tail of the epididymis, with the efferent ductules forming the head (fig. 1-4, right). The remaining portion of the mesonephric duct forms the vas (ductus) deferens. Vestigial remnants of the cranial portion of the mesonephric duct may persist as the appendix epididymis (figs. 1-4, 1-5). AMH, a glycoprotein produced by the fetal Sertoli cells and a member of the transforming growth factor-β superfamily of growth factors, causes the müllerian (paramesonephric) duct to regress by apoptosis as early as day 51. The action of AMH is unilateral on the side of its production. A small remnant of the müllerian duct often persists on the anterior-superior surface of the testis, near the head of the epididymis, as the appendix testis (figs. 1-4, right; 1-5).

The descent of the testis begins at about the 7th month of gestation, at which time the gonad occupies a retroperitoneal position in the iliac fossa. In animal models, normal descent requires both an intact androgen receptor as well as expression of an insulin-like growth

factor, INSL3, without which there is impaired development of the gubernaculum (40). Enlargement of the caudal end of the gubernaculum through mitotic activity and the generation of hyaluronic acid (the "swelling reaction") is critical to testicular descent (41). As the testes move caudally toward the embryonic scrotal swellings, two outpouchings of the peritoneal cavity, the vaginal processes, protrude through the inguinal canal into the twin scrotal sacs. Both testes follow this pathway but remain retroperitoneal and localize within the scrotum. Obliterative changes subsequently occur in the upper portions of the vaginal processes, whereas the caudal-most portions of these processes continue to invest the testes as the tunicae vaginalis. Incomplete obliteration of the processus vaginalis permits intrascrotal leakage of peritoneal fluid and the formation of a hydrocele.

Anatomy

The adult testis is normally located in one of two testicular compartments within the scrotum. It is ovoid, has an average weight of 19 to 20 g (42), measures approximately 4.0

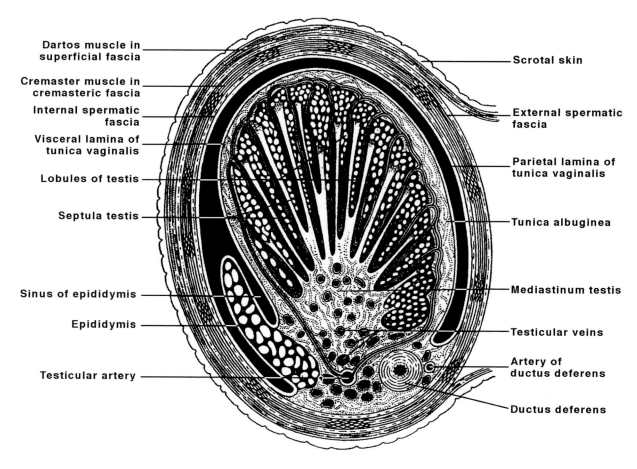

Dartos muscle in superficial fascia

Cremaster muscle in cremasteric fascia

Internal spermatic fascia

Visceral lamina of tunica vaginalis

Lobules of testis

Septula testis

Sinus of epididymis

Epididymis

Testicular artery

Scrotal skin

External spermatic fascia

Parietal lamina of tunica vaginalis

Tunica albuginea

Mediastinum testis

Testicular veins

Artery of ductus deferens

Ductus deferens

Figure 1-6

ANATOMY OF TESTIS

Cross sectional diagram of testicular anatomy at the level of the mediastinum testis. The space between the parietal and visceral layers of the tunica vaginalis is accentuated. (Fig.8.38 from Romanes GJ, ed. Cunningham's textbook of anatomy, 12th ed. Oxford: Oxford University Press, 1981:555.)

to 5.0 x 2.5 x 3.0 cm, and is surrounded, over most of its area, by a peritoneal sac, the tunica vaginalis. A small amount of serous fluid may be present in the space of the tunica vaginalis. The tunica albuginea is a tough, fibrous coating that invests the testis; its external surface is lined by the peritoneal-derived mesothelium that constitutes the visceral layer of the tunica vaginalis (fig. 1-6). The epididymis is closely applied to the testicular surface, with the epididymal head present superomedially and the tail posterolaterally (fig. 1-5).

The testicular parenchyma is homogeneous and light tan, consisting of densely packed seminiferous tubules arranged in poorly defined lobules separated by thin fibrous septa (fig. 1-7). The terminal portions of the seminiferous tubules empty into the tubuli recti (or straight tubules), which then connect with the tubules of the rete testis at the testicular hilum. Although a portion of the rete testis tubules intermingles with the structures of the testicular parenchyma near the hilum, the majority of the rete testis is surrounded by an intratesticular extension of dense fibrous tissue of the tunica albuginea at the testicular hilum; this combination of rete testis and fibrous tissue constitutes the mediastinum testis (fig. 1-6).

The rete testis tubules anastomose with 15 to 20 efferent ductules (or ductuli efferentes), which penetrate the tunica albuginea and coil to form

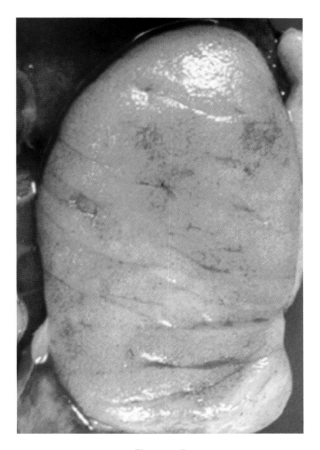

Figure 1-7

NORMAL GROSS APPEARANCE OF TESTIS

This normal testis from a prepubertal boy who had paratesticular rhabdomyosarcoma shows the usual light tan appearance with poorly defined lobules.

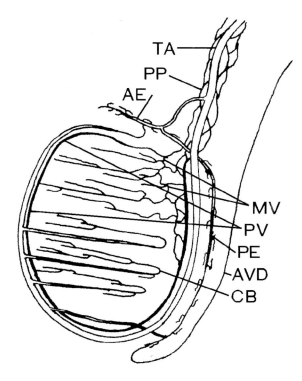

Figure 1-8

VASCULAR SUPPLY OF TESTIS

Schematic diagram of the arterial supply and venous drainage of the testis. See the text for details. (AE = anterior epididymal artery, AVD = artery of the vas deferens, CB = centripetal artery branch, MV = mediastinal venous plexus, PE = posterior epididymal artery, PP = pampiniform venous plexus, PV = peripheral veins, TA = testicular artery.) (Fig. 22-2 from Wheeler JE. Anatomy, embryology and physiology of the testis and its ducts. In: Hill GS, ed. Uropathology, New York: Churchill-Livingstone, 1989:937.)

the head of the epididymis (figs. 1-4, 1-5). These tubules are in continuity with the epididymal duct of the body and tail, which in turn drains into the vas (ductus) deferens. The vas deferens exits the scrotum through the inguinal canal as one of the structures of the spermatic cord. Vestigial tubular structures include the appendix testis (figs. 1-4, 1-5), derived from the regressed müllerian duct; the appendix epididymis (figs. 1-4, 1-5), derived from the cranial portion of the mesonephric duct; the ductuli aberrantes (vas aberrans of Haller) (fig. 1-5), derived from mesonephric remnants; and the paradidymis (figs. 1-4, 1-5), derived from the caudal portion of the mesonephric tubules (the paragenital tubules).

The major arterial supply to the testis is derived from the testicular artery (also known as the internal spermatic artery), which most commonly originates from the aorta, slightly inferior to the renal artery. It passes through the inguinal ring with the other structures of the spermatic cord. As the testicular artery approaches the testis, it gives off two branches to supply the head (the anterior epididymal artery) and the body and tail (the posterior epididymal artery) of the epididymis, and often further subdivides into two or three branches to penetrate the tunica albuginea of the posterior testis (fig. 1-8). These branches then run along the surface of the testis, giving off penetrating branches at intervals (centripetal arterial branches) to supply the testicular parenchyma (fig. 1-8). They cannot be visualized through the tunica albuginea, and, since there is a risk of vascular damage to the testis in performing testicular biopsies, these procedures are usually directed at the anterosuperior aspect of the testis, an area least likely to contain a surface arterial branch. The artery of the vas deferens provides a second source of blood to the testis. It is derived as a branch of the superior vesical artery, supplies the vas deferens, and may anastomose with the main testicular artery or the posterior epididymal branch of the testicular artery.

The venous drainage of the testis occurs through a series of small veins that interconnect and exit the testis as four to eight branches at the mediastinum. Other small veins may run beneath the tunica albuginea and connect with the venous branches at the mediastinum testis. These venous structures then form a convoluted mass of veins, the pampiniform plexus, which invests the testicular artery in the spermatic cord (fig. 1-8). Eventually, anastomoses occur and reduce the number of veins to one on the right side and one or two on the left side. The right testicular vein usually empties into the inferior vena cava slightly below the ostium of the right renal vein. The left testicular vein(s) most commonly drains into the left renal vein. The difference in the venous drainage between the right and left testis, with increased hydrostatic pressure on the left side due to its perpendicular anastomosis with the renal vein, is a frequently cited explanation for the predominance of left-sided varicoceles when that disorder is unilateral.

Histology

The visceral layer of the tunica vaginalis consists of a layer of flattened mesothelium on a supporting basement membrane that is applied to the external aspect of the compact, sparsely cellular fibrous tissue of the tunica albuginea. The densely collagenous portion of the tunica albuginea is typically about 0.5-mm thick in adults. Ducts, nerves, and vessels enter and exit the testis at its posterior aspect where the tunica albuginea is thickened and forms the mediastinum testis. The innermost aspect of the tunica albuginea, the tunica vasculosa, consists of loose connective tissue containing vessels; this is continuous with the fibrous septa that divide the testis into lobules containing one to four convoluted seminiferous tubules. The

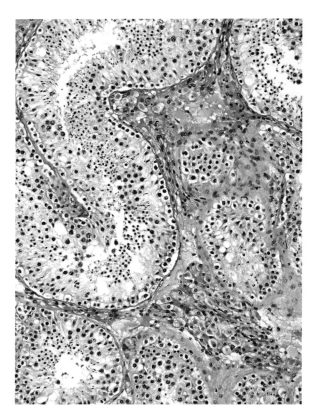

Figure 1-9

NORMAL HISTOLOGY OF ADULT TESTIS

Clusters of Leydig cells (lower, mid-right), small vessels, and spindle-shaped stromal cells are present in the interstitium between seminiferous tubules, which show active spermatogenesis with germ cells and Sertoli cells.

septa converge at the mediastinum. An average testis is subdivided into 200 to 300 such lobules, with a total testicular content of 400 to 600 seminiferous tubules, each 30- to 80-cm long. The estimated total combined length of the seminiferous tubules in both testes is 300 to 980 meters (43). Small blood vessels, lymphatics, scattered macrophages, testosterone-producing interstitial (Leydig) cells, and spindle-shaped stromal cells are present between the seminiferous tubules (fig. 1-9).

Each seminiferous tubule is surrounded by a thin layer of connective tissue and a well-defined basement membrane, which separate the seminiferous epithelium from the underlying connective tissue, the lamina propria of the testis. Three to five layers of flattened myoid cells in the lamina propria surround the tubules and

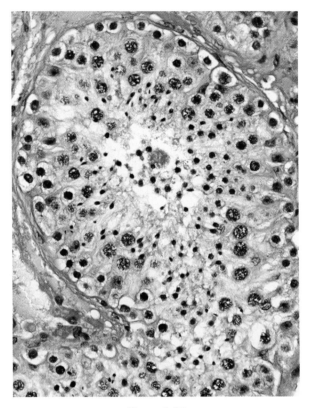

Figure 1-10

NORMAL HISTOLOGY OF ADULT TESTIS

At high magnification, a normal seminiferous tubule shows basally arranged spermatogonia and a patchy distribution of Sertoli cells. The Sertoli cells have prominent nucleoli (mid to lower left). There are primary spermatocytes with the characteristic meiotic chromatin; spermatids and spermatozoa are seen near the lumen.

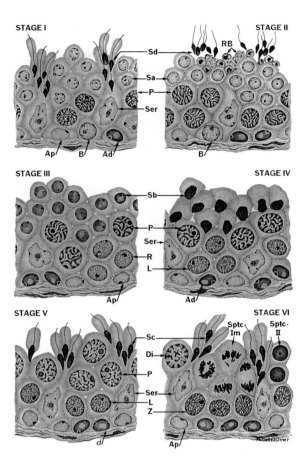

Figure 1-11

SPERMATOGENESIS

Different cell types in the seminiferous tubules during different stages of spermatogenesis. Sertoli cells (Ser); type A spermatogonia (Ap and Ad); type B spermatogonia (B); primary spermatocytes in stages of meiosis (R = resting, L = leptotene, Z = zygotene, P = pachytene, Di = diplotene, Sptc Im = division); secondary spermatocytes (Sptc II); spermatids (Sa, Sb, Sc, and Sd), and residual bodies (RB). (Fig. 3 from Clermont Y. The cycle of the seminiferous epithelium in man. Am J Anat 1963;112:39.)

promote movement of spermatozoa into the ductal system of the testis by contractile activity. The seminiferous epithelium is composed of two basic cell types: the Sertoli cells and the various spermatogenic cells (fig. 1-10).

Sertoli cells have an elongated, triangular contour and extend the entire thickness of the seminiferous epithelium, from the basement membrane to the luminal surface (fig. 1-11). In hematoxylin and eosin (H&E)-stained preparations, Sertoli cells have ill-defined, lightly eosinophilic cytoplasm; nuclei with fine chromatin; and moderate-sized, round nucleoli. Notches in the nuclear membrane are common (fig. 1-11) (44). Ultrastructurally, Sertoli cells have extremely intricate cytoplasmic processes (fig. 1-12) that completely surround the adjacent

spermatogenic cells. A distinctive ultrastructural feature in human Sertoli cells of postpubertal subjects is the presence of long, spindle-shaped inclusions in the basal and perinuclear aspects of the cytoplasm, known as Charcot-Böttcher filaments or inclusion bodies (fig. 1-13). Adjacent Sertoli cells are joined by long tight junctions where the membranes undergo fusion; this resultant structure is considered to be responsible for the maintenance of a blood-testis barrier (34). Lipid droplets and a well-developed

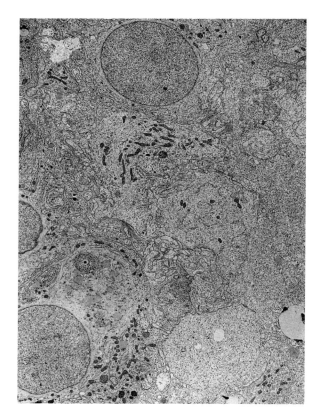

Figure 1-12

SERTOLI CELLS

Electron micrograph of Sertoli cells shows intricate, interdigitating cytoplasmic processes. The cell at the bottom left has numerous lipid droplets and annulate lamellae.

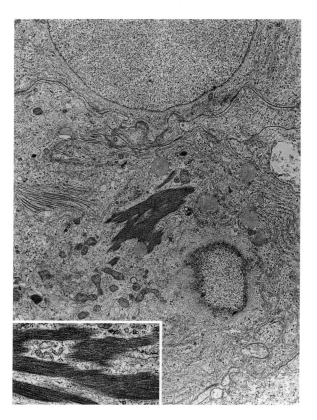

Figure 1-13

SERTOLI CELLS

Sertoli cell with prominent, juxtanuclear Charcot-Böttcher filaments, cytoplasmic lipid droplets, and cisternae of smooth and rough endoplasmic reticulum. Inset: The characteristic parallel arrangement of Charcot-Böttcher filaments is shown.

smooth endoplasmic reticulum are consistent with the steroid hormone synthesizing capacity of Sertoli cells (fig. 1-13). Sertoli cells, in addition to providing a "nurturing" function for the maturing germ cell population, are also phagocytic and may contain fragments of degenerated germ cells.

The spermatogonia are the first cells of spermatogenesis and occupy a basal position in the seminiferous tubules, adjacent to the basement membrane. Two types of spermatogonia are described: type A cells, which serve as self-renewing stem cells, and type B cells, which are derived from the mitotic division of type A spermatogonia but which later differentiate, after additional mitotic divisions, to more mature spermatogenic cells, primary spermatocytes (44). Type A spermatogonia have an ovoid nucleus, one or two nucleoli adjacent to the

nuclear membrane, finely granular chromatin, and generally pale cytoplasm (fig. 1-11). Type B spermatogonia have a more rounded nucleus, clumps of peripheral nuclear chromatin, and a single central nucleolus (fig. 1-11) (44).

The primary spermatocytes are tetraploid cells that occupy the cell layers just luminal to the basal layer of spermatogonia and participate in meiotic division to give rise to the distinctive, filamentous chromatin patterns of a prolonged prophase (fig. 1-11). The product of the first meiotic division of a primary spermatocyte is the secondary spermatocyte, which contains a diploid amount of DNA but a haploid number of chromosomes. These cells are rarely observed in sections because they rapidly undergo a second meiotic division to form the haploid spermatids, the early forms of which they closely resemble. The early spermatid is recognized on the luminal aspect of the primary spermatocyte layer as a round cell with finely granular, pale chromatin and a nuclear diameter of about 6 μm (fig. 1-11). Spermatids gradually transform, in the process of spermiogenesis, into spermatozoa as the nuclear chromatin condenses and the nucleus becomes oval to pear-shaped (fig. 1-11). A given cross section of a seminiferous tubule may not show complete spermatogenesis because of a wave-like pattern of maturation that occurs within the seminiferous tubules. Examination of many cross sections is therefore necessary before a conclusion concerning pathologic maturation arrest is indicated, and, indeed, some investigators conclude that "maturation arrest" is actually an artifact of this pattern in patients with hypospermatogenesis (45).

The interstitium of the testis comprises the space between the seminiferous tubules, and is occupied by blood vessels, lymphatics, loose connective tissue with fibrocytes, mast cells, peritubular myoid cells, and Leydig cells. Leydig cells are normally few in number from just after the neonatal period to puberty, at which time they proliferate and become numerous. Leydig cells characteristically occur in clusters and vary from round or polygonal to ovoid. They have a round nucleus with a central nucleolus and eosinophilic, sometimes vacuolated, cytoplasm that, in postpubertal patients, often contains lipochrome pigment or Reinke crystals. The latter are intracytoplasmic rod-shaped crystals measuring up to 20 μm (fig. 1-14). They have characteristic geometric configurations on ultrastructural examination (fig. 1-15) and contain proteins and glycosylated proteins, but their precise functional significance, if any, remains unclear. Immunohistochemical study has localized nestin, an intermediate filament protein expressed in non-neoplastic stem cells and embryonic cells of mesenchymal and neuroectodermal lineage, to Reinke crystals (46). Large numbers of vesicles of smooth endoplasmic reticulum, mitochondria with tubular cristae, and lipid droplets, all of which are characteristics of steroid hormone-producing cells, occupy the cytoplasm of Leydig cells (fig. 1-15). Leydig cells synthesize testosterone and other steroid hormones. In addition to occurring in

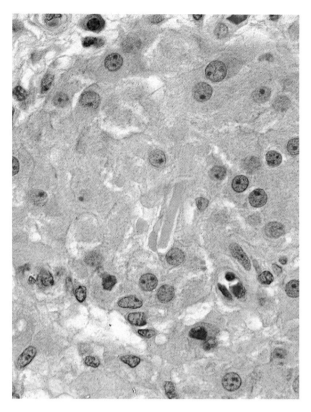

Figure 1-14

LEYDIG CELLS

Leydig cells are clustered in the testicular interstitium. Round, eccentrically placed nuclei; round nucleoli; and abundant eosinophilic cytoplasm are seen. There are rod-shaped, intracytoplasmic Reinke crystals with surrounding retraction artifact (center).

the interstitium between seminiferous tubules, Leydig cells may also be seen in the testicular mediastinum, within the tunica albuginea, and in the paratesticular soft tissues, including those associated with the epididymis and vas deferens. Such "ectopic" Leydig cells are often associated with small nerves (fig. 1-16) (47).

The straight tubules (tubuli recti) are lined by cuboidal epithelium and lack the Sertoli cells characteristic of the seminiferous tubules. They run a short distance to empty into the branching channels of the rete testis, which, for the most part, are invested by the dense connective tissue of the mediastinum testis (fig. 1-17), although occasional tubules of the rete testis are present among the seminiferous tubules adjacent to the testicular mediastinum. The tubules of the

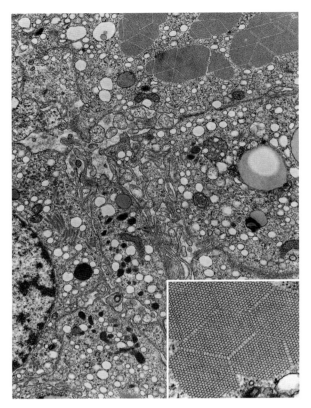

Figure 1-15

LEYDIG CELLS

A cluster of Leydig cells shows prominent vesicles of smooth endoplasmic reticulum, lipid droplets, lysosomes, and characteristic geometric patterns of Reinke crystals. Inset: Striking periodicity of the Reinke crystals.

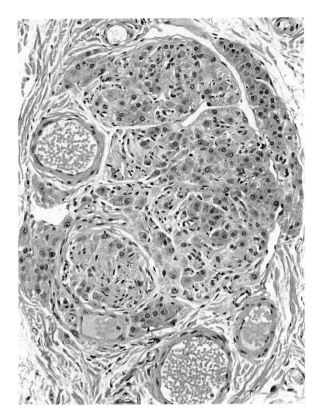

Figure 1-16

LEYDIG CELLS

Clusters of Leydig cells are present in the paratesticular soft tissues associated with small nerves. This is a normal finding.

Figure 1-17

RETE TESTIS

Branching tubules of the rete testis are set in the dense, hypocellular, fibrous stroma of the mediastinum testis.

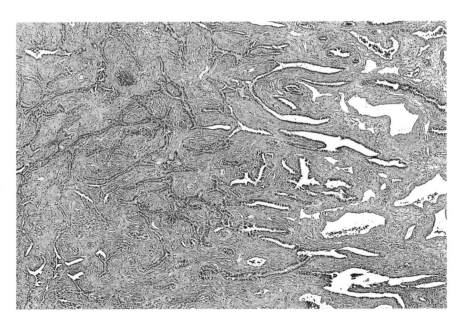

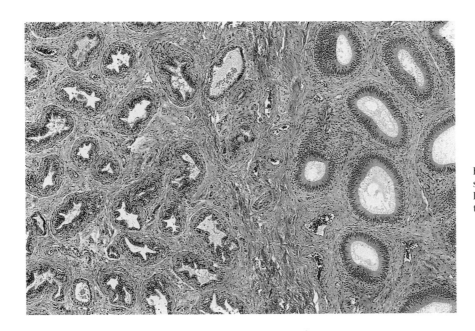

Figure 1-18

EPIDIDYMIS

The efferent ductules (left) have an undulating luminal surface unlike the straight luminal border of the epididymal tubules (right).

rete testis are lined by epithelium varying from cuboidal to columnar, with frequently grooved nuclei. Occasional tufts of the underlying connective tissue of the mediastinum testis project as epithelial-lined papillae into the lumens of the rete testis and are known as the chordae retis. The tubules of the rete testis empty into the efferent ductules, groups of 8 to12 tubular channels that are interposed between the rete testis and the epididymal tubules (fig. 1-18). These structures comprise part of the head of the epididymis and are lined by pseudostratified, columnar epithelium with foci of interspersed cuboidal epithelium, a pattern that produces a characteristic undulating luminal surface. Intra-cytoplasmic lipofuscin occurs in the epithelium of the efferent ductules. A small amount of circular smooth muscle is closely applied to the basal aspect of the epithelium of the efferent ductules, separated from it only by a basement membrane and scant connective tissue.

The efferent ductules empty into a highly convoluted tubule, the ductus epididymis, which forms the body and tail of the epididymis. Cross sections of the convoluted epididymal duct produce multiple profiles often referred to as epididymal tubules. These epididymal tubules are lined by two layers of cells: a basal layer of smaller cells with spherical nuclei and a luminal layer of tall columnar

cells (the principal cells) with elongated nuclei. Unlike the efferent ductules, the epididymal tubules have a smooth luminal surface that is punctuated by long stereocilia (fig. 1-19, left), long branching microvilli that are artifactually aggregated in routine histologic preparations. A few concentrically arranged smooth muscle cells invest this highly convoluted epididymal duct. Cribriform arrangements of the epithelium may sometimes occur (fig. 1-20). Periodic acid–Schiff (PAS)-positive intranuclear inclusions are present in the principal cells as well as the epithelium of the vasa deferentia and seminal vesicles. Other findings in the normal epididymis include cytoplasmic lipofuscin granules, foci of Paneth cell-like metaplasia (fig. 1-21), intranuclear cytoplasmic inclusions, and focal moderate to severe nuclear atypia (fig 1-19, right) (48–50).

The epididymal duct in turn joins the vas deferens at the tail of the epididymis. The epithelium of the vas deferens is similar to that of the epididymal duct, and stereocilia are visible along its luminal surface. Three thick layers of smooth muscle comprise the wall of the vas deferens: an innermost longitudinally oriented layer, a middle circular layer, and an outermost longitudinal layer. These are applied closely to the epithelium of the vas deferens, with only a thin layer of connective tissue separating them.

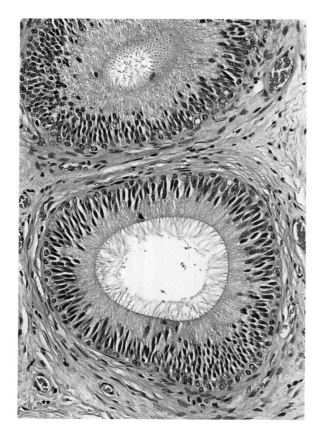 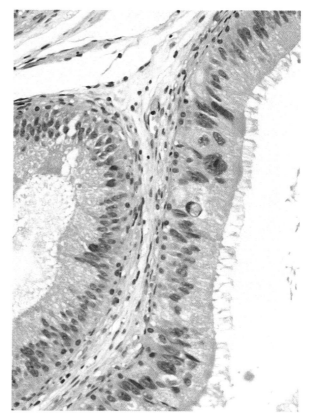

Figure 1-19

EPIDIDYMIS

Left: Epididymal tubules are lined by an innermost layer of tall columnar cells with luminal stereocilia and a much less conspicuous layer of basal cells.

Right: There is focal nuclear atypia, a normal variant.

Figure 1-20

EPIDIDYMIS

The epithelium is arranged in a cribriform pattern, a normal variant.

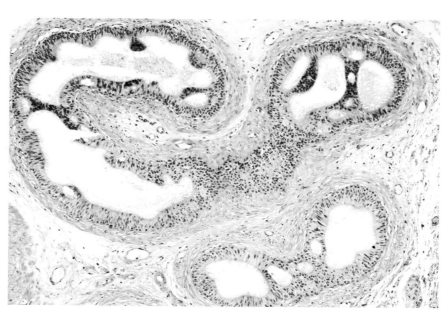

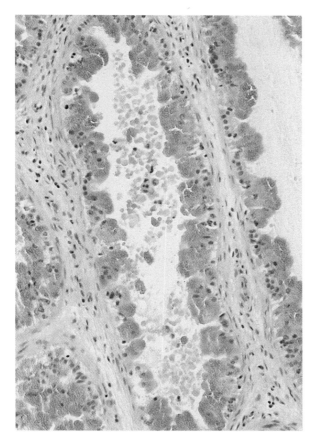

Figure 1-21

EPIDIDYMIS

The epithelial cells show Paneth-cell-like change, a normal variant.

Physiology

Testicular function is under the control of a number of hormones. Gonadotropin-releasing hormone (GnRH), secreted by the hypothalamus, stimulates the secretion of follicle-stimulating hormone (FSH) and luteinizing hormone (LH) from the anterior pituitary gland. FSH, in turn, causes the Sertoli cells to release androgen-binding protein (ABP), leading to high levels of androgen in the fluid of the seminiferous tubules. Local androgen then acts upon the Sertoli cells, permitting the maturation of spermatids embedded within their cytoplasm to spermatozoa. FSH also acts directly on Sertoli cells to aid in this maturation. It appears that the progression of spermatogonia to spermatids is androgen independent.

Testosterone is the principal androgenic hormone produced by the Leydig cells, although it often undergoes conversion to a more transcriptionally active form, dihydrotestosterone, in certain target cells. LH stimulates testosterone production and release from Leydig cells, and circulating testosterone and other androgens provide negative feedback for LH secretion from the pituitary gland.

In addition to AMH and ABP, Sertoli cells also secrete inhibins (inhibin A and inhibin B) which inhibit FSH secretion from the pituitary gland. Activins are related proteins formed by hetero and homo dimerization of the beta subunits found in inhibin A and inhibin B, and have a stimulatory effect on FSH secretion. Sertoli cells also contain aromatase, an enzyme that converts androgens to estrogens and is responsible for the estrogenic manifestations of some Sertoli cell neoplasms.

It is common for testicular germ cell tumors with a component of syncytiotrophoblast cells to produce human chorionic gonadotropin (hCG). hCG has LH-like and thyroid-stimulating hormone (TSH)-like activity. It therefore stimulates Leydig cells to proliferate and secrete testosterone, which is converted to estrogen in adipose tissue, resulting in gynecomastia in some cases. TSH-like activity may result in thyroid gland hyperplasia and thyrotoxicosis.

CLASSIFICATION

Table 1-1 provides a classification of testicular neoplasms and non-neoplastic lesions that may, either clinically or pathologically, mimic neoplasms. The classification of testicular germ cell tumors used in this text is a modification of the WHO classification, which, in turn, is derived largely from the work of Friedman and Moore (51), Dixon and Moore (52,53), Melicow (54), and Mostofi and Price (55). The fundamental tenet of this classification is that all of the different morphologic types of germ cell tumors are derived from neoplastic germ cells that differentiate along various pathways. The close association of virtually all of the morphologic types of germ cell tumors (except for spermatocytic seminoma and specialized forms of teratoma [dermoid cyst, carcinoid tumor]) with the lesion designated "intratubular germ cell neoplasia, unclassified" (see chapter 2), provides

Table 1-1

WHOᵃ-BASED CLASSIFICATION OF TESTICULAR AND PARATESTICULAR TUMORS AND TUMOR-LIKE LESIONS

Germ Cell Tumors
  Precursor lesions
    Intratubular germ cell neoplasia, unclassified
    Intratubular germ cell neoplasia, specific types
  Germ cell tumors of one histologic type
    Seminoma
      Variant: with syncytiotrophoblast cells
    Spermatocytic seminoma
      Variant: with sarcomatous component
    Embryonal carcinoma
    Yolk sac tumor (endodermal sinus tumor)
    Trophoblastic tumors
      Choriocarcinoma
      Placental site trophoblastic tumor
      Cystic trophoblastic tumor
      Unclassified
    Teratoma
      Variant: dermoid cyst
      Teratoma with a secondary malignant component
        (specify)
      Monodermal variants
        Carcinoid (pure and with teratomatous elements)
        Primitive neuroectodermal tumor
        Others
  Germ cell tumors of more than one histologic type
    Mixed germ cell tumors (specify individual com-
      ponents and estimate their amount as percentage
      of the tumor)
    Polyembryoma
    Diffuse embryoma
  Regressed ("burnt out") germ cell tumors
    Scar only
    Scar with intratubular germ cell neoplasia
    Scar with minor residual germ cell tumor
      (seminoma, teratoma or other)

Germ Cell-Sex Cord-Stromal Tumors
  Gonadoblastoma
  Unclassified

Sex Cord-Stromal Tumors
  Sertoli-stromal cell tumors
    Sertoli cell tumor
      Variants: large cell calcifying
        intratubular large cell hyalinizing
        sclerosing
    Sertoli-Leydig cell tumor
  Leydig cell tumor
  Granulosa-stromal cell tumors
    Granulosa cell tumor
    Variants: adult and juvenile
  Tumors in the fibroma-thecoma group
  Mixed
  Unclassified

Tumors of the Rete Testis
  Adenoma/Adenofibroma/Cystadenoma
  Carcinoma

Miscellaneous (including unclassified tumors and
    tumors of uncertain cell type)
  Tumors of ovarian epithelial type
  Squamous cell carcinoma
  Carcinosarcoma
  Others

Paratesticular Tumors (including tumors of the
    spermatic cord)ᵇ
  Tumors of ovarian epithelial type
    Papillary serous borderline tumor
    Serous carcinoma
    Mucinous cystadenoma
    Mucinous borderline tumor
    Mucinous carcinoma
    Endometrioid carcinoma
    Mullerian adenosarcoma
    Malignant mixed müllerian tumor
  Adenomatoid tumor
  Malignant mesothelioma
  Desmoplastic small round cell tumor
  Epididymal cystadenoma
  Epididymal carcinoma
  Melanotic neuroectodermal tumor (retinal anlage
    tumor)
  Benign (or locally aggressive) soft tissue-type tumors
    Fibromatous tumors
    Lipoma
    Vascular tumors
    Myoid gonadal stromal tumor
    Aggressive angiomyxoma
    Angiomyofibroblastoma-like tumor (cellular
      angiofibroma)
    Mammary-type myofibroblastoma
    Others
  Malignant soft tissue-type tumors
    Rhabdomyosarcoma
      Embryonal
      Variant: spindle cell
      Alveolar
    Liposarcoma
      Well-differentiated
      Pleomorphic
      Dedifferentiated
      Myxoid/round cell
    Leiomyosarcoma
    Others
  Miscellaneous
    Wilms tumor
    Squamous cell carcinoma
    Paraganglioma
    Juvenile xanthogranuloma

Hematopoietic and Lymphoid Tumors
  Lymphoma
  Multiple myeloma and plasmacytoma
  Leukemia and myeloid sarcoma

Table 1-1, continued

Secondary Tumors	Hydrocele-related changes
	Proliferative funiculitis (pseudosarcomatous myofibro-blastic proliferation)
Tumor-Like Lesions	Fibrous pseudotumor (fibromatous periorchitis, nod-ular periorchitis)
Leydig cell hyperplasia	Meconium periorchitis
Sertoli cell nodules	Mesothelial/histiocytic hyperplasia
Testicular tumor of the adrenogenital syndrome	Sclerosing lipogranuloma
Steroid cell nodules with other disorders	Abnormalities related to sexual precocity
Adrenal cortical rests	Idiopathic hypertrophy
Torsion/infarct (of testis, of appendix testis, of appendix epididymis)	Hyperplasia of the rete testis
	Epidermoid cyst
Hematoma/hematocele	Other cysts (parenchymal, rete, of tunics, epididymal)
Testicular appendages and Walthard cell nests	Cystic dysplasia
Orchitis/epididymitis	Microlithiasis
Infectious (bacterial, viral, granulomatous)	Spermatocele
Autoimmune/vasculitis	Sperm granuloma
Idiopathic granulomatous	Vasitis nodosa
Granulomatous epididymitis	Splenic-gonadal fusion
Sarcoidosis	Smooth muscle hyperplasia of the adnexa
Malakoplakia	Others
Rosai-Dorfman disease (sinus histiocytosis with massive lymphadenopathy)	

[a]WHO = World Health Organization.
[b]Some of these lesions may rarely be primary in the testis.

PATTERNS OF SPREAD AND METASTASIS IN TESTICULAR CANCER

convincing support for this viewpoint. It is furthermore apparent that many of the neoplasms have the capacity to transform to other germ cell tumor types, as discussed in chapter 2.

The tunica albuginea is a difficult barrier for testicular cancers to penetrate. Most testicular neoplasms extend into the paratesticular structures by way of the mediastinum testis, where the dense fibrous tissue of the tunica albuginea disperses into a loose admixture of fat, connective tissue, blood vessels, and nerves. Even this pathway is used uncommonly, with only 10 to 15 percent of malignant testicular tumors involving either the epididymis or spermatic cord (56). Extension into the rete testis is, however, common, and occurred in about 80 percent of seminomas in one series (57). Involvement of scrotal skin is an unusual and late event.

Most of the information regarding the distribution of metastases is derived from studies of patients with testicular germ cell tumors, which represent approximately 95 percent of primary malignant tumors of the testis. Malignant tumors other than germ cell tumors appear to have similar metastatic patterns, however (58). Metastases occur via either a lymphatic

or hematogenous route. Seminoma tends to spread by lymphatics, with hematogenous metastases usually occurring only late in the clinical course. Choriocarcinoma, on the other hand, has a proclivity for early dissemination through blood-borne routes, although nodal metastases also occur. The other nonseminomatous germ cell tumors show both lymphatic and hematogenous patterns of dissemination, with early metastases tending to be mainly lymphatic based, although childhood yolk sac tumor is an exception, with a proclivity for initial hematogenous metastases (59).

The sites of lymph node metastases depend upon the side of testicular involvement and the presence or absence of paratesticular extension. Neoplasms of the right testis tend first to metastasize to the interaortocaval, retroperitoneal lymph nodes at about the level of the second lumbar vertebral body (56), although precaval and right paracaval involvement may also occur (fig. 1-22). There is absence of both suprahilar nodal involvement and left para-aortic involvement below the inferior mesenteric artery in early retroperitoneal metastases from right-sided tumors (60). The left testis tends to first produce retroperitoneal nodal metastases in the left para-aortic region between the left ureter, left renal vein, aorta, and origin of the inferior mesenteric

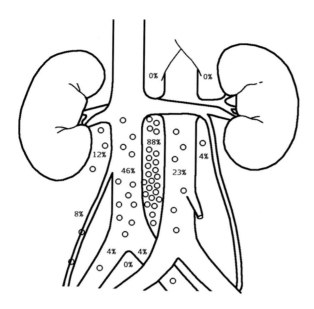

Figure 1-22

RETROPERITONEAL METASTASES

This diagram shows the distribution of retroperitoneal metastases in early stage II nonseminomatous germ cell tumors from right-sided testicular lesions. Most metastases occur in the interaortocaval and precaval areas. There is an absence of suprahilar involvement and left para-aortic involvement below the level of the inferior mesenteric artery. (Fig. 2 from Donohue JP. Metastatic pathways of nonseminomatous germ cell tumors. Semin Urol 1984;2:220.)

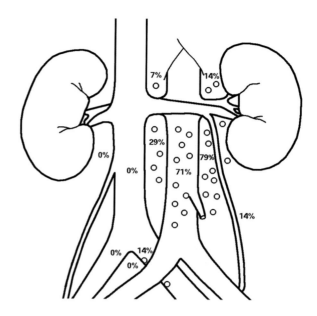

Figure 1-23

RETROPERITONEAL METASTASES

This diagram shows the distribution of retroperitoneal metastases in early stage II nonseminomatous germ cell tumors from left-sided testicular lesions. For left-sided lesions, most of the metastases occur in the left para-aortic and preaortic areas. There is an absence of precaval, right paracaval, and right iliac involvement. (Fig. 5 from Donohue JP. Metastatic pathways of nonseminomatous germ cell tumors. Semin Urol 1984;2:222.)

artery (fig. 1-23) (56). Preaortic involvement is also common, but there is an absence of right paracaval and precaval involvement. Unlike right-sided lesions, early left-sided tumors produce occasional suprahilar nodal metastases (60). Because of this tendency for selective site involvement in early stage disease, limited retroperitoneal dissections, tailored according to the laterality of the primary tumor, are feasible. This often permits retention of ejaculatory capability, in contrast to more extensive retroperitoneal dissections (61,62).

With more advanced disease, more widespread retroperitoneal involvement occurs. Suprahilar involvement occurs with right-sided lesions, and contralateral spread is seen. The likelihood of suprahilar spread increases greatly for left-sided lesions, as does interaortocaval and contralateral (precaval) involvement (60). As the volume of retroperitoneal tumor increases, retro-

grade metastases develop and iliac and inguinal nodal areas may become involved. Inguinal node involvement is also a consequence of extension of the primary tumor to the scrotal skin or prior inguinal or scrotal surgery. A trans-scrotal surgical approach in a patient with a possible testicular tumor is therefore contraindicated because of the consequent increase in the potential metastatic field. Involvement of the epididymis may lead to external iliac node involvement. Cephalad dissemination eventually involves mediastinal and supraclavicular nodes. In rare cases, mediastinal or supraclavicular metastases occur in the absence of clinical retroperitoneal involvement (55). If supraclavicular involvement occurs, it is the left supraclavicular area that is affected in 85 percent of the cases (63).

Distant organ metastases are usually the consequence of hematogenous spread, although some cases of gastrointestinal tract involvement

Table 1-2

**COMPARISON OF HISTOLOGIC TYPES OF PRIMARY TESTICULAR GERM CELL TUMORS
AND THE TYPES IDENTIFIED IN METASTASES AT AUTOPSY (PRECHEMOTHERAPY DATA)[a]**

| Primary Tumor | Autopsy Findings | | | |
	Seminoma (%)	Embryonal Carcinoma (%)	Teratoma (%)	Choriocarcinoma (%)
Seminoma (N = 23)	74	26	4	9
Embryonal carcinoma (N = 74)[b]	4	96	8	5
Teratoma (N = 16)[b]	0	63	63	25
Mixed germ cell tumors (N = 74)	0	80	42	30
Choriocarcinoma (N = 7)	0	0	0	100

[a]Data from: Dixon FJ, Moore RA. Testicular tumors: a clinicopathologic study. Cancer 1953;427-54.
[b]Pure or with seminoma.

result from direct spread of retroperitoneal metastases (64). In an autopsy study of patients with testicular germ cell tumors, 89 percent had pulmonary involvement, 73 percent had liver metastases, 31 percent had brain metastases, and 30 percent had bone metastases (65). In a clinical study, gastrointestinal involvement by metastases from testicular germ cell tumors occurred in only 3.6 percent of the patients (64). Choriocarcinoma is particularly prone to produce brain metastases and seminoma to produce bone metastases (65). The latter are also common with malignant Sertoli cell tumors (66).

An interesting and important aspect of testicular germ cell tumors is the marked tendency of metastatic lesions to show a different histology from that of the primary tumor. For example, a tumor that initially lacked a teratomatous component may show teratomatous elements in the metastatic deposits. This observation antedates the utilization of chemotherapy, as is shown in Table 1-2.

TUMOR STAGING

The staging of testicular tumors is based on the original work of Boden and Gibb (67), which divided the stages into purely testicular, retroperitoneal, and extraretroperitoneal. The current TNM system of the American Joint Committee on Cancer (AJCC) (Table 1-3) (68), which represents a refinement of both this approach and that of the International Union Against Cancer (UICC) (69), includes elaboration of each T, N, and M category and modification based on serologic information (S). T, N, M, and S categories are then grouped into stages 0 to III. The widespread use of this method is helpful in the assessment of interinstitutional results. Some authorities, however, feel that while the AJCC method provides a useful approach for nonseminomatous germ cell tumors, it is less helpful in determining meaningful staging subdivisions in patients with seminoma (70).

GROSS EXAMINATION

Orchiectomy specimens should be received fresh and dissected promptly. Many of the diagnostic problems in testicular neoplasia (especially the confusion of seminoma with embryonal carcinoma) can be attributed to delayed or incomplete fixation. If the testis is placed intact in fixative and sent to the pathology laboratory, a several-hour delay in dissection may result in suboptimal morphology since the testicular tunics do not permit ready access of fixative to the neoplasm. If for some reason it is not possible for a specimen to be evaluated promptly by a pathologist, it is preferable for the surgeon to bisect the specimen with a single sagittal cut before placing it in fixative and sending it to the laboratory. This approach is also suboptimal because it prevents the gross inspection of the intact, unfixed specimen by the pathologist and does not allow the harvesting of fresh tissues for ancillary studies. It may also cause difficulty in assessment if the neoplasm has grown through the tunica albuginea, since the tumor may bulge beyond the incision and protrude onto the surface of the tunica albuginea, although close inspection can usually resolve this problem.

Table 1-3

STAGING SYSTEM FOR TESTICULAR CANCER[a]

TNM system		Stage Grouping	
pTX	- Unknown status of testis	Stage 0	- Tis, N0, M0, S0
pT0	- No apparent primary (includes scars)	Stage IA	- T1, N0, M0, S0
pTis	- Intratubular tumor, no invasion	Stage IB	- T2-T4, N0, M0, S0
pT1	- Testis and epididymis only; no vascular invasion or penetration of tunica albuginea	Stage IS	- any T, N0, M0, S1-S3 (postorchiectomy)
pT2	- Testis and epididymis with vascular invasion or through tunica albuginea to involve tunica vaginalis	Stage IIA	- any T, N1, M0, S0-S1
		Stage IIB	- any T, N2, M0, S0-S1
pT3	- Spermatic cord	Stage IIC	- any T, N3, M0, S0-S1
pT4	- Scrotum	Stage IIIA	- any T, any N, M1a, S0-S1
		Stage IIIB	- any T, N1-N3, M0, S2
			any T, any N, M1a, S2
		Stage IIIC	- any T, N1-N3, M0, S3
pNX	- Unknown nodal status		any T, any N, M1a, S3
pN0	- No regional node involvement		any T, any N, M1b, any S
pN1	- Node mass or single nodes ≤ 2 cm; ≤ 5 nodes involved (no node > 2 cm)		
pN2	- Node mass >2 cm but <5 cm; or > 5 nodes involved, none > 5cm; or extranodal tumor		
pN3	- Node mass > 5 cm		
pMX	- Unknown status of distant metastases		
pM0	- No distant metastases		
pM1a	- Nonregional nodal or lung metastases		
pM1b	- Distant metastasis other than nonregional nodal or lung		

SX	- Unknown serum markers		
S0	- Normal serum markers		
	LDH[b]	hCG (mIU/ml)	AFP(ng/ml)
S1	- <1.5 x N &	<5,000 &	<1,000
S2	- 1.5-10 x N or	5,000-50,000 or	1,000-10,000
S3	- >10 x N or	>50,000 or	>10,000

[a]Adapted from reference 68. From the American Joint Committee on Cancer (AJCC).
[b]LDH (lactate dehydrogenase) levels expressed as elevations above upper limit of normal (N); AFP = alpha-fetoprotein; hCG = human chorionic gonadotropin.

A radical orchiectomy is performed for virtually all suspected testicular neoplasms because of the high probability that a testicular mass represents a malignant tumor. The specimen therefore consists of the testis and the surrounding tunica vaginalis, the paratesticular structures (epididymis and soft tissues), and a length of spermatic cord. External inspection of the tunica vaginalis should be performed for possible tumor penetration, followed by opening of the parietal layer of the tunica vaginalis testis. Any fluid present should be measured and described. The length of spermatic cord should be measured, serially cut at regular intervals, and inspected for gross evidence of neoplasm. The proximal cord margin should be separately submitted as one block and any abnormal-appearing areas submitted as additional blocks, or, if no grossly abnormal areas are apparent, a slice from the middle and distal cord submitted. These cassettes should be placed in fixative and submitted at the same time as the remainder of the specimen. It is best to take sections of the cord before incising the testis in order to avoid the common artifactual contamination of the cord (71). The parietal layer of the tunica vaginalis should then be removed, and the external aspect of the testis inspected and gently palpated, with any abnormalities noted.

The testis should be measured in three dimensions, weighed, and bisected in a sagittal plane from anterior to posterior toward the epididymal head. The cut surface of the neoplasm should be described, its relationship to the tunica albuginea noted, and its size recorded. Foci of hemorrhage and necrosis, translucent cartilage, cysts, fleshy encephaloid areas, and evidence of multifocality should be noted.

Special attention should be directed toward rete testis involvement, paratesticular extension at the mediastinum, or invasion through the tunica albuginea. Photographs and samples for electron microscopy, flow cytometry, molecular biologic, and karyotyping analyses may be obtained at this point, although these techniques are not required for diagnosis of most cases and are primarily for research purposes. Additional parallel cuts are then made at regular intervals, leaving the tunica albuginea intact to hold the specimen together.

The specimen is then placed in an adequate volume of fixative and allowed to fix thoroughly before the submission of additional blocks; overnight fixation is required for formalin. Ten percent neutral-buffered formalin is a satisfactory fixative but others may be used depending on individual preference. One study noted improved cytologic detail with more acidic fixatives (72). Adequate fixation is crucial since the distinction of seminoma from nonseminomatous germ cell tumors may primarily depend on cytologic features that may be obscured by poor tissue preservation.

Following fixation, any observations additional to those already made should be noted. Representative blocks of all of the different-appearing areas should be submitted, with a minimum number of one block for each centimeter of maximum tumor dimension. Foci with hemorrhage and necrosis should be represented in the sampling, as well as blocks to include the tunica albuginea and subjacent parenchyma. Generous sampling of tumor with adjacent testicular parenchyma is recommended since it is close to this interface that most of the involved lymphatics are found. For tumors with the gross appearance of seminoma, we recommend submission of at least 10 blocks of the neoplasm, even if it appears homogeneous, because of the possibility of detecting small foci of nonseminomatous elements that may alter the therapy. Small tumors should be entirely submitted. A representative section of the non-neoplastic testis and hilum should be submitted, as well as any areas of testicular scarring.

These are general guidelines, and tumors with an extremely variegated gross appearance may require more sections. In some situations more sections are required, such as in a patient who appears to have, on initial examination, a pure seminoma but who has an elevated serum alpha-fetoprotein (AFP) level (73). After the tumor is sampled, the epididymis should be incised by multiple cuts perpendicular to its long axis, any abnormalities noted, and an appropriate block submitted. Germ cell tumors, particularly seminoma and embryonal carcinoma, are friable, making knife implantation on tissue surfaces and into vascular spaces common (71); care during specimen dissection, with the use of clean instruments, reduces the frequency of this artifact, which may result in an erroneous diagnosis of extratesticular extension or vascular invasion.

The final pathology report, at the minimum, should provide a histologic classification of the neoplasm, an assessment of the presence or absence of lymphatic or blood vessel invasion, information regarding the local extent of the tumor (including the status of the spermatic cord margin and whether or not the rete testis is invaded), the greatest tumor dimension, and, for mixed germ cell tumors, an estimate of the percentage of the different tumor components. Additional information may be important depending upon the specific type of tumor, especially for the sex cord-stromal tumors where the assessment of malignant potential is often problematic and largely dependent upon features such as mitotic rate, degree of cytologic atypia, and presence of tumor necrosis.

FROZEN SECTION EXAMINATION

Frozen sections are not routinely required for the management of patients with testicular tumors since the neoplastic nature of the lesion is often evident preoperatively as a result of serum marker studies and testicular ultrasound, and orchiectomy is required for treatment. If there is clinical ambiguity concerning the neoplastic nature of a testicular mass, frozen section evaluation of a biopsy obtained by an inguinal approach may permit testicular conservation if a clearly benign lesion can be identified (74–76). This approach has been applied most frequently to epidermoid cysts (74,77,78), although biopsies for permanent sections of the surrounding testis should also be obtained to exclude intratubular germ cell neoplasia and ensure the diagnosis (79–81). A neoplasm that abuts the tunica albuginea or is entirely paratesticular is more likely to be benign (for example, an adenomatoid tumor) than an intraparenchymal mass, and enucleation of such a neoplasm on the basis of well-prepared frozen sections is justified. Frozen section is particularly likely to be beneficial in allowing conservative management in cases where the location and gross appearance of a mass are suggestive of a non-neoplastic process, such as fibromatous periorchitis (see chapter 8). It may also be employed when the patient's age, preoperative evaluation, or both, suggest the likelihood of an unusual, possibly benign neoplasm, as illustrated by a case of hemangioma treated conservatively (82). Testicular masses in children are more amenable to this approach than those in adults (83).

One study reported 70 testicular tumors diagnosed by biopsy and frozen section evaluation (84). This technique established the correct diagnosis in 81 percent of the cases, and a second biopsy established the correct diagnosis in an additional 11 percent. In four patients, no definite diagnosis was established at frozen section, and in one patient, a mature teratoma was misinterpreted as an epidermoid cyst, necessitating reoperation with orchiectomy. Another study of 94 cases reported two false negatives and three false positives (85). In our experience and that of others (86), it is often difficult to subcategorize germ cell tumors with total confidence, but subtyping does not affect surgical management.

CYTOLOGIC EXAMINATION

Although there are data to suggest that fine-needle aspiration cytology of testicular masses provides an accurate classification of most testicular tumors (87–89), cytology does not play a role in the diagnosis of primary testicular neoplasms. It may, however, be a feasible alternative to orchiectomy or more limited surgical excision in certain circumstances, including the recognition of relapse in children with acute lymphoblastic leukemia (90) or where there is good clinical or ultrasonographic evidence for adenomatoid tumor (91–93). Also, aspiration cytology of enlarged lymph nodes or visceral lesions is useful in confirming metastases (94). It should be emphasized that a negative result in this context does not exclude a metastasis because of the frequently focal nature of vi-

able, metastatic tumor (94). The distinction of seminoma from nonseminomatous germ cell tumors can generally be made in a reliable fashion (88,94,95), but it may not be possible to distinguish among the various forms of nonseminomatous germ cell tumor (94). Furthermore, cytologic examination alone may not permit differentiation of embryonal carcinoma or yolk sac tumor at metastatic sites from undifferentiated carcinoma or poorly differentiated adenocarcinoma of somatic origin (94).

EPIDEMIOLOGY

Most epidemiologic studies use medical records or death certificates as diagnostic sources and discuss "testicular cancer" in a generic sense. Because about 95 percent of primary malignant tumors of the testis are germ cell tumors, the results of these studies generally apply only to germ cell tumors and cannot be extrapolated to other primary testicular malignant tumors. When patients are less than 50 years of age, a generally pure germ cell tumor population can be expected. However, many of the tumors that occur in older patients and that account for the second peak of the bimodal distribution of "testicular cancer" (fig. 1-24) are not only not of germ cell origin but are often secondary, i.e., lymphomas or carcinomas that spread to the testis. In one study, 67 percent of malignant testicular tumors in patients over 70 years old were lymphomas (96). The sex cord-stromal tumors also represent a higher proportion of primary neoplasms in older patients. Epidemiologic studies of testicular germ cell tumors are therefore necessarily flawed if they include the older group of patients without pathologic verification of the nature of their neoplasms (96).

There is evidence that testicular cancers in childhood, although also predominantly of germ cell origin, are fundamentally different from postpubertal germ cell tumors since they are not associated with intratubular germ cell neoplasia of the unclassified type, are almost always of a pure histologic type, have different cytogenetic and molecular biologic features, and tend to pursue a more indolent course. Additionally, a higher proportion of testicular masses in children are either sex cord-stromal tumors or benign epidermoid cysts. The standard epidemiologic

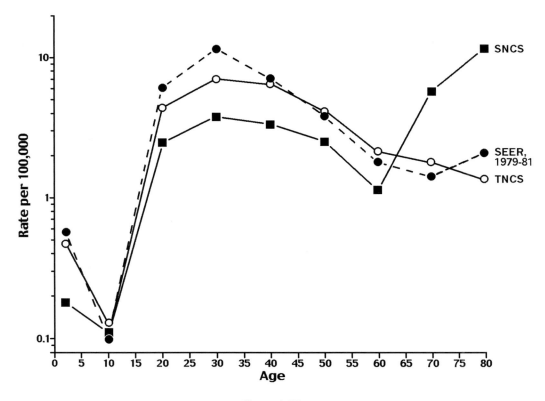

Figure 1-24

INCIDENCE OF TESTICULAR CANCER VERSUS AGE

Three studies examining the incidence of testicular cancer with age demonstrate a small peak in infancy, a nadir at 10 years, an increasing incidence following puberty, a second peak at roughly age 30 years, and a slow decline thereafter. In some studies another peak occurring in the elderly is not due to germ cell tumors but lymphomas and secondary malignancies. (SNCS = Second National Cancer Survey, TNCS = Third National Cancer Survey, SEER = Surveillance, Epidemiology, and End Results Program.) (Fig. 1 from Brown LM, Pottern LM, Hoover RN, Devesa SS, Aselton P, Flannery JT. Testicular cancer in the United States: trends in incidence and mortality. Int J Epidemiol 1986;15:165.)

observations on "testicular cancer" therefore do not apply to prepubertal patients.

Testicular cancer is uncommon, accounting for about 1 percent of malignant neoplasms in males, but it is the most frequent solid malignancy of young men from 15 to 44 years of age (97). The incidence of testicular cancer rises dramatically around puberty, peaks at about 30 years of age, and slowly declines to a nadir near age 60 years; after this, a second peak occurs in some studies in the 8th and 9th decades, mostly due to secondary neoplasms involving the testis (fig. 1-24). Although rare, germ cell tumors of typical type, usually seminomas, are occasionally seen in the elderly. Specific subtypes of testicular germ cell tumors tend to occur at different ages. Seminomas characteristically are seen in patients who are roughly 10 years

older than those with nonseminomatous germ cell tumors (40.5 years and 31.7 years, respectively [99]). Spermatocytic seminomas occur in an older population (average, 58.8 years [99]). Most epidemiologic studies, however, do not separately analyze the various subtypes.

The incidence of testicular cancer had significantly increased, doubling in some instances, in a number of European, North American, and Australasian countries from 1936 to 1976 (fig. 1-25) (96,100–110). In the last half of the 20th century, some countries had an increase of 2 to 5 percent per year, therefore experiencing a doubling of incidence every 15 to 25 years (fig. 1-25) (111). Some studies noted a leveling of this upward trend in European countries for those born during World War II, only to have the trend continue after the war (104,112). The

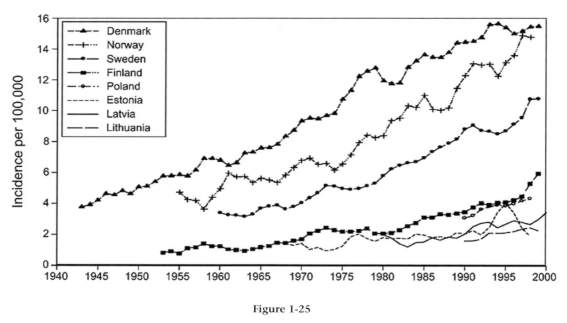

Figure 1-25

INCIDENCE OF TESTICULAR CANCER OVER TIME

An increasing incidence of germ cell tumors is evident in a number of European countries from 1945-2000. (Fig. 1 from Richiardi L, Bellocco R, Adami HO, et al. Testicular cancer incidence in eight Northern European countries: secular and recent trends. Cancer Epidemiol Biomarkers Prev 2004;13:2160.)

incidence may have peaked in Denmark (one of the countries with the highest rates), with a slight decline reported recently (107). One analysis demonstrated a world-wide increase in the incidence in both low-risk and high-risk populations and in age groups characteristically affected by seminomas and nonseminomatous germ cell tumors (113). This increase does not appear to apply to pediatric cases but only becomes manifest in adolescents (fig. 1-26) (114,115).

There are wide variations in the incidence of testicular cancer in different countries (Table 1-4). The overall annual incidence in the United States is 5 to 6 cases per 100,000 male population (98), whereas in Switzerland and Denmark it is about 10, in England about 5, in Japan about 1, and in China 0.4. Racial variations are apparent in the United States, with the highest rates in the white population (4.6 to 6.4 cases per year per 100,000 male population), followed by Hispanic (3.1 to 4.0 per 100,000), Japanese (2.3 per 100,000), African-American (0.5 to 1.6 per 100,000), and Chinese (1.0 per 100,000) (98). There is some evidence for the operation of environmental factors since Hispanics, Japanese, and Chinese men who migrate to the

United States have incidences intermediate between their country of origin and their county of adoption, although no effect of migration is seen in the African-American population (116). The only non-white race with a comparably high incidence of testicular cancer is the Maori population of New Zealand (117,118), although native Hawaiians, native Alaskans, and Native Americans have higher incidences than do other non-white populations (119).

Numerous studies have attempted to identify possible environmental or other etiologic agents in the development of testicular cancer. Several studies have documented an increased risk of testicular cancer in higher socioeconomic classes and in professional as opposed to manual workers (110,119–126). To what extent these data are skewed by the simultaneous operation of racial (genetic) factors is not clear. Such differences are nonetheless identifiable in cohorts from the early 20th century in England and Wales (124), among populations that would be expected to be fairly homogeneous. Increased risks have been identified in persons working in food manufacture and preparation and farming, and among draftsmen (121); in

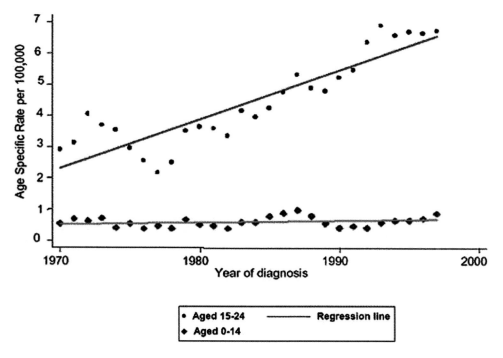

Figure 1-26

AGE-SPECIFIC RATES FOR TESTICULAR GERM CELL TUMORS BY YEAR OF DIAGNOSIS

This study, done in the north of England in patients 0 to 14 years of age and 15 to 24 years of age, showed that the younger group of patients experienced no significant increase in incidence of germ cell tumors from 1968 to 1999 in contrast to the post-pubertal group. (Fig. 2 from Xu Q, Pearce MS, Parker L. Incidence and survival for testicular germ cell tumor in young males: a report from the Northern Region Young Person's Malignant Disease Registry, United Kingdom. Urol Oncol 2007;25:34.)

sales and service workers, physicians, production supervisors, and motor vehicle mechanics (110); in professions with an exposure to heat, fertilizers, phenols, fumes, or smoke (127); in workers exposed to temperature extremes (128); in fire fighters (129); in electrical workers, foresters, fishermen, and paper and printing workers (120); in leather workers (130,131); in aircraft repairmen (132,133); in metal workers (134); and in police officers exposed to hand-held radar (135). Most such associations, however, remain weak and some are disputed (110), which has led to the conclusion that occupational status is not of major etiologic importance in testicular cancer (117,136).

Patients with acquired immunodeficiency syndrome (AIDS) (137–139) and those with other forms of immunosuppression (137) have an increased frequency of testicular germ cell tumors, disproportionately seminomas, that occur at a somewhat younger average age. Unlike many immunosuppression-related lymphomas,

however, Epstein-Barr virus (EBV) proteins and nucleic acids are not detected in tumor cells by immunohistochemical and in situ hybridization techniques, respectively (140). Other factors that have been linked to a possible increased risk for testis cancer include: single marital status (increasing the risk for nonseminomatous but not seminomatous tumors [141]), prior inguinal hernia (142–145) although some believe that the association with inguinal hernia represents a false positive association due to the confusion of cryptorchidism with hernia (116); past mumps orchitis (142,146); a history of a sexually-transmitted disease (147); exposure to estrogenic compounds in utero (148–150); a dizygotic twin (150); a maternal history of hyperemesis during gestation (151); neonatal jaundice (126); low or high birth weight (126); testicular atrophy with oligospermia and hypofertility (127); Down syndrome (152–156); Klinefelter syndrome (157); Marfan syndrome

Table 1-4

ANNUAL INCIDENCE OF TESTICULAR CANCER PER 100,000 MALE POPULATION[a]

Switzerland (Zurich)	10.1	Italy (North East)	3.9
Denmark	9.9	Canada (Quebec)	3.5
Norway	8.2	Israel (Jews)	3.3
France (Bas-Rhin)	7.9	Belgium (Flanders)	3.2
Austria (Tyrol)	7.5	USA (California, Los Angeles: Hispanic White)	3.1
Uruguay (Montevideo)	7.3	Finland	2.7
USA (Hawaii: White)	7.1	Spain (Murcia)	2.2
Germany (Saarland)	6.9	USA (Hawaii: Japanese)	2.2
UK (England, South & Western Regions)	6.1	Colombia (Cali)	1.9
UK (Scotland)	6.1	Japan (Hiroshima)	1.9
Iceland	5.8	Russia (St. Petersburg)	1.8
New Zealand	5.8	China (Hong Kong)	1.7
Slovenia	5.8	Brazil (Campinas)	1.4
USA (California, Los Angeles: Non-Hispanic White)	5.7	Singapore: Malay	1.4
USA (New Jersey: White)	5.5	USA (California, Los Angeles: Black)	1.4
Australia (Queensland)	5.4	USA (New Jersey: Black)	1.4
USA (Connecticut: White)	5.4	Japan (Osaka Prefecture)	1.2
Slovakia	5.2	Israel (Non-Jews)	1.1
UK (England)	5.1	Singapore (Chinese)	1.0
Australia (New South Wales)	5.1	India (Delhi)	0.8
Sweden	5.0	India (Mumbai)	0.8
The Netherlands	4.7	Algeria (Algiers)	0.7
Canada (Ontario)	4.4	Israel (Jews born in Africa or Asia)	0.7
Ireland	4.4	Viet Nam (Ho Chi Minh City)	0.6
France (Isere)	4.3	Korea (Seoul)	0.5
Poland (Warsaw)	4.2	China (Beijing)	0.4
Canada	4.2	Thailand (Bangkok)	0.4
Israel (Jews born in Europe or America)	4.0	Zimbabwe (Harare: African)	0.4
Italy (Torino)	4.0		

[a]Data from reference 98.

(153); dysplastic nevus syndrome (158); certain human leukocyte antigen (HLA) haplotypes (A-10, Bw35 [159]; Aw24 [for metastatic tumors] [160]; A3, Aw32, Aw33, B5, B7 [161]; B13, Bw-41 [162,163]; DR5 [161,164,165], and Dw7 [166]); ichthyosis (167); testicular trauma (146,147); maternal history of breast cancer (168); early puberty (125,143,168); tall stature (144,169); and exogenous hormone administration (170,171). There is an increased frequency of sarcoidosis in patients with testicular cancer, but the tumor usually occurs first (172). Sometimes, however, noncaseating granulomas reflect a reaction to tumor (usually seminoma) that may require careful inspection to identify.

An increased frequency of rare alleles of the variable-number-of-tandem-repeat regions flanking the *HRAS* oncogene has been demonstrated in testicular cancer patients, supporting a genetic factor (173), and linkage studies in familial cases have implicated a "testicular cancer risk gene" on Xq27 (174), although subsequent studies failed to identify this linkage (175). The association of testicular germ cell tumors with Klinefelter syndrome was not confirmed in another study (157), but there was a significant association of Klinefelter syndrome with mediastinal germ cell tumors (153), a finding supported in other studies (176). A protective effect has been associated with: exercise (143,144,147), a history of acne (149), and antenatal life during World War II (103,104,112). Four factors that have not been convincingly associated with testicular cancer are: tobacco use, alcohol use, radiation exposure, and prior vasectomy (117,147,177–180).

It is apparent that numerous associations with testicular cancer are described, but most are weak and inconsistent. There are, however, five well-established, positive associations with testicular cancer: 1) cryptorchidism, 2) a prior testicular germ cell tumor, 3) a family history of testicular germ cell tumor, 4) certain disorders of sex development (intersex syndromes), and 5) infertility.

Cryptorchidism

Cryptorchidism is strongly associated with testicular cancer (143). The frequency of past (corrected) or current cryptorchidism in patients with testicular germ cell tumors is between 3.5 and 14.5 percent of cases in various series (100,149,151,181–186), despite a low overall prevalence of cryptorchidism in the general population (in one study as low as 0.25 percent [187] and 2.7 percent in a case-control study [188]). The calculated increased risk for testicular cancer in patients with cryptorchidism has varied, mostly because of the variable estimates of its prevalence in the control population, from 2.5 to 35.0 times the noncryptorchid male population (116,142–145,151,182–184,187,189–192); the most credible prevalence is from 3.5 to 5.0 times elevated risk (145,184,190). The increased risk, however, does not become manifest before late adolescence, which is an appropriate time for possible screening (190).

Cryptorchidism likely shares predisposing maldevelopmental factors that are also important in the causation of testicular germ cell tumors (193). This is reflected by oligospermia in 15 to 25 percent of patients with unilateral cryptorchidism (194) and an increased frequency of other genitourinary anomalies in patients with testicular cancer, including ureteral duplication and ectopy, hypospadias, and ectopic kidney (145,195–197). The absence of a demonstrable

effect of orchidopexy in reducing the rate of testicular cancer in previously cryptorchid gonads (116,145,185,186,198) is another feature that favors a developmental basis for the increased risk associated with cryptorchidism. In the absence of cryptorchidism (127), the increased risk associated with testicular atrophy, hypofertility, and oligospermia may reflect dysembryogenesis. Several studies have documented that the increased risk is not limited to the cryptorchid testis, and the contralateral testis is also at increased risk (116,142,145,199,200), although to a lesser degree (119,142,145). Cryptorchidism and other genitourinary anomalies may indicate patients with a stronger genetic component for testicular germ cell tumors since such anomalies occur with increased frequency in patients with a familial history (188).

A higher proportion of seminomas occur in cryptorchid testes than in the general population (191,201,202), and the proportion of seminomas is greater for abdominal cryptorchid testes (89 percent) compared to inguinal testes (78 percent) (181). These figures contrast with the overall frequency of seminoma among germ cell tumors (50 percent) (99).

Because of the significantly increased risk of testicular cancer in patients with a history of cryptorchidism, testicular biopsies have been recommended for these at-risk patients (203). The presence of intratubular germ cell neoplasia of the unclassified type (IGCNU; carcinoma in situ) appears to be a reliable method of identifying patients at-risk, as only one testicular cancer developed when over 1,500 cryptorchid patients with negative testicular biopsies were followed for up to 8 years (203). On the other hand, invasive testicular germ cell tumors occur in at least 50 percent of patients with a positive biopsy for IGCNU who are followed for this length of time (6). The frequency of IGCNU in patients with cryptorchidism varied from 2 to 8 percent in different studies (203-206), which is an approximate four-fold increase over the general male population (206). A single-time postpubertal testicular biopsy appears to be sufficient for the identification of cryptorchid patients with IGCNU, but each testis should be biopsied (207). The suggested age for these biopsies is 18 to 20 years (207). At-risk patients cannot be reliably identified in the prepubertal period (208). Furthermore, the usual anterosuperior location of testicular biopsies may miss some cases of IGCNU in patients with cryptorchidism and severe atrophy of the seminiferous tubules (209); this study reported two patients in whom IGCNU was visualized only in intact tubules near the rete testis, and in whom a conventional biopsy would not have sampled the lesion, leading to a recommendation for posterior biopsies in cryptorchid patients who have an initial biopsy showing severe germ cell hypoplasia. Not all authorities agree that cryptorchid patients should be biopsied for the investigation of IGCNU (210).

Although orchidopexy, even at an early age, has not generally been shown to reduce the subsequent development of germ cell tumors in originally cryptorchid testes (116,145,185,198), some urologists feel that early orchidopexy may reduce the likelihood of subsequent infertility (211). The placement of the cryptorchid testis in the scrotum permits easier clinical assessment of the gonad if biopsy and prophylactic orchiectomy are not performed. One study, however, failed to show any difference in clinical stages of patients with corrected and uncorrected cryptorchidism in whom germ cell tumors developed (212).

Bilateral Testicular Germ Cell Tumors

Patients with a past or current testicular germ cell tumor are at increased risk for a contralateral testicular germ cell tumor (213–217). In two large series, the frequency of simultaneous or subsequent testicular cancer was 1.9 percent and 2.7 percent (218,219), but has ranged from 4 to 5 percent in other studies (216,220,221). Such frequencies correspond to an elevated risk more than 20 times higher than that of the general population (217,219). This risk is even greater if the second testis is cryptorchid or atrophic (222,223). In biopsies of the contralateral testis of patients with a history of testicular cancer, 4.5 to 5.7 percent were found to have IGCNU (215,222,224), but this frequency increased significantly (to 23 percent in one study [222]) when the opposite testis was either cryptorchid or atrophic (222,224,225). The interval between the two cancers is variable but can be lengthy; two studies reported that 50 percent of second germ cell tumors occur 3 to 5 years after the initial diagnosis (218,223). Because some second

tumors may not be diagnosed for more than a decade after the first, the average interval in one report was 8.8 years (226). One study claimed the risk of a second primary tumor was greater if the initial neoplasm was a nonseminomatous germ cell tumor rather than a seminoma (219). Although the histologic types of the two tumors in a given patient are often discordant (223), there is a tendency for patients with seminoma to have a second seminoma rather than a nonseminomatous tumor (218); a similar tendency is not apparent for nonseminomatous tumors (218). If a testicular cancer patient has a positive family history, the risk of bilaterality increases four-fold (227,228). There is also an increased frequency of bilateral tumors in patients with bilateral cryptorchidism and the occurrence of the first tumor at a young age (215). If the patient receives chemotherapy for the first tumor, the risk of a second tumor is decreased (214).

One way to identify patients with testicular cancer who are at risk for a second primary tumor is the examination of biopsies of the opposite testis for IGCNU. Such biopsies are positive for IGCNU in 5.4 percent of cases (229). Thirty percent of those with contralateral IGCNU already have a second tumor at the time of diagnosis of the IGCNU, and 50 percent of the remainder develop a second primary germ cell tumor within 5 years (229). None of 473 patients with testicular cancer who did not have IGCNU in a biopsy of the opposite testis had a second testicular cancer at follow-up of 12 to 96 months (229).

One study found a 93 percent frequency of codon 816 (exon 17) mutations in the *KIT* gene of bilateral testicular germ cell tumors but only a 1.3 percent frequency of the same mutation in unilateral tumors (230). This result suggested that analysis of the *KIT* gene in the index tumor may provide an effective means of identifying a high proportion of patients who will develop a second tumor. Other studies, however, failed to verify this result, finding restriction of *KIT* mutations to seminomas and also occurring in unilateral cases (231–233). At this time, therefore, mutational analysis remains unproven as a means to identify patients at risk for bilateral disease.

Familial Testicular Cancer

A case control study found a 2.2 percent frequency of testicular cancer in the first-degree male relatives of patients with testicular cancer, with the control population having a frequency of 0.4 percent (188), a six-fold increased risk (188,234). The risk for brothers is greater than the risk for fathers (227,235,236,238–240) or sons (236), an observation in keeping with linkage studies showing a positive association with a gene or genes on the X chromosome (174,237); other studies failed to verify this linkage (175). Additionally, there is an excessive risk of bilaterality with familial testis cancer, which occurs in 8.1 to 14.2 percent of cases (227,234,236), and a tendency for earlier age of onset compared to sporadic cases (236). Other observations include greater differences in the age of onset and less tendency for concordant histology as the genetic differences between the relatives become greater (i.e., from twins, to brothers, to fathers and sons) (227).

An increased frequency of cryptorchidism as well as inguinal hernias and hydroceles in the first-degree male relatives of patients with testis cancer supports an inherited tendency for urogenital malformations as a possible etiology for testicular cancer in these patients (188), although this observation has not been demonstrated in all studies (236). A genetic factor is also supported by the demonstration of an increased frequency of certain rare alleles associated with the *HRAS* proto-oncogene in patients with testicular germ cell tumors, especially those with bilateral occurrence or early age of onset (173). Germ-line mutations in the *p53* gene are not a component of the genetic predisposition to testicular cancer (241), despite the common occurrence of p53 overexpression, as detected by immunohistochemistry (241–250). One study failed to find any increase in nontesticular cancers in the families of patients with testicular cancer, supporting a lack of a generalized genetic cancer risk (251).

Disorders of Sex Development/ Intersex Syndromes

There are several disorders of sex development (intersex syndromes) that result in an increased risk for germ cell tumors, including certain forms of gonadal dysgenesis, true hermaphroditism, and the form of male pseudohermaphroditism due to the androgen insensitivity syndrome (252,253).

The term gonadal dysgenesis is somewhat ambiguous, but when applied to the testes, implies that they are not only abnormal morphologically (often showing severe regressive changes or "streak" morphology, possibly in conjunction with ovarian-type stroma) but also have failed to induce full masculinization of target organs and regression of müllerian structures. Substantial risk for the development of germ cell tumors is associated with gonadal dysgenesis in which the patients have an intact or portion of the Y chromosome. These disorders include: 46,XY pure gonadal dysgenesis (Swyer syndrome), in which bilateral streak gonads composed of ovarian-type stroma are present in a phenotypic female with infantile internal genitalia; mixed gonadal dysgenesis, in which the patients have combinations of a streak gonad and testis, female internal genitalia, and ambiguous external genitalia; and dysgenetic male pseudohermaphroditism in which bilaterally dysembryogenetic cryptorchid testes with hypoplastic tubules, sometimes with ovarian-type stroma, occur in patients with incompletely masculinized external genitalia and both müllerian and wolffian structures in the internal genitalia (253). Neoplasms are estimated to occur in 25 to 30 percent of patients with these syndromes, the most common of which is gonadoblastoma (253,254). Since neoplasms may develop during childhood, early gonadectomy is indicated. Gonadal biopsy may successfully identify patients with gonadal dysgenesis who are at risk; four phenotypic male children with 45,X/46,XY mixed gonadal dysgenesis had IGCNU identified on biopsy, leading to prophylactic orchiectomy (255). About 8 percent of children and adolescents with gonadal dysgenesis have IGCNU independent of a gonadoblastoma (256). An increased risk of germ cell tumor is also associated with true hermaphroditism, with IGCNU reported in a rare case (256) and malignant tumors in 2.6 percent of cases (253).

Male pseudohermaphrodites with androgen insensitivity syndrome lack fully functional androgen-binding receptors; they have maldescended testes with solid immature tubules, markedly decreased or absent germ cells, ovarian-type stroma, Leydig cell hyperplasia, and, frequently, hamartomatous nodules and

Sertoli cell adenomas (252,253,257,258). These patients also have a substantially increased frequency of malignant germ cell tumors, which occur in 5 to 10 percent (252,257,259,260). Most such tumors occur following pubescence, with the risk increasing substantially with age (259); a 22 percent frequency of malignant tumors is reported in patients older than 30 years (261). IGCNU may also be identified on gonadal biopsy (262).

Infertility

When analyzing patients with infertility, it is difficult to separate those who are infertile because of cryptorchidism or gonadal dysgenesis from those who are not. An association of male infertility with an increased risk of germ cell tumors is therefore expected, given the association of infertility with cryptorchidism and gonadal dysgenesis and the already discussed proclivity of patients with these disorders to develop testicular germ cell tumors. In support of this, one study found a 22 percent frequency of cryptorchidism in infertile patients with IGCNU (3). Some argue there is no clear evidence that infertility, in the absence of cryptorchidism, is significantly associated with an increased risk of testicular cancer (169). Two studies reported a frequency of IGCNU in subfertile men of 0.4 to 1.1 percent (222,263). Comparable figures appear in other studies (5,264,265). It is, therefore, apparent that patients with infertility as a whole are at increased risk for testicular germ cell tumors, especially if there is a history of cryptorchidism or testicular atrophy. Such patients are likely to have severe oligospermia or azoospermia.

GENERAL CLINICAL FEATURES

The clinical aspects of specific tumors are addressed in detail in the pertinent sections, but some general remarks are made here. Most patients with testicular tumors present with self-identified, palpable masses (generalized enlargement or distinct nodules) and less commonly, local pain (54), which was present in only 11 percent of the cases in one large series (266). It is not generally appreciated, however, that a substantial number of patients may have normal-sized or even smaller than normal testes (11 percent for those with seminomas [267]) because of the tendency for germ cell tumors to develop in atrophic testes and also because

of the occasional occurrence of spontaneous tumor regression ("burnt-out" germ cell tumors; see chapter 5). Furthermore, rare seminomas have a marked degree of intertubular growth, which does not cause either a discrete mass or significant testicular enlargement (268). Tumors that develop in cryptorchid testes, because of their inaccessibility to palpation, are also more likely to present with metastases and to be larger than those that develop in scrotal testes (54). The more aggressive tumors, especially choriocarcinoma, have a common tendency to disseminate prior to the perception of a mass. As a consequence, a number of patients present either secondary to the development of metastases in the absence of a clinically palpable mass (2 percent of cases in one study [266]). Sometimes tumors are identified incidentally in specimens obtained for other reasons, such as testicular biopsies conducted for the investigation of infertility or orchiectomy specimens removed prophylactically for longstanding cryptorchidism. In 6 percent of patients in one series (266), careful clinical palpation was able to detect small tumors in the absence of a self-identified testicular mass. Other rare forms of presentation have been reported, including a seminoma in an undescended testis that invaded the adjacent appendix and caused acute appendicitis (269) and massive tumor emboli resulting in sudden death (270,271).

The overwhelming majority of testicular tumors are of germ cell origin (95 percent [54]), typically occur in young adults, and are malignant but highly curable with current therapies. The right testis is affected more frequently than the left, with an approximate 5 to 4 ratio (54,272). Sex cord-stromal tumors are much less common and tend to occur over a wider age range than germ cell tumors, and, unlike germ cell tumors, are frequently benign. Germ cell tumors and sex cord-stromal tumors may exceptionally occur as apparent primary tumors in the paratesticular structures (273–275), although paratesticular involvement is much more common as direct spread or metastasis from primary testicular neoplasms.

Occasionally, patients present with endocrine manifestations, gynecomastia being the most common, which occur in approximately 4 percent of adults with a germ cell tumor (276). This usually reflects hCG production by a germ cell tumor, causing secondary Leydig cell hyperplasia, increased androgen production, and subsequent conversion of androgen to estrogen by aromatase in peripheral tissues. Because of the association with hCG production, gynecomastia, when due to a germ cell tumor, is seen in patients with tumors having a trophoblastic component (choriocarcinoma, seminoma, or embryonal carcinoma with syncytiotrophoblast cells). Thyrotoxicosis may also occur secondary to hCG production because of its TSH-like activity. Patients with metastatic choriocarcinoma and hyperthyroidism may have elevated levels of "molar" TSH, with normal levels of pituitary TSH, and gynecomastia may accompany hyperthyroidism in some instances (276).

Direct production of androgens and estrogens by tumors in the sex cord-stromal group may cause pseudoprecocity and gynecomastia (see chapter 6), respectively. Other manifestations have included exophthalmos (in patients with seminoma on an apparent paraneoplastic basis [277,278]), carcinoid syndrome (in five patients with apparently primary carcinoid tumors [279]), hyperandrogenism with polycythemia (a seminoma with syncytiotrophoblast cells and Leydig cell hyperplasia [280]), paraneoplastic hypercalcemia (seven patients with seminoma [281]), autoimmune hemolytic anemia (a seminoma [282]), Cushing syndrome (see chapters 6 to 8), and limbic encephalopathy (germ cell tumors [283–285]).

REFERENCES

1. Skakkebaek NE. Abnormal morphology of germ cells in two infertile men. Acta Pathol Microbiol Scand A 1972;80:374-8.
2. Skakkebaek NE. Possible carcinoma-in-situ of the testis. Lancet 1972;2:516-7.
3. Skakkebaek NE, Berthelsen JG, Visfeldt J. Clinical aspects of testicular carcinoma-in-situ. Int J Androl 1981;4(Suppl):153-60.
4. Muller J, Skakkebaek NE. Abnormal germ cells in maldescended testes: a study of cell density, nuclear size and deoxyribonucleic acid content in testicular biopsies from 50 boys. J Urol 1984;131:730-3.
5. Skakkebaek NE. Carcinoma in situ of the testis: frequency and relationship to invasive germ cell tumours in infertile men. Histopathology 1978;2:157-70.
6. Skakkebaek NE, Berthelsen JG, Giwercman A, Müller J. Carcinoma-in-situ of the testis: possible origin from gonocytes and precursor of all types of germ cell tumours except spermatocytoma. Int J Androl 1987;10:19-28.
7. Berthelsen JG, Skakkebaek NE, von der Maase H, Sorensen BL, Mogensen P. Screening for carcinoma in situ of the contralateral testis in patients with germinal testicular cancer. Br Med J (Clin Res Ed) 1982;285:1683-6.
8. Berthelsen JG, Skakkebaek NE. Value of testicular biopsy in diagnosing carcinoma in situ testis. Scand J Urol Nephrol 1981;15:165-8.
9. Ottesen AM, Skakkebaek NE, Lundsteen C, Leffers H, Larsen J, Rajpert-De Meyts E. High-resolution comparative genomic hybridization detects extra chromosome arm 12p material in most cases of carcinoma in situ adjacent to overt germ cell tumors, but not before the invasive tumor development. Genes Chromosomes Cancer 2003;38:117-25.
10. Eble JN, Sauter G, Epstein GI, Sesterhenn IA, eds. Pathology and genetics of tumours of the urinary system and male genital organs. Lyon: IARC Press; 2004.
11. Oosterhuis JW, Castedo SM, de Jong B, et al. Ploidy of primary germ cell tumors of the testis. Pathogenetic and clinical relevance. Lab Invest 1989;60:14-21.
12. El-Naggar AK, Ro JY, McLemore D, Ayala AG, Batsakis JG. DNA ploidy in testicular germ cell neoplasms: histogenetic and clinical implications. Am J Surg Pathol 1992;16:611-8.
13. de Jong B, Oosterhuis JW, Castedo SM, Vos A, te Meerman GJ. Pathogenesis of adult testicular germ cell tumors. A cytogenetic model. Cancer Genet Cytogenet 1990;48:143-67.
14. Lachman MF, Ricci A Jr, Kosciol C. DNA ploidy in testicular germ cell tumors: can an atypical seminoma be identified? Conn Med 1995;59:133-6.
15. Gibas Z, Prout GR, Pontes JE, Sandberg AA. Chromosome changes in germ cell tumors of the testis. Cancer Genet Cytogenet 1986;19:245-52.
16. Atkin NB, Baker MC. i(12p): specific chromosomal marker in seminoma and malignant teratoma of the testis? Cancer Genet Cytogenet 1983;10:199-204.

17. Samaniego F, Rodriguez E, Houldsworth J, et al. Cytogenetic and molecular analysis of human male germ cell tumors: chromosome 12 abnormalities and gene amplification. Genes Chrom Cancer 1990;1:289-300.

18. Bosl GJ, Dmitrovsky E, Reuter VE, et al. Isochromosome of the short arm of chromosome 12: clinically useful markers for male germ cell tumors. J Natl Cancer Inst 1989;81:1874-8.

19. Almstrup K, Hoei-Hansen CE, Nielsen JE, et al. Genome-wide gene expression profiling of testicular carcinoma in situ progression into overt tumours. Br J Cancer 2005;92:1934-41.

20. de Jong B, van Echten J, Looijenga LH, Geurts van Kessel A, Oosterhuis JW. Cytogenetics of the progression of adult testicular germ cell tumors. Cancer Genet Cytogenet 1997;95:88-95.

21. Oosterhuis JW, Looijenga LH. Testicular germ-cell tumours in a broader perspective. Nat Rev Cancer 2005;5:210-22.

22. Sohval AR, Churg J, Gabrilove JL Freiberg EK, Katz N. Ultrastructure of feminizing testicular Leydig cell tumors. Ultrastruc Pathol 1982;3:335-45.

23. Gier HT, Marion GB. Development of the mammalian testis. In: Johnson AD, Gomes WR, Vandmark NL, eds. The testis, vol. I. New York: Academic Press; 1970:1-42.

24. Gruenwald P. The development of the sex cords in the gonads of man and mammals. Am J Anat 1942;70:359-97.

25. Neville AM, Grigor KM. Structure, function and development of the human testis. In: Pugh RC, ed. Pathology of the testis. Oxford: Blackwell Scientific; 1976:1-37.

26. van Wagenen G, Simpson ME. Embryology of the ovary and testis: Homo sapiens and Macaca mulatta. New Haven: Yale University Press; 1965.

27. Wartenberg H. Differentiation and development of the testes. In: Burger H, de Kretser D, eds. The testis, 2nd ed. New York: Raven Press; 1989:67-118.

28. Sadler TW. Langman's medical embryology, 5th ed. Baltimore: Williams & Wilkins; 1985.

29. Carlson BM. Patten's foundations of embryology, 5th ed. New York: McGraw-Hill; 1988.

30. Park SY, Jameson JL. Minireview: transcriptional regulation of gonadal development and differentiation. Endocrinology 2005;146:1035-42.

31. Brennan J, Capel B. One tissue, two fates: molecular genetic events that underlie testis versus ovary development. Nat Rev Genet 2004;5:509-21.

32. Hollinshead WH. Textbook of anatomy, 3rd ed. Hagerstown, Maryland: Harper & Row; 1974.

33. Williams PL, Warwick R. Gray's anatomy, 36th ed. Philadelphia: W.B. Saunders; 1980.

34. Trainer TD. Histology of the normal testis. Am J Surg Pathol 1987;11:797-809.

35. Cormack DH. Ham's histology, 9th ed. Philadelphia: JB Lippincott; 1987.

36. Wheeler JE. Histology of the fertile and infertile testis. Monogr Pathol 1991;33:56-103.

37. Mattiske D, Kume T, Hogan BL. The mouse forkhead gene Foxc1 is required for primordial germ cell migration and antral follicle development. Develop Biol 2006;290:447-58.

38. Chuva de Sousa Lopes SM, van den DS, Carvalho RL et al. Altered primordial germ cell migration in the absence of transforming growth factor beta signaling via ALK5. Develop Biol 2005;284:194-203.

39. Nochomovitz LE, Orenstein JM. Adenocarcinoma of the rete testis: review and regrouping of reported cases and a consideration of miscellaneous entities. J Urogenit Pathol 1991;1:11-40.

40. Adham IM, Emmen JM, Engel W. The role of the testicular factor INSL3 in establishing the gonadal position. Mol Cell Endocrinol 2000;160:11-6.

41. Hutson JM, Hasthorpe S. Testicular descent and cryptorchidism: the state of the art in 2004. J Pediatr Surg 2005;40:297-302.

42. Giwercman A, Müller J, Skakkebaek NE. Prevalence of carcinoma in situ and other histopathological abnormalities in testes from 399 men who died suddenly and unexpectedly. J Urol 1991;145:77-80.

43. Lennox B, Ahmad KN, Mack WS. A method for determining the relative total length of the tubules in the testis. J Pathol 1970;102:229-38.

44. Clermont Y. The cycle of the seminiferous epithelium in man. Am J Anat 1963;112:35-51.

45. Guarch R, Pesce C, Puras A, Lazaro J. A quantitative approach to the classification of hypospermatogenesis in testicular biopsies for infertility. Hum Pathol 1992;23:1032-7.

46. Lobo MV, Arenas MI, Alonso FJ, et al. Nestin, a neuroectodermal stem cell marker molecule, is expressed in Leydig cells of the human testis and in some specific cell types from human testicular tumours. Cell Tissue Res 2004;316:369-76.

47. Halley JB. The infiltrative activity of Leydig cells. J Pathol Bacteriol 1961;81:347-53.

48. Mai KT. Cytoplasmic eosinophilic granular change of the ductal efferentes: a histological, immunohistochemical, and electron microscopic study. J Urol Pathol 1994;2:273-82.

49. Schned AR, Memoli VA. Coarse granular cytoplasmic change of the epididymis: an immunohistochemical and ultrastructural study. J Urol Pathol 1994;2:213-22.

50. Shah VI, Ro JY, Amin MB, Mullick S, Nazeer T, Ayala AG. Histologic variations in the epididymis: findings in 167 orchiectomy specimens. Am J Surg Pathol 1998;22:990-6.

51. Friedman NB, Moore RA. Tumors of the testis: a report on 922 cases. Milit Surgeon 1946;99:573-93.

52. Dixon FJ, Moore RA. Tumors of the male sex organs. Atlas of Tumor Pathology, 1st series, Fascicles 31b & 32. 1 ed. Washington, D.C.: Armed Forces Institute of Pathology; 1952.

53. Dixon FJ, Moore RA. Testicular tumors: a clinicopathologic study. Cancer 1953;6:427-54.

54. Melicow MM. Classification of tumors of testis: a clinical and pathological study based on 105 primary and 13 secondary cases in adults, and 3 primary and 4 secondary cases in children. J Urol 1955;73:547-74.

55. Mostofi FK, Price EB Jr. Tumors of the male genital system. Atlas of Tumor Pathology, 2nd Series, Fascicle 8. Washington D.C.: Armed Forces Institute of Pathology; 1973.

56. Morse MJ, Whitmore WF. Neoplasms of the testis. In: Walsh PC, Gittes RF, Perlmutter AD, Stamey TA, eds. Campbell's urology. Philadelphia: W.B. Saunders; 1986:1535-82.

57. Thackray AC, Crane WA. Seminoma. In: Pugh RC, ed. Pathology of the testis. Oxford: Blackwell Scientific; 1976:164-98.

58. Jacobsen GK. Malignant Sertoli cell tumors of the testis. J Urol Pathol 1993;1:233-55.

59. Grady RW, Ross JH, Kay R. Patterns of metastatic spread in prepubertal yolk sac tumor of the testis. J Urol 1995;153:1259-61.

60. Donohue JP. Metastatic pathways of non-seminomatous germ cell tumors. Semin Urol 1984;2:217-29.

61. Donohue JP, Thornhill JA, Foster RS, Rowland RG, Bihrle R. Primary retroperitoneal lymph node dissection in clinical stage A non-seminomatous germ cell testis cancer. Review of the Indiana University experience 1965-1989. Br J Urol 1993;71:326-35.

62. de Bruin MJ, Oosterhof GO, Debruyne FM. Nerve-sparing retroperitoneal lymphadenectomy for low stage testicular cancer. Br J Urol 1993;71:336-9.

63. Richie JP. Diagnosis and staging of testicular tumors. In: Skinner DG, Lieskovsky G, eds. Diagnosis and management of genitourinary cancer. Philadelphia: W.B. Saunders; 1988:498-507.

64. Sweetenham JW, Whitehouse JM, Williams CJ, Mead GM. Involvement of the gastrointestinal tract by metastases from germ cell tumors of the testis. Cancer 1988;61:2566-70.

65. Bredael JJ, Vugrin D, Whitmore WF Jr. Autopsy findings in 154 patients with germ cell tumors of the testis. Cancer 1982;50:548-51.

66. Young RH, Koelliker DD, Scully RE. Sertoli cell tumors of the testis, not otherwise specified: a clinicopathologic analysis of 60 cases. Am J Surg Pathol 1998;22:709-21.

67. Boden G, Gibb R. Radiotherapy and testicular neoplasms. Lancet 1951;2:1195-7.

68. American Joint Committee on Cancer. Testis. In: Edge SB, Byrd DR, Compton CC, Fritz AG, Greene FL, Trotti AI, eds. AJCC Cancer Staging Manual. Seventh ed. New York: Springer; 2010:469-78.

69. International Union Against Cancer. Sobin LH, Wittekind C, eds. TNM classification of malignant tumors, 5th ed. New York: Wiley-Liss; 1997.

70. Thomas G, Jones W, VanOosterom A, Kawai T. Consensus statement on the investigation and management of testicular seminoma 1989. Prog Clin Biol Res 1990;357:285-94.

71. Nazeer T, Ro JY, Kee KH, Ayala AG. Spermatic cord contamination in testicular cancer. Mod Pathol 1996;9:762-6. [French]

72. Krivosic I. [Specimen fixation in seminoma.] Ann Pathol 1993;13:45-7.

73. Nazeer T, Ro JY, Amato RJ, Park YW, Ordonez NG, Ayala AG. Histologically pure seminoma with elevated alpha-fetoprotein: a clinicopathologic study of ten cases. Oncol Rep 1998;5:1425-29.

74. Kressel K, Schnell D, Thon WF, Heymer B, Hartmann M, Altwein JE. Benign testicular tumors: a case for testis preservation? Eur Urol 1988; 15:200-4.

75. MacLennan GT, Quinonez GE, Cooley M. Testicular juvenile capillary hemangioma: conservative management with frozen-section examination. A case report. Can J Surg 1994;37:493-4.

76. Wegner HE, Herbst H, Loy V, Dieckmann KP. Testicular dermoid cyst in a 10-year-old child: case report and discussion of etiopathogenesis, diagnosis, and treatment. Urol Int 1995;54:109-11.

77. Kressel K, Hartmann M. [Nongerminal, benign testicular tumors--report of experiences.] Urologe [A] 1988;27:96-8. [German]

78. Buckspan M, Skeldon SC, Klotz PG, Pritzker KPH. Epidermoid cysts of the testicle. J Urol 1985;134:960-1.

79. Dieckmann KP, Loy V. Epidermoid cyst of the testis: a review of clinical and histogenetic considerations. Br J Urol 1994;73:436-41.

80. Heidenreich A, Zumbe J, Vorreuther R, Klotz T, Vietsch H, Engelmann UH. [Testicular epidermoid cyst: orchiectomy or enucleation resection?] Urologe A 1996;35:1-5. [German]

81. Manivel JC, Reinberg Y, Niehans GA, Fraley EE. Intratubular germ cell neoplasia in testicular teratomas and epidermoid cysts. Correlation with prognosis and possible biologic significance. Cancer 1989;64:715-20.

82. Slaughenhoupt BL, Cendron M, Al-Hindi HN, Wallace EC, Ucci A. Capillary hemangioma of the testis. J Urol Pathol 1996;4:283-8.

83. Valla JS, for the Group D'Etude en Urologie Pediatrique. Testis-sparing surgery for benign testicular tumors in children. J Urol 2001;165:2280-3.

84. Hermanek P. Frozen section diagnosis in tumors of the testis. Possibilities, limitations, indications. Pathol Res Pract 1981;173:54-65.

85. Connolly SS, D'Arcy FT, Bredin HC, Callaghan J, Corcoran MO. Value of frozen section analysis with suspected testicular malignancy. Urology 2006;67:162-5.

86. Elert A, Olbert P, Hegele A, Barth P, Hofmann R, Heidenreich A. Accuracy of frozen section examination of testicular tumors of uncertain origin. Eur Urol 2002;41:290-3.

87. Assi A, Patetta R, Fava C, Berti GL, Bacchioni AM, Cozzi L. Fine-needle aspiration of testicular lesions: report of 17 cases. Diagn Cytopathol 2000;23:388-92.

88. Balslev E, Francis D, Jacobsen GK. Testicular germ cell tumors. Classification based on fine needle aspiration biopsy. Acta Cytol 1990;34:690-4.

89. Garcia-Solano J, Sanchez-Sanchez C, Montalban-Romero S, Sola-Perez J, Perez-Guillermo M. Fine needle aspiration (FNA) of testicular germ cell tumours; a 10-year experience in a community hospital. Cytopathology 1998;9:248-62.

90. de Almeida MM, Chagas M, de Sousa JV, Mendonca ME. Fine-needle aspiration cytology as a tool for the early detection of testicular relapse of acute lymphoblastic leukemia in children. Diagn Cytopathol 1994;10:44-6.

91. Rege JD, Amarapurkar AD, Phatak AM. Fine needle aspiration cytology of adenomatoid tumor. A case report. Acta Cytol 1999;43:495-7.

92. Tewari R, Mishra MN, Salopal TK. The role of fine needle aspiration cytology in evaluation of epididymal nodular lesions. Acta Cytol 2007;51:168-70.

93. Manjunath GV, Nandini NM, Sunila. Fine needle aspiration cytology of adenomatoid tumour—a case report with review of literature. Indian J Pathol Microbiol 2005;48:503-4.

94. Highman WJ, Oliver RT. Diagnosis of metastases from testicular germ cell tumours using fine needle aspiration cytology. J Clin Pathol 1987;40:1324-33.

95. Caraway NP, Fanning CV, Amato RJ, Sneige N. Fine-needle aspiration cytology of seminoma: a review of 16 cases. Diagn Cytopathol 1995;12:327-33.

96. Pike MC, Chilvers CE, Bobrow LG. Classification of testicular cancer in incidence and mortality statistics. Br J Cancer 1987;56:83-5.

97. Brown LM, Pottern LM, Hoover RN, Devesa SS, Aselton P, Flannery JT. Testicular cancer in the United States: trends in incidence and mortality. Int J Epidemiol 1986;15:164-70.

98. Parkin DM, Whelan SL, Ferlay F, Teppo L, Thomas DB, eds. International Agency for Research on Cancer. Cancer incidence in five continents. Lyon: IARC Press; 2002.

99. Krag Jacobsen G, Barlebo H, Olsen J, et al. Testicular germ cell tumours in Denmark 1976-1980: pathology of 1058 consecutive cases. Acta Radiol Oncol 1984;23:239-47.

100. Schottenfeld D, Warshauer ME, Sherlock S, Zauber AG, Leder M, Payne R. The epidemiology of testicular cancer in young adults. Am J Epidemiol 1980;112:232-46.

101. Zheng T, Holford TR, Ma Z, Ward BA, Flannery J, Boyle P. Continuing increase in incidence of germ-cell testis cancer in young adults: experience from Connecticut, USA, 1935-1992. Int J Cancer 1996;65:723-9.

102. Osterlind A. Diverging trends in incidence and mortality of testicular cancer in Denmark, 1943-1982. Br J Cancer 1986;53:501-5.

103. Moller H. Clues to the aetiology of testicular germ cell tumours from descriptive epidemiology. Eur Urol 1993;23:8-13.

104. Wanderas EH, Tretli S, Fossa SD. Trends in incidence of testicular cancer in Norway 1955-1992. Eur J Cancer 1995;31A:2044-8.

105. Boyle P, Kaye SB, Robertson AG. Changes in testicular cancer in Scotland. Eur J Cancer Clin Oncol 1987;23:827-30.

106. Bray F, Richiardi L, Ekbom A, Pukkala E, Cuninkova M, Moller H. Trends in testicular cancer incidence and mortality in 22 European countries: continuing increases in incidence and declines in mortality. Int J Cancer 2006;118:3099-111.

107. Richiardi L, Bellocco R, Adami HO, et al. Testicular cancer incidence in eight northern European countries: secular and recent trends. Cancer Epidemiol Biomarkers Prev 2004;13:2157-66.

108. Agnarsson BA, Gudbjartsson T, Einarsson GV, et al. Testicular germ cell tumours in Iceland: a nationwide clinicopathological study. APMIS 2006;114:779-83.

109. Stone JM, Cruickshank DG, Sandeman TF, Matthews JP. Trebling of the incidence of testicular cancer in Victoria, Australia (1950-1985). Cancer 1991;68:211-9.

110. Pearce N, Sheppard RA, Howard JK, Fraser J, Lilley BM. Time trends and occupational differences in cancer of the testis in New Zealand. Cancer 1987;59:1677-82.

111. Adami HO, Bergstrom R, Mohner M, et al. Testicular cancer in nine northern European countries. Int J Cancer 1994;59:33-8.

112. Bergstrom R, Adami HO, Mohner M, et al. Increase in testicular cancer incidence in six European countries: a birth cohort phenomenon. J Natl Cancer Inst 1996;88:727-33.

113. Forman D, Moller H. Testicular cancer. Cancer Surv 1994;19-20:323-41.

114. Moller H, Jorgensen N, Forman D. Trends in incidence of testicular cancer in boys and adolescent men. Int J Cancer 1995;61:761-4.

115. Walsh TJ, Grady RW, Porter MP, Lin DW, Weiss NS. Incidence of testicular germ cell cancers in U.S. children: SEER program experience 1973 to 2000. Urology 2006;68:402-5.

116. Senturia YD. The epidemiology of testicular cancer. Br J Urol 1987;60:285-91.

117. Forman D, Gallagher R, Moller H, Swerdlow TJ. Aetiology and epidemiology of testicular cancer: report of consensus group. Prog Clin Biol Res 1990;357:245-53.

118. Wilkinson TJ, Colls BM, Schluter PJ. Increased incidence of germ cell testicular cancer in New Zealand Maoris. Br J Cancer 1992;65:769-71.

119. Swerdlow AJ. The epidemiology of testicular cancer. Eur Urol 1993;23 Suppl 2:35-8.

120. Swerdlow AJ, Skeet RG. Occupational associations of testicular cancer in south east England. Br J Indust Med 1988;45:225-30.

121. McDowall ME, Balarajan R. Testicular cancer mortality in England and Wales 1971-80: variations by occupation. J Epidemiol Comm Health 1986;40:26-9.

122. Ross RK, McCurtis JW, Henderson BE, Menck HR, Mack TM, Martin SP. Descriptive epidemiology of testicular and prostatic cancer in Los Angeles. Br J Cancer 1979;39:284-92.

123. Graham S, Gibson R, West D, Swanson M, Burnett W, Dayal H. Epidemiology of cancer of the testis in Upstate New York. J Natl Cancer Inst 1977;58:1255-61.

124. Davies JM. Testicular cancer in England and Wales: some epidemiological aspects. Lancet 1981;1:928-32.

125. Moller H, Skakkebaek NE. Risks of testicular cancer and cryptorchidism in relation to socio-economic status and related factors: case-control studies in Denmark. Int J Cancer 1996;66:287-93.

126. Akre O, Ekbom A, Hsieh CC, Trichopoulos D, Adami HO. Testicular nonseminoma and seminoma in relation to perinatal characteristics. J Natl Cancer Inst 1996;88:883-9.

127. Haughey BP, Graham S, Brasure J, Zielezny M, Sufrin G, Burnett WS. The epidemiology of testicular cancer in upstate New York. Am J Epidemiol 1989;130:25-36.

128. Zhang ZF, Vena JE, Zielezny M, et al. Occupational exposure to extreme temperature and risk of testicular cancer. Arch Environ Health 1995;50:13-8.

129. Bates MN, Lane L. Testicular cancer in fire fighters: a cluster investigation. N Z Med J 1995;108:334-7.

130. Marshall EG, Melius JM, London MA, Nasca PC, Burnett WS. Investigation of a testicular cancer cluster using a case-control approach. Int J Epidemiol 1990;19:269-73.

131. Center for Disease Control. Testicular cancer in leather workers—Fulton County, New York. MMWR 1989;38:105-6, 111-14.

132. Ducatman AM, Conwill DE, Crawl J. Germ cell tumors of the testicle among aircraft repairmen. J Urol 1986;136:834-6.

133. Foley S, Middleton S, Stitson D, Mahoney M. The incidence of testicular cancer in Royal Air Force personnel. Br J Urol 1995;76:495-6.

134. Rhomberg W, Schmoll HJ, Schneider B. High frequency of metalworkers among patients with seminomatous tumors of the testis: a case-control study. Am J Ind Med 1995;28:79-87.

135. Davis RL, Mostofi FK. Cluster of testicular cancer in police officers exposed to hand-held radar. Am J Ind Med 1993;24:231-3.

136. Van den Eeden SK, Weiss NS, Strader CH, Daling JR. Occupation and the occurrence of testicular cancer. Am J Indust Med 1991;19:327-37.

137. Leibovitch I, Baniel J, Rowland RG, Smith ER Jr, Ludlow JK, Donohue JP. Malignant testicular neoplasms in immunosuppressed patients. J Urol 1996;155:1938-42.

138. Wilson WT, Frenkel E, Vuitch F, Sagalowsky AI. Testicular tumors in men with human immunodeficiency virus. J Urol 1992;147:1038-40.

139. Powles T, Bower M, Daugaard G, et al. Multicenter study of human immunodeficiency virus-related germ cell tumors. J Clin Oncol 2003;21:1922-7.

140. Rajpert-De Meyts E, Hording U, Nielsen HW, Skakkebaek NE. Human papillomavirus and Epstein-Barr virus in the etiology of testicular germ cell tumours. APMIS 1994;102:38-42.

141. Newell GR, Spitz MR, Sider JG, Pollack ES. Incidence of testicular cancer in the United States related to marital status, histology, and ethnicity. J Natl Cancer Inst 1987;78:881-5.

142. Swerdlow AJ, Huttly SRA, Smith PG. Testicular cancer and antecedent disease. Br J Cancer 1987;55:97-103.

143. United Kingdom Testicular Cancer Study Group. Aetiology of testicular cancer: association with congenital abnormalities, age at puberty, infertility, and exercise. BMJ 1994;308:1393-9.

144. Gallagher RP, Huchcroft S, Phillips N, et al. Physical activity, medical history, and risk of testicular cancer (Alberta and British Columbia, Canada). Cancer Causes Control 1995;6:398-406.

145. Prener A, Engholm G, Jensen OM. Genital anomalies and risk for testicular cancer in Danish men. Epidemiology 1996;7:14-9.

146. Brown LM, Pottern LM, Hoover RN. Testicular cancer in young men: the search for causes of the epidemic increase in the United States. J Epidemiol Comm Health 1987;41:349-54.

147. UK Testicular Cancer Study Group. Social, behavioural and medical factors in the aetiology of testicular cancer: results from the UK study. Br J Cancer 1994;70:513-20.

148. Swerdlow AJ, Huttly SR, Smith PG. Prenatal and familial associations of testicular cancer. Br J Cancer 1987;55:571-7.

149. Depue RH, Pike MC, Henderson BE. Estrogen exposure during gestation and risk of testicular cancer. J Natl Cancer Inst 1983;71:1151-5.

150. Braun MM, Ahlbom A, Floderus B, Brinton LA, Hoover RN. Effect of twinship on incidence of cancer of the testis, breast, and other sites (Sweden). Cancer Causes Control 1995;6:519-24.

151. Henderson BE, Benton B, Jing J, Yu MC, Pike MC. Risk factors for cancer of the testis in young men. Int J Cancer 1979;23:598-602.

152. Braun DL, Green MD, Rausen AR, et al. Down's syndrome and testicular cancer: a possible association. Am J Pediat Hematol Oncol 1985;7:208-11.

153. Dexeus FH, Logothetis CJ, Chong C, Sella A, Ogden S. Genetic abnormalities in men with germ cell tumors. J Urol 1988;140:80-4.

154. Benson RC Jr, Beard CM, Kelalis PP, Kurland LT. Malignant potential of the cryptorchid testis. Mayo Clin Proc 1991;66:372-8.

155. Dieckmann KP, Rübe C, Henke RP. Association of Down's syndrome and testicular cancer. J Urol 1997;157:1701-4.

156. Satgé D, Sasco AJ, Curé H, Leduc B, Sommelet D, Vekemans MJ. An excess of testicular germ cell tumors in Down's syndrome: three case reports and a review of the literature. Cancer 1997;80:929-35.

157. Sogge MR, McDonald SD, Cofold PB. The malignant potential of the dysgenetic germ cell in Klinefelter's syndrome. Am J Med 1979;66:515-8.

158. Sigg C, Pelloni F. Dysplastic nevi and germ cell tumors of the testis - a possible further tumor in the spectrum of associated malignancies in dysplastic nevus syndrome. Dermatologica 1988;176:109-10.

159. Majsky A, Abrahamova J, Korinkova P, Bek V. HLA system and testicular germinative tumors. Oncology 1979;36:228-31.

160. Carr BI, Bach FH. Possible association between HLA-Aw24 and metastatic germ-cell tumours. Lancet 1979;1:1346-7.

161. Pollack MS, Vugrin D, Hennessy W, Herr HW, Dupont B, Whitmore WF Jr. HLA antigens in patients with germ cell cancers of the testis. Cancer Res 1982;42:2470-3.

162. Dieckmann KP, von Keyserlingk HJ. HLA association of testicular seminoma. Klin Wochenschr 1988;66:337-9.

163. Dieckmann KP, Klan R, Bunte S. HLA antigens, Lewis antigens, and blood groups in patients with testicular germ-cell tumors. Oncology 1993;50:252-8.

164. Kratzik C, Aiginger P, Kuzmits R, et al. HLA-antigen distribution in seminoma, HCG-positive seminoma and non-seminomatous tumours of the testis. Urol Res 1989;17:377-80.

165. Oliver RT. HLA phenotype and clinicopathological behaviour of germ cell tumours: possible evidence for clonal evolution from seminomas to nonseminomas. Int J Androl 1987;10:85-93.

166. DeWolf WC, Lange PH, Einarson ME, Yunis EJ. HLA and testicular cancer. Nature 1979;277:216-7.

167. Lykkesfeldt G, Bennett P, Lykkesfeldt AE, et al. Testis cancer. Ichthyosis constitutes a significant risk factor. Cancer 1991;67:730-4.

168. Moss AR, Osmond D, Bacchetti P, Torti FM, Gurgin V. Hormonal risk factors in testicular cancer: a case control study. Am J Epidemiol 1986;124:39-52.

169. Swerdlow AJ, Huttly SR, Smith PG. Testis cancer: post-natal hormonal factors, sexual behaviour and fertility. Int J Cancer 1989;43:549-53.

170. Neoptolemos JP, Locke TJ, Fossard DP. Testicular tumour associated with hormonal treatment for oligospermia. Lancet 1981;2:754.

171. Reyes FI, Faiman C. Development of a testicular tumour during cisclomiphene therapy. Can Med Assoc J 1973;109:502-6.

172. Rayson D, Burch PA, Richardson RL. Sarcoidosis and testicular carcinoma. Cancer 1998;83:337-43.

173. Ryberg D, Heimdal K, Fossa SD, Borresen AL, Haugen A. Rare Ha-ras1 alleles and predisposition to testicular cancer. Int J Cancer 1993;53:938-40.

174. Rapley EA, Crockford GP, Teare D, et al. Localization to Xq27 of a susceptibility gene for testicular germ-cell tumours. Nature Genet 2000;24:197-200.

175. Crockford GP, Linger R, Hockley S, et al. Genome-wide linkage screen for testicular germ cell tumour susceptibility loci. Hum Mol Genet 2006;15:443-51.

176. Nichols CR, Heerema NA, Palmer C, Loehrer PJ Sr, Williams SD, Einhorn LH. Klinefelter's syndrome associated with mediastinal germ cell neoplasms. J Clin Oncol 1987;5:1290-4.

177. Nienhuis H, Goldacre M, Seagroatt V, Gill L, Vessey M. Incidence of disease after vasectomy: a record linkage retrospective cohort study. BMJ 1992;304:743-6.

178. Hewitt G, Logan CJ, Curry RC. Does vasectomy cause testicular cancer? Br J Urol 1993;71:607-8.

179. Rosenberg L, Palmer JR, Zauber AG, et al. The relation of vasectomy to the risk of cancer. Am J Epidemiol 1994;140:431-8.

180. Moller H, Knudsen LB, Lynge E. Risk of testicular cancer after vasectomy: cohort study of over 73,000 men. BMJ 1994;309:295-9.

181. Halme A, Kellokumpu-Lehtinen P, Lehtonen T, Teppo L. Morphology of testicular germ cell tumours in treated and untreated cryptorchidism. Br J Urol 1989;64:78-83.

182. Lanson Y. Epidemiology of testicular cancers. Prog Clin Biol Res 1985;203:155-9.

183. Javadpour N, Bergman S. Recent advances in testicular cancer. Curr Prob Surg 1978;15(Feb):1-64.

184. Pottern LM, Brown LM, Hoover RN, et al. Testicular cancer risk among young men: role of cryptorchidism and inguinal hernia. J Natl Cancer Inst 1985;74:377-81.

185. Pike MC, Chilvers C, Peckham MJ. Effects of age at orchidopexy on risk of testicular cancer. Lancet 1986;1:1246-8.

186. Dow JA, Mostofi FK. Testicular tumors following orchiopexy. South Med J 1967;60:193-5.

187. Mostofi FK. Testicular tumors: epidemiologic, etiologic, and pathologic features. Cancer 1973;32:1186-201.

188. Tollerud DJ, Blattner WA, Fraser MC, et al. Familial testicular cancer and urogenital developmental anomalies. Cancer 1985;55:1849-54.

189. Brendler H. Cryptorchidism and cancer. Prog Clin Biol Res 1985;203:189-96.

190. Giwercman A, Grindsted J, Hansen B, Jensen OM, Skakkebaek NE. Testicular cancer risk in boys with maldescended testis: a cohort study. J Urol 1987;138:1214-6.

191. Miller A, Seljelid R. Histopathologic classification and natural history of malignant testis tumors in Norway, 1959-1963. Cancer 1971;28:1054-62.

192. Whitaker RH. Neoplasia in cryptorchid men. Semin Urol 1988;6:107-9.

193. Fram RJ, Garnick MB, Retik A. The spectrum of genitourinary abnormalities in patients with cryptorchidism, with emphasis on testicular carcinoma. Cancer 1982;50:2243-5.

194. Bar-Maor JA, Nissan S, Lernau OZ, Oren M, Levy E. Orchidopexy in cryptorchidism assessed by clinical, histologic and sperm examinations. Surg Gynecol Obstet 1979;118:855-9.

195. Sakashita S, Koyanagi T, Tsuji I, Arikado K, Matsuno T. Congenital anomalies in children with testicular germ cell tumor. J Urol 1980;124:889-91.

196. Li FP, Fraumeni JF Jr. Testicular cancers in children: epidemiologic characteristics. J Natl Cancer Inst 1972;48:1575-82.

197. Swerdlow AJ, Stiller CA, Wilson LM. Prenatal factors in the aetiology of testicular cancer: an epidemiological study of childhood testicular cancer deaths in Great Britain, 1953-73. J Epidemiol Comm Health 1982;36:96-101.

198. Batata MA, Chu FC, Hilaris BS, Whitmore WF, Golbey RB. Testicular cancer in cryptorchids. Cancer 1982;49:1023-30.

199. Johnson DE, Woodhead DM, Pohl DR, Robison JR. Cryptorchidism and testicular tumorigenesis. Surgery 1968;63:919-22.

200. Gilbert JB, Hamilton JB. Studies in malignant testis tumors: III - incidence and nature of tumors in ectopic testes. Surg Gynecol Obstet 1940;71:731-43.

201. Collins DH, Pugh RC. Classification and frequency of testicular tumours. Br J Urol 1964; 36(Suppl):1-11.

202. Morrison AS. Cryptorchidism, hernia, and cancer of the testis. J Natl Cancer Inst 1976;56:731-3.

203. Giwercman A, Muller J, Skakkebaek NE. Carcinoma in situ of the undescended testis. Semin Urol 1988;6:110-9.

204. Pedersen KV, Boiesen P, Zetter-Lund CG. Experience of screening for carcinoma-in-situ of the testis among young men with surgically corrected maldescended testes. Int J Androl 1987;10:181-5.

205. Krabbe S, Skakkebaek NE, Berthelsen JG, et al. High incidence of undetected neoplasia in maldescended testes. Lancet 1979;1:999-1000.

206. Giwercman A, von der Maase H, Skakkebaek NE. Epidemiological and clinical aspects of carcinoma in situ of the testis. Eur Urol 1993;23:104-10.

207. Giwercman A, Bruun E, Frimodt-Moller C, Skakkebaek NE. Prevalence of carcinoma in situ and other histopathologic abnormalities in testes of men with a history of cryptorchidism. J Urol 1989;142:998-1002.

208. Parkinson MC, Swerdlow AJ, Pike MC. Carcinoma in situ in boys with cryptorchidism: when can it be detected? Br J Urol 1994;73:431-5.

209. Nistal M, Codesal J, Paniagua R. Carcinoma in situ of the testis in infertile men. A histological, immunocytochemical, and cytophotometric study of DNA content. J Pathol 1989;159:205-10.

210. Oliver RT. Germ cell cancer of the testes. Curr Opin Oncol 1995;7:292-6.

211. Hezmall HP, Lipshultz LI. Cryptorchidism and infertility. Urol Clin North Am 1982;9:361-9.

212. Jones BJ, Thornhill JA, O'Donnell B, et al. Influence of prior orchiopexy on stage and prognosis of testicular cancer. Eur Urol 1991;19:201-3.

213. Reinberg Y, Manivel JC, Zhang G, Reddy PK. Synchronous bilateral testicular germ cell tumors of different histologic type: pathogenetic and practical implications of bilaterality in testicular germ cell tumors. Cancer 1991;68:1082-5.

214. Bokemeyer C, Schmoll HJ, Schoffski P, Harstrick A, Bading M, Poliwoda H. Bilateral testicular tumours: prevalence and clinical implications. Eur J Cancer 1993;29A:874-6.

215. Dieckmann KP, Loy V. Prevalence of bilateral testicular germ cell tumors and early detection by testicular intraepithelial neoplasia. Eur Urol 1993;23 Suppl 2:22-3.

216. Dieckmann KP, Loy PV, Buttner P. Prevalence of bilateral testicular germ cell tumours and early detection based on contralateral testicular intraepithelial neoplasia. Br J Urol 1993;71:340-5.

217. Colls BM, Harvey VJ, Skelton L, Thompson PI, Frampton CM. Bilateral germ cell testicular tumors in New Zealand: experience in Auckland and Christchurch 1978-1994. J Clin Oncol 1996;14:2061-5.

218. Kristianslund S, Fossa SD, Kjellevold K. Bilateral malignant testicular germ cell cancer. Br J Urol 1986;58:60-3.

219. Osterlind A, Berthelsen JG, Abildgaard N, et al. Incidence of bilateral testicular germ cell cancer in Denmark, 1960-84: preliminary findings. Int J Androl 1987;10:203-8.

220. Scheiber K, Ackermann D, Studer UE. Bilateral testicular germ cell tumors: a report of 20 cases. J Urol 1987;138:73-6.

221. Dieckmann KP, Boeckmann W, Brosig W, Jonas D, Bauer HW. Bilateral testicular germ cell tumors. Report of nine cases and review of the literature. Cancer 1986;57:1254-8.

222. Giwercman A, Berthelsen JG, Muller J, von der Maase H, Skakkebaek NE. Screening for carcinoma-in-situ of the testis. Int J Androl 1987;10:173-80.

223. Zingg EJ, Zehntner C. Bilateral testicular germ cell tumors. Prog Clin Biol Res 1985;203:673-80.

224. Loy V, Dieckmann KP. Prevalence of contralateral testicular intraepithelial neoplasia (carcinoma in situ) in patients with testicular germ cell tumour. Results of the German multicentre study. Eur Urol 1993;23:120-2.

225. Harland SJ, Cook PA, Fossa SD, et al. Risk factors for carcinoma in situ of the contralateral testis in patients with testicular cancer. An interim report. Eur Urol 1993;23:115-8.

226. Ware SM, Heyman J, Al-Askari S, Morales P. Bilateral testicular germ cell malignancy. Urology 1982;19:366-72.

227. Dieckmann KP, Becker T, Jonas D, Bauer HW. Inheritance and testicular cancer. Arguments based on a report of 3 cases and a review of the literature. Oncology 1987;44:367-77.

228. Hayakawa M, Mukai K, Nagakura K, Hata M. A case of simultaneous bilateral germ cell tumors arising from cryptorchid testes. J Urol 1986;136:470-2.

229. von der Maase H, Rorth M, Walbom-Jorgensen S, et al. Carcinoma in situ of contralateral testis in patients with testicular germ cell cancer: study of 27 cases in 500 patients. BMJ 1986;293:1398-401.

230. Looijenga LH, de Leeuw H, van Oorschot M, et al. Stem cell factor receptor (c-KIT) codon 816 mutations predict development of bilateral testicular germ-cell tumors. Cancer Res 2003;63:7674-8.

231. Sakuma Y, Sakurai S, Oguni S, Hironaka M, Saito K. Alterations of the c-kit gene in testicular germ cell tumors. Cancer Sci 2003;94:486-91.

232. Kemmer K, Corless CL, Fletcher JA, et al. KIT mutations are common in testicular seminomas. Am J Pathol 2004;164:305-13.

233. Biermann K, Göke F, Nettersheim D, et al. c-KIT is frequently mutated in bilateral germ cell tumours and down-regulated during progression from intratubular germ cell neoplasia to seminoma. J Pathol 2007;213:311-8.

234. Fuller DB, Plenk HP. Malignant testicular germ cell tumors in a father and two sons. Case report and literature review. Cancer 1986;58:955-8.

235. Westergaard T, Olsen JH, Frisch M, Kroman N, Nielsen JW, Melbye M. Cancer risk in fathers and brothers of testicular cancer patients in Denmark. A population-based study. Int J Cancer 1996;66:627-31.

236. Heimdal K, Olsson H, Tretli S, Flodgren P, Borresen AL, Fossa SD. Familial testicular cancer in Norway and southern Sweden. Br J Cancer 1996;73:964-9.

237. Rapley EA, Crockford GP, Easton DF, Stratton MR, Bishop DT, International Testicular Cancer Linkage Consortium. Localisation of susceptibility genes for familial testicular germ cell tumour. APMIS 2003;111:128-33.

238. Patel SR, Kvols LK, Richardson RL. Familial testicular cancer: report of six cases and review of the literature. Mayo Clin Proc 1990;65:804-8.

239. Forman D, Oliver RT, Brett AR, et al. Familial testicular cancer: a report of the UK family register, estimation of risk and an HLA class 1 sib-pair analysis. Br J Cancer 1992;65:255-62.

240. Dieckmann KP, Pichlmeier U. The prevalence of familial testicular cancer: an analysis of two patient populations and a review of the literature. Cancer 1997;80:1954-60.

241. Riou G, Barrois M, Prost S, Terrier MJ, Theodore C, Levine AJ. The p53 and mdm-2 genes in human testicular germ-cell tumors. Mol Carcinog 1995;12:124-31.
242. Bartkova J, Bartek J, Lukas J, et al. p53 protein alterations in human testicular cancer including pre-invasive intratubular germ-cell neoplasia. Int J Cancer 1991;49:196-202.
243. Heimdal K, Lothe RA, Lystad S, Holm R, Fossa SD, Borresen AL. No germline TP53 mutations detected in familial and bilateral testicular cancer. Genes Chrom Cancer 1993;6:92-7.
244. Peng HQ, Hogg D, Malkin D, et al. Mutations of the p53 gene do not occur in testis cancer. Cancer Res 1993;53:3574-8.
245. Ye DW, Zheng J, Qian SX, et al. p53 gene mutations in Chinese human testicular seminoma. J Urol 1993;150:884-6.
246. Ulbright TM, Orazi A, de Riese W, et al. The correlation of P53 protein expression with proliferative activity and occult metastases in clinical stage I non-seminomatous germ cell tumors of the testis. Mod Pathol 1994;7:64-8.
247. Fleischhacker M, Strohmeyer T, Imai Y, Slamon DJ, Koeffler HP. Mutations of the p53 gene are not detectable in human testicular tumors. Mod Pathol 1994;7:435-9.
248. Lewis DJ, Sesterhenn IA, McCarthy WF, Moul JW. Immunohistochemical expression of P53 tumor suppressor gene protein in adult germ cell testis tumors: clinical correlation in stage I disease. J Urol 1994;152:418-23.
249. Wu WJ, Kakehi Y, Habuchi T, et al. Allelic frequency of p53 gene codon 72 polymorphism in urologic cancers. Jpn J Cancer Res 1995;86:730-6.
250. Schenkman NS, Sesterhenn IA, Washington L, et al. Increased p53 protein does not correlate to p53 gene mutations in microdissected human testicular germ cell tumors. J Urol 1995;154:617-21.
251. Heimdal K, Olsson H, Tretli S, Flodgren P, Borresen AL, Fosså SD. Risk of cancer in relatives of testicular cancer patients. Br J Cancer 1996;73:970-3.
252. Rutgers JL. Advances in the pathology of intersex syndromes. Hum Pathol 1991;22:884-91.
253. Rutgers JL, Scully RE. Pathology of the testis in intersex syndromes. Semin Diagn Pathol 1987;4:275-91.
254. Hughesdon PE, Kumarasamy T. Mixed germ cell tumours (gonadoblastomas) in normal and dysgenetic gonads: case reports and review. Virchows Arch A Pathol Anat 1970;349:258-80.
255. Muller J, Skakkebaek NE, Ritzën M, Plöen L, Petersen KE. Carcinoma in situ of the testis in children with 45,X/46,XY gonadal dysgenesis. J Pediatr 1985;106:431-6.
256. Ramani P, Yeung CK, Habeebu SS. Testicular intratubular germ cell neoplasia in children and adolescents with intersex. Am J Surg Pathol 1993;17:1124-33.
257. Rutgers JL, Scully RE. The androgen insensitivity syndrome (testicular feminization): a clinicopathologic study of 43 cases. Int J Gynecol Pathol 1991;10:126-44.
258. Collins GM, Kim DU, Logrono R, Rickert RR, Zablow A, Breen JL. Pure seminoma arising in androgen insensitivity syndrome (testicular feminization syndrome): a case report and review of the literature. Mod Pathol 1993;6:89-93.
259. Manuel M, Katayama KP, Jones HW. The age of occurrence of gonadal tumors in intersex patients with a Y chromosome. Am J Obstet Gynecol 1976;124:293-306.
260. Morris JM. The syndrome of testicular feminization in male pseudohermaphrodites. Am J Obstet Gynecol 1953;65:1192-211.
261. Morris JM, Mahesh VB. Further observations on the syndrome, "testicular feminization". Am J Obstet Gynecol 1963;87:731-48.
262. Nogales FF Jr, Toro M, Ortega I, Fulwood HR. Bilateral incipient germ cell tumours of the testis in the incomplete testicular feminization syndrome. Histopathology 1981;5:511-5.
263. Gondos B, Migliozzi JA. Intratubular germ cell neoplasia. Semin Diagn Pathol 1987;4:292-303.
264. Pryor JP, Cameron KM, Chilton CP, et al. Carcinoma in situ in testicular biopsies in men presenting with infertility. Br J Urol 1983;55:780-4.
265. West AB, Butler MR, Fitzpatrick J, O'Brien A. Testicular tumors in subfertile men: report of 4 cases with implications for management of patients presenting with infertility. J Urol 1985;133:107-9.
266. Lewis LG. Testis tumors: report of 250 cases. J Urol 1948;59:763-72.
267. Thackray AC. Seminoma. Br J Urol 1964;36 (Suppl):12-27.
268. Henley JD, Young RH, Wade CL, Ulbright TM. Seminomas with exclusive intertubular growth: a report of 12 clinically and grossly inconspicuous tumors. Am J Surg Pathol 2004;28:1163-8.
269. Sarma DP, Weilbaecher TG, Hatem AA. Seminoma arising in undescended testis clinically presenting as acute appendicitis. J Surg Oncol 1986;31:44-7.
270. Saukko P, Lignitz E. [Sudden death caused by malignant testicular tumors.] Z Rechtsmed 1990;103:529-36. [German]
271. Aronsohn RS, Nishiyama RH. Embryonal carcinoma. An unexpected cause of sudden death in a young adult. JAMA 1974;229:1093-4.

272. Pugh RC. Testicular tumours—introduction. In: Pugh RC, ed. Pathology of the testis. Oxford: Blackwell Scientific; 1976:139-59.

273. Dichmann O, Engel U, Jensen DB, Bilde T. Juxtatesticular seminoma. Br J Urol 1990;66:324-5.

274. Leaf DN, Tucker GR 3rd, Harrison LH. Embryonal cell carcinoma originating in the spermatic cord: case report. J Urol 1974;112:285-6.

275. Srigley JR, Hartwick RW. Tumors and cysts of the paratesticular region. Pathol Annu 1990;25(Pt 2):51-108.

276. Scully RE. Testicular tumors with endocrine manifestations. In: DeGroot LJ, ed. Endocrinology. 3rd ed. Philadelphia: WB Saunders Co; 1995:2442-8.

277. Mann AS. Bilateral exophthalmos in seminoma. J Clin Endocrinol Metab 1967;27:1500-2.

278. Taylor JB, Solomon DH, Levine RE, Ehrlich RM. Exophthalmos in seminoma: regression with steroids and orchiectomy. JAMA 1978;240:860-1.

279. Zavala-Pompa A, Ro JY, El-Naggar A, et al. Primary carcinoid tumor of testis. Immunohistochemical, ultrastructural, and DNA flow cytometric study of three cases with a review of the literature. Cancer 1993;72:1726-32.

280. Reman O, Reznik Y, Casadevall N, et al. Polycythemia and steroid overproduction in a gonadotropin-secreting seminoma of the testis. Cancer 1991;68:2224-9.

281. da Silva MA, Edmondson JW, Eby C, Loehrer PJ. Humoral hypercalcemia in seminomas. Med Pediatr Oncol 1992;20:38-41.

282. Lundberg WB, Mitchell MS. Transient warm autoimmune hemolytic anemia and cryoglobulinemia associated with seminoma. Yale J Biol Med 1977;50:419-27.

283. Landolfi JC, Nadkarni M. Paraneoplastic limbic encephalitis and possible narcolepsy in a patient with testicular cancer: case study. Neurol Oncol 2003;5:214-6.

284. Burton GV, Bullard DE, Walther PJ, Burger PC. Paraneoplastic encephalopathy with testicular carcinoma: a reversible neurologic syndrome. Cancer 1988;62:2248-51.

285. Voltz R, Gultekin SH, Rosenfeld MR, et al. A serologic marker of paraneoplastic limbic and brain-stem encephalitis in patients with testicular cancer. N Engl J Med 1999;340:1788-95.

2 GERM CELL TUMORS: HISTOGENETIC CONSIDERATIONS AND INTRATUBULAR GERM CELL NEOPLASIA

HISTOGENESIS

Most germ cell tumors of the testis evolve from a common neoplastic precursor lesion, *intratubular germ cell neoplasia of the unclassified type* (IGCNU). In the past, two divergent pathways were postulated, one leading to seminoma and the second to embryonal carcinoma (1). While seminoma was considered an "end stage" neoplasm, embryonal carcinoma was felt to be capable of forming yolk sac tumor, teratoma, or choriocarcinoma. The existence of specific forms of intratubular germ cell neoplasia, however, supports the theory that an intratubular malignant germ cell may directly give rise to a number of germ cell tumor types (2). Furthermore, a number of additional findings (see below) provide convincing evidence that seminoma may transform to other germ cell tumor types, although Friedman and Moore (3) believed that seminomas evolved into embryonal carcinomas in their seminal study in 1946.

The frequent occurrence of nonseminomatous metastases at autopsy in patients who died subsequent to an orchiectomy that demonstrated only seminoma (see Table 1-2) is consistent with the concept that seminomas may evolve into other types of germ cell tumor (4,5). Additional evidence includes epithelial features of typical seminomas on ultrastructural examination (6) and the development of minor foci of yolk sac tumor in nodules of otherwise pure seminoma (7,8). Ultrastructural studies of xenografted tumors have identified cells with features intermediate between those of seminoma and yolk sac tumor (9).

A higher mean DNA content in seminomas than in nonseminomatous germ cell tumors indicates that embryonal carcinoma may evolve from seminoma as gene loss occurs, perhaps representing the loss of cancer suppressor genes with the resultant evolution to a more aggressive neoplasm (10–13). Karyotypic analyses lend credence to this hypothesis (12), demonstrating the common occurrence of a marker chromosome, isochromosome 12p (i[12p]), in seminomas and nonseminomatous germ cell tumors (14–23), which leads to an excessive copy number of genes derived from the short arm of chromosome 12. Over-representation of these genes occurs even in cases lacking i(12p) (20–22,24,25), with excess 12p considered very strong support for a diagnosis of germ cell tumor. The sharing of other cytogenic abnormalities by both seminomas and nonseminomatous tumors, including loss of chromosomes 4, 5, 11, 13, 18, and Y and gain of 7, 8 and X (in addition to 12) (26), provides additional support for a precursor role for seminoma.

Identical immunohistochemical staining patterns in IGCNU and seminomas supports a close relationship between the cells of these neoplastic processes (27–33). Similar ploidy patterns, cytogenetic findings, lectin binding patterns, and numbers of nucleolar organizer regions in IGCNU and seminoma provide additional support for this close relationship (11,12,34–37), and, because of the totipotential nature of the cells of IGCNU, implicate seminoma with a totipotential capacity. A key difference between seminoma and IGCNU, however, is that the latter lacks evidence of 12p amplification (38), which is now considered to be essential for the development of an invasive capacity, perhaps by suppressing apoptosis and allowing malignant germ cells to survive apart from Sertoli cells (39). One current hypothesis is that IGCNU cells represent the neoplastic counterpart to primordial germ cells or gonocytes, with malignant transformation induced by blocked maturation of the gonocyte by in utero exposure to substances, particularly those with estrogenic properties, that also cause testicular maldevelopment ("dysgenesis" in a broad sense) (26). Some support for this idea derives from the re-expression of fetal germ cell markers in IGCNU, including placental alkaline phosphatase (PLAP); the nuclear transcription factors OCT3/4, NANOG, and SALL4; and the

Figure 2-1

GERM CELL TUMOR HISTOGENESIS

This model shows benign tumors in green, more indolent tumors in yellow, intratubular tumors in orange, and malignant tumors in red. Seminoma plays a pivotal role in the formation of the common postpubertal tumors, all of which derive from intratubular germ cell neoplasia, unclassified type (IGCNU). The pediatric tumors, however, as well as spermatocytic seminoma and dermoid and epidermoid cysts do not form through IGCNU. (Fig. 47.2 from Ulbright TM, Berney DM. Testicular and paratesticular tumors. In: Mills SE, Reuter VE, Stoler M, Wick MR (eds): Sternberg's diagnostic surgical pathology, New York: Lippincott Williams & Wilkins, 2010:1947.)

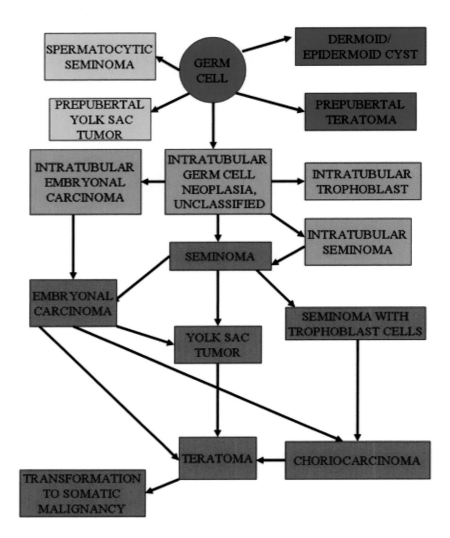

stem cell factor receptor, c-KIT (33,40–45). Gene expression profiles have demonstrated significant overlap in IGCNU and embryonic stem cells (46).

Not all testicular germ cell tumors follow this pathway. Those that occur in children as well as dermoid and epidermoid cysts (although the latter is not considered a germ cell tumor by some) and spermatocytic seminoma do not derive from IGCNU. The childhood germ cell tumors are hypothesized to arise from an embryonically earlier form of germ cell than the precursor to the usual adult tumors. This is supported by the partial erasure of genomic imprinting in them (47,48), in contrast to the more complete erasure in the adult forms (49). Furthermore, the pediatric tumors lack 12p amplification,

and this has also been verified for the rare dermoid cysts (unpublished observations, 2012). Spermatocytic seminoma also differs from the usual adult tumors by lacking IGCNU and 12p amplification, with its most frequent chromosomal change being gain of chromosome 9 (50). It is believed to derive from a more mature germ cell, a spermatogonium/spermatocyte, than the typical adult tumors and also to show a paternal pattern of genomic imprinting (26).

Because of these observations, the current histogenetic model of testicular germ cell tumors (fig. 2-1) places seminoma in a central role, often serving as a precursor. Embryonal carcinoma may arise from seminoma or as a derivative of its intratubular form. Other forms of germ cell tumor, including choriocarcinoma, teratoma, and yolk sac tumor, may arise either from seminoma or embryonal carcinoma or, rarely, even directly from IGCNU (for teratoma and yolk sac tumor), based on the occurrence of specific types of intratubular germ cell tumor. Intratubular seminoma may serve as a direct precursor to invasive seminomas and nonseminomas (51,52), but a similar role for intratubular embryonal carcinoma is less well-founded (52,53). Similarities in the chromosome composition of IGCNU and adjacent nonseminomatous tumors that contrast with the chromosome composition of seminoma and its associated IGCNU show that intratubular genetic transformation occurs prior to morphologic change (54,55). This explains many observations that are otherwise difficult to understand, including: the occurrence of seminoma with syncytiotrophoblastic cells and the demonstration of human chorionic gonadotropin (hCG) within seminoma-like cells (56,57); the presence of elevated serum alpha-fetoprotein (AFP) levels in some patients with apparently pure testicular seminoma (8,58); and the common identification of nonseminomatous metastases at autopsy in patients whose orchiectomy showed only seminoma (4,5).

Although the general inability of seminoma to grow in tissue culture or to be reproduced in animal experiments has hindered the laboratory investigation of its precursor role (59), such techniques have proved useful in the evaluation of the precursor role of embryonal carcinoma (60). Pierce et al. (61–63) demonstrated that embryonal carcinoma cells from mouse-derived testicular tumors differentiated into teratomatous structures. Cloning experiments showed that single embryonal carcinoma cells that were transplanted into the peritoneal cavity of mice differentiated into complex teratocarcinomas (embryonal carcinoma plus teratoma) (64). Furthermore, the overgrowth of teratocarcinomas maintained in vitro or in ascites by yolk sac tumor elements supports the differentiation of embryonal carcinoma into yolk sac tumor elements as well as teratomatous elements (63). The ability to form trophoblastic tissue from embryonal carcinoma was suggested by the development of uterine hyperplasia after heterotransplantation of a morphologically typical embryonal carcinoma into cortisone-treated ham-

sters (65). Clinical evidence shows that patients with pure embryonal carcinomas of the testis may have teratomatous metastases (66,67). These data provide convincing evidence for the precursor role of embryonal carcinoma in the formation of other germ cell tumor elements.

The spindle cell component of yolk sac tumor may form differentiated mesenchymal tissues, supporting its transformation to teratomatous elements (68). The close juxtaposition of yolk sac tumor and neuroectodermal structures and their frequent intimate admixture in metastatic lesions provide additional support for the capability of yolk sac tumor to form teratoma.

As suggested by these observations, germ cell tumors have greater morphologic plasticity than other forms of human neoplasms, allowing for a truly diverse combination of different elements. Table 2-1 provides a breakdown of the frequencies of different types of testicular germ cell tumors in four large series. Because of differences in nomenclature, it is not possible to provide information regarding some categories. It is apparent that seminomas and nonseminomatous tumors are of approximately equal frequency, with the heterogeneous mixed germ cell tumors constituting the great majority of nonseminomatous neoplasms.

INTRATUBULAR GERM CELL NEOPLASIA

Intratubular germ cell neoplasia consists of malignant germ cells growing within the seminiferous tubules. In its most common form, IGCNU, there is a basal proliferation of undifferentiated, atypical, enlarged germ cells with mostly clear cytoplasm which resemble the cells of seminoma. A classification of intratubular germ cell neoplasia is provided in Table 2-2.

Intratubular Germ Cell Neoplasia Unclassified

General Features. Skakkebaek (69,70) first described atypical germ cells in the testes of two infertile men in 1972 and speculated that they represented the preinvasive phase of testicular cancer. Ensuing work verified this hypothesis to the degree that such atypical germ cells are frequently termed, especially in Europe, "carcinoma in situ," although the term recommended at a consensus conference of pathologists at the University of Minnesota in 1980 was *intratubular germ cell neoplasia, unclassified type* (IGCNU)

Table 2-1

DISTRIBUTION OF TESTICULAR GERM CELL TUMORS IN FOUR SERIES[a]

	Jacobsen	von Hochstetter	Pugh	Teppo	Total
Seminoma	554	171	1082	63	1870 (48.3%)
classic	515	162	–	–	–
with STGCs[b]	–[c]	3	–	–	–
spermatocytic	13	6	–	–	–
"anaplastic"	26	–	–	–	–
NSGCTs (includes those mixed with S)	499[d]	153	1291	57	2000 (51.7%)
Pure NSGCTs	145	53	–	–	–
EC	109	35	–	–	–
PE	–	0	–	–	–
YST	3	5	53	–	–
T	31	13	–	–	–
mature	–	6	–	–	–
immature	–	6	–	–	–
"malignant"	–	1	–	–	–
CC	2	0	–	–	–
Mixed NSGCTs	352	100[e]	–	–	–
EC + T	90	33	–	–	–
S + T	21	7	–	–	–
S + EC + T	23	15	–	–	–
S + EC	58	24	–	–	–
CC + T	3	1	–	–	–
CC + EC + T	26	13	–	–	–
CC + EC + T + S	3	2	–	–	–
CC + EC	13	5	–	–	–
Others (including not assessable)	115	0	1238	–	–
Total	1053	324	2373	120	3870

[a]Adapted from references 154–157.
[b]Abbreviations: CC = choriocarcinoma; EC = embryonal carcinoma; NSGCTs = nonseminomatous germ cell tumors; PE = polyembryoma; S = seminoma; STGCs = syncytiotrophoblastic giant cells; T = teratoma; YST = yolk sac tumor.
[c]Not specifically assessed.
[d]2 NSGCTs were not further classified due to extensive necrosis.
[e]YST was not separately categorized as a component of mixed germ cell tumors.

Table 2-2

CLASSIFICATION OF INTRATUBULAR GERM CELL NEOPLASIA

Intratubular germ cell neoplasia, unclassified

Intratubular seminoma
    Usual
    Spermatocytic

Intratubular embryonal carcinoma

Intratubular germ cell neoplasia, other forms
    Seminoma with syncytiotrophoblast cells
    Syncytiotrophoblast cells
    Teratoma
    Yolk sac tumor

(71). This term was preferred because the intratubular malignant germ cells do not have epithelial properties (72–74), and the tumors they give rise to are not always carcinomas.

The evidence that IGCNU is a form of in situ neoplasia comes from several sources. Most importantly, patients with IGCNU who were followed developed invasive germ cell tumors at a high rate: 50 percent within 5 years of diagnosis (75), with few patients free of invasive tumor at 8 years (fig. 2-2). Rare patients, however, may not develop a tumor until 15 years or more after a biopsy showing IGCNU (76). IGCNU is found at a greater than expected frequency in populations that are known to be at increased risk for invasive germ cell tumors and is not

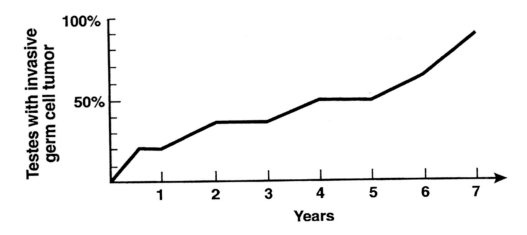

Figure 2-2

DEVELOPMENT OF INVASIVE TUMORS IN PATIENTS WITH IGCNU

Graph of the rate of development of invasive germ cell tumors in patients who had a preceding testicular biopsy positive for IGCNU. At 5 years, about 50 percent of the patients have developed invasive germ cell tumors, and only a small fraction remain free of invasive tumors by 7 years. (Data from: Skakkebaek NE, Berthelsen JG, Visfeldt J. Clinical aspects of testicular carcinoma-in-situ. Int J Androl 1981;4(suppl):153-162; reproduced from Ulbright TM. Neoplasms of the testis. In: Bostwick DG, Eble JN, eds: Urologic surgical pathology. St. Louis: Mosby; 1997:577.)

identified in control populations (77). The frequency of IGCNU in patients with a history of cryptorchidism is 2 to 8 percent (73,78–81); there is about a 5 percent frequency of IGCNU in the testis opposite one having a germ cell tumor (82–84); and 0.4 to 1.0 percent of patients with infertility have IGCNU (85–87), as do 68 percent of patients with gonadal dysgenesis (88), and about 25 percent of patients with androgen insensitivity (testicular feminization) syndrome (89). IGCNU is demonstrable in 8 percent of children and adolescents with gonadal dysgenesis but not in comparably young patients with the androgen insensitivity syndrome (90). Residual seminiferous tubules adjacent to invasive germ cell tumors show IGCNU in more than 90 percent of the cases (91–93), providing additional support for the precursor role of IGCNU, which, however, is not found with spermatocytic seminomas and pediatric germ cell tumors.

Special studies also support the neoplastic and precursor nature of IGCNU. Ploidy studies show that IGCNU is aneuploid (92,94). The cytogenetic abnormalities in IGCNU and the adjacent invasive germ cell tumor are similar (37,95,96), with shared allelic losses (97). Both IGCNU and the adjacent invasive testicular

germ cell tumor express a unique transcript of the platelet-derived growth factor alpha-receptor gene (98). IGCNU and seminoma have similar protein expression profiles that include c-KIT, OCT3/4, NANOG, PLAP, and the AP-2γ transcription factor (33,40,41,44,99–102).

IGCNU, in the absence of an invasive tumor, is asymptomatic and is usually a finding in a testicular biopsy performed for other indications or for screening purposes. The testis having IGCNU is often smaller than normal (measuring 10 to 12 mL in volume), and there is usually oligospermia (103). In screening studies for IGCNU, there is a much greater likelihood of a positive testicular biopsy in the presence of testicular atrophy (104,105).

Testicular biopsies are very sensitive for the detection of IGCNU. It is estimated that if IGCNU involves greater than 2 percent of the testicular volume, a single biopsy will detect more than 50 percent of the cases, and if IGCNU involves more that 10 percent of the testis, a single biopsy will detect all the cases (106). Another study calculated that one or two biopsy specimens 3 mm in diameter would detect virtually all cases (106). In support of this high sensitivity, only 1 patient among more that 1,500 with infertility and/or testicular maldescent and negative testicular biopsies developed testicular cancer on follow-up extending to 8 years (103). Because regressive tubular changes with obliterative sclerosis are typically more severe in the anterior testis, posterior biopsies near the rete testis permit better detection of IGCNU, especially if the testis is atrophic (107). Since IGCNU may be bilateral (one series reported IGCNU in both testes of one third of infertility patients who had positive biopsies [85]), sampling of both testes is advocated (86). Possible patients to consider for screening biopsies include: those with a history of testicular cancer; patients with somatosexual ambiguity and a Y chromosome; those with presumed extragonadal germ cell tumor (to evaluate the possibility it is a metastasis from a regressed testicular primary [see chapter 5]); and patients with cryptorchidism (76,103). Whether patients with oligospermic infertility merit biopsy is unclear (103). Many urologists take issue with the recommendation for biopsy of the contralateral testis in patients with a testicular germ cell tumor; they argue that the yield is low, the procedure potentially injurious, and the result, whether positive or negative, does not alter their plan for continued follow-up.

Biopsy in cryptorchid patients should be delayed until the postpubertal period since there does not appear to be a significant risk of invasive testicular cancer in this group prior to puberty, and the efficacy of screening at an earlier age is not established (103). IGCNU is not easily detectable in at-risk, cryptorchid boys who are prepubertal; most of these patients have some abnormal-appearing germ cells with an increased nuclear DNA content (108), but the clinical significance of such cells regarding risk for invasive germ cell tumor is not known, and their appearance is different from IGCNU (see next page).

Gross Findings. A testis harboring IGCNU may appear normal or atrophic. A firmer than usual character may be secondary to tubular shrinkage and intertubular fibrosis, particularly in cases of "burnt-out" germ cell tumor (see chapter 5) (109). If there is an associated germ cell tumor, the findings characteristic of that lesion are present.

Microscopic Findings. IGCNU consists of enlarged cells with clear cytoplasm that are aligned along the basal portion of the seminiferous tubules (fig. 2-3). The nuclei are polygonal,

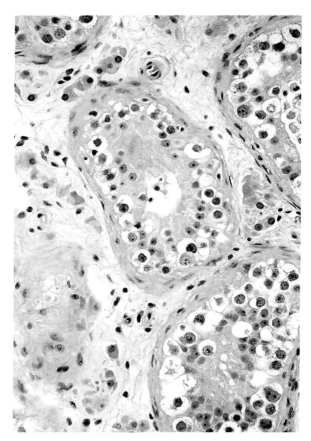

Figure 2-3

IGCNU

Clear cells with enlarged nuclei, some with flattened edges, are aligned along the basal aspect of the seminiferous tubules. These tubules lack spermatogenesis and have thickened basement membranes. Sertoli cells are present on the luminal aspect.

often with "squared-off" edges lending them a boxy appearance. They are significantly larger than those of spermatogonia (median of 9.7 μm versus 6.5 μm [103]), and have one or more prominent nucleoli (fig. 2-4). The nuclear membranes are thickened and irregular. Mitotic figures are present but usually not prominent and may be atypical. The cells are often distributed in a segmental fashion in the testis.

The seminiferous tubules involved by IGCNU are usually abnormal, frequently showing a decreased diameter, thickened peritubular basement membrane, and often, except in very early stages, absence of normal spermatogenic cells (figs. 2-3, 2-4). Sertoli cells, but not spermatogonia or more

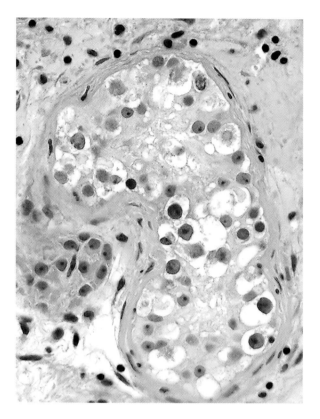

Figure 2-4

IGCNU

The malignant cells have clear or retracted cytoplasm and enlarged, "boxy" nuclei with one or more nucleoli. Spermatogenesis is absent.

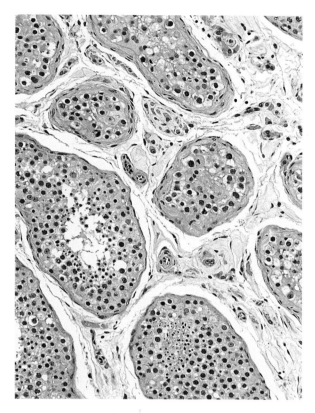

Figure 2-5

IGCNU

The neoplastic cells (top) are distributed in a patchy fashion, with adjacent normal tubules showing active spermatogenesis.

mature spermatogenic cells, are characteristically intermingled with IGCNU but show luminal displacement (fig. 2-3). If IGCNU is extensive, however, the Sertoli cells may be replaced. In some cases, there is a peritubular lymphoid infiltrate and, infrequently, an intratubular granulomatous reaction. Adjacent seminiferous tubules may be completely normal and show intact spermatogenesis (fig. 2-5). The Leydig cells appear normal but may be increased in number (fig. 2-6).

In the rare cases of possible neoplastic germ cells described in prepubertal patients, the atypical cells, rather than being basally located, are more randomly distributed within the tubules (fig. 2-7) (110). There is evidence, however, that such atypical germ cells in children, rather than being neoplastic, reflect "delayed maturation" of germ cells that may with low frequency progress to IGCNU (see Differential Diagnosis)

(111,112). When that happens, the typical adult pattern evolves as the patient ages (111).

It is common for IGCNU to extend into the ductal system of the testis, spreading in a pagetoid pattern into the rete testis (fig. 2-8) and occasionally into the epididymis or even the vas deferens (113,114). Especially in an atrophic testis, such spread can result in a palpable mass, even in the absence of an invasive component. Extensive IGCNU sometimes is associated with microscopic foci of invasive cells in the interstitium (fig. 2-9). While this has been termed, not unreasonably, "microinvasive germ cell tumor" (115,116), this is a term we do not use. In our opinion, the term "microinvasion" implies little or no capacity to metastasize, and that inability is not established for this lesion. To use "microinvasion" as it is employed in other organ systems (e.g., uterine cervix, ovary, vulva)

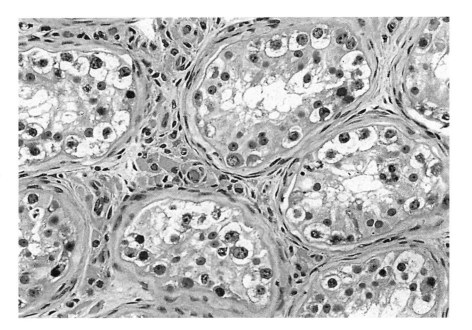

Figure 2-6

IGCNU

All of these tubules are involved.

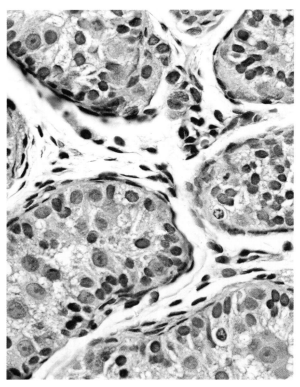

Figure 2-7

ATYPICAL INTRATUBULAR GERM CELLS IN A PREPUBERTAL TESTIS

Large, atypical germ cells with dense cytoplasm and prominent nucleoli in a random, often central distribution are present in immature seminiferous tubules.

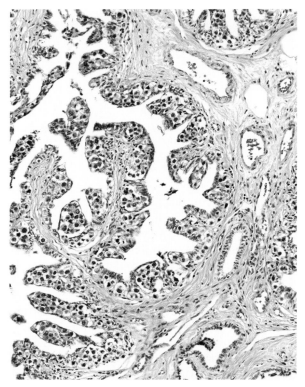

Figure 2-8

IGCNU IN RETE TESTIS

There is pagetoid-type spread of the characteristic cells beneath the epithelium of the rete testis.

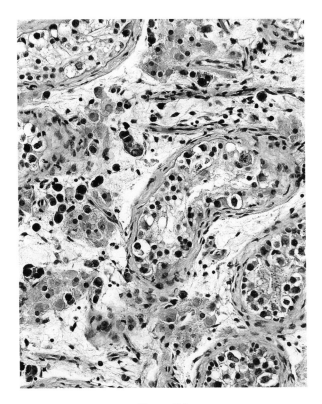

Figure 2-9

IGCNU WITH FOCI OF INTERTUBULAR SEMINOMA

Single and small clusters of seminoma cells, sometimes admixed with Leydig cells, are seen between tubules showing IGCNU.

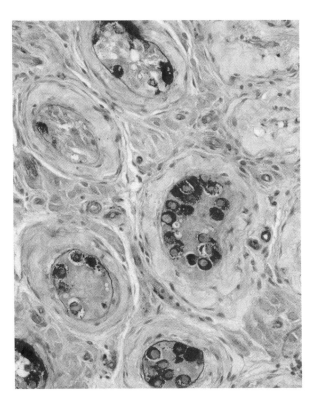

Figure 2-10

IGCNU

Intense periodic acid–Schiff (PAS) positivity is present in the neoplastic cells.

would require establishing the maximum amount of invasive tumor that could occur without producing metastasis. Since early invasion in the testis is often multifocal, this analysis would be very complex. Furthermore, it is well established that testicular germ cell tumors often undergo spontaneous regression so that no invasive tumor can be identified even in patients with widespread metastases. We therefore regard "microinvasive" foci of cells resembling those of IGCNU as small seminomas with intertubular growth, a concept further supported by the fact that such invasive cells have acquired the 12p abnormality that sets them apart from IGCNU.

Glycogen is readily demonstrated in most cases of IGCNU (fig. 2-10): one study reported periodic acid-Schiff (PAS) positivity in 46 of 47 (98 percent) cases (93). Although non-neoplastic spermatogonia and Sertoli cells may also contain glycogen (117), it is typically only in

small amounts, making PAS stains quite helpful for the detection of IGCNU. The silver staining technique for the demonstration of nucleolar organizer regions (AgNOR) is also efficacious in identifying IGCNU: in one study the AgNOR counts per cell for IGCNU ranged from 19 to 52, with no overlap in values for Sertoli cells or spermatogonia (range, 5 to 18) (118).

Immunohistochemical Findings. IGCNU has immunohistochemical properties similar to fetal germ cells. Markers of immature germ cells are therefore useful for its detection or confirmation, although some pediatric testes may exhibit delayed germ cell maturation (119), the long term significance of which is not yet clear, and this is a frequent finding in the gonads of patients with undervirilization syndrome (see Differential Diagnosis) (120).

Positivity for PLAP occurs in 83 to 98 percent of cases of IGCNU (28,117,121–123). It appears as membrane (predominantly) and cytoplasmic

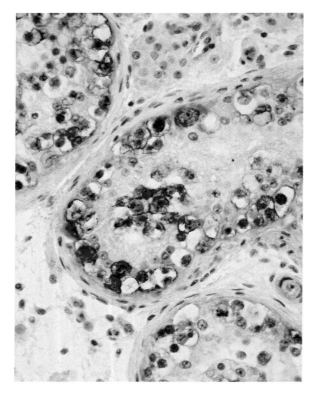

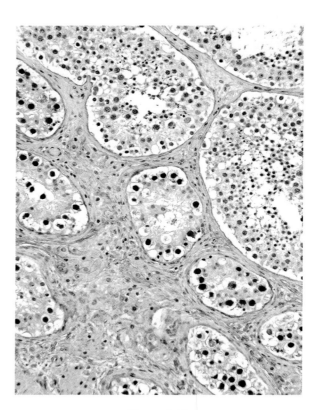

Figure 2-11

IGCNU

Staining with an antibody directed against placental alkaline phosphatase (PLAP) shows intense, predominantly membrane-associated positivity (PLAP immunostain).

Figure 2-12

IGCNU

The OCT3/4 antibody produces a strong nuclear signal.

reactivity (fig. 2-11). Non-neoplastic spermatogenic cells are almost always PLAP negative: only 4 of 469 (0.9 percent) testicular biopsies lacking IGCNU showed rare, isolated PLAP-positive spermatocytes (124). PLAP positivity is therefore very useful in confirming IGCNU if the light microscopic findings alone are not entirely diagnostic.

OCT3/4 is a nuclear transcription factor that is expressed in virtually all cases of IGCNU and is negative in non-neoplastic testicular parenchyma (33,44,125). It produces a strong nuclear signal that is easily detectable at low magnification (fig. 2-12). NANOG, another DNA-binding transcription factor, has similar staining properties to OCT3/4, although experience with it is limited (40,41). c-KIT (CD117) is positive in IGCNU in 83 to 96 percent of cases (126,127), showing a cytoplasmic membrane pattern of reactivity similar to that seen for PLAP (fig. 2-13). Limited c-KIT reactivity has, however,

also been described in non-neoplastic spermatogonia (127). Antibodies to M2A (D2-40, podoplanin) as well as monoclonal antibodies 43-9F and TRA-1-60 are very sensitive for identifying IGCNU (27,30,128–130). An antibody directed against glutathione-S-transferase π also marks IGCNU (29), and p53 is identifiable in a majority of cases (131). SALL4 is a very sensitive marker for IGCNU but is nonspecific as it also stains non-neoplastic germ cells (45).

Ultrastructural Findings. On ultrastructural examination, IGCNU cells have evenly dispersed nuclear chromatin lacking peripheral margination, complex central nucleoli, mitochondria with eccentric cristae, granular intermitochondrial matrix ("nuage"), annulate lamellae, sparse cisternae of rough endoplasmic reticulum, a high density of free ribosomes, generally abundant glycogen, and only loose intercellular attachment plaques (73,74,132–134). These

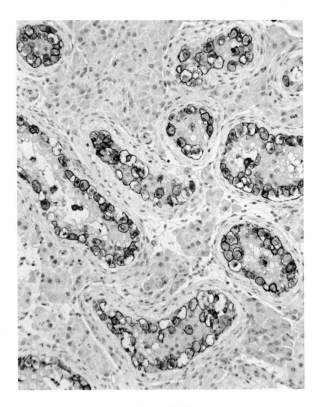

Figure 2-13

IGCNU

Staining for CD117 highlights the cytoplasmic membranes.

features are considered similar to those of pre-spermatogenic germ cells, including gonocytes. There is absence of the synaptinemal complexes that characterize spermatocytic differentiation (73). The ultrastructural features are essentially identical to those of seminoma (135).

Special Techniques. Microspectrophotometric methods have documented that the neoplastic cells of IGCNU are aneuploid (92,94). They have a similar distribution of AgNORs as seminoma (34). Despite the presence of 12p amplification, often as i(12p), in invasive germ cell tumors, IGCNU lacks 12p increase, the presence of which is thought to be important in the capacity of IGCNU to progress to an invasive tumor (95,136,137). Loss of expression of the tumor suppressor genes *PTEN* and *p18* also occurs in the transition of IGCNU to an invasive tumor (138,139). Although IGCNU strongly expresses c-KIT, an increased copy number of the *KIT* gene is absent, in contrast

to seminoma where such amplification occurs in about 20 percent of cases (140). IGCNU cells, in contrast to normal germ cells, do not express RNA-binding motif protein (141). About 50 percent of cases of IGCNU express the protein product of the cancer-testis gene *NY-ESO-1* (142). IGCNU cells commonly demonstrate loss of heterozygosity at numerous loci, which is also seen in invasive germ cell tumors (143). Comparative genomic hybridization analysis has shown similar patterns of gains and losses in IGCNU compared to seminoma, with more divergent results when comparing IGCNU to nonseminomatous tumors (144).

Differential Diagnosis. Some forms of intratubular neoplasia (see next section) may be confused with IGCNU. Intratubular seminoma is characterized by a total filling of the seminiferous tubules by seminoma cells (fig. 2-14), in contrast to IGCNU, where other cell types persist. Like IGCNU, its cells are intensely PAS reactive (fig. 2-14) and have identical immuno-staining properties.

Although most cases of intratubular spermatocytic seminoma show the prominent filling and distension of the seminiferous tubules by the usual polymorphous cell population (fig. 2-15), there are rare cases where the tumor cells are restricted to the base of the tubules (fig. 2-16), making them prone to misinterpretation as IGCNU. They, however, retain the round nuclear configuration of spermatocytic seminoma cells, often have the characteristic filamentous chromatin, do not mark with the usual IGCNU immunostains, and are associated with invasive spermatocytic seminoma.

Rarely, prepubertal testes have atypical germ cells with enlarged nuclei and abnormal chromatin that lack the basal orientation and, sometimes, the cytoplasmic clarity typical of IGCNU (see fig. 2-7). They have a random distribution in tubules lined by immature Sertoli cells. These cells may express the fetal germ cell markers also seen in IGCNU and may be analogous to what has been described as "delayed maturation" of germ cells in disorders of sex development (undervirilization) syndromes and trisomy 21 (120,145), although occurring outside of those contexts. One likely case did progress to diagnostic IGCNU and an invasive tumor (111), although this is infrequent based

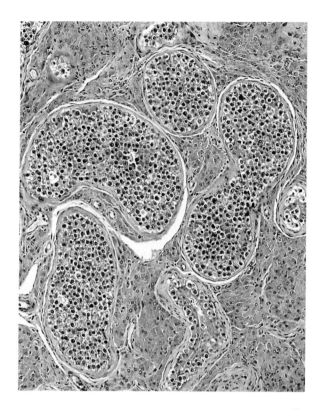
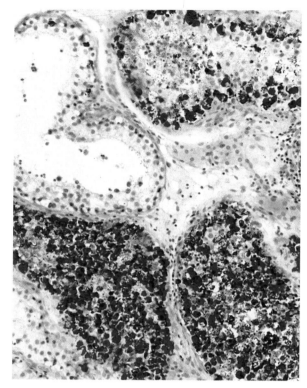

Figure 2-14

INTRATUBULAR SEMINOMA

Left: The seminiferous tubules are filled and expanded by seminoma cells.
Right: Intensely PAS-positive cells fill two tubules (bottom). The tubule at top right shows IGCNU.

Figure 2-15

INTRATUBULAR SPERMATOCYTIC SEMINOMA

The seminiferous tubules are filled and expanded by neoplastic germ cells that vary in size.

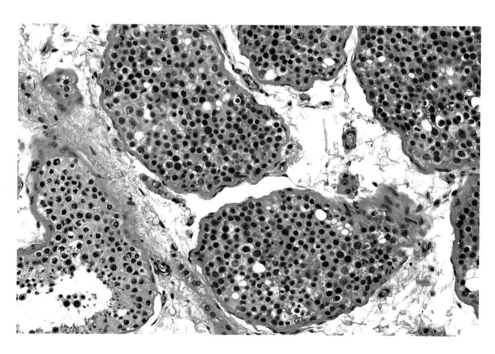

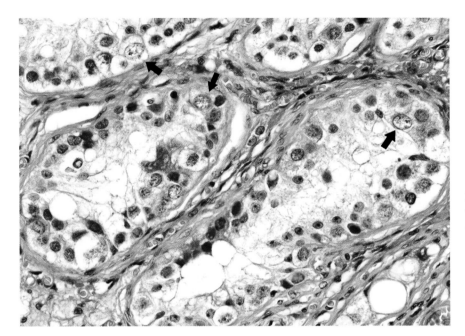

Figure 2-16

INTRATUBULAR SPERMATOCYTIC SEMINOMA

In this unusual case, the spermatocytic seminoma cells (arrows) are mostly present as a single layer near the base of the tubules, simulating IGCNU. They are significantly larger than adjacent spermatogonia and have cytologic features that differ from IGCNU.

on a study that found no germ cell tumors among 15 patients who had PLAP-positive germ cells "morphologically identical" to IGCNU in the prepubertal biopsies of their cryptorchid testes taken at orchiopexy and who were followed for a median of 21 years (112). Similar cells have on rare occasion been identified in seminiferous tubules adjacent to pediatric teratomas (146,147). The distinction of maturation-delayed atypical germ cells from IGCNU is important because of the high rate of progression of IGCNU to an invasive tumor. Such distinction is based on the prepubertal age of the patients, the random intratubular placement of the maturation-delayed atypical germ cells, and the diffuse distribution of these cells in the testis (as opposed to the often segmental distribution of IGCNU). The usual immunohistochemical markers in IGCNU do not have value in this context, and normal germ cells of young children (under 1.5 years) may retain immunoreactivity for IGCNU markers.

Other forms of atypical germ cells occur in the testes of both adults (fig. 2-17) and children (figs. 2-18, 2-19) and should be distinguished from IGCNU. Such cells may have single, enlarged hyperchromatic nuclei and occur in normal tubules with active spermatogenesis (fig. 2-17, left) or, more commonly, in atrophic tubules (fig 2-17, right). Some show prominent multinucleation (fig. 2-18) or there may be both mononucleated and multinucleated atypical germ cells (fig. 2-19). In all instances, however, they lack the "squared off" nuclear contours and nucleolar prominence of IGCNU cells and they do not stain for the usual IGCNU markers. Some feel that they are a manifestation of disturbed testicular development (testicular dysgenesis in a broad sense [148]) and therefore a manifestation of an increased risk for future germ cell tumor development. This is supported by the frequent finding of hypertrophic and multinucleated spermatogonia in the parenchyma adjacent to germ cell tumors of adults (149). The magnitude of such risk, however, is not known and is probably low, and it is therefore important to distinguish such "non-IGCNU" atypical germ cells from IGCNU because of the known uniform progression of IGCNU to an invasive tumor.

Treatment and Prognosis. Because of the high frequency of progression to an invasive germ cell tumor, most patients with IGCNU undergo orchiectomy if it is unilateral and low-dose radiation if it is bilateral (although the latter causes sterility). Some patients with invasive testicular cancer who receive chemotherapy have regression of contralateral IGCNU, but the reappearance of IGCNU in an occasional patient following chemotherapy casts doubt on the efficacy of this treatment (103,150–152).

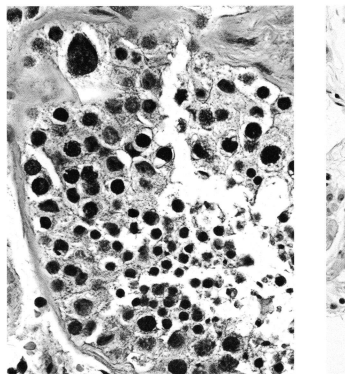
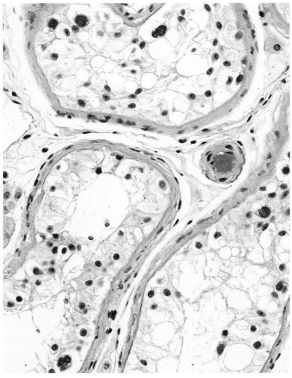

Figure 2-17

ATYPICAL INTRATUBULAR GERM CELLS IN ADULT TESTIS

Left: A single cell with an enlarged, hyperchromatic nucleus is present in a tubule with intact spermatogenesis.
Right: Scattered atypical germ cells, some multinucleated, are present in atrophic tubules.

Figure 2-18

**ATYPICAL INTRATUBULAR
GERM CELLS IN
PREPUBERTAL TESTIS**

This cryptorchid testis contains
intratubular atypical germ cells
with large, hyperchromatic and
multiple nuclei that are often
centrally located.

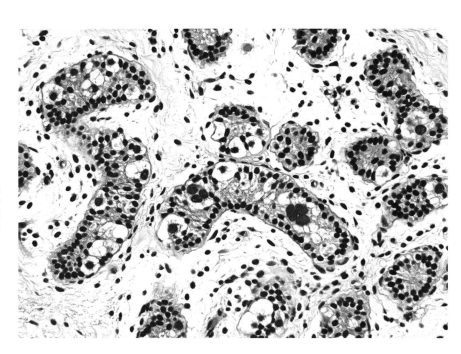

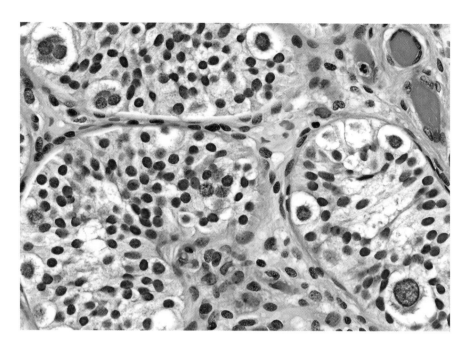

Figure 2-19

ATYPICAL INTRATUBULAR GERM CELLS IN PREPUBERTAL TESTIS

Mononucleated and multinucleated atypical germ cells are seen in immature tubules.

Other Forms of Intratubular Germ Cell Neoplasia

In most cases, intratubular neoplasia of other forms occurs simultaneously with an invasive germ cell tumor of the same type, and hence these are additionally covered in the sections dealing with the specific form of invasive tumor. *Intratubular seminoma* (fig. 2-14) occurs with approximately equal frequency adjacent to seminomas and nonseminomas, a finding that has been advanced as an argument for it, like IGCNU, having a precursor role rather than deriving from tubular invasion by seminoma (51). Rare cases of intratubular seminoma may provoke a prominent granulomatous reaction (figs. 2-20, 2-21), making the identification of tumor cells difficult, a process that can be aided, however, by appropriate immunostains. *Intratubular spermatocytic seminoma* usually distends the seminiferous tubules with the characteristic polymorphous population of cells that typifies the invasive tumor (fig. 2-15). It is often prominent, and we have never identified it in the absence of an invasive tumor. In rare cases, characteristic round, intermediate-sized cells with filamentous chromatin of intratubular spermatocytic seminoma have a basilar distribution (fig. 2-16).

Intratubular embryonal carcinoma has the cytologic features of that neoplasm (fig. 2-22).

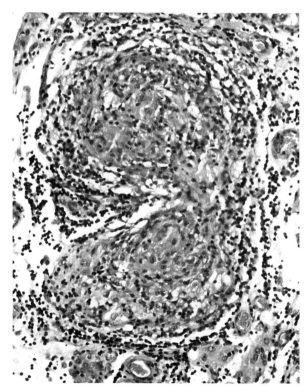

Figure 2-20

INTRATUBULAR SEMINOMA WITH GRANULOMATOUS REACTION

The tubules are filled with epithelioid histiocytes; seminoma cells are inconspicuous.

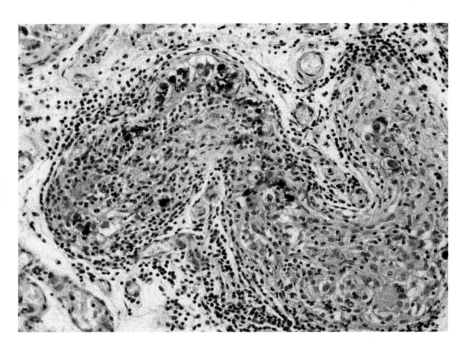

Figure 2-21

INTRATUBULAR SEMINOMA WITH GRANULOMATOUS REACTION

A stain for PLAP highlights the neoplastic germ cells (anti-PLAP immunostain). (Courtesy of Dr. F. Algaba, Barcelona, Spain.)

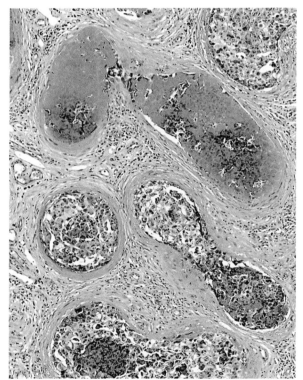

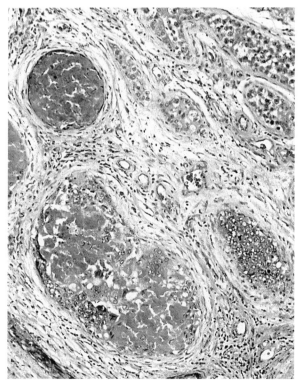

Figure 2-22

INTRATUBULAR EMBRYONAL CARCINOMA

Left: The tubules are distended by the typical pleomorphic cells with crowded nuclei. Central necrosis is seen.
Right: In this case, intratubular embryonal carcinoma is associated with intratubular seminoma (top right).

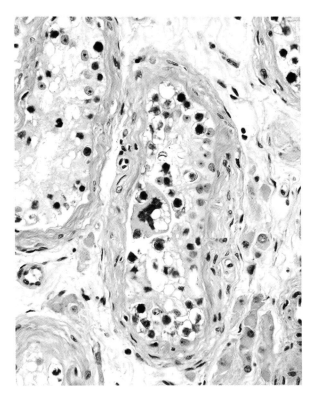

Figure 2-23

INTRATUBULAR SYNCYTIOTROPHOBLAST CELL

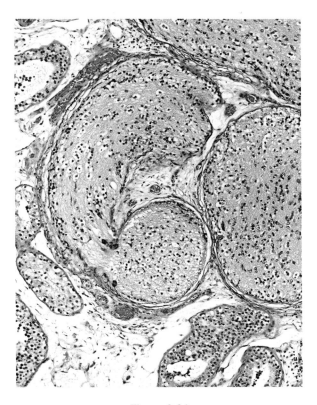

Figure 2-24

INTRATUBULAR TERATOMA

Neuroectodermal tissue distends the seminiferous tubules in a testis that also had invasive teratoma.

It usually fills and expands the seminiferous tubules and often shows extensive necrosis, producing a comedocarcinoma-like appearance, with occasional calcification. Intratubular syncytiotrophoblast cells are frequent (17 percent) adjacent to invasive seminomas and less frequent (4 percent) adjacent to nonseminomatous tumors (fig. 2-23) (153). We have seen rare examples of *intratubular teratoma* (fig. 2-24).

Rare *intratubular yolk sac tumors* are reported (2), but we are not aware of an intratubular choriocarcinoma.

Two or more forms of intratubular germ cell neoplasia may coexist, usually IGCNU with either intratubular seminoma or intratubular embryonal carcinoma. Less commonly, intratubular seminoma occurs with intratubular embryonal carcinoma (fig. 2-22).

REFERENCES

1. Pierce GB, Abell MR. Embryonal carcinoma of the testis. Pathol Annu 1970;4:27-60.
2. Mostofi FK, Sesterhenn IA. Pathology of germ cell tumors of testes. Prog Clin Biol Res 1985;203:1-34.
3. Friedman NB, Moore RA. Tumors of the testis: a report on 922 cases. Milit Surgeon 1946;99:573-93.
4. Bredael JJ, Vugrin D, Whitmore WF Jr. Autopsy findings in 154 patients with germ cell tumors of the testis. Cancer 1982;50:548-51.
5. Johnson DE, Appelt G, Samuels ML, Luna M. Metastases from testicular carcinoma. Study of 78 autopsied cases. Urology 1976;8:234-9.
6. Talerman A. A mixed germ cell-sex cord stromal tumor of the ovary in a normal female infant. Obstet Gynecol 1972;40:473-8.
7. Czaja JT, Ulbright TM. Evidence for the transformation of seminoma to yolk sac tumor, with histogenetic considerations. Am J Clin Pathol 1992;97:468-77.
8. Raghavan D, Sullivan AL, Peckham MJ, Neville AM. Elevated serum alphafetoprotein and seminoma: clinical evidence for a histologic continuum? Cancer 1982;50:982-9.
9. Monaghan P, Raghavan D, Neville M. Ultrastructure of xenografted human germ cell tumors. Cancer 1982;49:683-97.
10. Oosterhuis JW, Castedo SM, de Jong B, et al. Ploidy of primary germ cell tumors of the testis. Pathogenetic and clinical relevance. Lab Invest 1989;60:14-21.
11. El-Naggar AK, Ro JY, McLemore D, Ayala AG, Batsakis JG. DNA ploidy in testicular germ cell neoplasms: histogenetic and clinical implications. Am J Surg Pathol 1992;16:611-8.
12. de Jong B, Oosterhuis JW, Castedo SM, Vos A, te Meerman GJ. Pathogenesis of adult testicular germ cell tumors. A cytogenetic model. Cancer Genet Cytogenet 1990;48:143-67.
13. Lachman MF, Ricci A Jr, Kosciol C. DNA ploidy in testicular germ cell tumors: can an atypical seminoma be identified? Conn Med 1995;59:133-6.
14. Gibas Z, Prout GR, Pontes JE, Sandberg AA. Chromosome changes in germ cell tumors of the testis. Cancer Genet Cytogenet 1986;19:245-52.
15. Atkin NB, Baker MC. i(12p): specific chromosomal marker in seminoma and malignant teratoma of the testis? Cancer Genet Cytogenet 1983;10:199-204.
16. Samaniego F, Rodriguez E, Houldsworth J. Cytogenetic and molecular analysis of human male germ cell tumors: chromosome 12 abnormalities and gene amplification. Genes Chrom Cancer 1990;1:289-300.
17. Bosl GJ, Dmitrovsky E, Reuter VE, et al. Isochromosome of the short arm of chromosome 12: clinically useful markers for male germ cell tumors. J Natl Cancer Inst 1989;81:1874-8.
18. Delozier-Blanchet CD, Walt H, Engel E, Vuagnat P. Cytogenetic studies of human testicular germ cell tumours. Int J Androl 1987;10:69-77.
19. Vos A, Oosterhuis JW, de Jong B, Buist J, Schraffordt Koops H. Cytogenetics of carcinoma in situ of the testis. Cancer Genet Cytogenet 1990;46:75-81.
20. Geurts van Kessel A, Suijkerbuijk RF, Sinke RJ, Looijenga L, Oosterhuis JW, de Jong B. Molecular cytogenetics of human germ cell tumours: i(12p) and related chromosomal anomalies. Eur Urol 1993;23:23-8.
21. Sandberg AA, Meloni AM, Suijkerbuijk RF. Reviews of chromosome studies in urological tumors. III. Cytogenetics and genes in testicular tumors. J Urol 1996;155:1531-56.
22. Smolarek TA, Blough RI, Foster RS, Ulbright TM, Palmer CG, Heerema NA. Identification of multiple chromosome 12 abnormalities in human testicular germ cell tumors by two-color fluorescence in situ hybridization (FISH). Genes Chromosomes Cancer 1995;14:252-8.
23. van Echten J, Oosterhuis JW, Looijenga LH, et al. No recurrent structural abnormalities apart from i(12p) in primary germ cell tumors of the adult testis. Genes Chromosomes Cancer 1995;14:133-44.
24. Atkin NB, Fox MF, Baker MC, Jackson Z. Chromosome 12-containing markers, including two dicentrics, in three i(12p)-negative testicular germ cell tumors. Genes Chromosomes Cancer 1993;6:218-21.
25. Parrington JM, West LF, Heyderman E. Chromosome analysis of parallel short-term cultures from four testicular germ-cell tumors. Cancer Genet Cytogenet 1994;75:90-102.
26. Oosterhuis JW, Looijenga LH. Testicular germ-cell tumours in a broader perspective. Nat Rev Cancer 2005;5:210-22.
27. Giwercman A, Marks A, Bailey D, Baumal R, Skakkebaek NE. M2A—a monoclonal antibody as a marker for carcinoma-in-situ germ cells of the human adult testis. Acta Pathol Microbiol Immunol Scand [A] 1988;96:667-70.

28. Jacobsen GK, Norgaard-Pedersen B. Placental alkaline phosphatase in testicular germ cell tumours and carcinoma-in-situ of the testis: an immunohistochemical study. Acta Pathol Microbiol Immunol Scand [A] 1984;92:323-9.

29. Klys HS, Whillis D, Howard G, Harrison DJ. Glutathione S-transferase expression in the human testis and testicular germ cell neoplasia. Br J Cancer 1992;66:589-93.

30. Giwercman A, Andrews PW, Jorgensen N, Muller J, Graem N, Skakkebaek NE. Immunohistochemical expression of embryonal marker TRA-1-60 in carcinoma in situ and germ cell tumors of the testis. Cancer 1993;72:1308-14.

31. Koide O, Iwai S, Baba K, Iri H. Identification of testicular atypical germ cells by an immunohistochemical technique for placental alkaline phosphatase. Cancer 1987;60:1325-30.

32. Niehans GA, Manivel JC, Copland GT, Scheithauer BW, Wick MR. Immunohistochemistry of germ cell and trophoblastic neoplasms. Cancer 1988;62:1113-23.

33. Jones TD, Ulbright TM, Eble JN, Cheng L. OCT4: A sensitive and specific biomarker for intratubular germ cell neoplasia of the testis. Clin Cancer Res 2004;10:8544-7.

34. Delahunt B, Mostofi FK, Sesterhenn IA, Ribas JL, Avallone FA. Nucleolar organizer regions in seminoma and intratubular malignant germ cells. Mod Pathol 1990;3:141-5.

35. Malmi R, Söderström KO. Lectin histochemistry of embryonal carcinoma. APMIS 1991;99:233-43.

36. de Graaff WE, Oosterhuis JW, de Jong B, et al. Ploidy of testicular carcinoma in situ. Lab Invest 1992;66:166-8.

37. van Echten J, van Gurp RJ, Stoepker M, Looijenga LH, de Jong J, Oosterhuis W. Cytogenetic evidence that carcinoma in situ is the precursor lesion for invasive testicular germ cell tumors. Cancer Genet Cytogenet 1995;85:133-7.

38. Rosenberg C, van Gurp RJ, Geelen E, Oosterhuis JW, Looijenga LH. Overrepresentation of the short arm of chromosome 12 is related to invasive growth of human testicular seminomas and nonseminomas. Oncogene 2000;19:5858-62.

39. Looijenga LH, Zafarana G, Grygalewicz B, et al. Role of gain of 12p in germ cell tumour development. APMIS 2003;111:161-71.

40. Hart AH, Hartley L, Parker K, et al. The pluripotency homeobox gene NANOG is expressed in human germ cell tumors. Cancer 2005;104:2092-8.

41. Hoei-Hansen CE, Almstrup K, Nielsen JE, et al. Stem cell pluripotency factor NANOG is expressed in human fetal gonocytes, testicular carcinoma in situ and germ cell tumours. Histopathology 2005;47:48-56.

42. Lu D, Medeiros LJ, Eskenazi AE, Abruzzo LV. Primary follicular large cell lymphoma of the testis in a child. Arch Pathol Lab Med 2001;125:551-4.

43. Honecker F, Stoop H, de Krijger RR, Chris Lau YF, Bokemeyer C, Looijenga LH. Pathobiological implications of the expression of markers of testicular carcinoma in situ by fetal germ cells. J Pathol 2004;203:849-57.

44. Looijenga LH, Stoop H, de Leeuw HP, et al. POU5F1 (OCT3/4) identifies cells with pluripotent potential in human germ cell tumors. Cancer Res 2003;63:2244-50.

45. Cao D, Li J, Guo CC, Allan RW, Humphrey PA. SALL4 is a novel diagnostic marker for testicular germ cell tumors. Am J Surg Pathol 2009;33:1065-1077.

46. Almstrup K, Hoei-Hansen CE, Wirkner U, et al. Embryonic stem cell-like features of testicular carcinoma in situ revealed by genome-wide gene expression profiling. Cancer Res 2004;64:4736-43.

47. Bussey KJ, Lawce HJ, Himoe E, et al. SNRPN methylation patterns in germ cell tumors as a reflection of primordial germ cell development. Genes Chromosomes Cancer 2001;32:342-52.

48. Schneider DT, Schuster AE, Fritsch MK, et al. Multipoint imprinting analysis indicates a common precursor cell for gonadal and nongonadal pediatric germ cell tumors. Cancer Res 2001;61:7268-76.

49. Sievers S, Alemazkour K, Zahn S, et al. IGF2/H19 imprinting analysis of human germ cell tumors (GCTs) using the methylation-sensitive single-nucleotide primer extension method reflects the origin of GCTs in different stages of primordial germ cell development. Genes Chromosomes Cancer 2005;44:256-64.

50. Rosenberg C, Mostert MC, Schut TB, et al. Chromosomal constitution of human spermatocytic seminomas: comparative genomic hybridization supported by conventional and interphase cytogenetics. Genes Chromosomes Cancer 1998;23:286-91.

51. Berney DM, Lee A, Shamash J, et al. The association between intratubular seminoma and invasive germ cell tumors. Hum Pathol 2006;37:458-61.

52. Lau SK, Weiss LM, Chu PG. Association of intratubular seminoma and intratubular embryonal carcinoma with invasive testicular germ cell tumors. Am J Surg Pathol 2007;31:1045-9.

53. Berney DM, Lee A, Randle SJ, Jordan S, Shamash J, Oliver RT. The frequency of intratubular embryonal carcinoma: implications for the pathogenesis of germ cell tumours. Histopathology 2004;45:155-61.

54. Oosterhuis JW, Gillis AJ, van Putten WJ, de Jong B, Looijenga LH. Interphase cytogenetics of carcinoma in situ of the testis. Numeric analysis of the chromosomes 1, 12 and 15. Eur Urol 1993;23:16-21.

55. Jones MA, Young RH, Srigley JR, Scully RE. Paratesticular serous papillary carcinoma. A report of six cases. Am J Surg Pathol 1995;19:1359-65.

56. Boseman FT, Giard RW, Kruseman AC, Knijenenburg G, Spaander PJ. Human chorionic gonadothropin and alpha-fetoprotein in testicular germ cell tumors: a retrospective immunohistochemical study. Histopathology 1980;4:673-84.

57. Mostofi FK. Pathology of germ cell tumors of testis: a progress report. Cancer 1980;45:1735-54.

58. Javadpour N. Significance of elevated serum alpha fetoprotein (AFP) in seminoma. Cancer 1980;45:2166-8.

59. Damjanov I. Spontaneous and experimental testicular tumors in animals. In: Talerman A, Roth LM, eds. Pathology of the testis and its adnexa. New York: Churchill Livingstone; 1986:193-206.

60. Damjanov I, Solter D. Experimental teratoma. Curr Top Pathol 1974;59:69-130.

61. Pierce GB Jr, Dixon FJ Jr, Verney EL. Teratocarcinogenic and tissue-forming potentials of cell types comprising neoplastic embryoid bodies. Lab Invest 1960;9:583-602.

62. Pierce GB Jr, Dixon FJ Jr. Testicular teratomas: I. Demonstration of teratogenesis by metamorphosis of multipotential cells. Cancer 1959;12:573-83.

63. Pierce GB Jr, Verney EL. An in vitro and in vivo study of differentiation in teratocarcinomas. Cancer 1961;14:1017-29.

64. Kleinsmith LJ, Pierce GB. Multipotentiality of single embryonal carcinoma cells. Cancer Res 1964;24:1544-51.

65. Pierce GB Jr, Dixon FJ Jr, Verney EL. The biology of testicular cancer: II. Endocrinology of transplanted tumors. Cancer Res 1958;18:204-6.

66. Willis GW, Hajdu SI. Histologically benign teratoid metastasis of testicular embryonal carcinoma: report of five cases. Am J Clin Pathol 1973;59:338-43.

67. Moran CA, Travis WD, Carter D, Koss MN. Metastatic mature teratoma in lung following testicular embryonal carcinoma and teratocarcinoma. Arch Pathol Lab Med 1993;117:641-4.

68. Michael H, Ulbright TM, Brodhecker CA. The pluripotential nature of the mesenchyme-like component of yolk sac tumor. Arch Pathol Lab Med 1989;113:1115-9.

69. Skakkebaek NE. Abnormal morphology of germ cells in two infertile men. Acta Pathol Microbiol Scand [A] 1972;80:374-8.

70. Skakkebaek NE. Possible carcinoma-in-situ of the undescended testis. Lancet 1972;2:516-7.

71. Scully RE. Intratubular germ cell neoplasia (carcinoma in situ). What it is and what should be done about it. Lesson 17. In: Fraley EE, ed. World urology update series, Vol. 1. Princeton: Continuing Professional Education Center; 1982:1-8.

72. Mostofi FK, Sesterhenn IA, Davis CJ Jr. Immunopathology of germ cell tumors of the testis. Semin Diagn Pathol 1987;4:320-41.

73. Gondos B, Migliozzi JA. Intratubular germ cell neoplasia. Semin Diagn Pathol 1987;4:292-303.

74. Sigg C, Hedinger C. Atypical germ cells of the testis. Comparative ultrastructural and immunohistochemical investigations. Virchows Arch [A] 1984;402:439-50.

75. Skakkebaek NE, Berthelsen JG, Muller J. Carcinoma-in-situ of the undescended testis. Urol Clin North Am 1982;9:377-85.

76. Giwercman A, von der Maase H, Skakkebaek NE. Epidemiological and clinical aspects of carcinoma in situ of the testis. Eur Urol 1993;23:104-10.

77. Giwercman A, Müller J, Skakkebaek NE. Prevalence of carcinoma in situ and other histopathological abnormalities in testes from 399 men who died suddenly and unexpectedly. J Urol 1991;145:77-80.

78. Krabbe S, Skakkebaek NE, Berthelsen JG, et al. High incidence of undetected neoplasia in maldescended testes. Lancet 1979;1:999-1000.

79. Giwercman A, Muller J, Skakkebaek NE. Carcinoma in situ of the undescended testis. Semin Urol 1988;6:110-9.

80. Pedersen KV, Bolesen P, Zetter Lund CG. Experience of screening for carcinoma-in-situ of the testis among young men with surgically corrected maldescended testes. Int J Androl 1987;10:181-5.

81. Giwercman A, Bruun E, Frimodt-Moller C, Skakkebaek NE. Prevalence of carcinoma-in-situ and other histopathologic abnormalities in testes of men with a history of cryptorchidism. J Urol 1989;142:998-1002.

82. von der Maase H, Rorth M, Walbom-Jorgensen S, et al. Carcinoma in situ of contralateral testis in patients with testicular germ cell cancer: study of 27 cases in 500 patients. Br Med J (Clin Res Ed) 1986;293:1398-401.

83. Berthelsen JG, Skakkebaek NE, von der Maase H, Sorensen BL, Mogensen P. Screening for carcinoma in situ of the contralateral testis in patients with germinal testicular cancer. Br Med J (Clin Res Ed) 1982;285:1683-6.

84. Mumperow E, Lauke H, Holstein AF, Hartmann M. Further practical experiences in the recognition and management of carcinoma in situ of the testis. Urol Int 1992;48:162-6.

85. Skakkebaek NE. Carcinoma in situ of the testis: frequency and relationship to invasive germ cell tumours in infertile men. Histopathology 1978;2:157-70.

86. Pryor JP, Cameron KM, Chilton CP, et al. Carcinoma in situ in testicular biopsies in men presenting with infertility. Br J Urol 1983;55:780-4.

87. West AB, Butler MR, Fitzpatrick J, O'Brien A. Testicular tumors in subfertile men: report of 4 cases with implications for management of patients presenting with infertility. J Urol 1985;133:107-9.

88. Slowikowska-Hilczer J, Romer TE, Kula K. Neoplastic potential of germ cells in relation to disturbances of gonadal organogenesis and changes in karyotype. J Androl 2003;24:270-8.

89. Muller J, Skakkebaek NE. Testicular carcinoma in situ in children with the androgen insensitivity (testicular feminisation) syndrome. Br Med J (Clin Res Ed) 1984;288:1419-20.

90. Ramani P, Yeung CK, Habeebu SS. Testicular intratubular germ cell neoplasia in children and adolescents with intersex. Am J Surg Pathol 1993;17:1124-33.

91. Jacobsen GK, Henriksen OB, von der Maase H. Carcinoma in situ of testicular tissue adjacent to malignant germ-cell tumors: a study of 105 cases. Cancer 1981;47:2660-2.

92. Skakkebaek NE. Atypical germ cells in the adjacent "normal" tissue of testicular tumours. Acta Pathol Microbiol Scand A 1975;83:127-30.

93. Coffin CM, Ewing S, Dehner LP. Frequency of intratubular germ cell neoplasia with invasive testicular germ cell tumors. Histologic and immunocytochemical features. Arch Pathol Lab Med 1985;109:555-9.

94. Muller J, Skakkebaek NE, Lundsteen C. Aneuploidy as a marker for carcinoma-in-situ of the testis. Acta Pathol Microbiol Scand A 1981;89:67-8.

95. Summersgill B, Osin P, Lu YJ, Huddart R, Shipley J. Chromosomal imbalances associated with carcinoma in situ and associated testicular germ cell tumours of adolescents and adults. Br J Cancer 2001;85:213-20.

96. Gillis AJ, Looijenga LH, de Jong B, Oosterhuis JW. Clonality of combined testicular germ cell tumors of adults. Lab Invest 1994;71:874-8.

97. Faulkner SW, Leigh DA, Oosterhuis JW, Roelofs H, Looijenga LH, Friedlander ML. Allelic losses in carcinoma in situ and testicular germ cell tumours of adolescents and adults: evidence suggestive of the linear progression model. Br J Cancer 2000;83:729-36.

98. Mosselman S, Looijenga LH, Gillis AJ, et al. Aberrant platelet-derived growth factor alpha-receptor transcript as a diagnostic marker for early human germ cell tumors of the adult testis. Proc Natl Acad Sci U S A 1996;93:2884-8.

99. Pauls K, Jager R, Weber S, et al. Transcription factor AP-2gamma, a novel marker of gonocytes and seminomatous germ cell tumors. Int J Cancer 2005;115:470-7.

100. Jones TD, Ulbright TM, Eble JN, Cheng L. OCT4 staining in testicular tumors: a sensitive and specific marker for seminoma and embryonal carcinoma. Am J Surg Pathol 2004;28:935-40.

101. Leroy X, Augusto D, Leteurtre E, Gosselin B. CD30 and CD117 (c-kit) used in combination are useful for distinguishing embryonal carcinoma from seminoma. J Histochem Cytochem 2002;50:283-5.

102. Tanner CO. Tumors of the testicle: with analysis of one hundred original cases. Surg Gynecol Obstet 1922;35:565-72.

103. Giwercman A, Skakkebaek NE. Carcinoma-in-situ (gonocytoma-in-situ) of the testis. In: Burger H, de Kretser D, eds. The testis, 2 ed. New York: Raven Press; 1989:475-91.

104. Loy V, Dieckmann KP. Prevalence of contralateral testicular intraepithelial neoplasia (carcinoma in situ) in patients with testicular germ cell tumour. Results of the German multicentre study. Eur Urol 1993;23:120-2.

105. Harland SJ, Cook PA, Fossä SD, et al. Risk factors for carcinoma in situ of the contralateral testis in patients with testicular cancer. An interim report. Eur Urol 1993;23:115-8.

106. Berthelsen JG, Skakkebaek NE. Value of testicular biopsy in diagnosing carcinoma in situ testis. Scand J Urol Nephrol 1981;15:165-8.

107. Nistal M, Codesal J, Paniagua R. Carcinoma in situ of the testis in infertile men. A histological, immunocytochemical, and cytophotometric study of DNA content. J Pathol 1989;159:205-10.

108. Muller J, Skakkebaek NE. Abnormal germ cells in maldescended testes: a study of cell density, nuclear size and deoxyribonucleic acid content in testicular biopsies from 50 boys. J Urol 1984;131:730-3.

109. Balzer BL, Ulbright TM. Spontaneous regression of testicular germ cell tumors: an analysis of 42 cases. Am J Surg Pathol 2006;30:858-65.

110. Skakkebaek NE, Berthelsen JG, Giwercman A, Müller J. Carcinoma-in-situ of the testis: possible origin from gonocytes and precursor of all types of germ cell tumours except spermatocytoma. Int J Androl 1987;10:19-28.

111. Muller J, Skakkebaek NE, Nielsen OH, Graem N. Cryptorchidism and testis cancer. Atypical infantile germ cells followed by carcinoma in situ and invasive carcinoma in adulthood. Cancer 1984;54:629-34.

112. Engeler DS, Hosli PO, John H, et al. Early orchiopexy: prepubertal intratubular germ cell neoplasia and fertility outcome. Urology 2000;56:144-148.

113. Perry A, Wiley EL, Albores-Saavedra J. Pagetoid spread of intratubular germ cell neoplasia into rete testis: a morphologic and histochemical study of 100 orchiectomy specimens with invasive germ cell tumors. Hum Pathol 1994;25:235-9.

114. Lee AH, Theaker JM. Pagetoid spread into the rete testis by testicular tumours. Histopathology 1994;24:385-9.

115. Klein FA, Melamed MR, Whitmore WF Jr. Intratubular malignant germ cells (carcinoma in situ) accompanying invasive testicular germ cell tumors. J Urol 1985;133:413-5.

116. von Eyben FE, Jacobsen GK, Rorth M, von der Maase H. Microinvasive germ cell tumour (MGCT) adjacent to testicular germ cell tumours. Histopathology 2004;44:547-54.

117. Manivel JC, Jessurun J, Wick MR, Dehner LP. Placental alkaline phosphatase immunoreactivity in testicular germ cell tumors. Am J Surg Pathol 1987;11:21-9.

118. Muller M, Lauke H, Hartmann M. The value of the AgNOR staining method in identifying carcinoma in situ testis. Pathol Res Pract 1994;190:429-35.

119. Fan R, Ulbright TM. Does intratubular germ cell neoplasia unclassified type exist in prepubertal, cryptorchid testes? Fetal Pediat Pathol 2012;31:21-4.

120. Cools M, van Aerde K, Kersemaekers AM, et al. Morphological and immunohistochemical differences between gonadal maturation delay and early germ cell neoplasia in patients with undervirilization syndromes. J Clin Endocrinol Metab 2005;90:5295-303.

121. Hustin J, Collettee J, Franchimont P. Immunohistochemical demonstration of placental alkaline phosphatase in various states of testicular development and in germ cell tumours. Int J Androl 1987;10:29-35.

122. Beckstead JH. Alkaline phosphatase histochemistry in human germ cell neoplasms. Am J Surg Pathol 1983;7:341-9.

123. Burke AP, Mostofi FK. Intratubular malignant germ cells in testicular biopsies: clinical course and identification by staining for placental alkaline phosphatase. Mod Pathol 1988;1:475-9.

124. Burke AP, Mostofi FK. Placental alkaline phosphatase immunohistochemistry of intratubular malignant germ cells and associated testicular germ cell tumors. Hum Pathol 1988;19:663-70.

125. de Jong J, Stoop H, Dohle GR, et al. Diagnostic value of OCT3/4 for pre-invasive and invasive testicular germ cell tumours. J Pathol 2005;206:242-9.

126. Rajpert-De Meyts E, Skakkebaek NE. Expression of the c-kit protein product in carcinoma-in-situ and invasive testicular germ cell tumours. Int J Androl 1994;17:85-92.

127. Izquierdo MA, Van der Valk P, Van Ark-Otte J, et al. Differential expression of the c-kit proto-oncogene in germ cell tumours. J Pathol 1995;177:253-8.

128. Giwercman A, Lindenberg S, Kimber SJ, Andersson T, Müller J, Skakkebaek NE. Monoclonal antibody 43-9F as a sensitive immunohistochemical marker of carcinoma in situ of human testis. Cancer 1990;65:1135-42.

129. Bailey D, Marks A, Stratis M, Baumal R. Immunohistochemical staining of germ cell tumors and intratubular malignant germ cells of the testis using antibody to placental alkaline phosphatase and a monoclonal anti-seminoma antibody. Mod Pathol 1991;4:167-71.

130. Marks A, Sutherland DR, Bailey D, et al. Characterization and distribution of an oncofetal antigen (M2A antigen) expressed on testicular germ cell tumours. Br J Cancer 1999;80:569-78.

131. Bartkova J, Bartek J, Lukas J, et al. p53 protein alterations in human testicular cancer including pre-invasive intratubular germ-cell neoplasia. Int J Cancer 1991;49:196-202.

132. Nielsen H, Nielsen M, Skakkebaek NE. The fine structure of possible carcinoma-in-situ in the seminiferous tubules in the testis of four infertile men. Acta Pathol Microbiol Scand A 1974;82:235-48.

133. Gondos B, Berthelsen JG, Skakkebaek NE. Intratubular germ cell neoplasia (carcinoma in situ): a preinvasive lesion of the testis. Ann Clin Lab Sci 1983;13:185-92.

134. Albrechtsen R, Nielsen MH, Skakkebaek NE, Wewer U. Carcinoma in situ of the testis. Some ultrastructural characteristics of germ cells. Acta Pathol Microbiol Immunol Scand [A] 1982;90:301-3.

135. Holstein AF, Körner F. Light and electron microscopical analysis of cell types in human seminoma. Virchows Arch [A] 1974;363:97-112.

136. Ottesen AM, Skakkebaek NE, Lundsteen C, Leffers H, Larsen J, Rajpert-De Meyts E. High-resolution comparative genomic hybridization detects extra chromosome arm 12p material in most cases of carcinoma in situ adjacent to overt germ cell tumors, but not before the invasive tumor development. Genes Chrom Cancer 2003;38:117-25.

137. Rosenberg C, van Gurp RJ, Geelen E, Oosterhuis JW, Looijenga LH. Overrepresentation of the short arm of chromosome 12 is related to invasive growth of human testicular seminomas and nonseminomas. Oncogene 2000;19:5858-62.

138. Di Vizio D, Cito L, Boccia A, et al. Loss of the tumor suppressor gene PTEN marks the transition from intratubular germ cell neoplasias (IT-GCN) to invasive germ cell tumors. Oncogene 2005;24:1882-94.

139. Bartkova J, Thullberg M, Rajpert-De Meyts E, Skakkebaek NE, Bartek J. Cell cycle regulators in testicular cancer: loss of p18INK4C marks progression from carcinoma in situ to invasive germ cell tumours. Int J Cancer 2000;85:370-5.

140. McIntyre A, Summersgill B, Grygalewicz B, et al. Amplification and overexpression of the KIT gene is associated with progression in the seminoma subtype of testicular germ cell tumors of adolescents and adults. Cancer Res 2005;65:8085-9.

141. Schreiber L, Lifschitz-Mercer B, Paz G, et al. Lack of RBM expression as a marker for carcinoma in situ of prepubertal dysgenetic testis. J Androl 2003;24:78-84.

142. Satie AP, Rajpert-De Meyts E, Spagnoli GC, et al. The cancer-testis gene, NY-ESO-1, is expressed in normal fetal and adult testes and in spermatocytic seminomas and testicular carcinoma in situ. Lab Invest 2002;82:775-80.

143. Faulkner SW, Leigh DA, Oosterhuis JW, Roelofs H, Looijenga LH, Friedlander ML. Allelic losses in carcinoma in situ and testicular germ cell tumours of adolescents and adults: evidence suggestive of the linear progression model. Br J Cancer 2000;83:729-36.

144. Looijenga LH, Rosenberg C, van Gurp RJ, et al. Comparative genomic hybridization of microdissected samples from different stages in the development of a seminoma and a nonseminoma. J Pathol 2000;191:187-92.

145. Cools M, Honecker F, Stoop H, et al. Maturation delay of germ cells in fetuses with trisomy 21 results in increased risk for the development of testicular germ cell tumors. Hum Pathol 2006;37:101-11.

146. Stamp IM, Barlebo H, Rix M, Jacobsen GK. Intratubular germ cell neoplasia in an infantile testis with immature teratoma. Histopathology 1993;22:69-72.

147. Renedo DE, Trainer TD. Intratubular germ cell neoplasia (ITGCN) with p53 and PCNA expression and adjacent mature teratoma in an infant testis. An immunohistochemical and morphologic study with a review of the literature. Am J Surg Pathol 1994;18:947-52.

148. Hoei-Hansen CE, Holm M, Rajpert-De Meyts E, Skakkebaek NE. Histological evidence of testicular dysgenesis in contralateral biopsies from 218 patients with testicular germ cell cancer. J Pathol 2003;200:370-4.

149. Nistal M, Gonzalez-Peramato P, Regadera J, Serrano A, Tarin V, De Miguel MP. Primary testicular lesions are associated with testicular germ cell tumors of adult men. Am J Surg Pathol 2006;30:1260-8.

150. von der Maase H, Giwercman A, Müller J, Skakkebaek NE. Management of carcinoma-in-situ of the testis. Int J Androl 1987;10:209-20.

151. Bottomley D, Fisher C, Hendry WF, Horwich A. Persistent carcinoma in situ of the testis after chemotherapy for advanced testicular germ cell tumours. Br J Urol 1990;66:420-4.

152. von der Maase H, Meinecke B, Skakkebaek NE. Residual carcinoma-in-situ of contralateral testis after chemotherapy. Lancet 1988;1:477-8.

153. Berney DM, Lee A, Shamash J, Oliver RT. The frequency and distribution of intratubular trophoblast in association with germ cell tumors of the testis. Am J Surg Pathol 2005;29:1300-3.

154. Jacobsen GK, Barlebo H, Olsen J, et al. Testicular germ cell tumours in Denmark 1976-1980: pathology of 1058 consecutive cases. Acta Radiol Oncol 1984;23:239-47.

155. von Hochstetter AR, Hedinger CE. The differential diagnosis of testicular germ cell tumors in theory and practice: a critical analysis of two major systems of classification and review of 389 cases. Virchows Arch [A] 1982;396:247-77.

156. Teppo L. Malignant testicular tumours in Finland. Acta Pathol Microbiol Scand 1969;75:18-26.

157. Pugh RC. Testicular tumours—introduction. In: Pugh RC, ed. Pathology of the testis. Oxford: Blackwell Scientific; 1976:139-59.

3 GERM CELL TUMORS: SEMINOMAS

SEMINOMA (TYPICAL FORM)

Definition. *Seminoma* is a malignant germ cell tumor composed of fairly uniform primitive cells, typically with pale to clear cytoplasm, well-defined borders, and nuclei that often have one or more prominent nucleoli. It almost always has delicate fibrous septa, an associated lymphoid infiltrate, and sometimes a granulomatous inflammatory response.

General Features. Seminoma was first authoritatively described by Chevassu in 1906 (1) and is the most common germ cell tumor of the testis, representing about 50 percent of cases (2,3). It occurs at an average age of 40.5 years (2), which is 5 to 10 years older than for those with nonseminomatous tumors (2,4). It is almost never is seen in children less than 10 years of age (5,6), except for those with a disorder of sex development (intersex disorder), and is uncommon in adolescents. Among 720 seminomas examined by the British Testicular Tumour Panel (7), 1 percent occurred in patients 19 years of age or younger, 13 percent in those 20 to 29 years, 65 percent in those 30 to 49 years, 19 percent in those 50 to 70 years, and 1 percent in those older than 70 years (7).

The epidemiology and risk factors are similar to those of other testicular germ cell tumors (see chapter 1). Some patients have an increased frequency of human leukocyte antigen (HLA) types DR5 (8) and Bw41 (9). An increased frequency of seminomas has been reported among very tall men (10). Some studies report a higher proportion of seminomas associated with cryptorchidism (11). A high frequency of testicular germ cell tumors, disproportionately seminomas, has been reported in patients with the acquired immunodeficiency syndrome (AIDS), as well as other forms of immunosuppression (12,13). It is important to distinguish seminoma from the other testicular tumors because of different treatments.

Clinical Features. Seminoma affects the right testis more often than the left (54 percent versus 46 percent) (7). Bilateral involvement, usually asynchronous, occurs in about 2 percent of patients. Most patients present with a self-identified testicular mass, occasionally associated with an ill-defined, aching sensation in the scrotum, inguinal area, or lower abdomen. Acute pain occurs in approximately 10 percent, and may result in a delayed diagnosis due to a clinical impression of epididymo-orchitis (14). About 2.5 percent of patients have the initial symptoms secondary to metastatic disease (15,16), most commonly lumbar back pain due to retroperitoneal metastases, but gastrointestinal bleeding, bone pain, dyspnea, cough, a supraclavicular mass, neurological manifestations, and lower extremity edema are also presenting symptoms (14). A mass is not always apparent clinically in such cases, which disproportionately have undergone regression (17) or have prominent intertubular growth (18) compared to cases with palpable tumors.

Although serum human chorionic gonadotropin (hCG) levels are elevated in 7 to 25 percent of patients with seminomas (19–24), levels are typically sufficiently low that gynecomastia is uncommon (25,26). Some patients present with infertility and have a small seminoma identified on testicular biopsy. Occasional tumors are occult and found in orchiectomy specimens done for cryptorchidism. Current or surgically corrected cryptorchidism is identified in 10 to 30 percent of patients with seminoma (2,7). Rarely, exophthalmos, apparently on a paraendocrine basis (27,28), or one of the following, is a presenting feature: hypercalcemia (29), autoimmune hemolytic anemia (30), polycythemia (31,32), limbic or brainstem encephalopathy (33–35), and membranous glomerulonephritis (36). About 75 percent of patients present with clinical disease limited to the testis, 20 percent have retroperitoneal involvement, and 5 percent have supradiaphragmatic or organ metastases (37). The metastases, however, are usually asymptomatic (2).

Alpha-fetoprotein (AFP) levels are not generally elevated (38,39); if a significantly elevated serum AFP is identified in a patient with apparently pure seminoma of the testis, it likely indicates a histologically undetected non-seminomatous element, perhaps in metastases. Modest AFP elevations may reflect liver disease, including metastatic involvement (40), and occasionally have also been found in patients with pure seminomas of the testis, for unclear reasons, without apparent effect on the biologic behavior (41).

In clinical stage I disease, 10 percent of patients have elevated serum hCG levels, which rise to over 25 percent with metastatic seminoma (39,42); serum from the testicular vein yields elevated levels in 80 percent of patients (43). In some cases, hCG production may be detectable only as an elevated beta subunit (21). It is rare for levels to exceed more than 1,000 IU/L. Elevated hCG usually correlates with histologically identifiable syncytiotrophoblast cells (see below). Some have suggested that hCG elevations in seminoma worsen the prognosis (44,45), but this is not proven (19,46).

Elevated serum levels of the enzyme lactate dehydrogenase (LDH) also occur in patients with seminoma, but this is an insensitive marker, occurring in only 82 percent of patients with advanced disease, according to one review (44). It is also nonspecific in that 7 of 37 patients who were disease free after treatment had elevated LDH levels. Furthermore, patients with benign testicular lesions may also show elevated serum LDH (44).

Most seminomas secrete placental-like alkaline phosphatase (PLAP), detectable in 33 to 91 percent of stage I patients and in 40 to 75 percent of patients with metastatic seminoma (39). The levels decline following eradication of the tumor (47). False-positive elevation of PLAP, however, occurs in patients who are heavy smokers, but may be distinguishable from tumor PLAP by the use of different antibodies (48). Elevated neuron-specific enolase (NSE) levels may occur in seminoma patients; in one study, only 1 of 54 patients with testicular germ cell tumors who were clinically disease free had an elevated NSE, whereas 8 of 11 patients with metastatic seminoma had high serum NSE values (49). The lack of sensitivity and specificity of NSE limits its clinical utility (50).

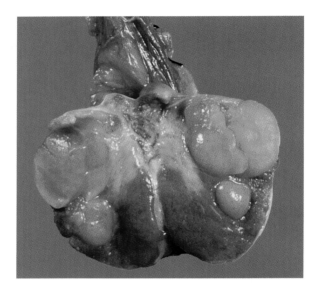

Figure 3-1

SEMINOMA

A lobulated and multinodular, light tan tumor bulges above the cut surface of the surrounding testis. The hemisection on the right shows two separate nodules, but these are seen to be in continuity on the left.

Gross Findings. Seminoma usually produces a symmetric, nondistorted enlargement of the testis. The average size is approximately 5 cm (2), although some exceed 10 cm. Of 261 clinical stage I seminomas, 61 percent were 2 to 6 cm (51). The tumor often totally replaces the testis (more than 50 percent of the cases in the experience of the British Testicular Tumour Panel [7]) or leaves only a compressed crescent of uninvolved parenchyma. The largest seminomas occur within intra-abdominal, maldescended testes because of their inaccessibility to palpation. In some patients with metastatic disease, no testicular enlargement is apparent; the testis is often atrophic and a scarred area, with or without residual microscopic foci of seminoma, is identified on histologic examination ("burnt-out" germ cell tumor; see chapter 5). Eleven percent of seminomas in the British series were in normal or smaller than normal testes (7). If gross testicular enlargement is present, prominent dilated veins may be identified on the surface of the tunica albuginea.

Most seminomas are solid, well-circumscribed, and lobulated to multinodular and bulge above the surrounding parenchyma (figs. 3-1, 3-2) but some are diffuse and smooth (figs. 3-3, 3-4). Sectioning may disclose two or more nodules, which connect in other planes (fig. 3-1), although truly separate nodules may, less commonly, also be seen (fig. 3-2). The tumors are usually soft, fleshy, and encephaloid (fig. 3-3), but may be firm and fibrous (fig. 3-4). The cut surface is commonly cream colored (fig. 3-3) to tan (fig. 3-1) to pale yellow (fig. 3-5) to pink. Intraparenchymal hemorrhage may rarely cause a red discoloration (fig. 3-6). Punctate foci of hemorrhage may indicate the presence of syncytiotrophoblastic giant cells (fig. 3-7) (52). Yellow foci of infarct-like necrosis, outlined by narrow bands of hemorrhage, are common (figs. 3-7, 3-8), and occasional tumors, particularly large ones, are extensively necrotic. Tumors with predominant or exclusive intertubular growth may show no gross abnormality or manifest as firm areas or discolored foci with respect to the surrounding parenchyma (18). About 90 percent of seminomas are grossly confined to the testis, with the remainder extending either through the mediastinum into the adjacent soft tissue, or the epididymis, or rarely, the tunica albuginea (53).

Microscopic Findings. On low power examination, the cells are arranged in more or less diffuse sheets (fig. 3-9), but closer inspection typically shows thin fibrous septa (fig. 3-10). The fibrous septa impart a nested (fig. 3-11) to

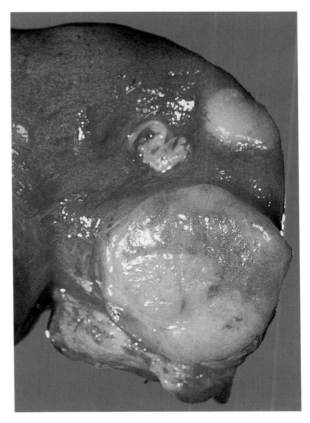

Figure 3-2

SEMINOMA

Two light tan nodules are seen.

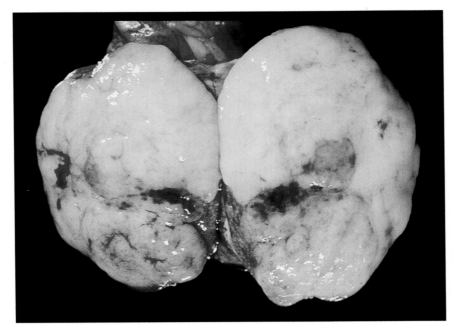

Figure 3-3

SEMINOMA

A fleshy, cream-colored tumor shows focal hemorrhage.

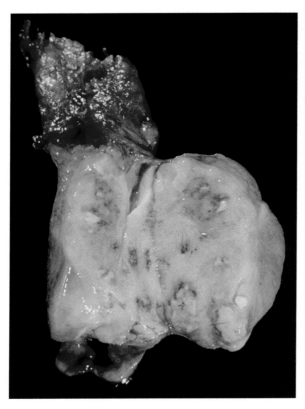

Figure 3-4

SEMINOMA

The white streaks in this diffuse tumor reflect extensive fibrosis in a case that prominently involved the epididymis. (Fig. 2.2 from Young RH, Scully RE. Testicular tumors. Chicago: ASCP Press; 1990:15.)

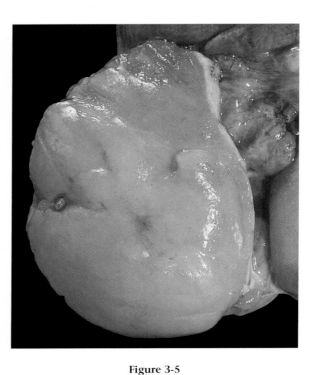

Figure 3-5

SEMINOMA

A light yellow-tan tumor replaces the testicular parenchyma.

Figure 3-6

SEMINOMA

Hemorrhage into the tumor nodules produces a beefy red appearance. (Fig. 2.4 from Young RH, Scully RE. Testicular tumors. Chicago: ASCP Press; 1990:16.)

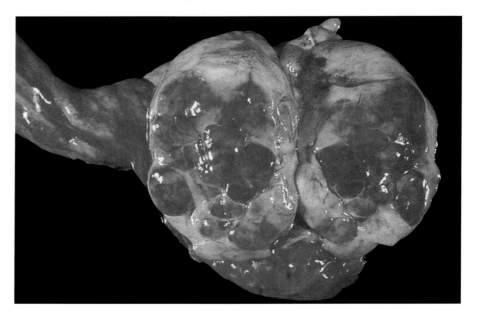

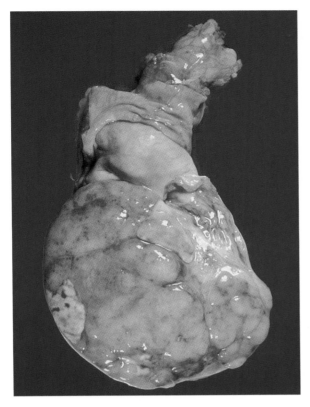

Figure 3-7

SEMINOMA

Punctate foci of hemorrhage and foci of necrosis are apparent on the cut surface of this seminoma. Lobulation is prominent. (Fig. 5 from Ulbright TM, Roth LM. Testicular and paratesticular tumors. In: Sternberg SS, ed. Diagnostic surgical pathology, New York: Raven Press; 1994:1894.)

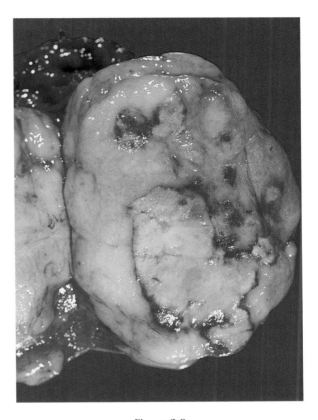

Figure 3-8

SEMINOMA

Variably sized yellow zones of necrosis are focally rimmed by hemorrhage.

Figure 3-9

SEMINOMA

This tumor has a diffuse, sheet-like pattern. A sprinkling of lymphocytes is seen even at this low power.

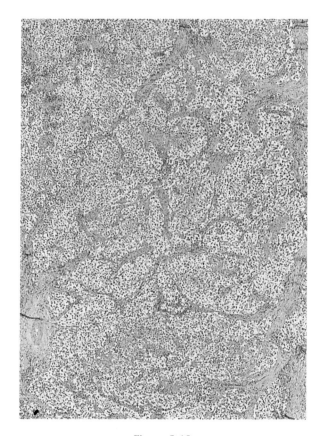

Figure 3-10

SEMINOMA

Typical thin, delicate septa with scattered lymphocytes are seen.

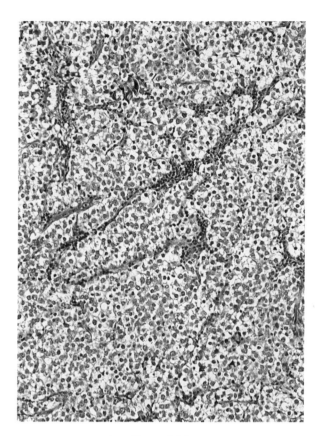

Figure 3-11

SEMINOMA

The fibrous trabeculae separate the tumor into nests of varying sizes and shapes.

nodular pattern (fig. 3-12), or they may delineate small groups of tumor cells, resulting in an alveolar pattern (fig. 3-13). The septal framework characteristic of this tumor is often highlighted by a lymphocytic infiltrate that varies from a light sprinkling (fig. 3-10) to a heavy infiltrate (fig. 3-14). Prominent fibrous tissue may separate individual nodules (fig. 3-15). Smaller nests (fig. 3-16), clusters (fig. 3-17), and individual seminoma cells in a dense, sometimes hyalinized stroma (fig. 3-18) may also occur. Many cases show cords (fig. 3-19) or, less commonly, trabecular arrangements of tumor cells (fig. 3-17). In rare cases, the tumor cells exhibit a solid (figs. 3-16, 3-20) or hollow tubular pattern (fig. 3-21) (54,55). Tubular patterns are often associated with microcystic arrangements (56), having either irregular spaces (fig. 3-22) or, less often, round, regular spaces (fig. 3-23). Edema fluid may or may not be identified in such

spaces (fig. 3-24). A pseudoglandular pattern is a variant of this process (fig. 3-25).

Although most tumors obliterate the underlying testicular parenchyma, it is common to find foci of intertubular growth with tubular preservation (fig. 3-26) (57), especially at the periphery. Seminoma cells may be mixed with Leydig cells in areas with intertubular growth (fig. 3-27). Some small seminomas have an exclusive intertubular growth pattern (fig. 3-28) and, rarely, such growth is conspicuous in large tumors. Tumors with exclusive intertubular growth are susceptible to being overlooked, although many have a lymphocytic infiltrate that draws attention to the tumor cells (fig. 3-29), and their common association with intratubular germ cell neoplasia, unclassified type (IGCNU) is also helpful. Tumors with exclusive intertubular growth are often not grossly visible (57).

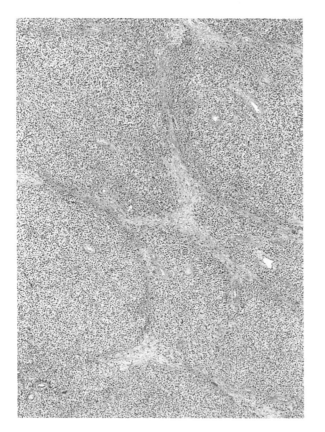

Figure 3-12

SEMINOMA

A multinodular pattern with fibrous bands is present.

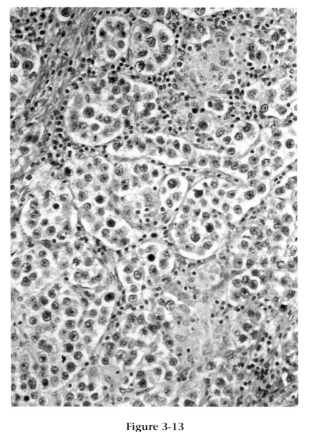

Figure 3-13

SEMINOMA

A solid alveolar pattern is created by thin septa around small nests of cells.

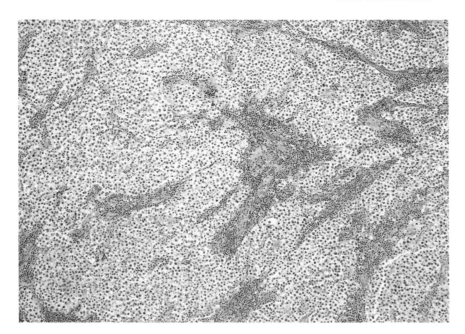

Figure 3-14

SEMINOMA

A dense lymphocytic infiltrate is centered on fibrous septa.

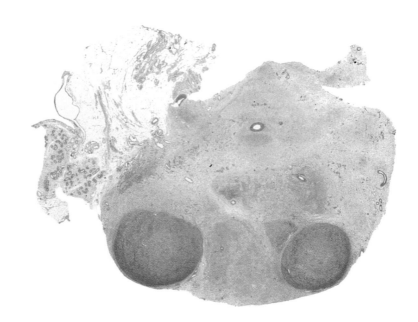

Figure 3-15

SEMINOMA

Two distinct nodules are present in a scarred parenchyma.

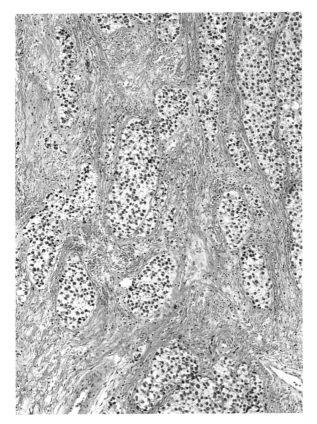

Figure 3-16

SEMINOMA

Prominent fibrous stroma compartmentalizes the tumor into nests and solid pseudotubules.

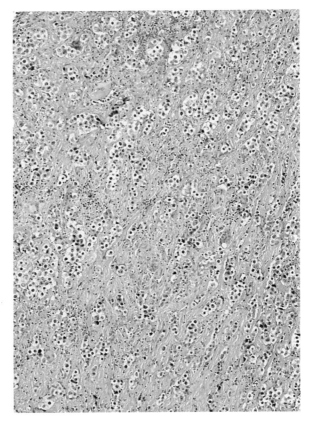

Figure 3-17

SEMINOMA

Extensive fibrous stroma separates small clusters and trabeculae of tumor cells.

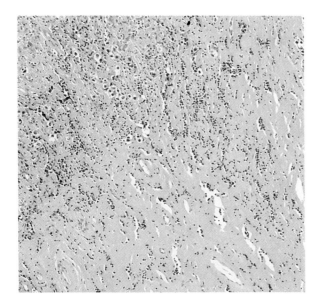

Figure 3-18

SEMINOMA

There is extensive scarring. Many lymphocytes and few seminoma cells are seen.

Figure 3-19

SEMINOMA

The tumor cells are growing in cords.

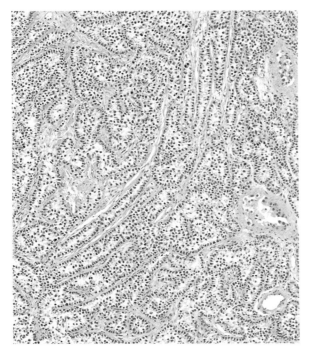

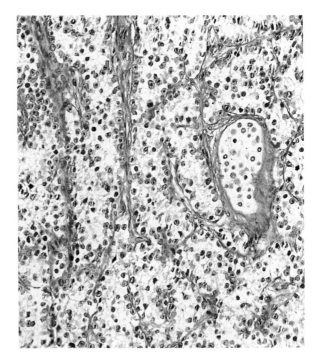

Figure 3-20

SEMINOMA

Left: A tubular pattern is created by central discohesion and a palisade-like arrangement of cells at the periphery of broad, anastomosing cords. Distinction from a Sertoli cell tumor is important in cases of this type.

Right: High-power view of the same case shows the typical cytologic features of seminoma cells.

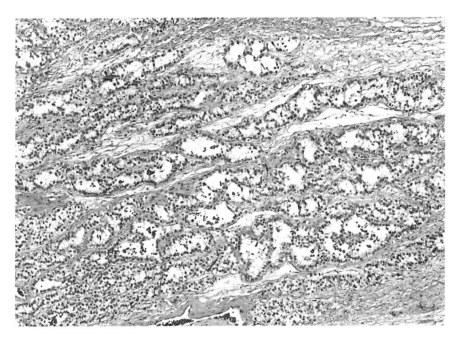

Figure 3-21

SEMINOMA

Distinct hollow tubules are present.

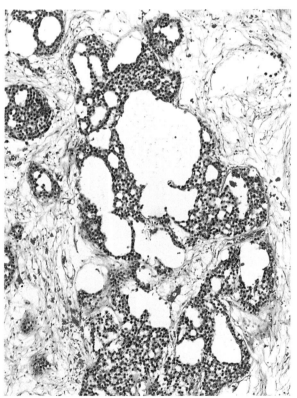

Figure 3-22

SEMINOMA

Irregular microcystic spaces form a cribriform arrangement of tumor cells.

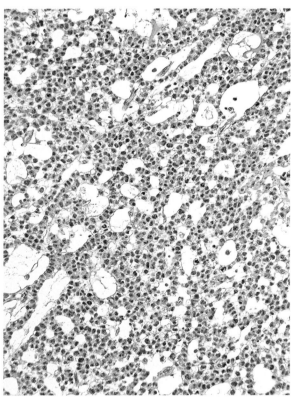

Figure 3-23

SEMINOMA

Regular gland-like spaces are present.

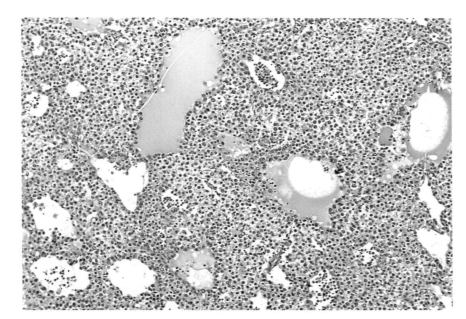

Figure 3-24

SEMINOMA

The spaces have eosinophilic fluid.

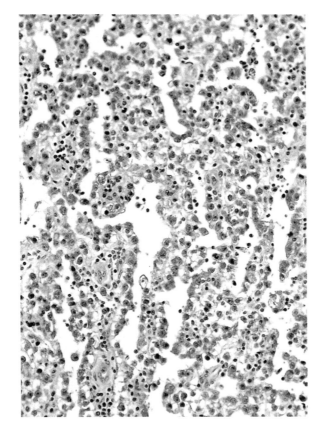

Figure 3-25

SEMINOMA

A pseudoglandular pattern is seen.

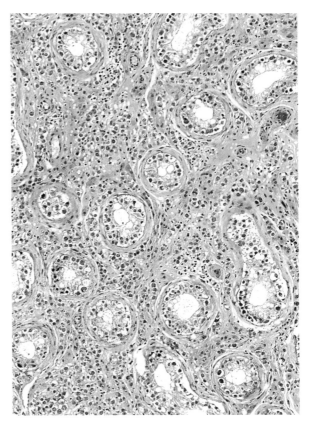

Figure 3-26

SEMINOMA

The tumor cells grow between preserved seminiferous tubules.

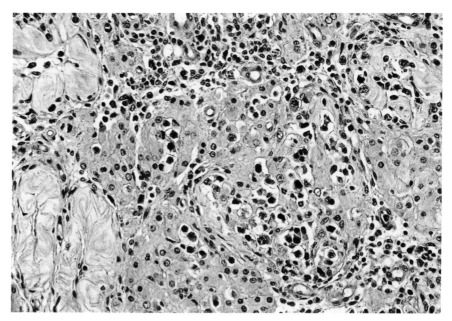

Figure 3-27

SEMINOMA

There is intertubular growth with seminoma cells within clusters of Leydig cells.

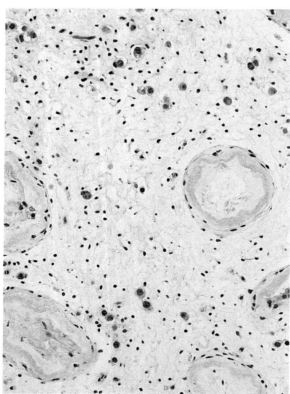

Figure 3-28

SEMINOMA

Scattered tumor cells are in the widened interstitium of an atrophic, cryptorchid testis. This tumor was grossly inapparent.

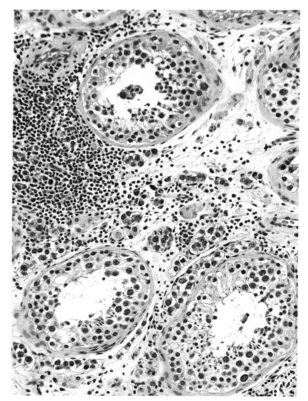

Figure 3-29

SEMINOMA

Small clusters of intertubular tumor cells are associated with a lymphocytic infiltrate.

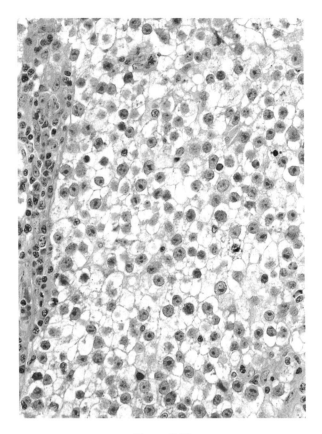

Figure 3-30

SEMINOMA

The tumor cells have abundant clear cytoplasm, well-defined cytoplasmic borders, evenly spaced nuclei (some of which have "squared-off" edges), and prominent central nucleoli.

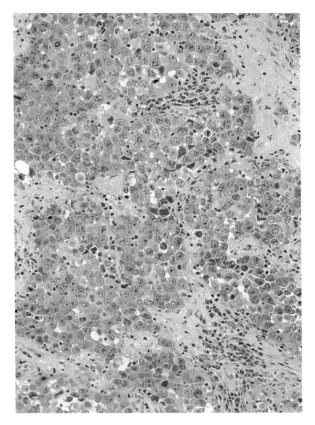

Figure 3-31

SEMINOMA

The cytoplasm is densely eosinophilic and the nuclei are more pleomorphic than in most seminomas.

Seminoma cells are round to polygonal and usually have clear or pale to lightly eosinophilic, granular cytoplasm and distinct cytoplasmic membranes in well-fixed specimens (fig. 3-30). In some cases, however, there are foci with eosinophilic to amphophilic cytoplasm (figs. 3-31, 3-32), and this occurs diffusely on rare occasion. The tumor cells are 15 to 25 μm in diameter. The nuclei are large and central or slightly eccentric, with granular chromatin, usually one or more prominent nucleoli, and an irregularly thickened nuclear membrane (fig. 3-33). In some cases with more densely staining cytoplasm, eccentric nuclei result in a plasmacytoid appearance, although a perinuclear hof is lacking (fig. 3-32). The nuclear membrane is typically somewhat flattened rather than perfectly round,

yielding a "squared-off" nuclear configuration (fig. 3-33). Another useful feature is the generally uniform distribution of nuclei within neoplastic islands such that the nuclei are separated from each other by roughly equivalent amounts of cytoplasm (fig. 3-30), in contrast to the overlapping nuclei of embryonal carcinoma.

In adequately fixed specimens, a useful diagnostic feature in many cases is the distinctly visible cytoplasmic membranes that separate adjacent neoplastic cells (figs. 3-30, 3-33); this feature contrasts with the syncytial arrangement that typifies embryonal carcinoma in which cytoplasmic borders are indistinct (see figs. 4-7, 4-20). Poor fixation, however, may produce a syncytial appearance in seminomas (fig. 3-34). The clear cytoplasm reflects an abundant amount of glycogen that usually is demonstrable as

Figure 3-32

SEMINOMA

Dense, amphophilic to eosinophilic cytoplasm and eccentric nuclei cause a plasmacytoid appearance, although perinuclear hofs are absent.

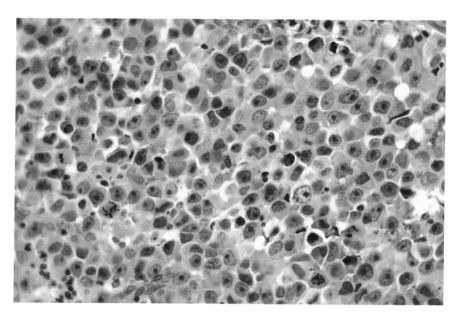

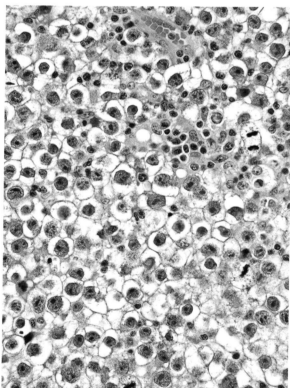

Figure 3-33

SEMINOMA

The tumor cells show the classic cytologic features of clear cytoplasm, distinct cytoplasmic membranes, and polygonal nuclei that have one or more prominent nucleoli and occasional flattened edges.

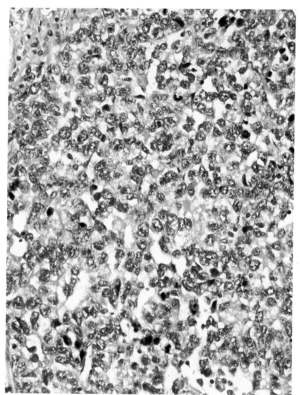

Figure 3-34

SEMINOMA

Poor fixation results in the loss of membrane definition, a syncytial appearance, and nuclear crowding. These features may cause confusion with the solid pattern of embryonal carcinoma.

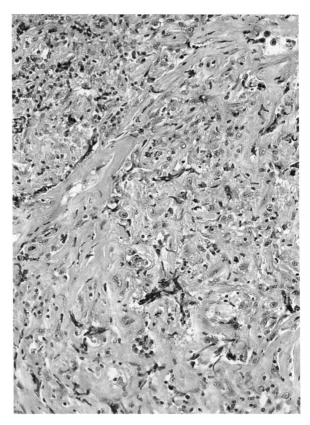

Figure 3-35

SEMINOMA

Diffuse reactivity with the periodic acid–Schiff (PAS) stain corresponds to abundant intracytoplasmic glycogen.

Figure 3-36

SEMINOMA

Many tumor cells have been compressed into darkly staining thread-like forms in a fibrotic stroma. (Fig. 2.22 from Young RH, Scully RE. Testicular tumors. Chicago: ASCP Press; 1990:25.)

granular, periodic acid–Schiff (PAS)-positive, diastase-labile deposits (fig. 3-35).

In some seminomas the nuclei have a smudgy appearance, with loss of chromatin detail. Seminomas are also susceptible to compression artifact, sometimes appearing as densely staining thread-like forms (fig. 3-36). In some tumors, this "squeeze" artifact is extensive (fig. 3-37); a lymphocytic and granulomatous reaction is helpful in recognizing these cases, as are appropriate immunostains.

Rare morphologic variants include tumors in which the cells have a focal signet ring morphology (58) caused by empty-appearing cytoplasmic vacuoles that compress the nuclei to a crescent shape (fig. 3-38); in one case this feature was prominent in much of the tumor (fig. 3-39). Rarely, the tumor cells focally assume a spindle cell configuration (fig. 3-40), a finding

previously noted by Thackray and Crane in the series of the British Testicular Tumour Panel and Registry (7).

Almost all seminomas contain a lymphocytic infiltrate, which is heavy in 20 to 25 percent (7,53). Lymphocytes are absent in only 1 percent of cases (51), and such absence should call into question the diagnosis, although such cases occur. The lymphocytes vary from a delicate sprinkling (see fig. 3-10), to numerous clusters (fig. 3-41), to dense aggregates (fig. 3-42). Lymphoid follicles occur in up to 18 percent of cases (fig. 3-43). Lymphocytes often are most prominent in a perivascular distribution and hence are most conspicuous in the fibrous septa (see fig. 3-14), but they are also irregularly scattered, at least to a limited extent, among the seminoma

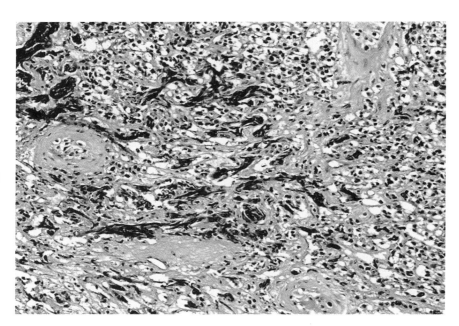

Figure 3-37

SEMINOMA

Prominent "squeeze" artifact is seen.

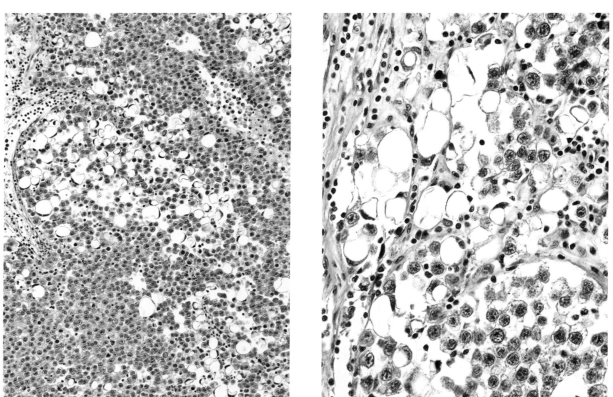

Figure 3-38

SEMINOMA

Left: Some tumor cells have empty-appearing cytoplasmic vacuoles that compress the nuclei, causing a signet ring cell appearance.

Right: A higher-magnification view shows the empty-appearing vacuoles that compress the nuclei.

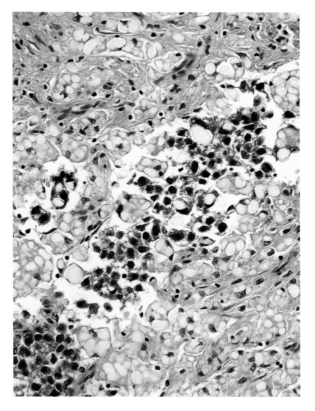

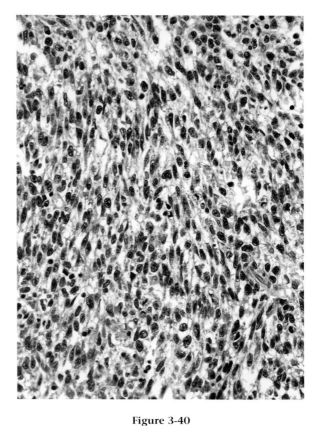

Figure 3-39

SEMINOMA

Some of the tumor cells have a signet cell ring appearance. There are also numerous vacuolated histiocytes.

Figure 3-40

SEMINOMA

This rare case shows foci of spindle-shaped tumor cells, which had the typical immunohistochemical properties of seminoma cells.

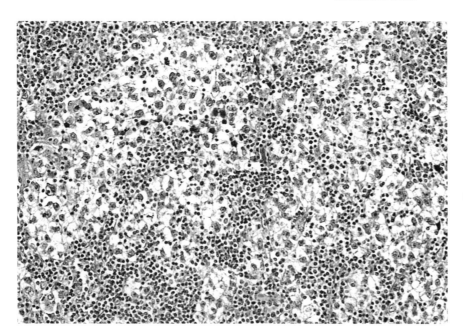

Figure 3-41

SEMINOMA

There is a striking lymphoid infiltrate.

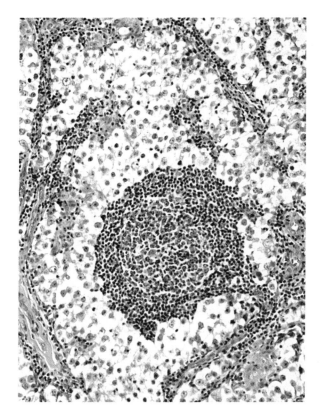

Figure 3-42

SEMINOMA

A lymphoid aggregate is seen. (Fig. 2.14 from Young RH, Scully RE. Testicular tumors. Chicago: ASCP Press; 1990:21.)

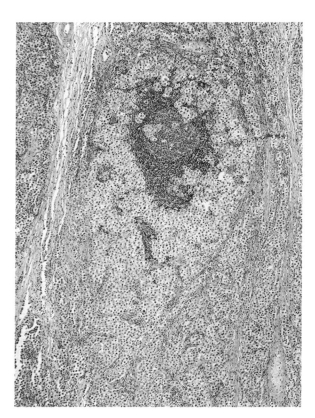

Figure 3-43

SEMINOMA

A lymphoid follicle with a germinal center is present.

cells away from the septa (fig. 3-41). At scanning magnification, aggregates of lymphocytes may be the first clue to a small focus of seminoma, especially those with an intertubular pattern (see fig. 3-29). Most lymphocytes mark as T cells (59-64), and many have gamma/delta receptors and appear to play a role in granuloma formation (65). Occasionally, plasma cells and eosinophils are identified in the infiltrate. Prominent lymphocytic infiltrates have been correlated with a better prognosis (66,67), an observation perhaps related to ultrastructural studies demonstrating damaged seminoma cells associated with the lymphoid component (64).

A granulomatous reaction occurs in 50 to 60 percent of seminomas (51,53). It varies from a light, scattered infiltrate of epithelioid histiocytes, to irregular clusters of such cells, to discrete well-defined granulomas (fig. 3-44). In

some cases there may be Langhans-type giant cells (fig. 3-45). The presence of an extensive granulomatous reaction, sometimes with a heavy lymphoid infiltrate, may mask the underlying seminoma cells (fig. 3-46) and cause a misdiagnosis of granulomatous orchitis (see Differential Diagnosis and chapter 8).

Foci of necrosis are common (fig. 3-47) and may be extensive; they occur in about half of the cases and are striking in about 10 percent (7,51). Necrosis generally occurs as discrete foci of the coagulative type, with ghost-like remnants of seminoma cells typically identifiable within the necrotic, eosinophilic zones. Recognition of a necrotic septal framework and small cells consistent with necrotic lymphocytes may help in the diagnosis, as may appropriate immunostains (68).

Seminomas often focally fill and distend seminiferous tubules (*intratubular seminoma*)

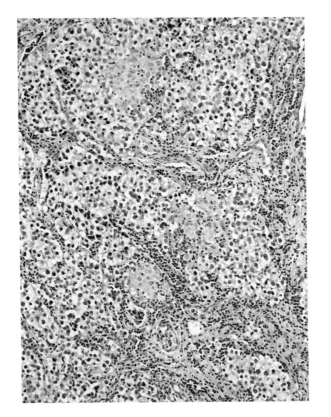

Figure 3-44

SEMINOMA

There are scattered aggregates of epithelioid histiocytes.

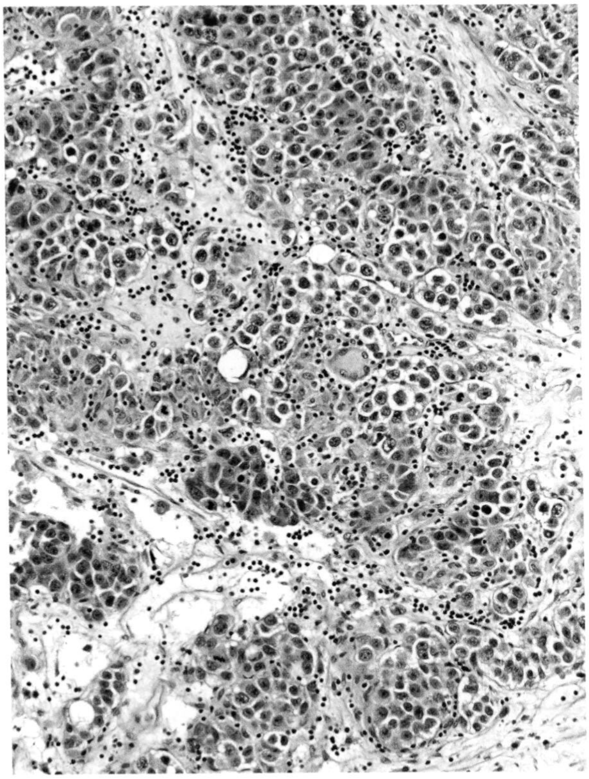

Figure 3-45

SEMINOMA

Occasional Langhans-type giant cells are present.

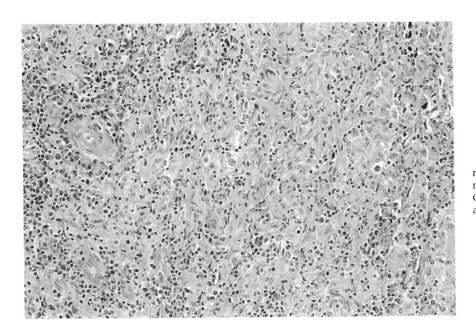

Figure 3-46

SEMINOMA

An extensive granulomatous reaction in a seminoma masks many of the neoplastic cells. Only rare scattered tumor cells are apparent.

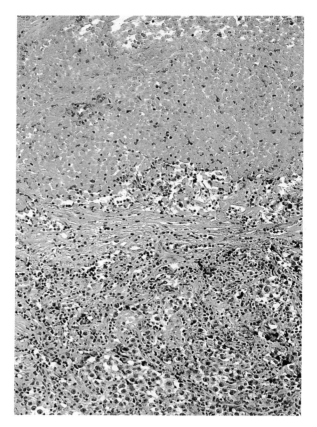

Figure 3-47

SEMINOMA

Necrosis is apparent within the tumor. Ghost outlines of seminoma cells can still be seen in the necrotic region.

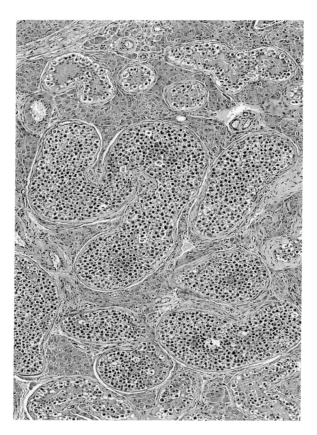

Figure 3-48

SEMINOMA

Intratubular seminoma (adjacent to invasive seminoma [not shown]) fills and distends the seminiferous tubules. Adjacent tubules show the typical pattern of intratubular germ cell neoplasia of the unclassified type (IGCNU). The Leydig cells are hyperplastic.

(fig. 3-48). Dixon and Moore (66) identified intratubular growth in 24 percent of their cases. This phenomenon, or its precursor, IGCNU, may extend into the rete testis where the tumor cells percolate between the rete epithelial cells in a pagetoid fashion (fig. 3-49) (69), thereby enlarging the rete and sometimes causing a clinical mass (fig. 3-50). Involvement of the rete by invasive seminoma occurs in more than 40 percent of cases (51). In tumors that provoke a marked granulomatous reaction, there may also be a prominent intratubular granulomatous response (fig. 3-51).

Dystrophic calcification may occur within scarred or necrotic foci. Rarely, ossification occurs within the fibrous stroma of seminomas (fig. 3-52) (70). Intratubular calcification in the form of microliths, small psammoma body-like structures, is common adjacent to seminomas

(and other germ cell tumor types) and is considered a marker of increased risk for germ cell tumor development (71–73). The testicular parenchyma adjacent to seminomas (and other germ cell tumors in postpubertal patients) is almost always atrophic, with shrunken seminiferous tubules having thickened basement membranes and diminished numbers of germ cells, many with a "Sertoli cell only" appearance or completely hyalinized (fig. 3-53). IGCNU is found in about 90 percent of cases. Collections of hyperplastic Leydig cells are also seen.

The mitotic activity of seminomas is variable but usually brisk, and tends to be greatest at the periphery of lobules where DNA synthesis is greatest (74). In the past, a high mitotic

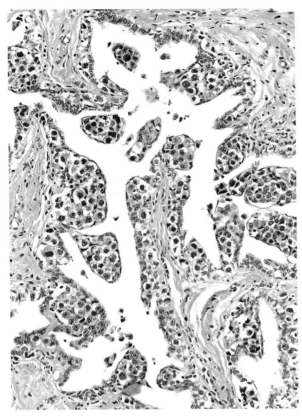

Figure 3-49

IGCNU IN SEMINOMA

IGCNU cells extend into the rete testis, with intact rete testis epithelium on the luminal aspect.

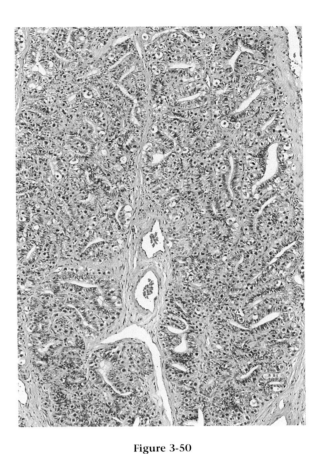

Figure 3-50

IGCNU IN SEMINOMA

There is prominent intra-rete extension of IGCNU, with expansion of the rete testis. The enlarged rete caused a palpable mass.

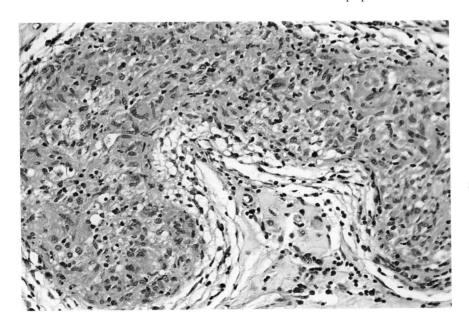

Figure 3-51

SEMINOMA

There is a marked intratubular granulomatous reaction.

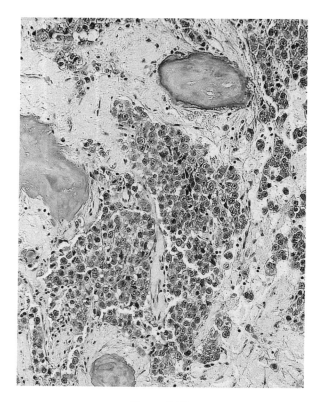

Figure 3-52

SEMINOMA

Ossification has occurred in a tumor with extensive stromal sclerosis.

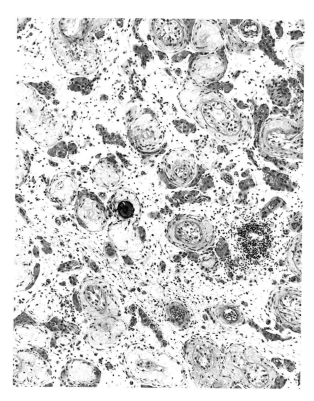

Figure 3-53

PARENCHYMA ADJACENT TO SEMINOMA

The tubules are atrophic, with a "Sertoli cell only" pattern and thickened basement membranes. An intratubular microlith and clusters of Leydig cells are seen. Intratubular germ cell neoplasia is absent, as is often the case in foci of severe atrophy.

rate (3 or more mitotic figures per high-power field) was used as a criterion for the recognition of an "anaplastic" subcategory of seminoma (53,75), a subset we, and most others, do not recognize. More recent studies cast doubt on the value of mitotic activity as a criterion for the recognition of aggressively behaving seminomas (76,77), since most show a "high" mitotic rate (78), a situation that led some to revise the "anaplastic" criterion to an average of 6 or more mitotic figures per high-power field. The lack of correlation of mitotic activity with prognosis in seminoma, however, argues against even this criterion. Similar findings in classic and "anaplastic" seminomas by ultrastructure, immunohistochemistry, and lectin-binding analyses provide further evidence against the validity of this category (77,79,80). There remain, nonetheless, rare seminomas with either focal or more diffuse pleomorphism than is typical, often with denser cytoplasm and greater nuclear

crowding (see fig. 3-31). Such tumors have been termed *atypical seminomas*, and in one study presented at a higher clinical stage than non-atypical seminomas (81). In our opinion, such tumors are likely in transition from seminoma to embryonal carcinoma in what is undoubtedly a multistep process. Our own approach is to regard these tumors as within the spectrum of seminoma unless there is clear-cut epithelial differentiation in the form of papillae or glands, or the tumor shows distinct cytokeratin (AE1/AE3) and CD30 reactivity that contrasts with weaker or absent reactivity in the morphologically typical seminoma foci of the same neoplasm.

Syncytiotrophoblast cells are seen in 4 to 7 percent of seminomas by routine light microscopy (51,82), but immunostains directed against hCG highlight cells with syncytiotrophoblastic

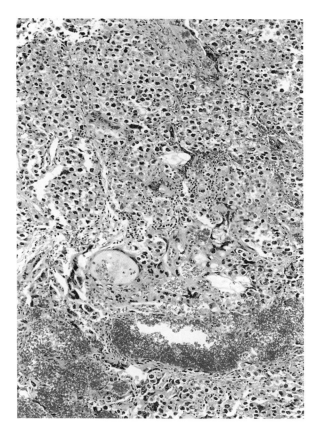

Figure 3-54

SEMINOMA

Prominent syncytiotrophoblastic cells and focal hemorrhage are intermingled with seminoma cells.

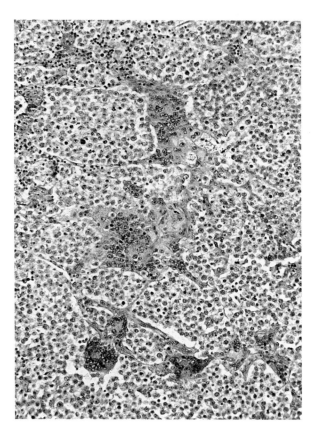

Figure 3-55

SEMINOMA

Scattered syncytiotrophoblastic cells, some with mulberry-like nuclei, are seen.

differentiation in 20 to 25 percent of cases (82,83). Sometimes punctate hemorrhagic foci or even blood lakes, surrounded by the syncytiotrophoblast cells, are seen (fig. 3-54) and are a clue to the diagnosis. In other cases, however, there is no associated hemorrhage (fig. 3-55). The syncytiotrophoblast cells are variable in appearance. They sometimes appear as classic syncytiotrophoblasts with abundant cytoplasm, several or numerous hyperchromatic nuclei, and intracytoplasmic lacunae (fig. 3-56) that may be cystically dilated (fig. 3-57). More commonly, they appear as multinucleated giant cells lacking lacunae (fig. 3-55). In some instances, the cells have relatively scant cytoplasm and contain "mulberry-like" aggregates of nuclei (fig. 3-55). Some hCG-positive cells are uninucleated and easily blend with the background of seminoma cells; some represent intermediate trophoblast

cells and are occasionally human placental lactogen (HPL) reactive (84). Most frequently, syncytiotrophoblast cells are scattered in a multifocal fashion in the tumor, tending to localize in small clusters adjacent to capillaries. An admixture with mononucleated trophoblast cells is lacking. Intratubular syncytiotrophoblast cells are identified in the parenchyma adjacent to 17 percent of seminomas upon careful examination (fig. 3-58) (85). When trophoblastic elements are identified in seminoma, their presence should be noted in the diagnosis as "seminoma with syncytiotrophoblast cells" or "seminoma with trophoblastic elements." The absence of choriocarcinoma should also be explicitly stated.

Clinically relevant features to assess include the presence or absence of lymphovascular space and rete testis invasion, and tunica vaginalis penetration. As mentioned in chapter 1, pathologic stage

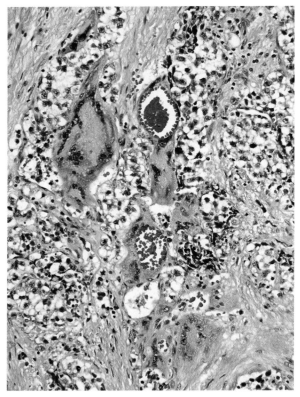

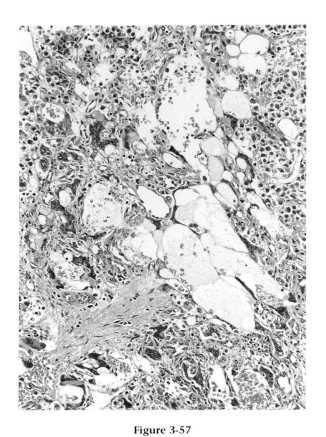

Figure 3-56

SEMINOMA

Syncytiotrophoblast cells have blood-filled lacunae.

Figure 3-57

SEMINOMA

The syncytiotrophoblast cells have cystically dilated intracytoplasmic lacunae.

Figure 3-58

INTRATUBULAR SYNCYTIOTROPHOBLAST CELL IN A SEMINOMA

(Courtesy of Dr. D. M. Berney, London, UK.)

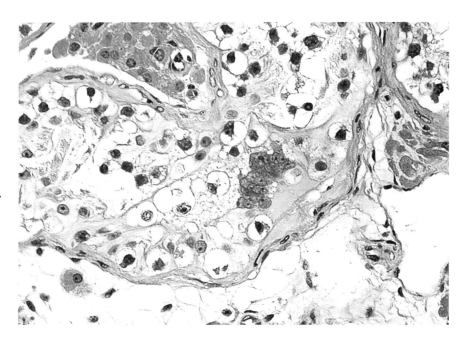

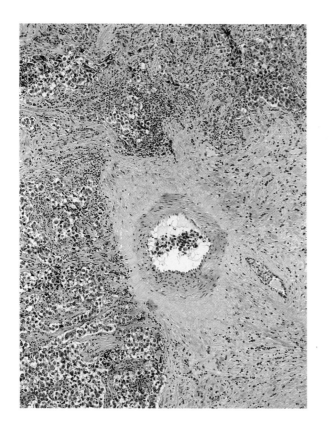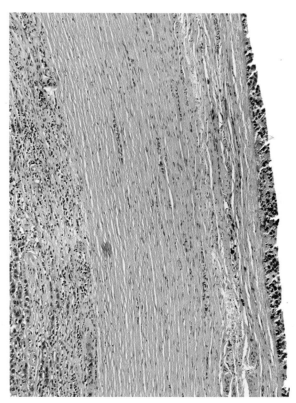

Figure 3-59

SEMINOMA

Left: "Floating" seminoma cells occupy a small fraction of a vessel seen in cross section; this represents implantation artifact.

Right: Tumor cells have been "buttered on" tissue surfaces.

T1 tumors lack both lymphovascular invasion and tunica vaginalis penetration, whereas stage T2 tumors have at least one of them. Artifactual implantation of tumor cells into the lumens of vessels and on tissue surfaces may mimic true invasion, and is common in seminomas because of their high cellularity and stromal-poor nature. Additionally, intratubular tumor may be confused with intravascular tumor. Implantation of tumor cells can be minimized but not altogether prevented by meticulous handling of the specimen, taking sections of the spermatic cord prior to incision of the tumor, and carefully cleaning the knife blade during tumor sectioning. Artifactually implanted tumor cells in vessels do not conform to the shape of the vessel and are not associated with thrombotic material; instead the tumor cells have a "floating" appearance, sometimes only occupying a fraction of the

lumen (fig. 3-59). These findings contrast with true vascular invasion, where tumor emboli fill and conform to vessel shapes, and may have fibrin attaching them to the walls. Also, vascular space implantation is usually associated with tissue implantation, which is recognizable as loosely cohesive cells that are "buttered on" the external aspect of tissues or deeper into tissue crevices (fig. 3-59) (86). Intratubular tumor may be admixed with residual Sertoli cells or non-neoplastic spermatogenic cells, and lacks an endothelial cell component.

Immunohistochemical Findings. A summary of immunostains that are helpful in the diagnosis of seminoma and other germ cell tumors is shown in Table 3-1. The most useful currently available markers for seminoma are OCT3/4, PLAP, c-KIT (CD117), and SOX17. Of these, OCT3/4 has the greatest sensitivity, staining

Table 3-1

POTENTIALLY USEFUL IMMUNOSTAINS IN GERM CELL TUMORS

	Keratin AE1/3	PLAP[a]	OCT 3/4	NANOG	c-KIT	Glypican 3	AFP	hCG	CD30	SALL4	SOX2	SOX17
IGCNU[a]	neg	pos	pos	pos	pos	neg	neg	neg	neg	pos	neg	pos
Seminoma (classic)	var	pos	pos	pos	pos	neg	neg	neg	neg	pos	neg	pos
Spermatocytic seminoma	neg	neg[b]	neg	neg	var	neg	neg	neg	neg	pos	neg	neg
Embryonal carcinoma	pos	pos	pos	pos	neg	var	var	neg	pos	pos	pos	neg
Yolk sac tumor	pos	pos	neg	neg	var[c]	pos	var	neg	neg	pos	neg	var
Choriocarcinoma	pos	pos	neg	neg	neg	pos	neg	pos	neg	var	neg	neg

[a]Abbreviations: PLAP = placental-like alkaline phosphate; AFP = alpha-fetoprotein; hCG = human chorionic gonadotropin; IGCNU = intratubular germ cell neoplasia, unclassified; pos = positive; var = variable; neg = negative.
[b]Rare positivity in individual and small groups of tumor cells.
[c]Solid pattern often positive.

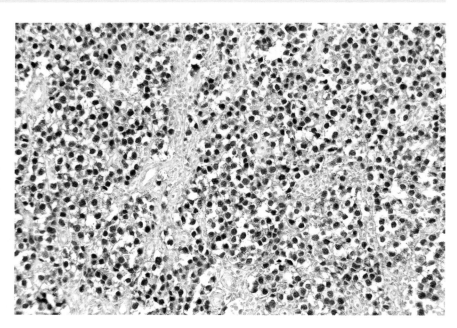

Figure 3-60

SEMINOMA

An immunostain directed against the OCT3/4 transcription factor produces strong nuclear staining.

all of 55 seminomas in two studies (87,88) and is specific for seminoma and embryonal carcinoma among all testicular tumors (87,88). It produces a diffuse nuclear reaction pattern (fig. 3-60), and we have found preservation of nuclear reactivity in totally necrotic seminomas, highlighting the "ghost" nuclei (fig. 3-61).

Anti-PLAP highlights PLAP in a diffuse and membrane-accentuated pattern in 87 to 98 percent of seminomas (fig. 3-62) (89–92). PLAP positivity, however, may also be seen in other germ cell tumors, where it tends to be more focal and cytoplasmic (93), and in some nongerm cell tumors, including adenocarcinomas of the lung, ovarian carcinomas, and endometrial carcinomas (94). The liver isoenzyme of alkaline phosphatase has been demonstrated in seminomas but not the intestinal form (95).

Staining for c-KIT (CD117) produces a membrane pattern of reactivity in 90 to 100 percent of seminomas that is identical to that seen with PLAP (fig. 3-63) (96,97). Positivity for c-KIT, however, also occurs in 40 percent of spermatocytic seminomas (98), 60 percent of solid pattern yolk sac tumors (99), and a variety of nongerm cell tumors, including gastrointestinal stromal tumors, papillary carcinoma of the thyroid, chromophobe renal cell carcinoma, and others.

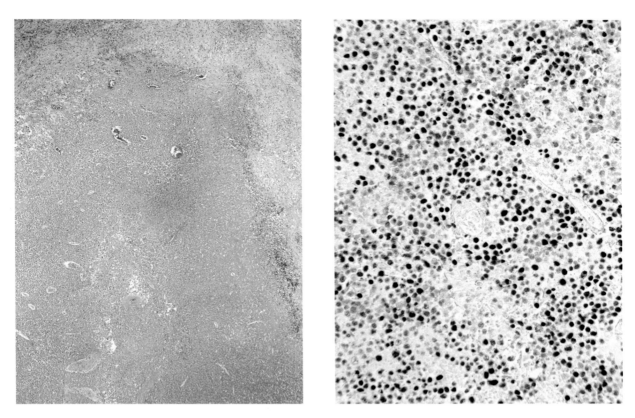

Figure 3-61

SEMINOMA

A totally necrotic tumor (left) still produces a strong nuclear reaction for OCT3/4 (right).

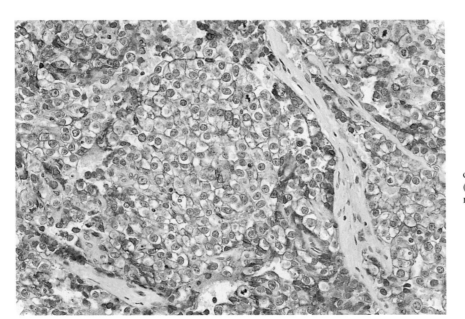

Figure 3-62

SEMINOMA

An immunostain for placental-like alkaline phosphatase (PLAP) shows the characteristic membranous pattern.

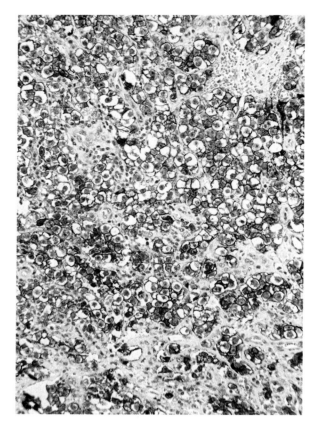

Figure 3-63

SEMINOMA

An immunostain for cKIT (CD117) highlights the cytoplasmic membranes of the tumor cells.

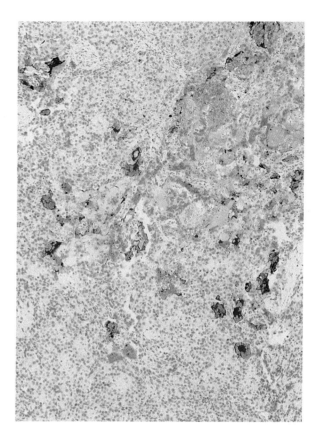

Figure 3-64

SEMINOMA

Prominent syncytiotrophoblast cells are highlighted by an immunostain for human chorionic gonadotropin (hCG).

Antibodies to SOX17 are sensitive for seminoma, staining the nuclei of 94 to 100 percent of cases and negative in embryonal carcinomas, but they also stain yolk sac tumors (100,101). Podoplanin is positive in virtually all seminomas and negative in embryonal carcinoma (102,103). It, however, is also positive in mesothelioma, vascular tumors, and some papillary renal cell carcinomas and lung carcinomas. Recently, MAGEC2, one of the "testis-cancer" antigens, has been reported as positive in the nuclei of 94 percent of seminomas and, like SOX17, negative in embryonal carcinomas (101). SALL4 is uniformly positive in seminomas but also stains numerous other germ cell tumor types (104).

As noted previously, 7 to 25 percent of pure seminomas are associated with an elevated serum level of hCG. Immunostaining usually discloses positivity for hCG in syncytiotrophoblast cells (fig. 3-64), although some hCG positivity occurs in cells that are not recognizable as syncytiotrophoblasts by routine light microscopy (82), suggesting that there is incomplete trophoblastic differentiation or differentiation to intermediate trophoblast in such cases (84). Immunopositivity for hCG in seminomas has ranged from 5 to 24 percent (82,83,91,105,106). Trophoblastic cells are also typically strongly cytokeratin reactive, in contrast to seminoma cells.

Cytokeratin filaments are not abundant in the majority of seminomas, and there are contradictory results concerning the frequency of keratin positivity. This is likely due to the specificity of the antibodies and the utilization of different methodologies for antigen retrieval. Reports of cytokeratin positivity range from 0 to 73 percent

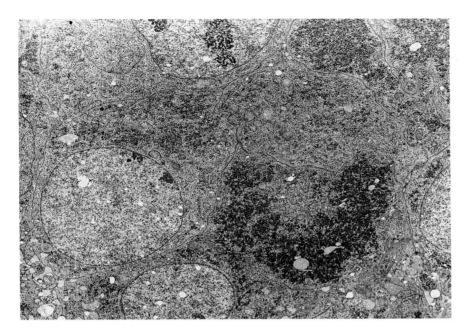

Figure 3-65

SEMINOMA

The seminoma cells have smooth, closely apposed cytoplasmic membranes, abundant glycogen particles, polarization of cytoplasmic organelles, and nuclei with evenly dispersed chromatin. A "meandering" nucleolus is seen in the cell at the top.

(107–113), with staining usually occurring in isolated cells or small clusters, although some otherwise typical seminomas have been diffusely positive (91,109,111). Cytokeratins (CK) 8 and 18 may be identified in seminomas (114), with the usual absence of CK19 (109,115), although scant amounts of CK19 were found in 5 of 26 seminomas using frozen sections (113). CK19, on the other hand, is common in embryonal carcinomas (115). CK7 is positive in 41 percent of seminomas but only 5 percent have more than 10 percent reactive tumor cells (116). Seminomas associated with borderline serum AFP elevations may disproportionately express CK7 (41). CK4 and CK17, more characteristic of stratified and complex glandular epithelia, are identified in rare seminomas, as are desmin and neurofilament protein (113). CK8, CK18, and CK19 are readily demonstrated in the syncytiotrophoblast cells of seminomas (113).

Seminomas are characteristically positive for vimentin but usually in only a small percentage of the tumor cells (108,109,112), although widespread staining occurred in 6 of 26 cases in one study (113). LDH, ferritin, and NSE are positive in most seminomas but are nonspecific (91,117,118). Alpha-1-antitrypsin and Leu-7 are positive in 5 percent and 14 percent of cases (91), respectively, whereas angiotensin-converting enzyme was positive in all of 20 germino-

mas (119). Focal positivity for CD30 occurs in a minority of cases (120).

Unlike yolk sac tumor and some embryonal carcinomas, stains for AFP are negative in seminoma (Table 3-1) (91,121,122). Epithelial membrane antigen (EMA) is also negative in seminoma, as it is in the great majority of embryonal carcinomas and yolk sac tumors (91,94).

A useful panel for the diagnosis of seminoma includes OCT3/4, AE1/AE3 cytokeratin, CD30, and EMA. Positivity for OCT3/4 and negativity for the other three markers is specific for seminoma.

Ultrastructural Findings. On ultrastructural examination, seminoma cells are closely apposed, with smooth or undulating cell membranes (fig. 3-65). Primitive junctions, most commonly consisting of electron-dense thickenings of the membranes of adjacent cells, are occasionally identified (123). Such junctions lack well-developed inserting filaments. In some seminomas, more differentiated, epithelial-type junctions and specializations are found. In these cases, rare tight junctional complexes are identified, with well-defined desmosomes, as adjacent cells form abortive extracellular lumens with short projecting microvilli (80,124,125). Complex interdigitating cell membranes may be identified (126). Seminomas displaying epithelial differentiation on ultrastructural

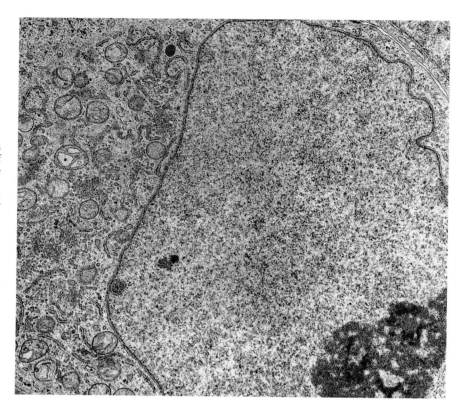

Figure 3-66

SEMINOMA

A portion of a seminoma cell shows polarization of cytoplasmic organelles. These consist of small mitochondria, short stacks of Golgi-like membranes, single strands of rough endoplasmic reticulum, scattered free ribosomes, and a small lysosome. The nucleolus is typically complex, and there is a primitive cell junction at the upper right. The chromatin is evenly dispersed.

examination ("seminoma with early carcinomatous features") retain a typical light microscopic morphology and clinical behavior (124).

The cytoplasm is primitive. Variable amounts of rosettes of glycogen are identified, from sparse to superabundant (fig. 3-65) (127). Organelles are usually polarized to one side of the cell (figs. 3-65, 3-66) and consist of mitochondria with tubulovesicular cristae and clear matrices; occasional granular, membrane-bound, lysosome-like bodies; annulate lamellae; and cisternae of rough and smooth endoplasmic reticulum (fig. 3-66). Free ribosomes and polysomes are dispersed in the cytoplasm, and Golgi bodies may be apparent (fig. 3-66). Occasional droplets of lipid are also present (127).

The nuclei are round and regular with evenly dispersed, finely granular chromatin. Heterochromatin clumps are sparse. The nucleoli are large and consist of complex, "wandering" strands of electron-dense fibrillar material (figs. 3-65, 3-66) (124).

Cytologic Findings. Fine needle aspiration cytology of metastases may be helpful in confirming tumor spread or in establishing a diagnosis in patients with occult testicular tumors (128). Seminomas, in aspirated, smeared preparations, consist of loose clusters, occasional sheets, and single cells (fig. 3-67) (128–131). The cytoplasm is fragile, and the smearing technique may produce long cytoplasmic tails between groups of cells (fig. 3-68) (130). An important diagnostic feature is a background of cytoplasmic debris that contains glycogen, yielding a striped or "tigroid" staining pattern between the preserved cellular elements in air-dried smears (figs. 3-67, 3-68) (128,131,132). This tigroid background is not commonly identified in other types of tumors (132), and is probably present in only a minority of seminoma specimens (128). The cells are generally 15 to 20 μm in diameter (in air-dried preparations) (129) and have round to oval nuclei with fine chromatin and one or more prominent nucleoli (129,130). The "squared-off" configuration of the nuclei is apparent in many cases (fig. 3-69). A moderate amount of cytoplasm is present, as well as variably prominent vacuoles (fig. 3-70), corresponding to cytoplasmic glycogen (129). The cytoplasmic borders are well defined (130). Admixed lymphocytes,

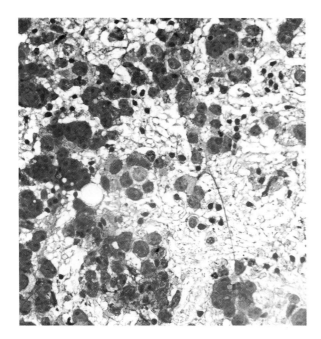

Figure 3-67

SEMINOMA

Fine-needle aspiration specimen shows loose clusters and occasional single tumor cells admixed with scattered lymphocytes. The background has the characteristic "tigroid" appearance (Diff-Quik stain).

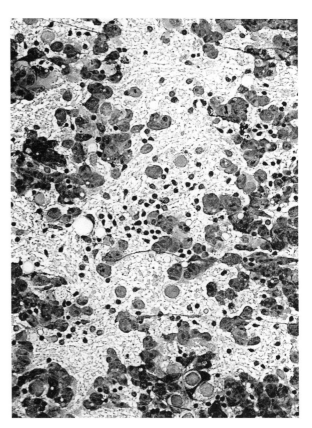

Figure 3-68

SEMINOMA

Air-dried preparation of a needle-aspirated seminoma shows small groups and single tumor cells with frequent lymphocytes. The background consists of cytoplasmic remnants admixed with nonstaining glycogen, yielding the striped pattern. There are two long cytoplasmic "tails" at the center (Diff-Quik stain).

plasma cells, and epithelioid cells (fig. 3-71) are common (128–130), but these may be less prominent than in tissue sections (128,131).

Special Techniques. Analysis of the DNA content of seminomas has shown a mean value of 1.6 to 1.8 times the normal diploid amount, which is significantly higher than in nonseminomas (mean, 1.4 times the normal) (133,134). This is further reflected in cytogenetic studies that demonstrate modal chromosome numbers of 63 to 112, with characteristic chromosomes either over or under represented (135–138). Isochromosome 12p (i[12p]) is commonly identified, and cases lacking it often have other forms of chromosome 12p amplification (135,139). The higher ploidy values for seminomas supports the view that nonseminomatous tumors evolve from seminomas as a consequence of chromosome loss (133,134,140). This is further supported by loss of heterozygosity studies demonstrating allelic losses in embryonal carcinoma compared to seminoma (141). Seminomas commonly show global DNA hypomethylation,

like IGCNU, contrasting with nonseminomas, a finding supporting a pathogenesis from primordial germ cells that have undergone erasure of deoxycytidine residues (142,143). In keeping with this, microarray studies have found lower expression of DNA methyltransferases in IGCNU and seminomas than in the nonseminomatous germ cell tumors (144). Loss of *PTEN*, a tumor suppressor gene, may play a role in the transition from IGCNU to seminoma (145).

Progression from IGCNU to seminoma likely depends on the amplification of genes on 12p, since i(12p) and other forms of 12p amplification are not identified in IGCNU except in some cases associated with an invasive tumor (146,147). It is not currently clear what genes

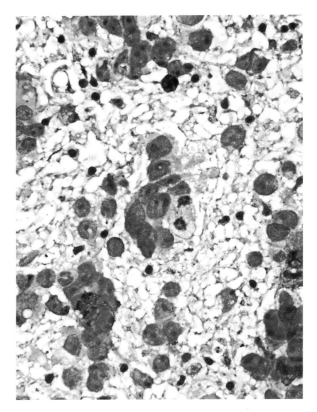

Figure 3-69

SEMINOMA

The "squared-off" nuclei are apparent in this cytologic preparation, especially in the cells at the center (Diff-Quik stain).

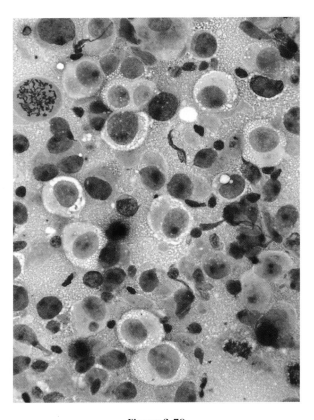

Figure 3-70

SEMINOMA

Tiny cytoplasmic vacuoles are present in some of the tumor cells (Diff-Quik stain).

Figure 3-71

SEMINOMA

An aggregate of epithelioid histiocytes is seen near the center in this cytologic preparation (Diff-Quik stain).

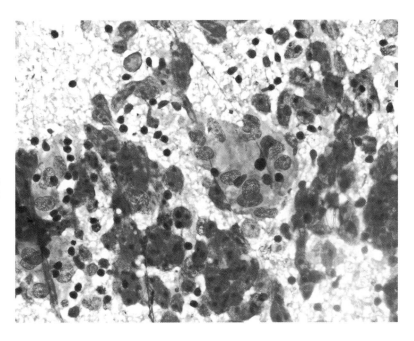

are critical for inducing invasion, but it is speculated that they likely suppress apoptosis, thereby permitting the survival of IGCNU cells apart from Sertoli cells (148). The antiapoptotic genes, *MCL1* and *survivin* (also known as *BIRC5*), are highly expressed in both seminomas and nonseminomas (149,150).

A number of molecular biologic changes have been found in seminomas, but it is not clear which are pathogenetically important. Seminomas lack FAS, a cell membrane receptor that activates an apoptotic pathway, but are positive for the FAS ligand (FASL) and FAS-associating phosphatase-1 (FAP-1), which blocks FAS and its downstream signaling. Because tumor infiltrating lymphocytes in seminomas express FAS but not FAP-1, the consequent induction of apoptosis in them by FASL may allow the seminoma to escape immune destruction (151). Loss of expression of CDKN2C (p18^{INK4C}) (152), increased cyclin E (152), and activation of CDKN2A (p16^{INK4a}) by hypermethylation (153) are reported, as is cyclin D2 expression (154).

Seminomas overexpress *PIWIL1* (*HIWI*), a gene that plays a putative role in stem cell renewal, and such overexpression is not identified in the nonseminomatous tumors (155). Activating exon 17 mutations of the *KIT* gene are seen in 9 to 19 percent of seminomas (156-159) and approximately 20 percent of seminomas have *KIT* gene amplification (157), unlike IGCNU (160), although virtually all seminomas overexpress KIT protein. FHIT protein, the product of a tumor suppressor gene, is frequently not expressed in seminoma and IGCNU (161) but is not inactivated by methylation (162). On the other hand, *RASSF1A*, a tumor suppressor gene, was inactivated by promoter hypermethylation in 4 of 10 seminomas (162). There is increased expression of *XIST*, a gene localized to the X chromosome, in seminomas but not in nonseminomatous germ cell tumors, although X chromosome gain is common in both (163); a role for genes on the X chromosome in testicular tumorigenesis is supported by the observed linkage of familial cases to Xq27 (163).

Other observations in seminoma include the absence of both RNA and protein expression of *NOTCH1* and its ligand, *JAG2* (164), *SMAD4* mutations with loss of protein function (165), the presence of DAZl1 protein (166), the usual

expression of *MAGE* genes (167), *RAS* gene mutations (168), MYCN expression (169–171), and FGF4 expression (172). Although TP53 overexpression is often reported in seminomas, it does not correlate with gene mutation.

Analysis of proliferative activity in seminomas, using the monoclonal antibody Ki-67, has demonstrated positive immunostaining in 50 to 80 percent of the cellular population, which, however, did not correlate with the degree of lymphoid reaction or the tumor volume (173). Such labeling was generally homogeneously distributed throughout the tumor. In contrast, thymidine labeling analysis of proliferative activity in seminomas has shown uniform labeling of small tumors but selective peripheral labeling in more advanced seminomas, with a mean labeling index of 11.6 percent (74,174).

Differential Diagnosis. Seminoma is most often confused with the solid pattern of embryonal carcinoma. In well-fixed preparations, they usually can be readily differentiated; however, seminoma is very susceptible to poor fixation, leading to loss of cytoplasm, poorly defined cell borders, and nuclear juxtaposition, all of which are features suggesting embryonal carcinoma (175). For this reason, it is crucial to institute procedures to assure prompt, well-fixed material. In good preparations, seminoma has round to polygonal, relatively regular nuclei; the nuclei are usually separated from each other by uniform amounts of cytoplasm, and cellular borders are typically well defined. Embryonal carcinoma has more irregularly shaped, vesicular nuclei that appear to overlap in routine histopathologic sections, and the cellular borders are frequently poorly defined. The cytoplasm of embryonal carcinomas is more frequently amphophilic to basophilic. A prominent granulomatous and lymphoid reaction favors seminoma, although occasional embryonal carcinomas are associated with a similar reaction. Embryonal carcinomas lack the characteristic delicate fibrous septa of seminoma but may have similar broad fibrous bands. The presence of true gland and papillae formation excludes seminoma. For those uncommon tumors that have ambiguous features, a selected immunohistochemical panel can assist. There is differential expression of c-KIT and SOX17 (both positive in seminoma) as well as CD30,

AE1/AE3 cytokeratin, and SOX2 (all negative or mostly negative in seminoma), with opposite reactivities in embryonal carcinoma (Table 3-1).

Yolk sac tumor with a solid pattern may mimic seminoma. Usually, however, solid yolk sac tumor is intermingled with other, more diagnostic patterns that permit this distinction with relative ease (99). Solid foci in yolk sac tumor usually do not have the typical fibrovascular septa and associated lymphocytes of seminoma. The cells in solid yolk sac tumor are more variable in size than in seminoma, with a significant number of smaller cells (99). Hyaline globules and intercellular basement membrane are absent or rare in seminoma and frequent in yolk sac tumor (99,176). Microcystic seminoma may mimic microcystic yolk sac tumor; the key to its distinction is that the cells lining the microcysts retain the typical cytomorphology of seminoma cells rather than having the frequently flattened contours seen in yolk sac tumor (56). An immunohistochemical panel consisting of OCT3/4, AE1/AE3 cytokeratin, glypican 3, and AFP facilitates the distinction from yolk sac tumor (Table 3-1). AFP reactivity in yolk sac tumor, however, is patchy and therefore may not be visualized in a limited sample. The differential with spermatocytic seminoma is discussed with that entity.

Malignant lymphomas may be confused with seminoma. Patients with malignant lymphoma are usually older, with a mean age of about 60 years (177–183). Lymphomas of the testis are more frequently bilateral (178,180–184), are usually associated with extratesticular disease (183), and often have a striking intertubular pattern of growth deep within the neoplasm (180,181,183,185), a feature much less conspicuous in most seminomas. On high-power examination, lymphoma cells often show twisted or angulated nuclei, and there is a tendency for the cell population to be more variable in size than in seminoma. The cytoplasm of lymphoma cells is generally less well-defined and not as clear as in seminoma, with occasional exceptions. Most seminomas are associated with residual IGCNU, which is absent in lymphomas. Leukocyte common antigen (LCA; CD45) and CD20 mark a high percentage of lymphomas but are not identified in seminomas (91); other lymphoid markers can be employed if needed

(91,183). OCT3/4 and PLAP are positive in seminoma but not lymphoma (87,94).

Rare seminomas composed of closely packed, solid tubules resemble Sertoli cell tumors (54,55). Some Sertoli cell tumors have a diffuse growth pattern, often with an associated lymphocytic infiltrate, and resemble seminoma (186). Differentiation depends upon the recognition of the typical cytology of seminoma cells, which contrasts with the smaller, often more irregular nuclei of Sertoli cells. Additionally, seminomas show more frequent mitotic figures, usually have abundant cytoplasmic glycogen rather than the large amounts of lipid expected for a Sertoli cell tumor with clear cytoplasm, and are associated with IGCNU (54,55,186). OCT3/4, PLAP, and SALL4 are positive in seminoma and inhibin is negative, whereas the first three are negative in Sertoli cell tumor and inhibin is variably positive.

Rarely, a marked granulomatous reaction in seminoma makes neoplastic cells difficult to identify and confusion with granulomatous orchitis can occur. Careful high-power examination identifies seminoma cells; PAS stains, and OCT3/4 and PLAP immunostains highlight them.

Treatment and Prognosis. Most seminomas are extremely sensitive to radiation and chemotherapy. The TNM system has not proved as useful in the stratification of seminoma patients into relevant treatment categories as it has for nonseminoma patients, and a modified Royal Marsden classification (see Table 1-3), with the addition of a stage IID category (maximum diameter, over 10 cm), has been advocated for seminoma (187). For seminomas that are clinically confined to the testis, many patients receive radiation therapy after orchiectomy, which in the past was directed at the ipsilateral inguinal and iliac nodes and the periaortic and pericaval lymph nodes to the level of the diaphragm. Usually about 30 Gy are delivered in fractionated doses over a 3-week interval, resulting in a cure rate of 95 percent or better (188–192). Equivalent results for clinical stage I or IIA seminoma (Royal Marsden system) can be achieved by radiation to a reduced field, omitting the pelvic sites (193). Although recurrences are unusual, most develop outside of the radiated field, in the mediastinum (190,194), cervical lymph nodes, or lungs (195), and almost always within 3 years of treatment.

In the past, surveillance was considered a less appealing option for clinical stage I seminomas than nonseminomatous tumors because of the excellent results with radiation, with little morbidity, and the absence of reliable tumor markers for the detection of recurrence in seminomas. However, surveillance saves roughly 87 percent of patients with early stage seminoma from radiation and its possible complications (196). A number of studies of surveillance management of clinical stage I seminoma patients have shown cause-specific survival rates in excess of 99 percent, with relapse rates of 15 to 20 percent and successful treatment of almost all patients who relapse (197). Vascular space invasion of the testicular primary indicates a subset of patients at increased risk for recurrence (198), although recurrences are present in about 10 percent of patients with no identifiable lymphovascular invasion (as opposed to 20 percent with it) (199). Tumor size beyond 4 cm and rete testis invasion correlated with increased risk for recurrence in a multivariate analysis (200).

Patients with seminoma metastatic to retroperitoneal sites (stage II or B) are most frequently treated according to the extent of the nodal involvement. For patients with less bulky disease, many authorities continue to advocate radiation therapy, perhaps with additional doses to larger deposits. Survival rates in this group of patients, when so treated, is 90 to 96 percent (192,201,202). Patients with bulkier retroperitoneal disease (defined variably as greater than 5 cm, 6 cm, or 10 cm) are now treated with platinum-based chemotherapy regimens because of high recurrence rates with radiation. In a review of several series, there was an 8 percent recurrence rate with radiation of retroperitoneal disease between 5 and 10 cm in diameter, and a 35 percent recurrence rate for retroperitoneal masses exceeding 10 cm in diameter (203). Several studies that included both previously radiated patients as well as previously untreated patients indicate an 80 percent survival rate for this group, as well as for those with stage III (or C) disease. Surgery, beyond the original orchiectomy, does not confer any additional survival benefits (14,196). Surgical excision of residual masses 3 cm or more in size following chemotherapy of advanced stage seminoma has been advocated to determine the presence of persistent neoplasm and therefore the need for additional chemotherapy (45).

Dixon and Moore (66) found a 4 percent 2-year mortality rate in seminoma patients having a lymphoid stroma but a 12 percent 2-year mortality rate in patients whose tumors lacked a lymphoid stroma. Evenson et al. (67) corroborated this, but this correlation was not statistically significant. Vascular invasion was also associated with a worse survival rate (15.2 percent versus 5.6 percent 2-year mortality rate) (66). Some studies have implicated an elevated level of hCG as a poor prognostic feature of seminoma (22,44,45), an observation that correlates with the poor prognosis associated with Leydig cell hyperplasia originally identified by Dixon and Moore (66). Others, however, have failed to identify such a correlation (19,46,204) or with the presence of syncytiotrophoblast cells (83). Anaplastic seminoma is purportedly a seminoma with a more aggressive clinical course (205); as previously stated, we do not recognize this variant of seminoma and feel that aggressively behaving seminomas cannot be reliably identified in a prospective fashion with currently employed methods, including various immunohistochemical markers (206). We do recognize that some seminomas have increased pleomorphism, and many such "atypical seminomas" have been shown to present at higher tumor stage (81).

SPERMATOCYTIC SEMINOMA

Definition. *Spermatocytic seminoma* is a germ cell neoplasm composed of three morphologic varieties of cells that range from 6 to 100 μm in diameter. It lacks cytoplasmic glycogen and is rarely associated with a lymphocytic infiltrate or granulomatous reaction, in contrast to usual seminoma. It is always pure, except for rare cases with sarcomatous transformation.

General Features. Spermatocytic seminoma was described in 1946 by Masson (207), who believed it mimicked spermatogenesis based on its polymorphous cell population which resembles spermatogenic cells, including a meiotic-like chromatin pattern (see below). Some studies have supported its spermatocytic differentiation based on either ultrastructure features (208), immunohistochemical reactivities (209), or expression of meiosis I-related genes (210), although

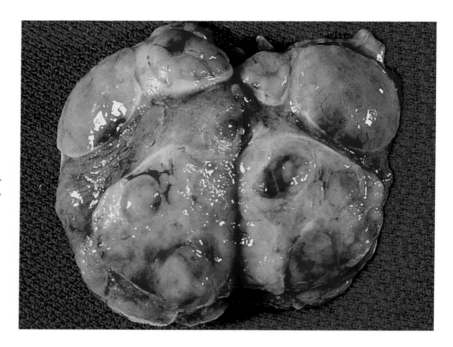

Figure 3-72

SPERMATOCYTIC SEMINOMA

The cut surface of this multinodular gray tumor has a glistening, mucoid quality.

meiotic-specific structures and haploid DNA values were not identified by others (211,212). Spermatocytic seminomas do not bind lectins that are ordinarily reactive for more advanced spermatogenic cells (213).

Spermatocytic seminoma represented 1.1 to 4.5 percent of seminomas in three series (2,214,215). Our experience supports the lower aspect of this range. It does not occur as a primary tumor in sites other than the testis. Its epidemiology is unclear. It is not strongly associated with cryptorchidism (214,216) and does not occur with IGCNU (217) or other forms of germ cell tumor, indicating a pathogenesis different from that of other germ cell tumors and typical seminoma.

Clinical Features. Spermatocytic seminoma tends to occur in older patients than usual seminoma. The average age in four series ranged from 52 to 59 years (2,214,215,218); nonetheless, 10 percent occur in patients less than 30 years of age, with rare cases in teenagers (215). Most patients present with painless testicular enlargement (214,218), but occasionally there is pain. Serum markers are negative in all cases. Bilaterality, usually asynchronous but occasionally synchronous, occurs in 9 percent of cases (214), and is accordingly more common than in other germ cell tumors. Rare spermatocytic seminomas undergo sarcomatous transformation (218–221). These patients typically have a

long history of painless testicular enlargement followed by the recent onset of pain and rapid growth (219,220). Occasionally, they present with metastatic disease (219).

Gross Findings. Spermatocytic seminomas have the same size range as typical seminomas (214). They are well circumscribed and sometimes multilobulated or multinodular (fig. 3-72). Occasionally, there are separate, multicentric nodules (207). They typically are soft, friable, and tan-gray, with an edematous to gelatinous cut surface (fig. 3-72), and may show cystic change. Foci of hemorrhage and necrosis may occur, especially in the larger tumors (fig. 3-73), but are generally not extensive. Cases with associated sarcoma (see below) are more apt to exhibit hemorrhage or necrosis, with solid, dull gray areas (219,220). Extension beyond the testis is rare in typical cases, but epididymal involvement has been reported (218,222).

Microscopic Findings. A multinodular (fig. 3-74) to diffuse pattern is apparent on scanning magnification; edema may also be striking on low power. Within the nodules, the neoplastic cells are usually arranged in sheets (fig. 3-75), but a typically scant but occasionally prominent fibrous stroma may separate them into nests or anastomosing islands (fig. 3-76). The characteristic fine fibrous septa of usual seminoma are lacking. Pools of pale to eosinophilic edema fluid

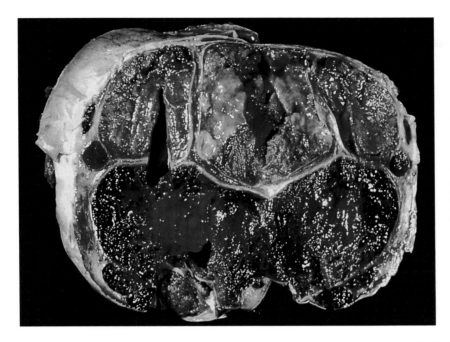

Figure 3-73

SPERMATOCYTIC SEMINOMA

Prominent fibrous septa subdivide a spermatocytic seminoma. There is extensive hemorrhage in the lower portion. (Fig. 2.28 from Young RH, Scully RE. Testicular tumors. Chicago: ASCP Press; 1990:28.)

may segregate the cells into clusters, trabeculae, and single cells (fig. 3-77), or accumulate in cysts (fig. 3-78) or pseudoglands (figs. 3-79, 3-80). Intertubular growth is seen on occasion (fig. 3-81). Spermatocytic seminoma almost always lacks a granulomatous reaction and usually has no or only a scant lymphoid infiltrate; rarely, however, there is a moderate lymphoid infiltrate (fig. 3-82), and we have seen a unique case that closely resembled typical seminoma in that a prominent granulomatous reaction and lymphoid infiltrate were present (fig. 3-83).

A polymorphous cell population is the hallmark of this tumor. There are three populations of neoplastic cells, resulting in a "tripartite" appearance. The cells are either small, averaging 6 to 8 µm in diameter; medium-sized ("intermediate cells"), averaging 15 to 20 µm in diameter; or giant, averaging 50 to 100 µm in diameter (figs. 3-84, 3-85). The medium-sized cells predominate, with the giant cells the least common. The small cells have a densely basophilic nucleus and a scant amount of eosinophilic to basophilic cytoplasm. These cells, which superficially resemble lymphocytes, are probably degenerate and, in contrast to lymphocytes, show no particular association with the stroma, unlike in typical seminoma, but are scattered randomly. The medium-sized (intermediate) cells have a round nucleus with finely granular chromatin

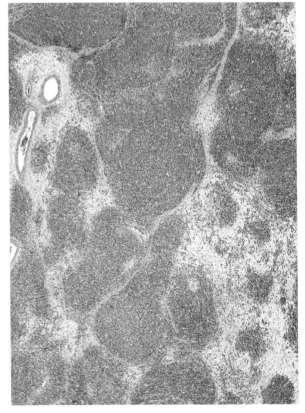

Figure 3-74

SPERMATOCYTIC SEMINOMA

This tumor has a prominent multinodular pattern.

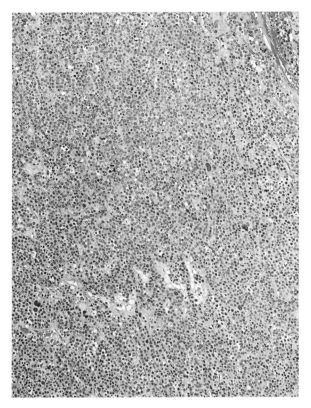

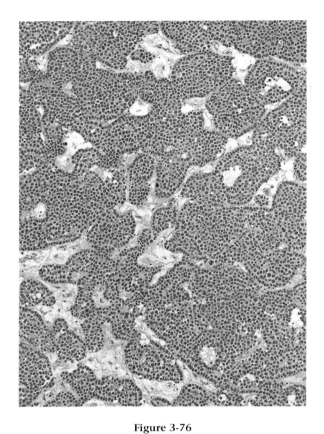

Figure 3-75

SPERMATOCYTIC SEMINOMA

A sheet-like pattern of growth is common.

Figure 3-76

SPERMATOCYTIC SEMINOMA

Anastomosing islands are interwoven with a loose fibrous stroma.

Figure 3-77

SPERMATOCYTIC SEMINOMA

Extensive intercellular edema causes a pattern of small nests, trabeculae, clusters, and single cells.

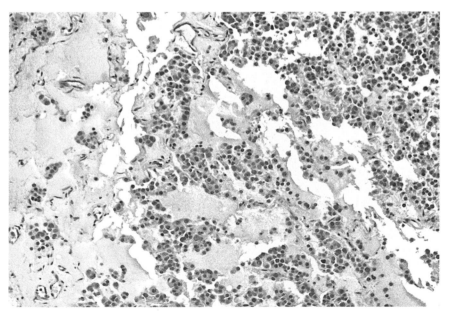

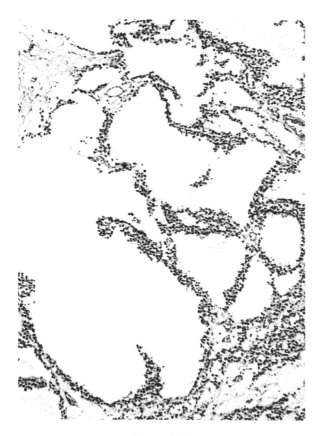

Figure 3-78

SPERMATOCYTIC SEMINOMA

Edema has resulted in a cystic pattern.

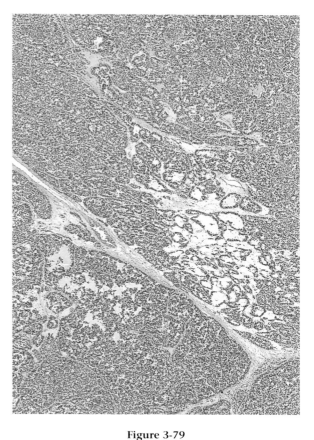

Figure 3-79

SPERMATOCYTIC SEMINOMA

Large nodules within which cells are arranged diffusely and show a focal pseudoglandular pattern.

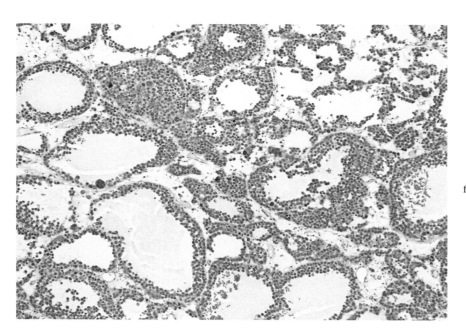

Figure 3-80

SPERMATOCYTIC SEMINOMA

Lightly eosinophilic edema fluid is present in pseudoglands.

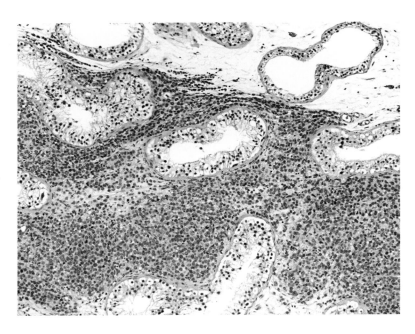

Figure 3-81

SPERMATOCYTIC SEMINOMA

There is prominent growth of tumor cells between seminiferous tubules.

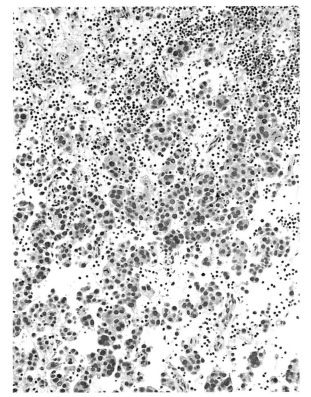

Figure 3-82

SPERMATOCYTIC SEMINOMA

Nests and cords of tumor cells are intermingled with a moderate lymphoid infiltrate; the latter is an unusual feature.

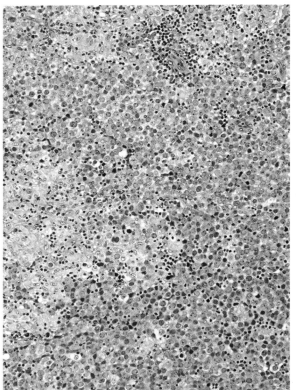

Figure 3-83

SPERMATOCYTIC SEMINOMA

This tumor has both a granulomatous reaction and lymphocytic infiltrate, findings the authors have seen together in only this case.

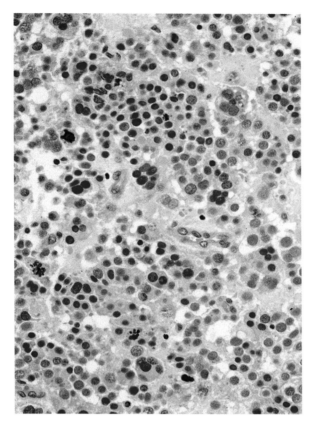

Figure 3-84

SPERMATOCYTIC SEMINOMA

The polymorphic population of neoplastic cells is characteristic of spermatocytic seminoma. Small cells with darkly staining nuclei and medium-sized cells with paler nuclei predominate; occasional multinucleated giant cells are also present.

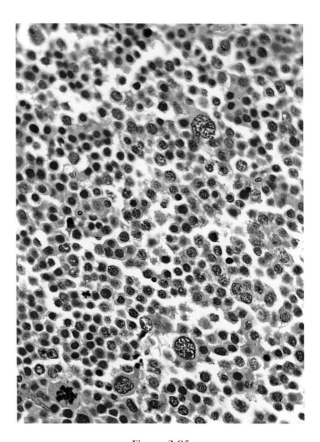

Figure 3-85

SPERMATOCYTIC SEMINOMA

The three cell types, small (superficially resembling lymphocytes), medium-sized, and larger with "spireme" type chromatin, are apparent.

and a modest amount of cytoplasm. The third and largest cells are uninucleated or multinucleated (fig. 3-86). They and the medium-sized cells may have distinctive filamentous or "spireme" chromatin, similar to primary spermatocytes in meiotic prophase (figs. 3-85, 3-86). The nucleoli are variably prominent in medium-sized and large cells. In all cell types, the intercellular borders are indistinct.

The mitotic rate of spermatocytic seminomas is often quite brisk and atypical mitoses may occur. There are usually many apoptotic tumor cells (fig. 3-87) (223). Glycogen is typically not demonstrable (218). Prominent intratubular growth is apparent in many cases, especially at the periphery of the tumor (fig. 3-86), and tubules that are greatly expanded by tumor may contrib-

ute to the multinodular appearance at scanning magnification. Intratubular tumor usually fills the tubules but in some cases is seen as only a layer or two of cells at the tubule periphery (fig. 3-88), potentially causing confusion with IGCNU, which is always absent (see chapter 2).

An *anaplastic variant of spermatocytic seminoma* has been described (224–226); this is characterized by a predominance of monomorphous cells with prominent nucleoli, thereby potentially causing confusion with usual seminoma or embryonal carcinoma (fig. 3-89) (224,225). Typical foci, however, are identified in these cases, and the immunohistochemistry, ultrastructure, and clinical course are typical for spermatocytic seminoma (224,225). In our opinion, such cases are part of the morphologic spectrum of spermatocytic seminoma since

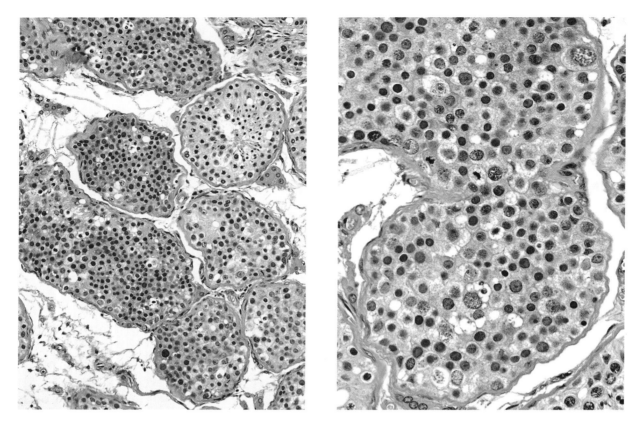

Figure 3-86

INTRATUBULAR SPERMATOCYTIC SEMINOMA

Left: Several tubules are distended by spermatocytic seminoma; one tubule shows normal spermatogenesis.
Right: The cell size is variable, the nuclei are round, and filamentous ("spireme") chromatin is present in a few of the larger cells.

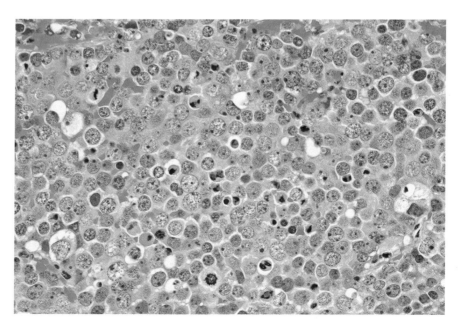

Figure 3-87

SPERMATOCYTIC SEMINOMA

Apoptotic tumor cells are numerous.

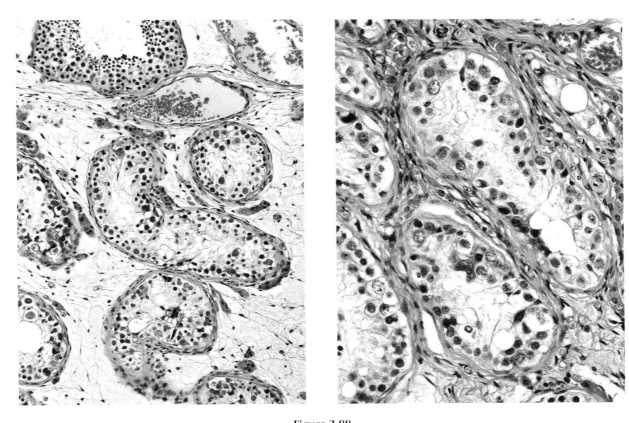

Figure 3-88

INTRATUBULAR SPERMATOCYTIC SEMINOMA

Left: The single spermatocytic seminoma cells at the base of the seminiferous tubules mimic IGCNU.
Right: Higher magnification of the same case.

nucleoli are of variable prominence in this neoplasm, and there may be areas lacking the usual polymorphism in other cases.

In *spermatocytic seminomas with associated sarcoma* (approximately 6 percent of reported cases [216]), the sarcomatous component may be intimately intermingled with the spermatocytic seminoma (fig. 3-90) or, more commonly, grow in an apparent pure pattern and replace much of the underlying typical neoplasm. The sarcoma is frequently undifferentiated (227), consisting of primitive-appearing, oval to spindle-shaped cells arranged in sheets and fascicles (fig. 3-91). Two that we have seen had prominent tumor giant cells (fig. 3-92). At least six cases have shown rhabdomyoblastic differentiation (fig. 3-93) (219–221,228-230). Intratubular spermatocytic seminoma may be within or adjacent to the sarcoma (fig. 3-94).

Immunohistochemical Findings. Spermatocytic seminomas are nonreactive with antibodies directed against vimentin, actin, desmin, OCT3/4, AFP, hCG, carcinoembryonic antigen, leukocyte common antigen (LCA), and CD30 (Table 3-1) (87,88,218,231,232). Lack of PLAP reactivity has been reported in some studies (98,233), although others described positivity in rare cells (218,231,232). Cytokeratin immunostains are also usually negative, although occasional dot-like positivity may be seen with antibodies that react with CK18 (113,231). There is positivity for SCP1 (synaptonemal complex protein 1), SSX (synovial sarcoma on X chromosome), and XPA (xeroderma pigmentosum type A), in contrast to usual seminoma (209). SALL4, a general germ cell tumor marker, is positive (104), and c-KIT is positive in 50 to 60 percent of cases (98,226,234).

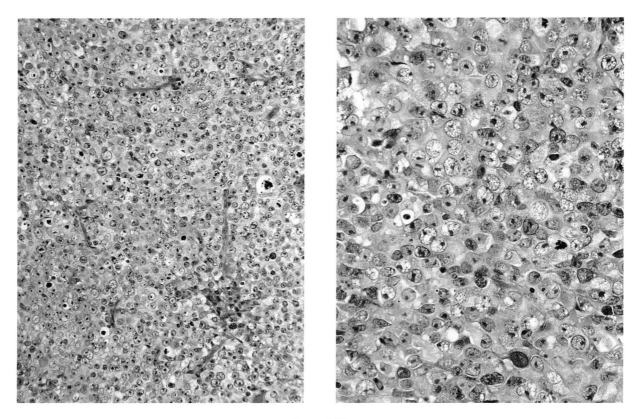

Figure 3-89

SPERMATOCYTIC SEMINOMA

Left: There is a diffuse proliferation of intermediate-sized cells with prominent nucleoli, a pattern referred to by some as an anaplastic variant.

Right: The cells have amphophilic cytoplasm, poorly defined cytoplasmic membranes, and round nuclei with prominent nucleoli. The dearth of large and small cells imparts a picture that may be confused with embryonal carcinoma.

Figure 3-90

SARCOMA WITH SPERMATOCYTIC SEMINOMA

Residual, poorly preserved spermatocytic seminoma (right) is adjacent to sarcoma. (Fig. 2.33 from Young RH, Scully RE. Testicular tumors. Chicago: ASCP Press; 1990:31.)

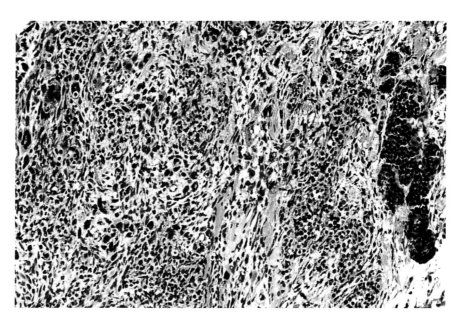

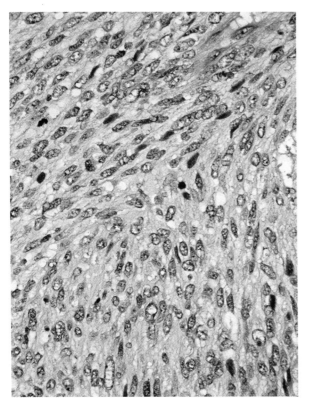

Figure 3-91

**SARCOMA ASSOCIATED WITH
SPERMATOCYTIC SEMINOMA**

This spindle cell sarcoma developed in a spermatocytic seminoma (not shown).

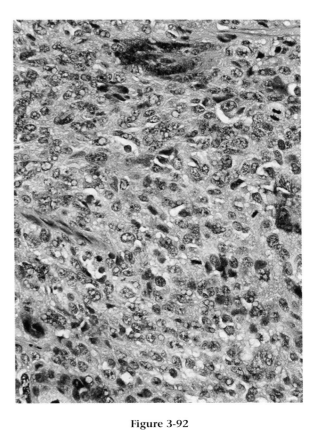

Figure 3-92

**SARCOMA ASSOCIATED WITH
SPERMATOCYTIC SEMINOMA**

Scattered tumor giant cells are seen. The spermatocytic seminoma is not shown in this image.

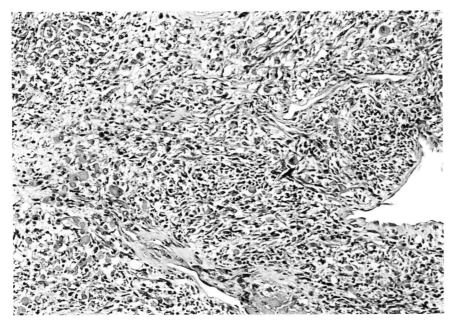

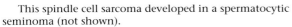

Figure 3-93

**RHABDOMYOSARCOMA
ASSOCIATED WITH
SPERMATOCYTIC SEMINOMA**

The spermatocytic seminoma is not shown in this image.

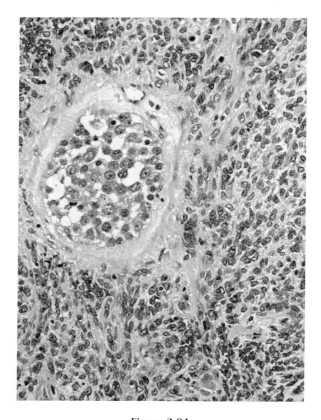

Figure 3-94

SARCOMA WITH SPERMATOCYTIC SEMINOMA

Intratubular spermatocytic seminoma is surrounded by sarcomatous growth. The growth had the features of embryonal rhabdomyosarcoma.

Ultrastructural Findings. Ultrastructural examination shows prominent nucleoli with dispersed nucleolonema and occasional chromosomes with a configuration similar to that of the leptotene stage of meiotic prophase, i.e., filamentous chromosomes with lateral chromatin fibrils (208). Another distinctive feature is the formation of intercellular bridges between adjacent cells, similar to those described in spermatocytic cells (fig. 3-95) (212). One study, however, failed to identify leptotene-type chromosomes or other meiotic-specific features (211); the presence of bridges between neoplastic cells was not considered specific for a meiotic cell (211). Macula adherens–type junctions are present between adjacent cells (fig. 3-95). The Golgi is variably prominent; there are scanty profiles of rough endoplasmic reticulum, numerous free ribosomes, scattered mitochondria, scant or absent glycogen, and a thin layer of basal lamina at the periphery of the cell nests (208,211).

Special Techniques. Studies of the DNA content in spermatocytic seminomas have frequently shown polyploid values (217,232,235), although some have been aneuploid, diploid, hyperdiploid, or peritriploid (211,217,232,236). It has been suggested that the cells form in cycles of polyploidization (98,237). No haploid values have been obtained, arguing against a true meiotic-phase neoplasm, a conclusion also supported by

Figure 3-95

SPERMATOCYTIC SEMINOMA

An intercellular bridge links two adjacent cells of a spermatocytic seminoma. Intercellular junctions are seen at left and center. Small, round mitochondria are numerous.

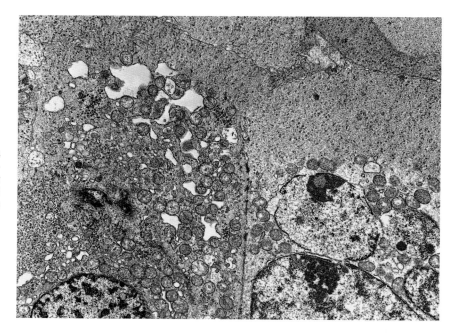

Table 3-2

COMPARISON OF THE CLINICAL AND PATHOLOGIC FEATURES
OF SPERMATOCYTIC SEMINOMA AND TYPICAL SEMINOMA[a]

Features	Spermatocytic Seminoma	Typical Seminoma
Proportion of germ cell tumors	0.5%	40 to 50%
Sites	testis only	testis, ovary (dysgerminoma), mediastinum, pineal, retroperitoneum
Association with cryptorchidism	no	yes
Bilaterality	9%	2%
Association with other forms of germ cell tumor	no	yes
Association with IGCNU[b]	no	yes
Intercellular edema	common	uncommon
Composition	3 cell types, with denser cytoplasm, round nuclei	1 cell type (except for occasional syncytiotrophoblasts), often clear cytoplasm, less regular nuclei
Stroma	usually scanty	often prominent
Edema	often conspicuous	rare
Lymphoid reaction	rare to absent	prominent
Granulomas	rare	often prominent
Sarcomatous transformation	occasional	absent
Glycogen	absent to scant	abundant
OCT3/4 staining	absent	diffusely positive
PLAP staining	absent to scant	prominent
hCG staining	absent	present in 10%
Metastases	rare	common

[a]Modified from Table 5 from Ulbright TM, Roth LM. Testicular and paratesticular neoplasms. In: Sternberg SS, ed. Diagnostic surgical pathology. New York: Raven Press; 1994:1885-1947 and references 227 and 229.
[b]IGCNU = intratubular germ cell neoplasia, unclassified; hCG = human chorionic gonadotropin; PLAP = placental-like alkaline phosphatase.

morphometric analysis (238) but contradicted by molecular studies showing expression of genes characteristic of the prophase of meiosis I (210). The most consistent cytogenetic finding is gain of chromosome 9, and it has been suggested that the *DMRT1* gene located on 9p plays a role in the pathogenesis of this tumor (210).

Differential Diagnosis. The major entity in the differential diagnosis is typical seminoma, with which it is often confused (222,239). Table 3-2 lists many of the features useful in the differentiation (222,240). Immunostains for OCT3/4 and PLAP are helpful in problematic cases.

The anaplastic variant of spermatocytic seminoma, because of its monomorphic appearance and nucleolar prominence, may be confused with solid embryonal carcinoma. Sampling discloses the typical "tripartite" morphology of spermatocytic seminoma. The nuclei of spermatocytic seminoma cells are more regularly round than those of embryonal carcinoma, and spermatocytic seminoma lacks the glands or papillae that may occur in embryonal carcinoma. IGCNU does not occur in spermatocytic seminoma but is common adjacent to embryonal carcinoma. OCT3/4 and AE1/AE3 cytokeratin are diffusely positive in embryonal carcinoma but negative in spermatocytic seminoma

Lymphoma is another consideration (239). The cells of lymphomas are usually less diverse; the nuclei tend to be less round, with frequent indentations. Lymphomas typically exhibit more prominent intertubular growth, whereas intratubular growth, common in spermatocytic seminoma, is rare in lymphoma. Bilateral involvement is more common in lymphoma, and most lymphomas are associated with extratesticular disease, which is virtually never true of spermatocytic seminoma. Immunostains for LCA (CD45) or other lymphoid markers are conclusive in problematic cases.

Treatment and Prognosis. The prognosis of patients with pure spermatocytic seminoma is excellent; there are only two well-documented, pathologically verified cases of pure spermatocytic seminoma that metastasized (to retroperitoneal lymph nodes) (216,241,242) among several hundred spermatocytic seminomas in the literature. For this reason, patients with

spermatocytic seminoma are managed by orchiectomy, without adjuvant therapy. Patients with anaplastic spermatocytic seminoma have a benign course, additional evidence that it is not a distinct clinicopathologic entity.

The excellent prognosis of pure spermatocytic seminoma contrasts with the poor prognosis of patients with spermatocytic seminoma with sarcomatous dedifferentiation. Five of nine patients are known to have died of metastasis of the sarcomatous component, most commonly to the lungs (219–221).

REFERENCES

1. Chevassu M. Tumeurs du testicule: Thèse pour le doctorat en médecine. Paris: G. Steinheil; 1906.
2. Jacobsen GK, Barlebo H, Olsen J, et al. Testicular germ cell tumours in Denmark 1976-1980. Pathology of 1058 consecutive cases. Acta Radiol Oncol 1984;23:239-47.
3. von Hochstetter AR, Hedinger CE. The differential diagnosis of testicular germ cell tumors in theory and practice: a critical analysis of two major systems of classification and review of 389 cases. Virchows Arch [A] 1982;396:247-77.
4. Friedman NB, Moore RA. Tumors of the testis: a report on 922 cases. Milit Surgeon 1946;99:573-93.
5. Perry C, Servadio C. Seminoma in childhood. J Urol 1980;124:932-3.
6. Kay R. Prepubertal testicular tumor registry. J Urol 1993;150:671-4.
7. Thackray AC, Crane WA. Seminoma. In: Pugh RC, ed. Pathology of the testis. Oxford: Blackwell Scientific; 1976:164-98.
8. Oliver RT. HLA phenotype and clinicopathological behaviour of germ cell tumours: possible evidence for clonal evolution from seminomas to nonseminomas. Int J Androl 1987;10:85-93.
9. Dieckmann KP, von Keyserlingk HJ. HLA association of testicular seminoma. Klin Wochenschr 1988;66:337-9.
10. Swerdlow AJ, Huttly SR, Smith PG. Testis cancer: post-natal hormonal factors, sexual behaviour and fertility. Int J Cancer 1989;43:549-53.
11. Halme A, Kellokumpu-Lehtinen P, Lehtonen T, Teppo L. Morphology of testicular germ cell tumours in treated and untreated cryptorchidism. Br J Urol 1989;64:78-83.
12. Leibovitch I, Baniel J, Rowland RG, Smith ER Jr, Ludlow JK, Donohue JP. Malignant testicular neoplasms in immunosuppressed patients. J Urol 1996;155:1938-42.
13. Wilson WT, Frenkel E, Vuitch F, Sagalowsky AI. Testicular tumors in men with human immunodeficiency virus. J Urol 1992;147:1038-40.
14. Morse MJ, Whitmore WF. Neoplasms of the testis. In: Walsh PC, Gittes RF, Perlmutter AD, Stamey TA, eds. Campbell's urology. Philadelphia: WB Saunders; 1986:1535-82.
15. Pugh RC. Testicular tumours—introduction. In: Pugh RC, ed. Pathology of the testis. Oxford: Blackwell Scientific; 1976:139-59.
16. Nilsson S, Anderstrom C, Hedelin H, Unsgaard B. Signs and symptoms of adult testicular tumours. Int J Androl 1981;4(Suppl):146-52.
17. Balzer BL, Ulbright TM. Spontaneous regression of testicular germ cell tumors: an analysis of 42 cases. Am J Surg Pathol 2006;30:858-65.
18. Henley JD, Young RH, Wade CL, Ulbright TM. Seminomas with exclusive intertubular growth: a report of 12 clinically and grossly inconspicuous tumors. Am J Surg Pathol 2004;28:1163-8.
19. Scheiber K, Mikuz G, Frommhold H, Bartsch G. Human chorionic gonadotropin positive seminoma: is this a special type of seminoma with a poor prognosis? Prog Clin Biol Res 1985;203:97-104.

20. Javadpour N. The role of biologic tumor markers in testicular cancer. Cancer 1980;45:1755-61.
21. Mann K, Siddle K. Evidence for free beta-subunit secretion in so-called human chorionic gonadotropin-positive seminoma. Cancer 1988;62:2378-82.
22. Dieckmann KP, Due W, Bauer HW. Seminoma testis with elevated serum beta-HCG—a category of germ cell cancer between seminoma and non-seminoma. Int Urol Nephrol 1989;21:175-84.
23. Javadpour N. Tumor markers in testicular cancer—an update. Prog Clin Biol Res 1985;203:141-54.
24. Chisolm GG. Tumour markers in testicular tumours. Prog Clin Biol Res 1985;203:81-91.
25. Yamashiro T, Iraha Y, Kamiya H, Nakayama T, Unten S, Murayama S. Testicular seminoma presenting with mediastinal lymphadenopathy and gynecomastia. Radiat Med 2007;25:303-5.
26. Hernes EH, Harstad K, Fossa SD. Changing incidence and delay of testicular cancer in southern Norway (1981-1992). Eur Urol 1996;30:349-57.
27. Taylor JB, Solomon DH, Levine RE, Ehrlich RM. Exophthalmos in seminoma: regression with steroids and orchiectomy. JAMA 1978;240:860-1.
28. Mann AS. Bilateral exophthalmos in seminoma. J Clin Endocrinol Metab 1967;27:1500-2.
29. da Silva MA, Edmondson JW, Eby C, Loehrer PJS. Humoral hypercalcemia in seminomas. Med Pediatr Oncol 1992;20:38-41.
30. Lundberg WB, Mitchell MS. Transient warm autoimmune hemolytic anemia and cryoglobulinemia associated with seminoma. Yale J Biol Med 1977;50:419-27.
31. Kaito K, Otsubo H, Usui N, Kobayashi M. Secondary polycythemia as a paraneoplastic syndrome of testicular seminoma. Ann Hematol 2004;83:55-7.
32. Reman O, Reznik Y, Casadevall N, et al. Polycythemia and steroid overproduction in a gonadotropin-secreting seminoma of the testis. Cancer 1991;68:2224-9.
33. Wingerchuk DM, Noseworthy JH, Kimmel DW. Paraneoplastic encephalomyelitis and seminoma: importance of testicular ultrasonography. Neurology 1998;51:1504-7.
34. Bennett JL, Galetta SL, Frohman LP, et al. Neuro-ophthalmologic manifestations of a paraneoplastic syndrome and testicular carcinoma. Neurology 1999;52:864-7.
35. Burton GV, Bullard DE, Walther PJ, Burger PC. Paraneoplastic encephalopathy with testicular carcinoma. A reversible neurologic syndrome. Cancer 1988;62:2248-51.
36. Schneider BF, Glass WF, Brooks CH, Koenig KG. Membranous glomerulonephritis associated with testicular seminoma. J Int Med 1995;237:599-602.
37. Smith RH. Testicular seminoma. In: Skinner DG, Lieskovsky G, eds. Diagnosis and management of genitourinary cancer. Philadelphia: W.B. Saunders; 1988:215-34.
38. Yamamoto H, Ruden U, Stahle E, et al. Pattern of seminoma tissue markers and deletions. Int J Cancer 1987;40:615-9.
39. Rustin GJ, Vogelzang NJ, Sleijfer DT, Nisselbaum JN. Consensus statement on circulating tumour markers and staging patients with germ cell tumours. Prog Clin Biol Res 1990;357:277-84.
40. Javadpour N. Management of seminoma based on tumor markers. Urol Clin North Am 1980;7:773-81.
41. Nazeer T, Ro JY, Amato B, Park YW, Ordonez NG, Ayala AG. Histologically pure seminoma with elevated alpha-fetoprotein: a clinicopathologic study of ten cases. Oncol Rep 1998;5:1425-29.
42. Ro JY, Dexeus FH, El-Naggar A, Ayala AG. Testicular germ cell tumor. Clinically relevant pathologic findings. Pathol Annu 1991;26(Pt 2):59-87.
43. Mumperow E, Hartmann M. Spermatic cord beta-human chorionic gonadotropin levels in seminoma and their clinical implications. J Urol 1992;147:1041-3.
44. Fossä A, Fossä SD. Serum lactate dehydrogenase and human chorionic gonadotropin in seminoma. Br J Urol 1989;63:408-15.
45. Motzer RJ, Bosl GJ, Geller NL, et al. Advanced seminoma: the role of chemotherapy and adjuvant surgery. Ann Int Med 1988;108:513-8.
46. Schwartz BF, Auman R, Peretsman SJ et al. Prognostic value of BHCG and local tumor invasion in stage I seminoma of the testis. J Surg Oncol 1996;61:131-3.
47. Tucker DF, Oliver RT, Travers P, Brodmer WF. Serum marker potential of placental alkaline phosphatase-like activity in testicular germ cell tumours evaluated by H17E2 monoclonal antibody assay. Br J Cancer 1985;51:631-9.
48. Koshida K, Stigbrand T, Munck-Wikland E, Hisazumi H, Wahren B. Analysis of serum placental alkaline phosphatase activity in testicular cancer and cigarette smokers. Urol Res 1990;18:169-73.
49. Kuzmits R, Schernthaner G, Krisch K. Serum neuron-specific enolase: a marker for response to therapy in seminoma. Cancer 1987;60:1017-21.
50. Gross AJ, Dieckmann KP. Neuron-specific enolase: a serum tumor marker in malignant germ-cell tumors? Eur Urol 1993;24:277-8.
51. Jacobsen GK, von der Maase H, Specht L, et al. Histopathological features in stage I seminoma treated with orchidectomy only. J Urol Pathol 1995;3:85-94.
52. Jacobsen GK, Talerman A. Atlas of germ cell tumours. Copenhagen: Munksgaard; 1989.

53. Mostofi FK, Price EB Jr. Tumors of the male genital system. Atlas of Tumor Pathology, 2nd Series, Fascicle 8. Washington D.C.: Armed Forces Institute of Pathology; 1973.

54. Young RH, Finlayson N, Scully RE. Tubular seminoma. Report of a case. Arch Pathol Lab Med 1989;113:414-6.

55. Zavala-Pompa A, Ro JY, El-Naggar AK, et al. Tubular seminoma: an immunohistochemical and DNA flow cytometric study of four cases. Am J Clin Pathol 1994;102:397-401.

56. Ulbright TM, Young RH. Seminoma with tubular, microcystic and related patterns: a study of 28 cases of unusual morphologic variants that often cause confusion with yolk sac tumor. Am J Surg Pathol 2005;29:500-5.

57. Henley JD, Young RH, Wade CL, Ulbright TM. Seminomas with exclusive intertubular growth: a report of 12 clinically and grossly inconspicuous tumors. Am J Surg Pathol 2004;28:1163-8.

58. Ulbright TM, Young RH, Ulbright TM, Young RH. Seminoma with conspicuous signet ring cells: a rare, previously uncharacterized morphologic variant. Am J Surg Pathol 2008;32:1175-81.

59. Bell DA, Flotte TJ, Bhan AK. Immunohistochemical characterization of seminoma and its inflammatory cell infiltrate. Hum Pathol 1987;18:511-20.

60. Strutton GM, Gemmell E, Seymour GJ, Walsh MD, Lavin MF, Gardiner RA. An immunohistological examination of inflammatory cell infiltration in primary testicular seminomas. Aust N Z J Surg 1989;59:169-72.

61. Wilkins BS, Williamson JM, O'Brien CJ. Morphological and immunohistological study of testicular lymphomas. Histopathology 1989;15:147-56.

62. Bentley AJ, Parkinson MC, Harding BN, Bains RM, Lantos PL. A comparative morphological and immunohistochemical study of testicular seminomas and intracranial germinomas. Histopathology 1990;17:443-9.

63. Akaza H, Kobayashi K, Umeda T, Niijima T. Surface markers of lymphocytes infiltrating seminoma tissue. J Urol 1980;124:827-8.

64. Wei YQ, Hang ZB, Liu KF. In situ observation of inflammatory cell-tumor cell interaction in human seminomas (germinomas): light, electron microscopic, and immunohistochemical study. Hum Pathol 1992;23:421-8.

65. Zhao X, Wei YQ, Kariya Y, Teshigawara K, Uchida A. Accumulation of gamma/delta T cells in human dysgerminoma and seminoma: roles in autologous tumor killing and granuloma formation. Immunol Invest 1995;24:607-18.

66. Dixon FJ, Moore RA. Tumors of the male sex organs. Atlas of Tumor Pathology, 1st series, Fascicles 31b & 32. 1 ed. Washington, D.C.: Armed Forces Institute of Pathology; 1952.

67. Evensen JF, Fosså SD, Kjellevold K, Lien HH. Testicular seminoma: histological findings and their prognostic significance for stage II disease. J Surg Oncol 1987;36:166-9.

68. Miller JS, Lee TK, Epstein JI, et al. The utility of microscopic findings and immunohistochemistry in the classification of necrotic testicular tumors: a study of 11 cases. Am J Surg Pathol 2009;33:1293-8.

69. Perry A, Wiley EL, Albores-Saavedra J. Pagetoid spread of intratubular germ cell neoplasia into rete testis: a morphologic and immunohistochemical study of 100 orchiectomy specimens with invasive germ cell tumors. Hum Pathol 1994;25:235-9.

70. Kahn DG. Ossifying seminoma of the testis. Arch Pathol Lab Med 1993;117:321-2.

71. Martin B, Turbiana JM. Significance of scrotal calcifications detected by sonography. J Clin Ultrasound 1988;16:545-52.

72. Grantham JG, Charboneau JW, James EM, et al. Testicular neoplasms: 29 tumors studied by high-resolution US. Radiology 1988;157:775-80.

73. Miller FN, Rosairo S, Clarke JL, Sriprasad S, Muir GH, Sidhu PS. Testicular calcification and microlithiasis: association with primary intratesticular malignancy in 3,477 patients. Eur Urol 2007;17:363-9.

74. Rabes HM. Proliferation of human testicular tumours. Int J Androl 1987;10:127-37.

75. Mostofi FK. Testicular tumors: epidemiologic, etiologic, and pathologic features. Cancer 1973;32:1186-201.

76. Zuckman MH, Williams G, Levin HS. Mitosis counting in seminoma: an exercise of questionable significance. Hum Pathol 1988;19:329-35.

77. Suzuki T, Sasano H, Aoki H, et al. Immunohistochemical comparison between anaplastic seminoma and typical seminoma. Acta Pathol Jap 1993;43:751-7.

78. von Hochstetter AR. Mitotic count in seminomas—an unreliable criterion for distinguishing between classical and anaplastic types. Virchows Arch [A] 1981;390:63-9.

79. Kosmehl H, Langbein L, Katenkamp D. Lectin histochemistry of human testicular germ cell tumors. Neoplasma 1989;36:29-39.

80. Janssen M, Johnston WH. Anaplastic seminoma of the testis: ultrastructural analysis of three cases. Cancer 1978;41:538-44.

81. Tickoo SK, Hutchinson B, Bacik J, et al. Testicular seminoma: a clinicopathologic and immunohistochemical study of 105 cases with special reference to seminomas with atypical features. Int J Surg Pathol 2002;10:23-32.

82. Mostofi FK, Sesterhenn IA. Pathology of germ cell tumors of testes. Prog Clin Biol Res 1985;203:1-34.

83. von Hochstetter AR, Sigg C, Saremaslani P, Hedinger C. The significance of giant cells in human testicular seminomas. A clinicopathological study. Virchows Arch [A] 1985;407:309-22.

84. Manivel JC, Niehans G, Wick MR, Dehner LP. Intermediate trophoblast in germ cell neoplasms. Am J Surg Pathol 1987;11:693-701.

85. Berney DM, Lee A, Shamash J, Oliver RT. The frequency and distribution of intratubular trophoblast in association with germ cell tumors of the testis. Am J Surg Pathol 2005;29:1300-3.

86. Nazeer T, Ro JY, Kee KH, Ayala AG. Spermatic cord contamination in testicular cancer. Mod Pathol 1996;9:762-6.

87. Looijenga LH, Stoop H, de Leeuw HP, et al. POU5F1 (OCT3/4) identifies cells with pluripotent potential in human germ cell tumors. Cancer Res 2003;63:2244-50.

88. Jones TD, Ulbright TM, Eble JN, Cheng L. OCT4 staining in testicular tumors: a sensitive and specific marker for seminoma and embryonal carcinoma. Am J Surg Pathol 2004;28:935-40.

89. Manivel JC, Jessurun J, Wick MR, Dehner LP. Placental alkaline phosphatase immunoreactivity in testicular germ cell tumors. Am J Surg Pathol 1987;11:21-9.

90. Uchida T, Shimoda T, Miyata H, et al. Immunoperoxidase study of alkaline phosphatase in testicular tumor. Cancer 1981;48:1455-62.

91. Niehans GA, Manivel JC, Copland GT, Scheithauer BW, Wick MR. Immunohistochemistry of germ cell and trophoblastic neoplasms. Cancer 1988;62:1113-23.

92. Hustin J, Collettee J, Franchimont P. Immunohistochemical demonstration of placental alkaline phosphatase in various states of testicular development and in germ cell tumours. Int J Androl 1987;10:29-35.

93. Burke AP, Mostofi FK. Placental alkaline phosphatase immunohistochemistry of intratubular malignant germ cells and associated testicular germ cell tumors. Hum Pathol 1988;19:663-70.

94. Wick MR, Swanson PE, Manivel JC. Placental-like alkaline phosphatase reactivity in human tumors: an immunohistochemical study of 520 cases. Hum Pathol 1987;18:946-54.

95. Brehmer-Andersson E, Ljungdahl-Stahle E, Koshida K, Yamamoto H, Stigbrand T, Wahren B. Isoenzymes of alkaline phosphatases in seminomas: an immunohistochemical and biochemical study. APMIS 1990;98:977-82.

96. Izquierdo MA, Van der Valk P, Van Ark-Otte J, et al. Differential expression of the c-kit proto-oncogene in germ cell tumours. J Pathol 2004;177:253-8.

97. Leroy X, Augusto D, Leteurtre E, Gosselin B. CD30 and CD117 (c-kit) used in combination are useful for distinguishing embryonal carcinoma from seminoma. J Histochem Cytochem 2002;50:283-5.

98. Kraggerud SM, Berner A, Bryne M, Pettersen EO, Fossa SD. Spermatocytic seminoma as compared to classical seminoma: an immunohistochemical and DNA flow cytometric study. APMIS 1999;107:297-302.

99. Kao CS, Idrees MT, Young RH, Ulbright TM. Solid pattern yolk sac tumor: a morphologic and immunohistochemical study of 52 cases. Am J Surg Pathol 2012;36:360-7.

100. Nonaka D. Differential expression of SOX2 and SOX17 in testicular germ cell tumors. Am J Clin Pathol 2009;131:731-6.

101. Bode PK, Barghorn A, Fritzsche FR et al. MAGEC2 is a sensitive and novel marker for seminoma: a tissue microarray analysis of 325 testicular germ cell tumors. Mod Pathol 2011;24:829-35.

102. Bailey D, Marks A, Stratis M, Baumal R. Immunohistochemical staining of germ cell tumors and intratubular malignant germ cells of the testis using antibody to placental alkaline phosphatase and a monoclonal anti-seminoma antibody. Mod Pathol 1991;4:167-71.

103. Idrees M, Saxena R, Cheng L, Ulbright TM, Badve S. Podoplanin, a novel marker for seminoma: A comparison study evaluating immunohistochemical expression of podoplanin and OCT3/4. Ann Diagn Pathol 2010;14:331-6.

104. Cao D, Li J, Guo CC, Allan RW, Humphrey PA. SALL4 is a novel diagnostic marker for testicular germ cell tumors. Am J Surg Pathol 2009;33:1065-77.

105. Jacobsen GK, Jacobsen M. Alpha-fetoprotein (AFP) and human chorionic gonadotropin in testicular germ cell tumours: a prospective immunohistochemical study. Acta Pathol Microbiol Scand [A] 1983;91:165-76.

106. Boseman FT, Giard RW, Kruseman AC, Knijenenburg G, Spaander PJ. Human chorionic gonadothropin and alpha-fetoprotein in testicular germ cell tumors: a retrospective immunohistochemical study. Histopathology 1980;4:673-84.

107. Battifora H, Sheibani K, Tubbs RR, Kopinski MI, Sun TT. Antikeratin antibodies in tumor diagnosis: distinction between seminoma and embryonal carcinoma. Cancer 1984;54:843-8.

108. Feitz WF, Debruyne FM, Ramaekers FC. Intermediate filament proteins as specific markers in normal and neoplastic testicular tissue. Int J Androl 1987;10:51-6.

109. Denk H, Moll R, Weybora W, et al. Intermediate filaments and desmosomal plaque proteins in testicular seminomas and non-seminomatous germ cell tumours as revealed by immunohistochemistry. Virchows Arch [A] 1987;410:295-307.

110. Düe W, Loy V. Evidence of interepithelial seminoma spread into the rete testis by immunostaining of paraffin sections with antibodies against cytokeratin and vimentin. Urol Res 1988;16:389-93.

111. Eglen DE, Ulbright TM. The differential diagnosis of yolk sac tumor and seminoma: usefulness of cytokeratin, alpha-fetoprotein, and alpha-1-antitrypsin immunoperoxidase reactions. Am J Clin Pathol 1987;88:328-32.

112. Miettinen M, Virtanen I, Talerman A. Intermediate filament proteins in human testis and testicular germ-cell tumors. Am J Pathol 1985;120:402-10.

113. Fogel M, Lifschitz-Mercer B, Moll R, et al. Heterogeneity of intermediate filament expression in human testicular seminomas. Differentiation 1990;45:242-9.

114. Moll R, Franke WW, Schiller DL, Geiger B, Krepler R. The catalog of human cytokeratins: patterns of expression in normal epithelia, tumors, and cultured cells. Cell 1982;31:11-4.

115. Bartkova J, Rejthar A, Bartek J, Kovarik J. Differentiation patterns in testicular germ-cell tumours as revealed by a panel of monoclonal antibodies. Tumor Biol 1987;8:45-56.

116. Cheville JC, Rao S, Iczkowski KA, Lohse CM, Pankratz VS. Cytokeratin expression in seminoma of the human testis. Am J Clin Pathol 2000;113:583-8.

117. Murakami SS, Said JW. Immunohistochemical localization of lactate dehydrogenase isoenzyme 1 in germ cell tumors of the testis. Am J Clin Pathol 1984;81:293-6.

118. Jacobsen GK, Jacobsen M. Ferritin (FER) in testicular germ cell tumours: an immunohistochemical study. Acta Pathol Microbiol Scand [A] 1983;91:177-81.

119. Saint-Andre JP, Alhenc-Gelas F, Rohmer V, Chretien MF, Bigorgne JC, Corvol P. Angiotensin-1-converting enzyme in germinomas. Hum Pathol 1988;19:208-13.

120. Hittmair A, Rogatsch H, Hobisch A, Mikuz G, Feichtinger H. CD30 expression in seminoma. Hum Pathol 1996;27:1166-71.

121. Jacobsen GK, Jacobsen M, Clausen PP. Distribution of tumor-associated antigens in the various histologic components of germ cell tumors of the testis. Am J Surg Pathol 1981;5:257-66.

122. Caillaud JM, Bellet D, Carlu C, Droz JP. Immunohistochemistry of germ cell tumors of the testis: study of hCG and AFP. Prog Clin Biol Res 1985;203:139-40.

123. Roth LM, Gillespie JJ. Pathology and ultrastructure of germinal neoplasia of the testis. In: Einhorn LH, ed. Testicular tumors: management and treatment. New York: Masson; 1980:1-28.

124. Srigley JR, Mackay B, Toth P, Ayala A. The ultrastructure and histogenesis of male germ neoplasia with emphasis on seminoma with early carcinomatous features. Ultrastruc Pathol 1988;12:67-86.

125. Min KW, Scheithauer BW. Pineal germinomas and testicular seminoma: a comparative ultrastructural study with special references to early carcinomatous transformation. Ultrastruc Pathol 1990;14:483-96.

126. Pierce GB Jr. Ultrastructure of human testicular tumors. Cancer 1966;19:1963-83.

127. Koide O, Iwai S. An ultrastructural study on germinoma cells. Acta Pathol Jap 1981;31:755-66.

128. Caraway NP, Fanning CV, Amato RJ, Sneige N. Fine-needle aspiration cytology of seminoma: a review of 16 cases. Diagn Cytopathol 1995;12:327-33.

129. Akhtar M, Ali MA, Huq M, Bakry M. Fine needle aspiration biopsy of seminoma and dysgerminoma: cytologic, histologic, and electron microscopic correlations. Diagn Cytopathol 1990;6:99-105.

130. Highman WJ, Oliver RT. Diagnosis of metastases from testicular germ cell tumours using fine needle aspiration cytology. J Clin Pathol 1987;40:1324-33.

131. Koss LG, Zajicek J. Aspiration biopsy. In: Koss LG, ed. Diagnostic cytology and its histopathologic basis. 4th ed. Philadelphia: J.B. Lippincott; 1992:1234-402.

132. Baslev E, Francis D, Jacobsen GK. Testicular germ cell tumors: classification based on fine needle aspiration biopsy. Acta Cytol 1990;34:690-4.

133. Oosterhuis JW, Castedo SM, de Jong B, et al. Ploidy of primary germ cell tumors of the testis. Pathogenetic and clinical relevance. Lab Invest 1989;60:14-21.

134. El-Naggar AK, Ro JY, McLemore D, Ayala AG, Batsakis JG. DNA ploidy in testicular germ cell neoplasms: histogenetic and clinical implications. Am J Surg Pathol 1992;16:611-8.

135. Castedo SM, de Jong B, Oosterhuis JW, et al. Cytogenetic analysis of ten human seminomas. Cancer Res 1989;49:439-43.

136. van Echten J, Oosterhuis JW, Looijenga LH, et al. No recurrent structural abnormalities apart from i(12p) in primary germ cell tumors of the adult testis. Genes Chromosomes Cancer 1995;14:133-44.

137. Looijenga LH, Oosterhuis JW. Pathogenesis of testicular germ cell tumours. Rev Reprod 1999;4:90-100.

138. Looijenga LH, Rosenberg C, van Gurp RJ, et al. Comparative genomic hybridization of microdissected samples from different stages in the development of a seminoma and a non-seminoma. J Pathol 2000;191:187-92.

139. Castedo SM, de Jong B, Oosterhuis JW, et al. i(12p)-negative testicular germ cell tumors. A different group? Cancer Genet Cytogenet 1988;35:171-8.

140. Damjanov I. Is seminoma a relative or a precursor of embryonal carcinoma? Lab Invest 1989;60:1-3.

141. Faulkner SW, Leigh DA, Oosterhuis JW, Roelofs H, Looijenga LH, Friedlander ML. Allelic losses in carcinoma in situ and testicular germ cell tumours of adolescents and adults: evidence suggestive of the linear progression model. Br J Cancer 2000;83:729-36.

142. Netto GJ, Nakai Y, Nakayama M, et al. Global DNA hypomethylation in intratubular germ cell neoplasia and seminoma, but not in non-seminomatous male germ cell tumors. Mod Pathol 2008;21:1337-44.

143. Zhang C, Kawakami T, Okada Y, Okamoto K. Distinctive epigenetic phenotype of cancer testis antigen genes among seminomatous and nonseminomatous testicular germ-cell tumors. Genes Chromosomes Cancer 2005;43:104-12.

144. Almstrup K, Hoei-Hansen CE, Nielsen JE, et al. Genome-wide gene expression profiling of testicular carcinoma in situ progression into overt tumours. Br J Cancer 2005;92:1934-41.

145. Di Vizio D, Cito L, Boccia A, et al. Loss of the tumor suppressor gene PTEN marks the transition from intratubular germ cell neoplasias (IT-GCN) to invasive germ cell tumors. Oncogene 2005;24:1882-94.

146. Ottesen AM, Skakkebaek NE, Lundsteen C, Leffers H, Larsen J, Rajpert-De Meyts E. High-resolution comparative genomic hybridization detects extra chromosome arm 12p material in most cases of carcinoma in situ adjacent to overt germ cell tumors, but not before the invasive tumor development. Genes Chromosomes Cancer 2003;38:117-25.

147. Rosenberg C, van Gurp RJ, Geelen E, Oosterhuis JW, Looijenga LH. Overrepresentation of the short arm of chromosome 12 is related to invasive growth of human testicular seminomas and nonseminomas. Oncogene 2000;19:5858-62.

148. Looijenga LH, Zafarana G, Grygalewicz B, et al. Role of gain of 12p in germ cell tumour development. APMIS 2003;111:161-71.

149. Sano M, Nakanishi Y, Yagasaki H, et al. Overexpression of anti-apoptotic Mcl-1 in testicular germ cell tumours. Histopathology 2005;46:532-9.

150. Weikert S, Schrader M, Krause H, Schulze W, Muller M, Miller K. The inhibitor of apoptosis (IAP) survivin is expressed in human testicular germ cell tumors and normal testes. Cancer Lett 2005;223:331-7.

151. Kersemaekers AM, van Weeren PC, Oosterhuis JW, Looijenga LH. Involvement of the Fas/FasL pathway in the pathogenesis of germ cell tumours of the adult testis. J Pathol 2002;196:423-9.

152. Bartkova J, Thullberg M, Rajpert-De Meyts E, Skakkebaek NE, Bartek J. Cell cycle regulators in testicular cancer: loss of p18INK4C marks progression from carcinoma in situ to invasive germ cell tumours. Int J Cancer 2000;85:370-5.

153. Chaubert P, Guillou L, Kurt AM, et al. Frequent p16INK4 (MTS1) gene inactivation in testicular germ cell tumors. Am J Pathol 1997;151:859-65.

154. Houldsworth J, Reuter V, Bosl GJ, Chaganti RS. Aberrant expression of cyclin D2 is an early event in human male germ cell tumorigenesis. Cell Growth Differ 1997;8:293-9.

155. Qiao D, Zeeman AM, Deng W, Looijenga LH, Lin H. Molecular characterization of hiwi, a human member of the piwi gene family whose overexpression is correlated to seminomas. Oncogene 2002;21:3988-99.

156. Sakuma Y, Sakurai S, Oguni S, Hironaka M, Saito K. Alterations of the c-kit gene in testicular germ cell tumors. Cancer Sci 2003;94:486-91.

157. Bennett AK, Ulbright TM, Ramnani DM, Young RH, Mills SE. Immunohistochemical expression of calretinin, CD99, and alpha-inhibin in Sertoli and Leydig cells and their lesions, emphasizing large cell calcifying Sertoli cell tumor. Mod Pathol 2005;18:128A.

158. Coffey J, Linger R, Pugh J, et al. Somatic KIT mutations occur predominantly in seminoma germ cell tumors and are not predictive of bilateral disease: report of 220 tumors and review of literature. Genes Chromosomes Cancer 2008;47:34-42.

159. Sakuma Y, Matsukuma S, Yoshihara M, et al. Mutations of c-kit gene in bilateral testicular germ cell tumours in Japan. Cancer Lett 2008;259:119-26.

160. McIntyre A, Summersgill B, Grygalewicz B, et al. Amplification and overexpression of the KIT gene is associated with progression in the seminoma subtype of testicular germ cell tumors of adolescents and adults. Cancer Res 2005;65:8085-9.

161. Eyzaguirre E, Gatalica Z. Loss of Fhit expression in testicular germ cell tumors and intratubular germ cell neoplasia. Mod Pathol 2002;15:1068-72.

162. Honorio S, Agathanggelou A, Wernert N, Rothe M, Maher ER, Latif F. Frequent epigenetic inactivation of the RASSF1A tumour suppressor gene in testicular tumours and distinct methylation profiles of seminoma and nonseminoma testicular germ cell tumours. Oncogene 2003;22:461-6.

163. Kawakami T, Okamoto K, Sugihara H, et al. The roles of supernumerical X chromosomes and XIST expression in testicular germ cell tumors. J Urol 2003;169:1546-52.

164. Hayashi T, Yamada T, Kageyama Y, Kihara K. Expression failure of the notch signaling system is associated with the pathogenesis of testicular germ cell tumor. Tumour Biol 2004;25:99-105.

165. Devouassoux-Shisheboran M, Mauduit C, Tabone E, Droz JP, Benahmed M. Growth regulatory factors and signalling proteins in testicular germ cell tumours. APMIS 2003;111:212-24.

166. Lifschitz-Mercer B, Elliott DJ, Issakov J, et al. Localization of a specific germ cell marker, DAZL1, in testicular germ cell neoplasias. Virchows Archiv 2002;440:387-91.

167. Hara I, Hara S, Miyake H, et al. Expression of MAGE genes in testicular germ cell tumors. Urology 1999;53:843-7.

168. Mulder MP, Keijzer W, Verkerk A, et al. Activated ras genes in human seminoma: evidence for tumor heterogeneity. Oncogene 1989;4:1345-51.

169. Misaki H, Shuin T, Yao M, Kubota Y, Hosaka M. [Expression of myc family oncogenes in primary human testicular cancer.] Nippon Hinyokika Gakkai Zasshi 1989;80:1509-13. [Japanese]

170. Saksela K, Mäkelä TP, Alitalo K. Oncogene expression in small-cell lung cancer cell lines and a testicular germ-cell tumor: activation of the N-myc gene and decreased RB mRNA. Int J Cancer 1989;44:182-5.

171. Shuin T, Misaki H, Kubota Y, Yao M, Hosaka M. Differential expression of protooncogenes in human germ cell tumors of the testis. Cancer 1994;73:1721-7.

172. Yoshida T, Tsutsumi M, Sakamoto H, et al. Expression of the HST1 oncogene in human germ cell tumors. Biochem Biophys Res Comm 1988;155:1324-9.

173. Düe W, Dieckmann KP, Loy V. Immunohistological determination of proliferative activity in seminomas. J Clin Pathol 1988;41:304-7.

174. Rabes HM, Schmeller N, Hartmann A, Rattenhuber U, Carl P, Staehler G. Analysis of proliferative compartments in human tumors. II. Seminoma. Cancer 1985;55:1758-69.

175. Ulbright TM, Roth LM. Recent developments in the pathology of germ cell tumors. Semin Diagn Pathol 1987;4:304-19.

176. Ulbright TM, Roth LM, Brodhecker CA. Yolk sac differentiation in germ cell tumors. A morphologic study of 50 cases with emphasis on hepatic, enteric and parietal yolk sac features. Am J Surg Pathol 1986;10:151-64.

177. Nonomura N, Aozasa K, Ueda T, et al. Malignant lymphoma of the testis: histological and immunohistological study of 28 cases. J Urol 1989;141:1368-71.

178. Hamlin JA, Kagan AR, Friedman NB. Lymphomas of the testicle. Cancer 1972;29:1352-6.

179. Hayes MM, Sacks MI, King HS. Testicular lymphoma. A retrospective review of 17 cases. S Afr Med J 1983;64:1014-6.

180. Paladugu RR, Bearman RM, Rappaport H. Malignant lymphoma with primary manifestation in the gonad: a clinicopathologic study of 38 patients. Cancer 1980;45:561-71.

181. Turner RR, Colby TV, MacKintosh FR. Testicular lymphomas: a clinicopathologic study of 35 cases. Cancer 1981;48:2095-102.

182. Sussman EB, Hajdu SI, Lieberman PH, Whitmore WF. Malignant lymphoma of the testis: a clinicopathologic study of 37 cases. J Urol 1977;118:1004-7.

183. Ferry JA, Harris NL, Young RH, Coen J, Zietman A, Scully RE. Malignant lymphoma of the testis, epididymis, and spermatic cord. A clinicopathologic study of 69 cases with immunophenotypic analysis. Am J Surg Pathol 1994;18:376-90.

184. Duncan PR, Checa F, Gowing NF, McElwain TJ, Peckham MJ. Extranodal non-Hodgkin's lymphoma presenting in the testicle: a clinical and pathologic study of 24 cases. Cancer 1980;45:1578-84.

185. Talerman A. Primary malignant lymphoma of the testis. J Urol 1977;118:783-6.

186. Henley JD, Young RH, Ulbright TM. Malignant Sertoli cell tumors of the testis: a study of 13 examples of a neoplasm frequently misinterpreted as seminoma. Am J Surg Pathol 2002;26:541-50.

187. Thomas G, Jones W, VanOosterom A, Kawai T. Consensus statement on the investigation and management of testicular seminoma 1989. Prog Clin Biol Res 1990;357:285-94.

188. Hunter M, Peschel RE. Testicular seminoma. Results of the Yale University experience, 1964-1984. Cancer 1989;64:1608-11.

189. Babaian RJ, Zagars GK. Testicular seminoma: the M.D. Anderson experience: an analysis of pathological and patient characteristics, and treatment recommendations. J Urol 1988;139:311-4.

190. Fossä SD, Aass N, Kaalhus O. Radiotherapy for testicular seminoma Stage I: treatment results and long-term post irradiation morbidity in 365 patients. Int J Rad Oncol Biol Phys 1989;16:383-8.

191. Amichetti M, Fellin G, Bolner A, et al. Stage I seminoma of the testis: long term results and toxicity with adjuvant radiotherapy. Tumori 1994;80:141-5.

192. Vallis KA, Howard GC, Duncan W, Cornbleet MA, Kerr GR. Radiotherapy for stages I and II testicular seminoma: results and morbidity in 238 patients. Br J Radiol 1995;68:400-5.

193. Brunt AM, Scoble JE. Para-aortic nodal irradiation for early stage testicular seminoma. Clin Oncol 1992;4:165-70.

194. Speer TW, Sombeck MD, Parsons JT, Million RR. Testicular seminoma: a failure analysis and literature review. Int J Radiat Oncol Biol Phys 1995;33:89-97.

196. Horwich A, Dearnaley DP. Treatment of seminoma. Semin Oncol 1992;19:171-80.

197. Peckham M. Testicular cancer. Acta Oncol 1988;27:439-53.

198. Marks LB, Rutgers JL, Shipley WU, et al. Testicular seminoma: clinical and pathological features that may predict para-aortic lymph node metastases. J Urol 1990;143:524-7.

199. Horwich A, Alsanjari N, A'Hern R, Nicholls J, Dearnaley DP, Fisher C. Surveillance following orchidectomy for stage I testicular seminoma. Br J Cancer 1992;65:775-8.

200. Warde P, Specht L, Horwich A, et al. Prognostic factors for relapse in stage I seminoma managed by surveillance: a pooled analysis. J Clin Oncol 2002;20:4448-52.

201. Doornbos JF, Hussey DH, Johnson E. Radiotherapy for pure seminoma of the testis. Radiology 1975;116:401-4.

202. Thomas GM, Rider WD, Dembo AJ, et al. Seminoma of the testis: results of treatment and patterns of failure after radiation therapy. Int J Rad Oncol Biol Phys 1982;8:165-74.

203. Thomas G. Management of metastatic seminoma: role of radiotherapy. In: Horwich A, ed. Testicular cancer—clinical investigation and management. New York: Chapman & Hall; 1991:211-31.

204. Javadpour N. Human chorionic gonadotropin in seminoma. J Urol 1984;131:407.

205. Maier JG, Sulak MH, Mittemeyer BT. Seminoma of the testis: analysis of treatment success and failure. Am J Roentgenol Rad Ther Nucl Med 1968;102:596-602.

206. Gallegos I, Valdevenito JP, Miranda R, Fernandez C. Immunohistochemistry expression of P53, Ki67, CD30, and CD117 and presence of clinical metastasis at diagnosis of testicular seminoma. Appl Immunohistochem Mol Morphol 2011;19:147-52.

207. Masson P. Étude sur le séminome. Rev Can Biol 1946;5:361-87.

208. Rosai J, Khodadoust K, Silber I. Spermatocytic seminoma. II. Ultrastructural study. Cancer 1969;24:103-16.

209. Stoop H, van Gurp R, de Krijger R, et al. Reactivity of germ cell maturation stage-specific markers in spermatocytic seminoma: diagnostic and etiological implications. Lab Invest 2001;81:919-28.

210. Looijenga LH, Hersmus R, Gillis AJ, et al. Genomic and expression profiling of human spermatocytic seminomas: primary spermatocyte as tumorigenic precursor and DMRT1 as candidate chromosome 9 gene. Cancer Res 2006;66:290-302.

211. Talerman A, Fu YS, Okagaki T. Spermatocytic seminoma. Ultrastructural and microspectrophotometric observations. Lab Invest 1984;51:343-9.

212. Romanenko AM, Persidsky YV, Mostofi FK. Ultrastructure and histogenesis of spermatocytic seminoma. J Urol Pathol 1993;1:387-95.

213. Lee MC, Talerman A, Oosterhuis JW, Damjanov I. Lectin histochemistry of classic and spermatocytic seminoma. Arch Pathol Lab Med 1985;109:938-42.

214. Talerman A. Spermatocytic seminoma: clinicopathological study of 22 cases. Cancer 1980;45:2169-76.

215. Carriere P, Baade P, Fritschi L. Population based incidence and age distribution of spermatocytic seminoma. J Urol 2007;178:125-8.

216. Eble JN. Spermatocytic seminoma. Hum Pathol 1994;25:1035-42.

217. Muller J, Skakkebaek NE, Parkinson MC. The spermatocytic seminoma: views on pathogenesis. Int J Androl 1987;10:147-56.

218. Burke AP, Mostofi FK. Spermatocytic seminoma: a clinicopathologic study of 79 cases. J Urol Pathol 1993;1:21-32.

219. True LD, Otis CN, Delprado W, Scully RE, Rosai J. Spermatocytic seminoma of testis with sarcomatous transformation. A report of five cases. Am J Surg Pathol 1988;12:75-82.

220. Floyd C, Ayala AG, Logothetis CJ, Silva EG. Spermatocytic seminoma with associated sarcoma of the testis. Cancer 1988;61:409-14.

221. Matoska J, Talerman A. Spermatocytic seminoma associated with rhabdomyosarcoma. Am J Clin Pathol 1990;94:89-95.

222. Scully RE. Spermatocytic seminoma of the testis: a report of 3 cases and review of the literature. Cancer 1961;14:788-94.

223. Bishop EF, Badve S, Morimiya Y, Ulbright TM. Apoptosis in spermatocytic and usual seminomas: a light microscopic and immunohistochemical study. Mod Pathol 2007;20:1036-44.

224. Albores-Saavedra J, Huffman H, Alvarado-Cabrero I, Ayala AG. Anaplastic variant of spermatocytic seminoma. Hum Pathol 1996;27:650-5.

225. Lombardi M, Valli M, Brisigotti M, Rosai J. Spermatocytic seminoma: review of the literature and description of a new case of the anaplastic variant. Int J Surg Pathol 2011;19:5-10.

226. Dundr P, Pesl M, Povýsil C, et al. Anaplastic variant of spermatocytic seminoma. Pathol Res Pract 2007;203:621-624.

227. Trivedi P, Pasricha S, Gupta A. Spermatocytic seminoma associated with undifferentiated sarcoma: a rare case report. Indian J Pathol Microbiol 2011;54:138-140.

228. Menon S, Karpate A, Desai S. Spermatocytic seminoma with rhabdomyosarcomatous differentiation: a case report with a review of the literature. J Cancer Res Ther 2009;5:213-5.

229. Robinson A, Bainbridge T, Kollmannsberger C. A spermatocytic seminoma with rhabdomyosarcoma transformation and extensive metastases. Am J Clin Oncol 2007;30:440-1.

230. Chelly I, Mekni A, Gargouri MM, et al. [Spermatocytic seminoma with rhabdomyosarcomatous contingent.] Prog Urol 2006;16:218-20. [French]

231. Cummings OW, Ulbright TM, Eble JN, Roth LM. Spermatocytic seminoma: an immunohistochemical study. Hum Pathol 1994;25:54-9.

232. Dekker I, Rozeboom T, Delemarre J, Dam A, Oosterhuis JW. Placental-like alkaline phosphatase and DNA flow cytometry in spermatocytic seminoma. Cancer 1992;69:993-6.

233. Aguirre P, Scully RE, Dayal Y, DeLellis R. Placental-like alkaline phosphatase reactivity in germ cell tumors of the ovary and testis. Lab Invest 1985;52:2A.

234. Decaussin M, Borda A, Bouvier R, et al. [Spermatocytic seminoma. A clinicopathological and immunohistochemical study of 7 cases.] Ann Pathol 2004;24:161-6. [French]

235. Takahashi H. Cytometric analysis of testicular seminoma and spermatocytic seminoma. Acta Pathol Jap 1993;43:121-9.

236. Muller J, Skakkebaek NE, Nielsen OH, Graem N. Cryptorchidism and testis cancer. Atypical infantile germ cells followed by carcinoma in situ and invasive carcinoma in adulthood. Cancer 1984;54:629-34.

237. Takahashi H, Aizawa S, Konishi E, Furusato M, Kato H, Ashihara T. Cytofluorometric analysis of spermatocytic seminoma. Cancer 1993; 72:549-52.

238. Frasik W, Okon K, Sokolowski A. Polymorphism of spermatocytic seminoma. A morphometric study. Anal Cell Pathol 1994;7:195-203.

239. Rosai J, Silber I, Khodadoust K. Spermatocytic seminoma. I. Clinicopathologic study of six cases and review of the literature. Cancer 1969;24:92-102.

240. Damjanov I. Tumors of the testis and epididymis. In: Murphy WM, ed. Urological pathology. Philadelphia: W.B.Saunders; 1989:314-79.

241. Matoska J, Ondrus D, Hornák M. Metastatic spermatocytic seminoma. A case report with light microscopic, ultrastructural, and immunohistochemical findings. Cancer 1988;62:1197-201.

242. Steiner H, Gozzi C, Verdorfer I, Mikuz G, Bartsch G, Hobisch A. Metastatic spermatocytic seminoma—an extremely rare disease. Eur Urol 2006;49:183-6.

4 NONSEMINOMATOUS GERM CELL TUMORS

EMBRYONAL CARCINOMA

Definition. *Embryonal carcinoma* is a neoplasm composed of primitive-appearing, anaplastic epithelial cells arranged in solid, glandular, papillary, or tubular patterns.

General Features. Pure embryonal carcinoma accounted for 2.3 percent of testicular germ cell tumors in one referral series (1), and 10 percent of cases in a study of consecutive testicular germ cell tumors (see Table 2-1) (2). This contrasts with earlier series showing a frequency of 20 percent (3,4), a difference reflecting the more recent recognition of other tumor types, particularly yolk sac tumor, that were previously grouped with embryonal carcinoma. The frequency of pure embryonal carcinomas also depends on the extent of sampling so that minor foci of teratoma and yolk sac tumor, in particular, are not excluded. We believe that at most 5 percent of testicular tumors are pure embryonal carcinomas. Approximately 40 percent of all testicular germ cell tumors and 87 percent of nonseminomatous ones have an embryonal carcinoma component (1,2).

There is a tradition of permitting the inclusion of a minor amount of primitive mesenchyme in embryonal carcinomas and not regarding it as a teratomatous component (4,5), despite immunohistochemical evidence that it is a form of early teratomatous differentiation (6). This approach derives from the experience of the British Testicular Tumour Panel (7), which identified no difference in survival in patients with embryonal carcinoma, with or without a neoplastic stroma. More recently, however, teratomatous elements in the testis have been found to correlate highly with persistent teratoma in metastatic sites after chemotherapy, an indication for surgical resection (8). This different outcome reflects the development of highly effective chemotherapy and is the basis of our recommendation to classify neoplastic stroma in embryonal carcinoma as a teratomatous component.

Clinical Features. Embryonal carcinoma most commonly occurs in patients between 25 and 35 years of age, with an average age of 32 years (2). We are not aware of a bona fide case in a prepubertal boy who did not have a disorder of sex development; the youngest patients in two series of testicular tumors in children were 11 years of age (9,10), and the tumor is rare under 15 years. Approximately 80 percent of patients present with a testicular mass that may be associated with pain or discomfort. About 10 percent present with symptoms of metastatic disease, and another 10 percent with hormonal symptoms, usually gynecomastia. Rarely, patients with tumors composed in part of embryonal carcinoma present with sudden death due to pulmonary embolism (11,12). After clinical evaluation, only about 40 percent of patients with nonseminomatous tumors have disease limited to the testis at presentation; 40 percent have retroperitoneal involvement and 20 percent have supradiaphragmatic involvement or visceral organ spread (13). Sixty-six percent of pathologically staged patients with a tumor composed predominantly of embryonal carcinoma have metastases (14). The figures are probably similar for pure embryonal carcinoma.

Pure embryonal carcinoma is usually not associated with serum alpha-fetoprotein (AFP) elevation (1); reports to the contrary largely reflect unrecognized yolk sac tumor elements. There is, however, the potential for AFP elevation in morphologically pure embryonal carcinoma since an occasional case does show staining (see below). Elevation of serum human chorionic gonadotropin (hCG) is reported in 60 percent of patients with embryonal carcinoma (15), reflecting the frequent presence of syncytiotrophoblast cells (1). A similar proportion of patients with advanced stage embryonal carcinoma has

121

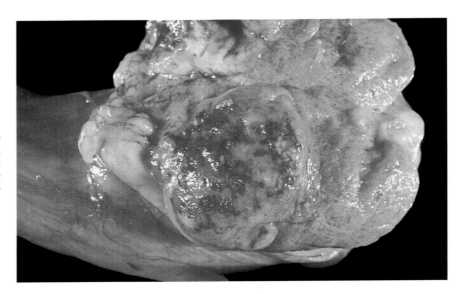

Figure 4-1

EMBRYONAL CARCINOMA

A tan, granular tumor nodule with foci of hemorrhage and necrosis bulges above the cut surface of the testis. The interface of the tumor with adjacent testis is ill-defined in areas.

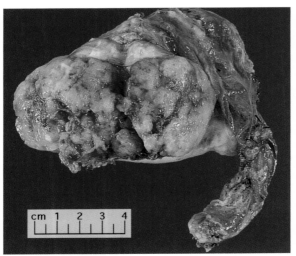

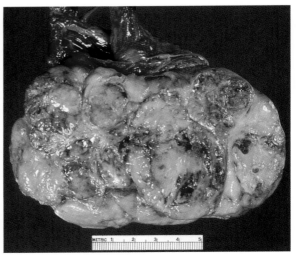

Figure 4-2

EMBRYONAL CARCINOMA

A white to pale pink, solid neoplasm with foci of hemorrhage and cystic degeneration is seen. (Courtesy of Dr. R. Harruff, Seattle, WA.)

Figure 4-3

EMBRYONAL CARCINOMA

This solid, yellow-tan tumor has patchy areas of hemorrhage and necrosis.

elevated serum lactate dehydrogenase (LDH) levels (16), and serum placental-like alkaline phosphatase (PLAP) may also be increased.

Gross Findings. Embryonal carcinoma typically forms a soft, pale gray to pink to tan, granular tumor. Foci of hemorrhage and necrosis may be prominent and frequent (figs. 4-1–4-3). Rarely, the tumor has a firm, fibrotic consistency, at least focally (fig. 4-4). Embryonal carcinomas are usually smaller than seminomas, averaging

about 2.5 cm in diameter (17). Additionally, they more frequently blend with the adjacent parenchyma, unlike the typically sharply demarcated seminoma. Local extension into the rete testis, epididymis, and beyond occurs in about 25 percent of the cases (fig. 4-5) (4,14).

Microscopic Findings. Embryonal carcinoma consists of cohesive groups of large cells that are arranged in several, often coexisting, patterns (fig. 4-6). Solid sheets of cells (fig. 4-7)

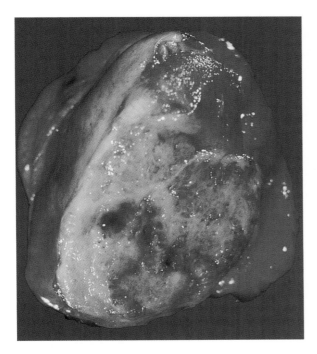

Figure 4-4

EMBRYONAL CARCINOMA

The white areas are firm, and microscopic examination showed prominent fibrosis. (Fig 3.2 from Young RH, Scully RE. Testicular tumors. Chicago: ASCP Press; 1990;48.)

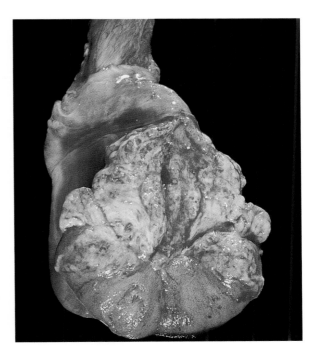

Figure 4-5

EMBRYONAL CARCINOMA

There is massive spread of tumor to the epididymis and paratesticular soft tissues.

often associated with foci of necrosis, both of individual cells and confluent areas, are common, as are glands that are round or, less often, elongated (fig. 4-8). Glands should be distinguished from degenerative spaces that may contain eosinophilic material. Papillae are less common than glands but still relatively frequent, with the tumor cells covering, in a radial fashion, a protruding core of fibrovascular tissue (fig. 4-9). When the vessels are prominent, a "pseudoendodermal sinus" pattern is produced (fig. 4-10) (18), but the tumor cells are larger and more pleomorphic than those of yolk sac tumor (see Yolk Sac Tumor and figs. 4-42, 4-45). Sometimes, papillary processes lack a stromal core and are composed of piled-up, carcinomatous epithelium (fig. 4-11).

The solid pattern is most common (100 percent), followed by the papillary/tubular (78 percent) and pseudoendodermal sinus (15 percent) patterns (18). What has been described as a "double-layered pattern," in our opinion, is the diffuse embryoma form of mixed germ cell tumor

composed of embryonal carcinoma and yolk sac tumor (see chapter 5; figs. 5-13, 5-15). Rarely, embryonal carcinoma forms blastocyst-like vesicles with a central cavity (fig. 4-12) (19).

It is common in the solid pattern to find darkly staining, degenerate-appearing, smudged cells. These are particularly prominent at the periphery of cell groups (figs. 4-7, 4-13) and may be confused with syncytiotrophoblast cells, resulting in a misdiagnosis of choriocarcinoma. Friedman and Moore (3), noting the tendency of the smudged cells to "apply" themselves to adjacent cells, called this the *appliqué pattern of embryonal carcinoma*. The lymphoid infiltrate and granulomatous reaction associated with seminoma are not usually prominent features of embryonal carcinoma but are identified in occasional cases (fig. 4-14, 4-15), as is a prominent fibrous stroma (fig. 4-16), correlating with the occasionally firm texture (fig. 4-4).

The tumor cells are usually polygonal, but in glandular foci, the lining cells are cuboidal (fig. 4-17) to columnar (fig. 4-18). The usually

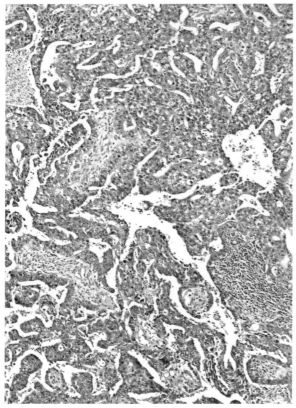

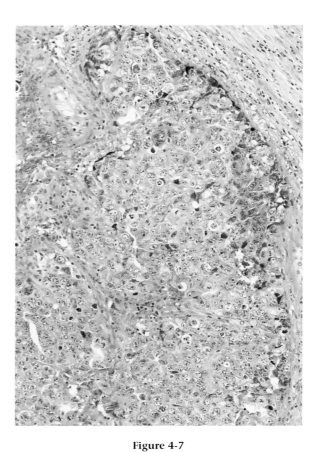

Figure 4-6

EMBRYONAL CARCINOMA

This tumor has a typical heterogeneous appearance with glandular, papillary, and solid patterns.

Figure 4-7

EMBRYONAL CARCINOMA

This tumor has a solid pattern with rare glands. Dark-staining, smudged cells are at the periphery.

Figure 4-8

EMBRYONAL CARCINOMA

The glands are round and elongated.

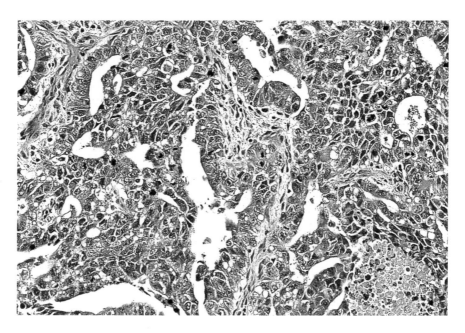

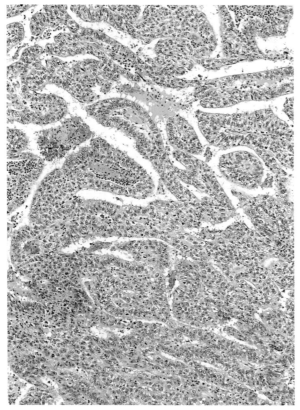

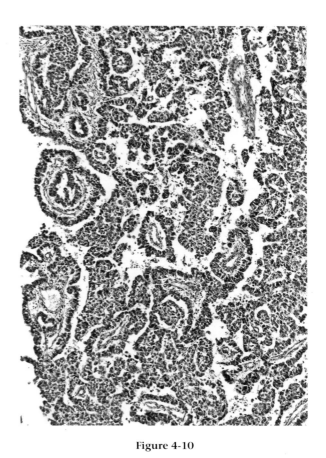

Figure 4-9

EMBRYONAL CARCINOMA

The tumor forms papillae with a radial arrangement of neoplastic cells on fibrovascular cores.

Figure 4-10

EMBRYONAL CARCINOMA

This papillary pattern creates a "pseudoendodermal sinus" appearance.

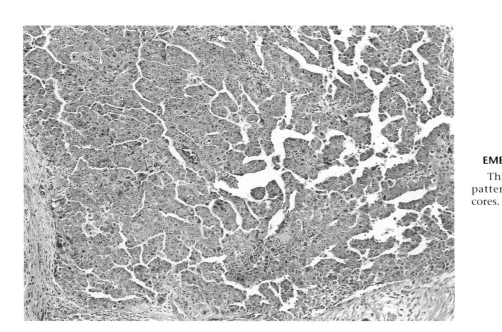

Figure 4-11

EMBRYONAL CARCINOMA

This tumor has a papillary pattern lacking fibrovascular cores.

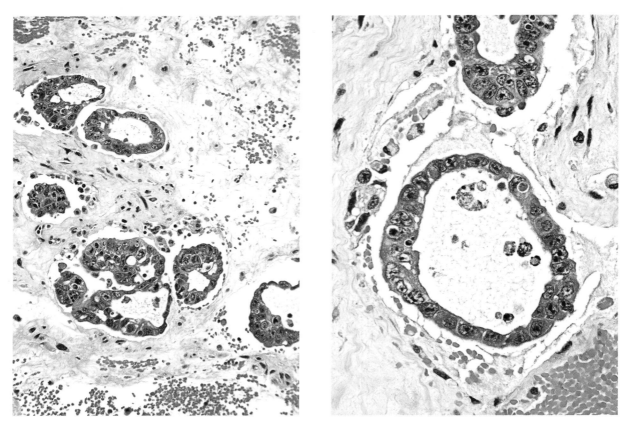

Figure 4-12

EMBRYONAL CARCINOMA

Left: The tumor forms blastocyst-like structures.
Right: The cells lining the vesicle of the blastocyst-like structure have the characteristic cytomorphology of embryonal carcinoma.

Figure 4-13

EMBRYONAL CARCINOMA

The appliqué pattern results from degenerate change at the periphery of a cellular lobule and imparts a "biphasic" appearance that may mimic choriocarcinoma.

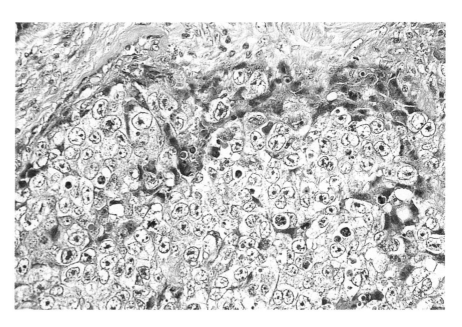

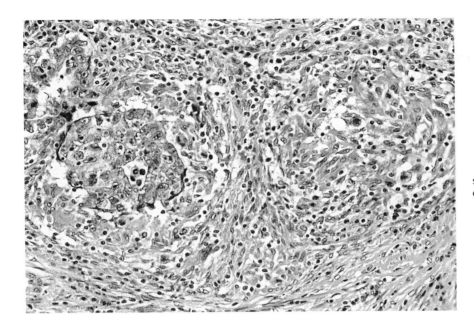

Figure 4-14

EMBRYONAL CARCINOMA

A granulomatous reaction surrounds clusters of tumor cells.

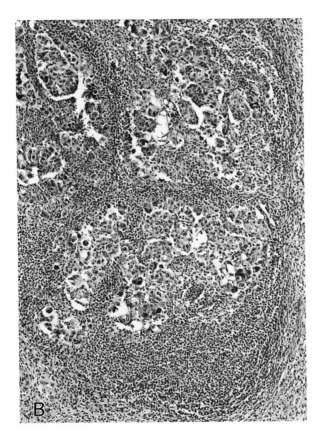

Figure 4-15

EMBRYONAL CARCINOMA

This tumor has a striking lymphocytic infiltrate.

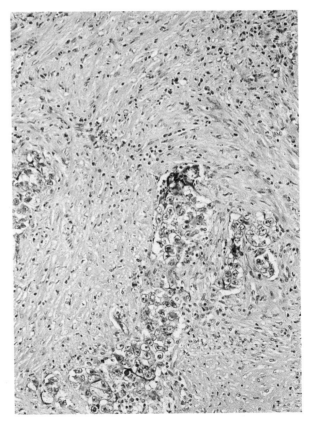

Figure 4-16

EMBRYONAL CARCINOMA

Prominent stromal fibrosis is present.

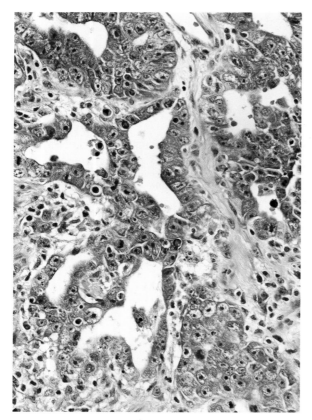

Figure 4-17

EMBRYONAL CARCINOMA

The glands are lined by cuboidal cells.

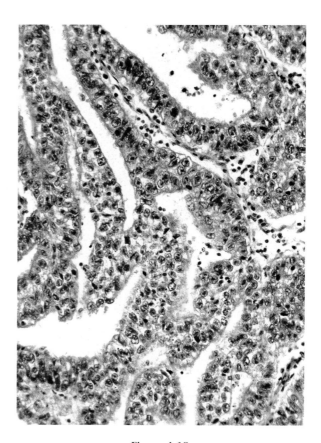

Figure 4-18

EMBRYONAL CARCINOMA

This glandular pattern has columnar tumor cells.

abundant cytoplasm is slightly granular and varies from basophilic (fig. 4-19) to amphophilic to eosinophilic (fig. 4-20) or even clear. Cytoplasmic borders cannot usually be appreciated in light microscopic sections, especially in neoplasms with a solid pattern that have a syncytial appearance. In semi-thin plastic sections, the cell borders are more easily identified, and the nuclei are discrete. The nuclei are large and vesicular, with irregular, coarsely clumped chromatin and prominent parachromatin clearing. The nuclear shape is generally polygonal, but frequently there are deep clefts and irregular contours. One or more very large nucleoli are present (figs. 4-19, 4-20). Often the crowded nuclei appear to abut or overlap each other (figs. 4-19, 4-20). The mitotic rate is high.

Syncytiotrophoblast cells are very common in embryonal carcinoma if assiduously searched for (fig. 4-21). They may be seen randomly

among tumor cells or in the stroma adjacent to aggregates of embryonal carcinoma. Just as with the appliqué pattern, they should not lead to the diagnosis of choriocarcinoma.

It is common to find intratubular embryonal carcinoma at the periphery of tumor nodules (fig. 4-22). Such foci are often extensively necrotic, with darkly staining masses of degenerated, intraluminal neoplastic cells (fig. 4-23). The residual intact nuclei frequently have a smudged appearance, and there is often dystrophic calcification.

Invasion of either lymphatic or blood vessels is common and is an important feature for identifying patients being considered for "surveillance only" protocols. The true frequency of vascular invasion is unclear because most of the studies have assessed mixed germ cell tumors; for instance, one study identified vascular invasion in 29 of 45 (64 percent) of nonseminomatous

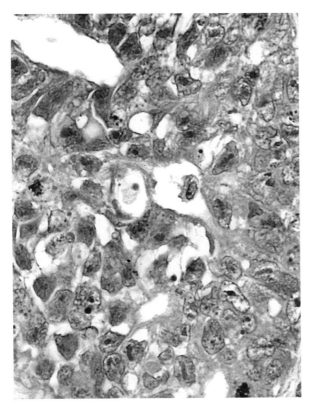

Figure 4-19

EMBRYONAL CARCINOMA

There are pleomorphic, crowded, irregularly shaped, vesicular nuclei with large, central nucleoli. The basophilic cytoplasm has indistinct borders.

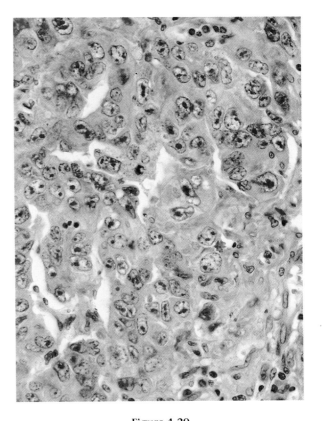

Figure 4-20

EMBRYONAL CARCINOMA

The pleomorphic nuclei have huge nucleoli and abut one another. The cytoplasm is eosinophilic to amphophilic and lacks distinct membranes.

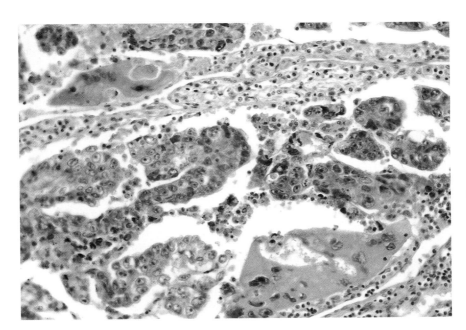

Figure 4-21

EMBRYONAL CARCINOMA

Two syncytiotrophoblast cells are present.

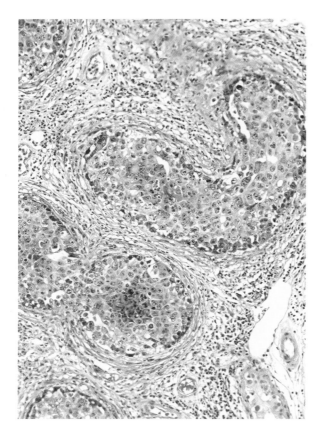

Figure 4-22

EMBRYONAL CARCINOMA

The tubules are expanded by mostly viable tumor cells with focal central necrosis.

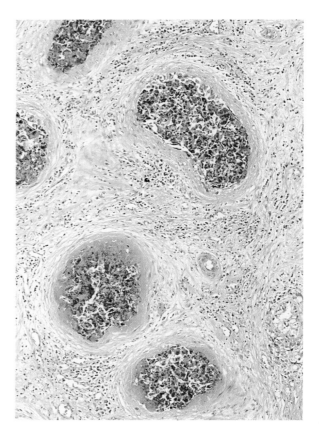

Figure 4-23

EMBRYONAL CARCINOMA

This focus of intratubular embryonal carcinoma is mostly necrotic, with nuclear fragments admixed with eosinophilic coagulum.

germ cell tumors of different stages (20). In our experience with nonseminomatous germ cell tumors, the angioinvasive element is disproportionately embryonal carcinoma. Such vascular invasion is often most easily identified in the surrounding non-neoplastic testis (fig. 4-24). Artifactual implantation of tumor cells into vascular spaces may mimic vascular invasion (although it is more common in cases of seminoma), but has loosely associated tumor cells dispersed randomly ("floating") in the lumen (fig. 4-25) rather than the cohesive groups that conform to the shape of the vessel that are the hallmark of true invasion (fig. 4-24). The association of true vascular invasion in some cases with thrombotic material is also helpful (21). The additional association of artifactual vascular implants with simultaneous implants

on tissue surfaces ("buttered on" artifact) also helps in the interpretation (fig. 4-26) (22). Retraction artifact, induced by fixation, may be misinterpreted as vascular space involvement but lacks an endothelial lining. Vascular invasion may also be mimicked by intratubular tumor, but the identification of residual Sertoli cells confirms an intratubular location in some cases. Intratubular tumor is more commonly extensively necrotic than intravascular tumor. Seminiferous tubules with intratubular tumor tend to have a more uniform diameter and are nonbranching, whereas vessels with tumor are less uniform in size and more frequently branching. Immunostaining for endothelial cell markers can resolve this dilemma if the routine light microscopic features are ambiguous.

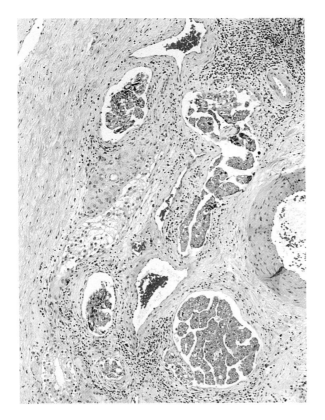

Figure 4-24

EMBRYONAL CARCINOMA

Cohesive groups of intravascular tumor cells conform to the shape of the vessels.

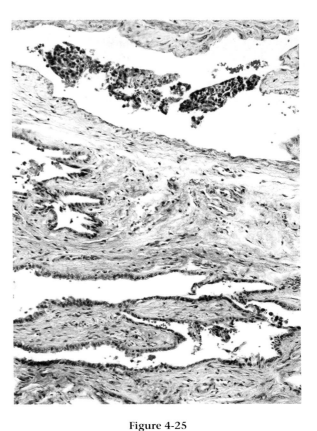

Figure 4-25

**EMBRYONAL CARCINOMA WITH
VASCULAR PSEUDOINVASION**

There are loose clusters of tumor cells "floating" in the lumen of a vessel (top). Smaller clusters are present in the rete testis (bottom).

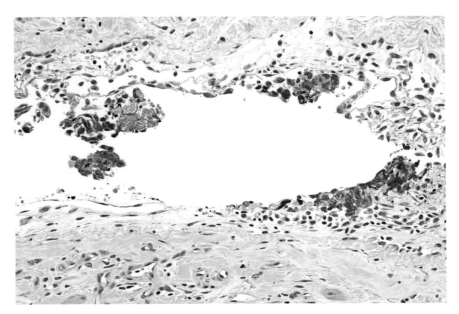

Figure 4-26

**EMBRYONAL CARCINOMA
WITH TUMOR IMPLANTATION**

Clumps of artifactually implanted tumor cells are distributed along the surface in a tissue crevice. This finding results from carry-over of tumor fragments from instruments used in specimen dissection and is commonly seen in many cellular germ cell tumors.

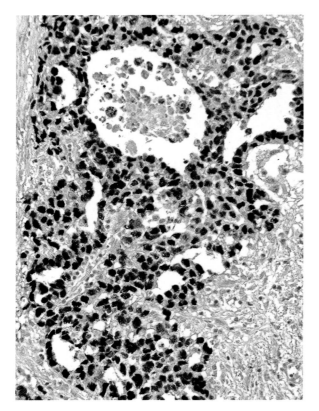

Figure 4-27

EMBRYONAL CARCINOMA

There is strong nuclear staining for OCT3/4.

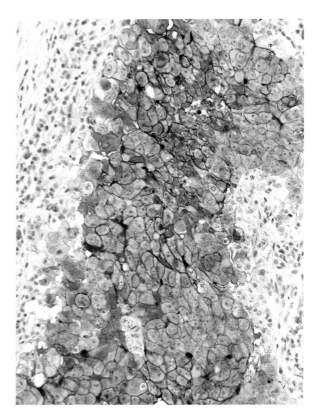

Figure 4-28

EMBRYONAL CARCINOMA

There is positivity in the cytoplasmic membranes for CD30.

Immunohistochemical Findings. Two of the most useful immunohistochemical markers for embryonal carcinoma are OCT3/4 and CD30. Of these, OCT3/4 is more sensitive and specific, staining the nuclei of virtually all embryonal carcinomas (23,24) and sometimes showing weak cytoplasmic reactivity (fig. 4-27). The staining pattern is similar in seminomas, however, but it is rarely identified in other neoplasms. Positivity for OCT3/4 occurred in 2 of 145 (1.4 percent) nonsmall cell carcinomas of the lung, 1 of 50 (2 percent) clear cell carcinomas of the kidney, and none of any other neoplasm among 3,000 nongerm cell tumors (23).

Diffuse CD30 reactivity occurs in 84 to 93 percent of embryonal carcinomas (25,26), highlighting the cytoplasmic membranes of the tumor cells (fig. 4-28). It is negative, or, at most, only focally positive, in seminomas (25–28). A number of other neoplasms, however, may be CD30 reactive, including lymphoma, undifferentiated nasopharyngeal carcinoma, melanoma, and benign and malignant mesenchymal tumors (29–32), although in many instances such staining is focal and nonmembranous, in contrast to that seen in embryonal carcinoma.

SOX2 has also proved valuable in the recognition of embryonal carcinoma and its distinction from seminoma. In three studies, all of the embryonal carcinomas showed nuclear positivity for SOX2 and all seminomas were negative (33–35). Teratoma, however, may also be positive for SOX2, particularly the primitive neuroectodermal elements (34,35)

Much of the reported AFP positivity in embryonal carcinoma probably represents admixed yolk sac tumor elements, but some typical embryonal carcinomas do stain (36,37). The staining frequency varies from 8 to 33 percent (38,39) and occurs more often in the embryonal carcinoma

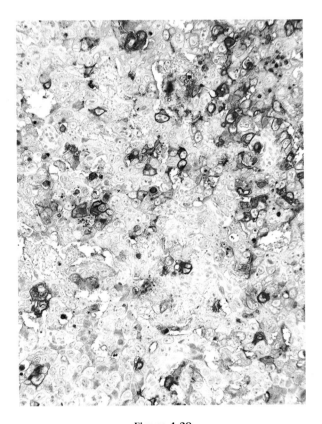

Figure 4-29

EMBRYONAL CARCINOMA

There is patchy cytoplasmic and membrane reactivity for placental-like alkaline phosphatase.

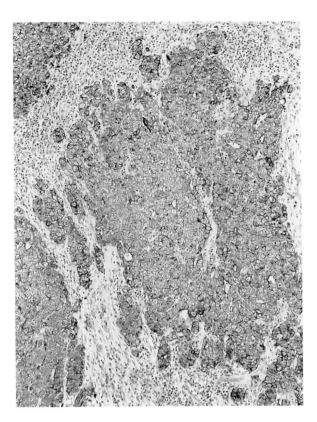

Figure 4-30

EMBRYONAL CARCINOMA

Diffuse positive staining occurs with a wide-spectrum anticytokeratin preparation (AE1/AE3).

component of mixed germ cell tumors than in pure cases (39,40), perhaps indicating early transformation to yolk sac tumor in these neoplasms. Positivity occurs most commonly in scattered cells of the solid pattern.

PLAP positivity occurs in 86 to 97 percent of embryonal carcinomas (38,41,42). It is often more focal than in seminoma, with both cytoplasmic and membrane positivity (fig. 4-29) (42).

Most embryonal carcinomas stain for pancytokeratins (AE1/AE3 and CAM5.2) (fig. 4-30) as well as cytokeratins (CK) 8, 18, and 19. Occasional cases also stain for CK4 and CK17 (38,43,44). Most do not react with epithelial membrane antigen (EMA) (38). SALL4 produces uniform nuclear staining in embryonal carcinoma as well as in many other germ cell tumors (45).

Several other antigens may be found in embryonal carcinoma but are diagnostically less useful. LDH-1 is positive in over 50 percent

of cases (46), and ferritin in 88 percent (47). Monoclonal antibody 43-9F is strongly reactive in 87 percent of cases, with weak or absent reactivity in seminomas, choriocarcinomas, and most yolk sac tumors (48). Embryonal carcinomas are strongly positive for p53 in 5 to 50 percent of the cell population, contrasting with weaker and more focal positivity in seminomas (49,50). Alpha-1-antitrypsin, Leu-7, vimentin, and human placental lactogen (HPL) are demonstrated in a small percentage of cases (38,39). Embryonal carcinomas are negative for carcinoembryonic antigen (CEA), and beta-hCG is demonstrable only in intermingled syncytiotrophoblast cells (38), which also stain for alpha-inhibin (51,52).

Ultrastructural Findings. Ultrastructural examination shows small, extracellular luminal spaces in solid patterns of tumor (fig. 4-31) and larger, more distinctive luminal spaces in overtly

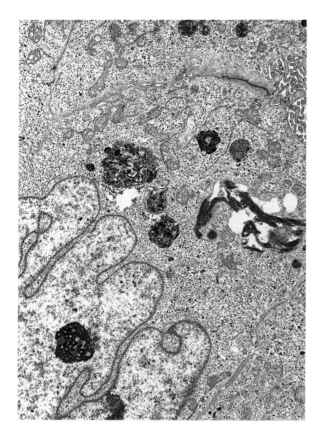

Figure 4-31

EMBRYONAL CARCINOMA

This electron micrograph shows the formation of a luminal space bordered by microvilli (upper right). A long tight junction is adjacent to the lumen. The nucleus has intricate folds, and the cytoplasm contains granular lysosomal bodies (telolysosomes), small mitochondria, and scattered glycogen granules.

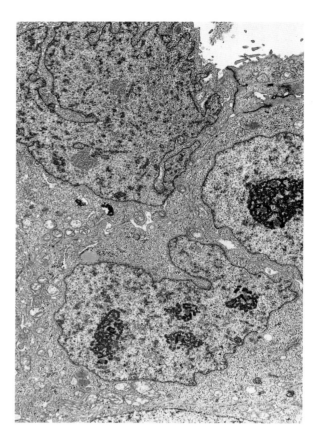

Figure 4-32

EMBRYONAL CARCINOMA

This glandular pattern has a luminal space (upper right), with well-defined junctional complexes. The nuclei are complexly folded and have large, intricate nucleoli. The cytoplasm contains round mitochondria and scattered glycogen granules.

glandular patterns (fig. 4-32) (53). Stubby microvilli project into the luminal spaces (fig. 4-31), and tight junctional complexes with well-defined desmosomes are present between cells abutting a lumen (figs. 4-31, 4-32) (54). The tight junctions of these complexes are frequently long; this feature has proved useful in the differentiation of glandular pattern embryonal carcinoma from somatic-type adenocarcinoma derived from teratomatous elements (55).

The cytoplasm of embryonal carcinoma cells is more complex than that seen in seminoma, with abundant numbers of ribosomes, frequent arrays of glycogen, and a much more prominent Golgi apparatus and rough endoplasmic reticulum (53). Mitochondria are numerous

and telolysosomes are prominent (fig. 4-31). Scattered lipid droplets are present. Basement membrane often surrounds nests of cells. The nuclei are irregular, with deep indentations, clumps of heterochromatin, and large nucleoli with a "complex meandering appearance" (figs. 4-31, 4-32) (53). Intranuclear cytoplasmic inclusions may be identified.

Cytologic Findings. In preparations derived from aspirated tumors, embryonal carcinoma appears as tight clusters of pleomorphic epithelium (fig. 4-33) (56). A sheet-like, papillary, or ball-like arrangement may occur (57). Nuclear and cytoplasmic borders may be blurred (56,57). The nuclei are irregularly shaped and pleomorphic, with clumped, unevenly distributed

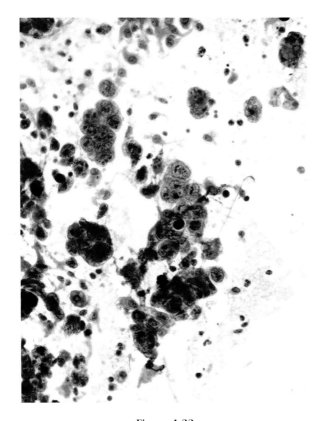

Figure 4-33

EMBRYONAL CARCINOMA

In this preparation from a needle aspirate, the cells are arranged in tight clusters, with scattered individual tumor cells. Ill-defined cytoplasm, pleomorphic overlapping nuclei, and prominent multiple nucleoli are seen.

chromatin and one or more prominent nucleoli (57,58). A branching, "right-angle" capillary network may be identified, with the tumor cells forming tight clusters along the branching capillaries (56). A "tigroid" background, as seen in seminomas, is not identified (56). The cohesive nature of aspirates of embryonal carcinoma further differentiates it from the more dissociated cellular elements derived from seminoma.

Special Techniques. Ploidy analysis of embryonal carcinomas yields a mean DNA value 1.43 times the diploid control, a result significantly less than that obtained for seminomas (1.66 times diploid). Nonseminomatous tumors, including embryonal carcinomas, most commonly have single aneuploid stem lines with ploidy values in the triploid range (59). These data support the hypothesis that embryonal

carcinomas may arise from seminomas secondary to gene loss (60).

Cytogenetic analysis of embryonal carcinomas confirms the presence of isochromosome 12p in many cases (61), and tumors lacking it have other forms of 12p amplification (62). "Disarray" of 12p or "multifocal 12p" on fluorescent in situ hybridization studies correlates with advanced pathologic stage disease (63). Because of the association of germ cell tumors with characteristic cytogenetic anomalies of chromosome 12, genetic analyses may aid in the diagnosis of ambiguous carcinomas in extragenital sites. Four of eight patients with poorly differentiated carcinomas involving midline structures had abnormalities of chromosome 12, consistent with germ cell tumors (64). Commonly overexpressed genes derived from 12p include *CCND2, SLC2A3 (GLUT3), PHB2 (REA), PYROXD1 (FLJ22028), DPPA3 (STELLA), CD9, GAPDH, GDF3, NANOG,* and *TEAD4* (65-67); oncogene candidates include *BRCC3, FOS, MLLT11, NES,* and *RAC1;* and possibly pathogenetically important putative cancer suppressor genes include *INTS6 (DDX26), ERCC5, FZD4, NME4, OPT*N, and *RBI.* In contrast to seminoma, embryonal carcinoma overexpresses several core "stemness" genes including *LEFTY2 (EBAF), TDGFI,* and *SOX2* (65); other overexpressed genes include *POU5F1 (OCT4), GAL, DPPA4,* and *NALP3* (68). Allelic loss at 3q27-q28 is a common finding in embryonal carcinomas (69), which also more frequently demonstrate methylation of certain gene promoters than do seminomas (70). Gene expression profiles of embryonal carcinomas show significant overlap with those of embryonic stem cells (71).

In keeping with a stem cell capacity, human embryonal carcinomas express certain globoseries carbohydrate surface antigens (so-called stage-specific embryonic antigens [SSEA]), which correspond to primitive embryonic development (SSEA-3) but do not express the more mature phenotype (SSEA-1) (72). Spontaneous differentiation to syncytiotrophoblast cells (73) and, after exposure to retinoic acid, to cells expressing neurofilament proteins, is described in tissue culture. Both muscle differentiation and neural differentiation were detected immunohistochemically in tumors produced by injecting cultured embryonal carcinoma into mice (74). These data support the capacity of embryonal carcinoma to differentiate into other forms of germ cell tumor.

Differential Diagnosis. Most embryonal carcinomas are easily recognized, but occasionally they are confused with seminoma or yolk sac tumor. The differentiation of typical and spermatocytic seminomas from embryonal carcinoma is discussed in chapter 3. A diagnosis of yolk sac tumor is justifiable only when one of the many distinctive patterns of yolk sac tumor is identified (see Yolk Sac Tumor below). Embryonal carcinomas lack these patterns and, although the solid and papillary patterns may be confused with yolk sac tumor, embryonal carcinomas have cells with larger nuclei and greater nuclear pleomorphism. These features, and associated patterns, help distinguish the two tumors, including cases of embryonal carcinoma with the "pseudoendodermal sinus" pattern. The common hyaline globules and basement membrane deposits of yolk sac tumors are not seen with any regularity in embryonal carcinomas (75). Immunostains are helpful: embryonal carcinomas are OCT3/4 and CD30 positive, in contrast to yolk sac tumor (23–25); glypican 3, on the other hand, is positive in yolk sac tumors and rarely seen in embryonal carcinomas (76,77).

Solid embryonal carcinomas with degenerate cells (the appliqué pattern; figs. 4-7, 4-13) may resemble choriocarcinoma but lack the well-defined, biphasic pattern of classic choriocarcinoma. Immunostains for hCG resolve this differential diagnosis. Immunostaining for OCT3/4 is also diagnostic: it is negative in choriocarcinoma and positive in embryonal carcinoma.

Large cell lymphoma, particularly with an immunoblastic phenotype, can be confused with embryonal carcinoma, and additionally anaplastic large cell or natural killer cell lymphoma with a prominent intratubular growth pattern may mimic embryonal carcinoma with an intratubular component (see fig. 7-112) (78). Patients with lymphoma are usually older, may have bilateral testicular involvement, and more commonly have paratesticular spread. The intertubular growth pattern of many lymphomas is not a feature of embryonal carcinoma, which destroys tubules and usually shows distinct epithelial differentiation. Intratubular germ cell neoplasia, unclassified (IGCNU), is usually present in the seminiferous tubules adjacent to embryonal carcinomas but not in lymphomas. Immunostains for cytokeratins and OCT3/4 are strongly positive in embryonal carcinoma and negative in lymphomas, whereas leukocyte common antigen is positive in many lymphomas and negative in embryonal carcinoma. Other lymphoid markers may be helpful in specific lymphoma subtypes, with the majority expressing CD20. CD30 is not useful since it may be identified in both embryonal carcinoma and anaplastic large cell lymphoma, although EMA reactivity favors the latter.

Metastatic carcinoma to the testis may simulate embryonal carcinoma. Patients with metastases are usually older, may have a history of prior cancer, and occasionally have bilateral involvement (79). Intertubular growth may be conspicuous (79), unlike embryonal carcinoma. The absence of IGCNU in metastases contrasts with its usual presence in embryonal carcinoma. Some metastatic carcinomas grow prominently in the tubules, with comedo-like necrosis, so this finding, frequent in embryonal carcinoma, is nonspecific.

Treatment and Prognosis. Embryonal carcinomas are not separated from other nonseminomatous germ cell tumors in current treatment strategies, and these general comments concerning therapy are applicable to most nonseminomatous germ cell tumors. The treatment of tumors clinically limited to the testis usually takes one of two approaches: either retroperitoneal lymph node dissection (RPLND), preferentially nerve sparing (80), or close follow-up (surveillance management) (81). Patients who have RPLND and lack nodal involvement (pathologic stage I disease) may then be followed without the need for adjuvant therapy (82). Approximately 10 percent of such patients relapse on follow-up (83), at which time they receive cisplatin-based chemotherapy. This approach achieves a greater than 98 percent overall cure rate (82,83). If positive lymph nodes are found on RPLND, patients are either followed or given chemotherapy, depending upon factors such as patient reliability and extent of involvement (84), with a breakpoint for the latter being pathologic stage N1 versus pathologic stage N2 disease (see Table 1-3, chapter 1) (83). A 98 to 100 percent survival rate can be anticipated (82,83).

Another approach for patients lacking clinical evidence of tumor spread beyond the testis is careful follow-up without immediate additional treatment after orchiectomy. For patients managed by "surveillance only," about 30 percent develop recurrences (85–87). Most patients with tumors that recur are those who, although clinical stage I, had occult metastases in the retroperitoneal lymph nodes (pathologic stage II). Careful pathologic examination of the orchiectomy specimen permits stratification of patients into low- and high-risk groups for either occult retroperitoneal metastases or recurrences on follow-up. The most important factors for recurrence appear to be either a substantial amount of embryonal carcinoma or the presence of lymphovascular invasion in the primary tumor. Various studies have reported a number of high-risk features, some of them obviously overlapping, including: vascular/lymphatic invasion (14,20,85–98), advanced local tumor stage (88,92,93,99), or various proportions or volumes of embryonal carcinoma with respect to other germ cell tumor elements (86–92,95,96,98,100–104). High S-phase values (101,105), high proliferation indices (Ki-67) (103), and tumor DNA indices in the hypertetraploid to hyperpentaploid range (106,107) also correlate with increased risk in clinical stage I patients, as do preorchiectomy serum AFP values of 80 ng/mL or greater (91) and an abnormal decline in serum AFP following orchiectomy (94). The overall disease-free survival rate achieved in several surveillance-only protocols for clinical stage I nonseminomatous patients was 97 percent, with 72 percent of patients not requiring treatment after orchiectomy (86).

Most patients in the United States who are treated at specialized centers and who have known retroperitoneal involvement of limited extent (6 cm or less [82]) receive RPLND, with either close follow-up (followed by full course chemotherapy if recurrence develops) or a short course of adjuvant therapy (82). Adjuvant treatment may be reserved for those with pN2 disease, with follow-up alone for those with pN1 status, since over 50 percent of the former relapse without adjuvant chemotherapy but only 17 percent of the latter (83). The overall survival rate in this group of patients is 98 percent or better with these methods (82,83,108).

For patients with advanced-stage, nonseminomatous germ cell tumors (i.e., bulky retroperitoneal disease or distant metastases), the standard treatment is initial cisplatin-based, multi-drug chemotherapy followed by surgical resection, if necessary, of residual masses. Treatment results in an overall survival rate of 70 to 80 percent for patients who present with advanced-stage disease (109,110). The nature of the residual mass in postchemotherapy resections influences the subsequent treatment and prognosis (111). The presence of viable-appearing, nonteratomatous germ cell tumor in the completely resected residual masses following chemotherapy identifies a group of patients who are at high risk for relapse (42 percent in one series [112]).

Numerous studies have been performed to identify patients with advanced-stage, nonseminomatous germ cell tumors who have a good prognosis or poor prognosis. The results, while showing some inconsistencies, are generally in agreement that the important prognostic factors include estimates of the extent of disseminated disease and the degree of elevation of serum markers (113–115). Thus, 99 percent of patients with disseminated, nonseminomatous germ cell tumors classified as "minimal" in extent achieve complete clinical remission compared to 89 percent with "moderate" extent disease and only 57 percent with "advanced" extent disease (110). Using such methods, patients with disseminated nonseminomatous testicular germ cell tumors can often be classified into good prognosis and poor prognosis categories, and treatment may be adjusted accordingly (116).

Therapies developed since the last quarter of the 20th century have resulted in an overall cure rate in excess of 90 percent for patients with testicular germ cell tumors (117). Analysis of the data presented by Dixon and Moore in the early 1950s (17) shows an overall 5-year survival rate of 60 percent, but a 5-year survival rate of only 30 percent for those with nonseminomatous germ cell tumors, in contrast to the current survival rates for nonseminomatous germ cell tumors in excess of 90 percent (82). The reduction in the overall death rate from testicular cancer is primarily due to the reduction in the death rate for those with nonseminomatous tumors (118).

YOLK SAC TUMOR

Definition. *Yolk sac tumor* is a malignant germ cell neoplasm that differentiates to form structures typical of the embryonic yolk sac, allantois, and extraembryonic mesenchyme (119,120).

General Features. Teilum identified this tumor by noting the resemblance of certain of its structures to extraembryonic mesoderm (119) and, his most seminal discovery, the close homology between the "glomerulus-like" structures of yolk sac tumor and the endodermal sinuses of the rat placenta (120). He also noted its association with other germ cell tumors (121) and its resemblance to structures of the extraembryonic fetal membranes, including the yolk sac and allantois. Additional evidence in support of Teilum's views occurred when AFP was localized both to the embryonic yolk sac as well as to yolk sac tumors (122).

Yolk sac tumor is the most common testicular tumor of children, representing 48 to 62 percent of cases in two registries of prepubertal testicular tumors (123,124) and occurring about twice as frequently as teratoma, the next most common tumor (123,124). It occurs at a median age of 16 to 20 months (123,124), with a range of 3 months to 8 years (123). Up to 75 percent of patients are younger than 2 years of age and rarely are any beyond 4 years (124,125). In contrast to the juvenile granulosa cell tumor, it is rarely, if ever, congenital. When yolk sac tumor occurs in a prepubertal child, it is almost always a pure neoplasm, whereas in postpubertal patients it is, with rare exceptions, one component of a mixed germ cell tumor.

The usual age range for postpubertal patients with a yolk sac tumor component in a mixed germ cell tumor is 15 to 40 years, but rare cases have been reported in the elderly (126,127). The reported frequency of yolk sac tumor with adult germ cell tumor depends upon the extent of sampling: extensive sampling discloses such a component in 44 percent of nonseminomatous germ cell tumors (128). Our experience with consultation material is similar to that of others (1) who found that yolk sac tumor was the most commonly overlooked component of testicular germ cell tumors, mostly because of its frequently focal and often subtle nature.

There is no association of childhood yolk sac tumor with cryptorchidism. Whereas the adult germ cell tumors are four or five times more common in whites than in African-Americans, the incidence of childhood yolk sac tumor is equal in both (129).

Clinical Features. The usual presentation is a painless testicular mass (130). Most children (85 to 94 percent) (131,132) have clinical stage I disease (i.e., no clinical, radiologic, or serologic evidence of metastatic disease). Similar data for adults with pure yolk sac tumors are not available because of their rarity. There is evidence that adults with a yolk sac tumor component in a mixed germ cell tumor have a higher frequency of pathologic stage I disease than do patients without such a component (95).

Yolk sac tumor is closely associated with elevated serum AFP. All 92 patients with a yolk sac tumor component had elevated serum AFP levels in one study (133), and 36 of 38 (95 percent) in another (134). Most elevations are substantial: hundreds to thousands of nanograms per milliliter (133). Significantly less elevated serum AFP is seen in patients with embryonal carcinoma (133). The correlation between elevated serum AFP and yolk sac tumor is a valuable method for monitoring the effects of therapy. It also serves to prompt further sectioning of a tumor if a yolk sac tumor is not found initially.

Gross Findings. Most yolk sac tumors are gray-white to tan to yellow, nonencapsulated but generally circumscribed tumors that often have a glistening, mucoid quality and frequently show cystic change on the cut surface (figs. 4-34, 4-35). Foci of hemorrhage and necrosis may be present and can be extensive, especially in postpubertal cases (fig. 4-36). The texture is usually soft but may be firm. Extratesticular extension is apparent in a minority of postpubertal cases (126,135).

Microscopic Findings. This diverse tumor has many patterns, the major ones usually coexisting (122,136). These include: 1) reticular (microcystic, vacuolated, honeycomb); 2) macrocystic; 3) endodermal sinus (perivascular, festoon); 4) papillary; 5) solid; 6) glandular-alveolar (including intestinal and endometrioid-like) (75,137,138); 7) myxomatous; 8) sarcomatoid (139); 9) polyvesicular vitelline; 10) hepatoid (75,140,141); and 11) parietal (75). Similar patterns are observed in both the pediatric and adult forms of the tumor (9).

The *reticular pattern*, the most common (fig. 4-37), has anastomosing, thin cords of tumor cells that enclose spaces often containing wispy, lightly eosinophilic mucoid secretion. A variant of this pattern occurs secondary to the development of large intracytoplasmic, empty-appearing vacuoles, resulting in a sieve-like or *microcystic pattern* (figs. 4-38, 4-39). Compression of the nuclei results in a lipoblast-like appearance (fig. 4-39). Occasionally, the cords of cells disperse as single spindle cells into the surrounding stroma (fig. 4-40). The stroma is often myxoid, and

such cases represent hybrids of the reticular and myxomatous patterns (see below). It is frequent to see reticular/microcystic patterns of yolk sac tumor intermingled with foci having a more solid appearance (fig. 4-41), but combinations

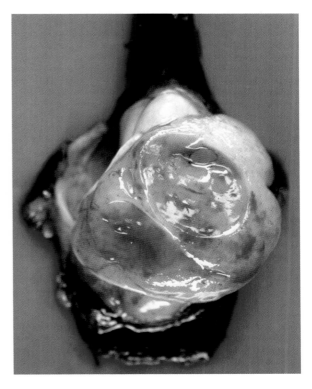

Figure 4-35

YOLK SAC TUMOR

A tan, focally cystic, circumscribed tumor in a 16-month-old.

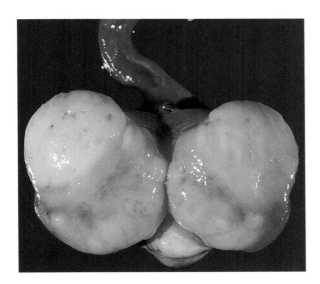

Figure 4-34

YOLK SAC TUMOR

A well-circumscribed tumor with a pale yellow, mucoid cut surface in a 4-month-old.

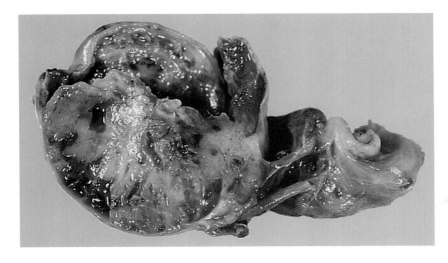

Figure 4-36

YOLK SAC TUMOR

A pure tumor in an adult shows gray tissue, hemorrhagic foci, and cystic degeneration. (Fig. 35 from Ulbright TM, Roth LM. Testicular and paratesticular tumors. In: Sternberg SS, ed. Diagnostic surgical pathology, New York: Raven Press; 1994:1910.)

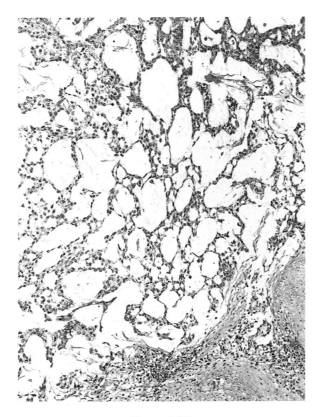

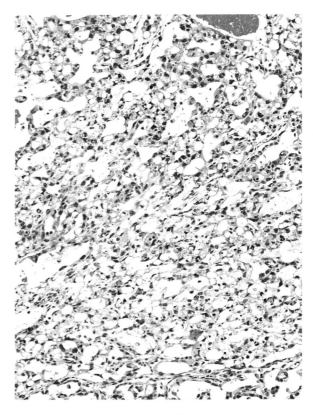

Figure 4-37

YOLK SAC TUMOR

The reticular pattern is created by anastomosing cords of tumor cells that enclose spaces containing wispy, eosinophilic secretions.

Figure 4-38

YOLK SAC TUMOR

A meshwork of small spaces creates a microcystic pattern.

Figure 4-39

YOLK SAC TUMOR

Vacuolated cells resembling lipoblasts and small cysts are present in this microcystic pattern.

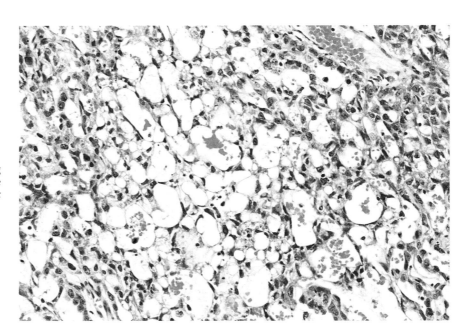

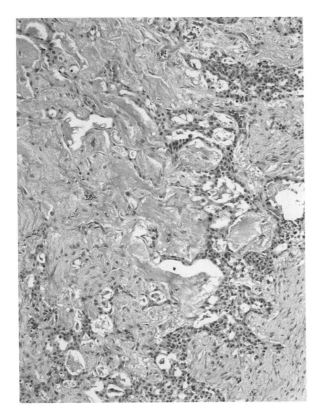

Figure 4-40

YOLK SAC TUMOR

Cords of cells extend from nests with microcysts into a myxoid stroma.

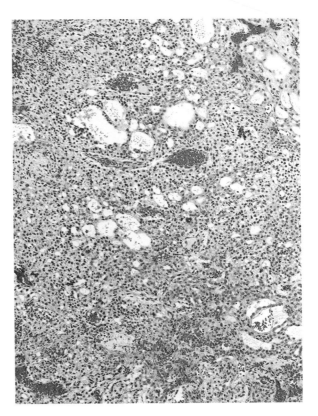

Figure 4-41

YOLK SAC TUMOR

Microcystic and solid patterns are admixed in a random fashion.

with endodermal sinus (fig. 4-42), glandular (fig. 4-43), and other patterns are also common. A *macrocystic pattern* is seen as microcysts become dilated or coalesce (fig. 4-44).

The *endodermal sinus pattern* of yolk sac tumor is the best known. It is classically characterized by a papillary core of fibrous tissue with a central small blood vessel that is ringed by a layer of malignant-appearing, cuboidal to columnar cells. This total structure is recessed into a small cystic space that is, in turn, lined by flattened tumor cells (fig. 4-45). These "Schiller-Duval bodies" or "glomeruloid bodies" may be cut longitudinally, resulting in an elongated structure (fig. 4-46). Oblique cuts of such structures may result in connective tissue cores that appear to be draped (festooned) by malignant epithelial cells (fig. 4-47). Abortive endodermal sinus structures, consisting of fibrovascular cores rimmed by malignant cells but not recessed into a well-defined

cystic space, are common and termed "atypical perivascular formations" (19). "Labyrinthine" spaces are a frequent feature of neoplasms with endodermal sinus formation (figs. 4-47, 4-48).

In the *papillary pattern*, small, irregularly shaped papillae, with (fig. 4-49) or without (fig. 4-50) fibrous cores, project into cystic spaces often containing many detached clusters of tumor cells (fig. 4-50). The tumor cells lining the papillae often have a low columnar to cuboidal profile, and a hobnail configuration of the nuclei may be present. Such papillae are sometimes superimposed on a festooned (endodermal sinus) type of arrangement (fig. 4-51).

The *solid pattern* consists of a sheet-like arrangement of polygonal tumor cells with lightly eosinophilic to clear cytoplasm, often well-defined cytoplasmic borders, and nonoverlapping nuclei with prominent to inconspicuous nucleoli (fig. 4-52). It is common to see occasional,

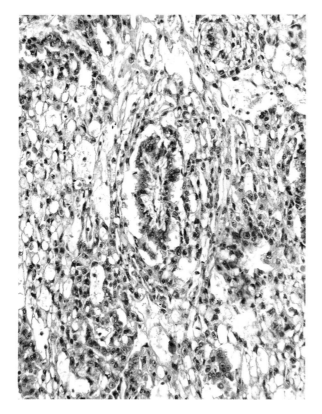

Figure 4-42

YOLK SAC TUMOR

An endodermal sinus-like structure is surrounded by a microcystic pattern.

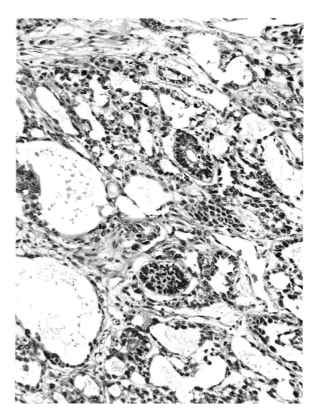

Figure 4-43

YOLK SAC TUMOR

Small glands are surrounded by microcysts.

Figure 4-44

YOLK SAC TUMOR

Microcystic and macrocystic patterns are seen.

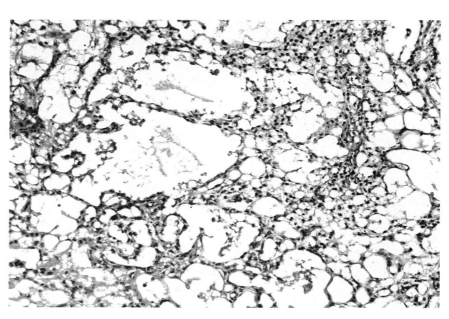

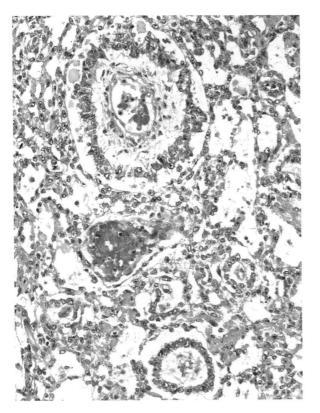

Figure 4-45

YOLK SAC TUMOR

There are anastomosing cords of cells and two endodermal sinus-like structures (Schiller-Duval bodies: the papillary structures lying in spaces and with central blood vessels in their stromal cores). There are also pink-staining basement membrane deposits.

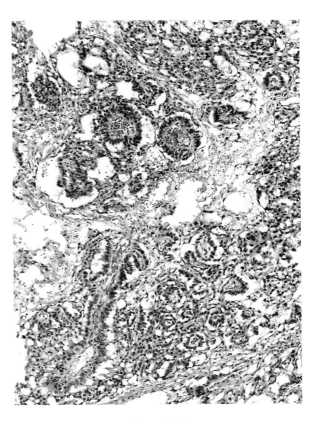

Figure 4-46

YOLK SAC TUMOR

Longitudinally (left bottom) and transversely sectioned endodermal sinus-like structures (Schiller-Duval bodies).

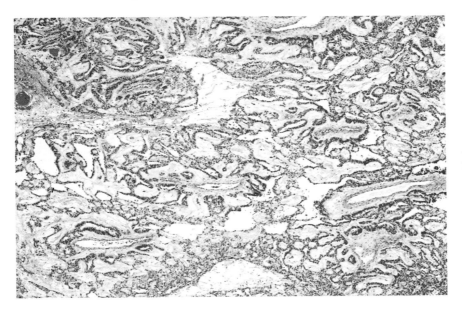

Figure 4-47

YOLK SAC TUMOR

Fibrous and fibrovascular cores are draped or "festooned" by malignant epithelium. Between the cores are interconnecting, irregular, "labyrinthine-like" spaces.

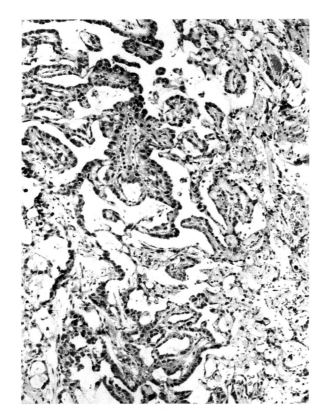

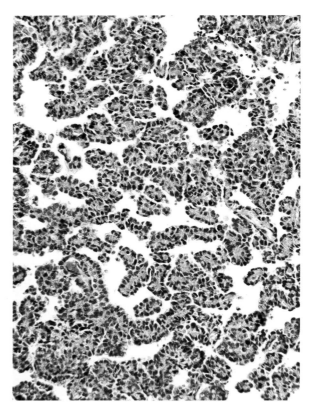

Figure 4-48

YOLK SAC TUMOR

Tangential and longitudinal sections of endodermal sinus-like structures are associated with a "labyrinthine-like" pattern of extracellular spaces.

Figure 4-49

YOLK SAC TUMOR

Slender papillae with fibrovascular cores are lined by cuboidal to low columnar tumor cells.

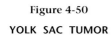

Figure 4-50

YOLK SAC TUMOR

Papillae lacking fibrovascular cores, rimmed by cells with scant cytoplasm and which sometimes have a "hobnail" nuclear arrangement, project into a cystic space. Clusters of exfoliated cells are present in the cyst.

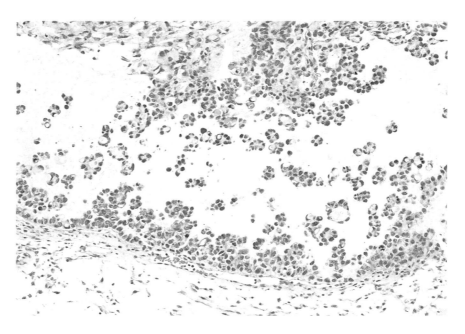

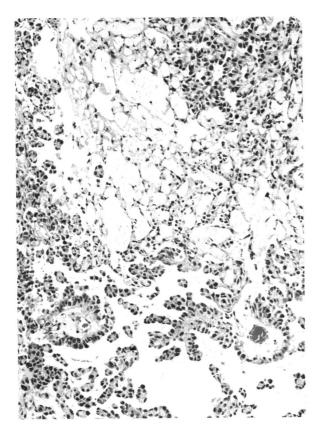

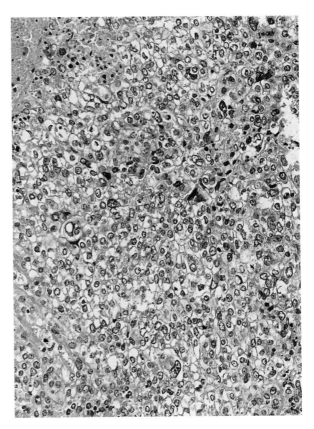

Figure 4-51

YOLK SAC TUMOR

On the right, papillary yolk sac tumor develops from well-defined endodermal sinus-like structures. A microcystic pattern is present in the center.

Figure 4-52

YOLK SAC TUMOR

Random pleomorphism and lack of fibrovascular septa (features that contrast with seminoma) are seen in this solid pattern.

randomly distributed tumor cells with larger nuclei (fig. 4-52). Often there is a prominent vascular network (fig. 4-53), and frequently there are focal microcysts (fig. 4-54). This pattern may be confused with seminoma, a differential diagnostic problem addressed in chapter 3. In some cases, the cells of solid pattern yolk sac tumor have a blastema-like appearance, being small and ovoid with hyperchromatic nuclei and scant cytoplasm (figs. 4-55, 4-56).

Glandular and *alveolar patterns* are common in yolk sac tumors but rarely occur in pure form. Glands often connect with cystic, alveolar-like spaces lined by flattened epithelium, resulting in overlap with the polyvesicular vitelline pattern (fig. 4-57) (see figs. 4-66–4-69). The glands often have enteric features consisting of pseudostratified columnar cells with eosinophilic cytoplasm and an apical brush border but, unlike many teratomatous glands, they lack a peripheral smooth muscle layer. A branching and anastomosing pattern is common (fig. 4-58), or more simple tubular glands are seen (figs. 4-59, 4-60). In some cases, the glandular component is prominent and complex (fig. 4-58). Such enteric-type glands were identified in 34 percent of yolk sac tumors in one series (75). The nuclei of the glands often appear less atypical than those of the adjacent nonglandular component. The glands may show basal cytoplasmic vacuolation reminiscent of early secretory phase endometrium (endometrioid-like) (fig. 4-61). Purely glandular yolk sac tumors of intestinal or endometrioid-like type occur rarely (fig. 4-61), sometimes with highly elevated serum AFP levels (138).

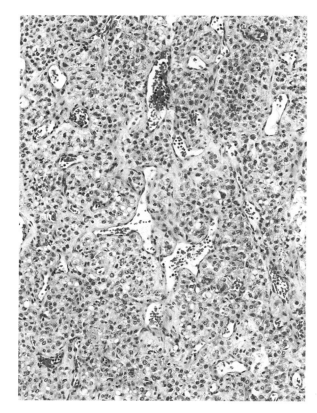

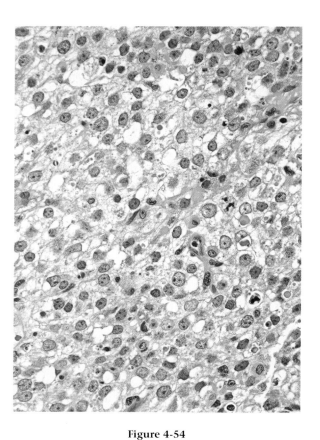

Figure 4-53

YOLK SAC TUMOR

A solid pattern with a prominent vascular network is seen. Foci of this type are nondiagnostic when viewed in isolation.

Figure 4-54

YOLK SAC TUMOR

This tumor has a mostly solid pattern with hyaline intra-cytoplasmic globules, a scant background of a few microcysts, and minimal extracellular basement membrane deposits.

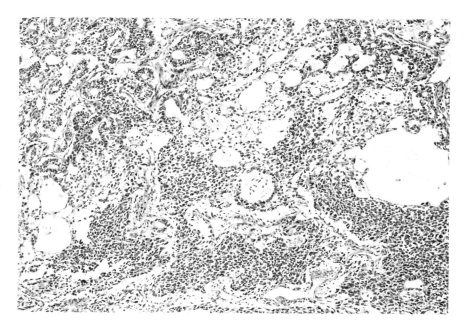

Figure 4-55

YOLK SAC TUMOR

Microcystic and solid patterns, the latter having a blastema-like appearance, are seen.

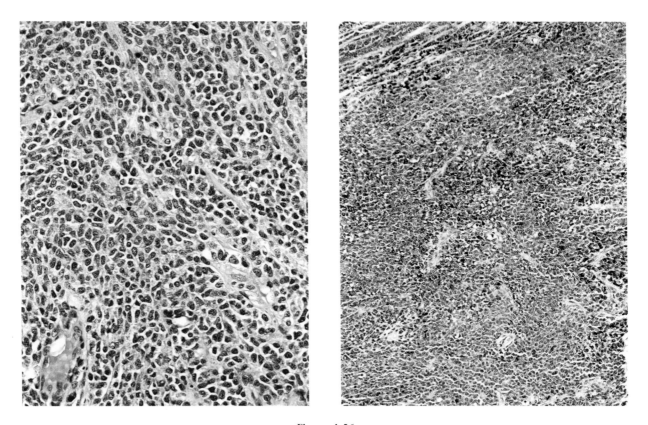

Figure 4-56

YOLK SAC TUMOR

Left: A solid pattern of blastema-like cells with oval to fusiform nuclei and scant cytoplasm is present in this tumor.
Right: An immunostain for alpha-fetoprotein (AFP) shows patchy reactivity in the same case.

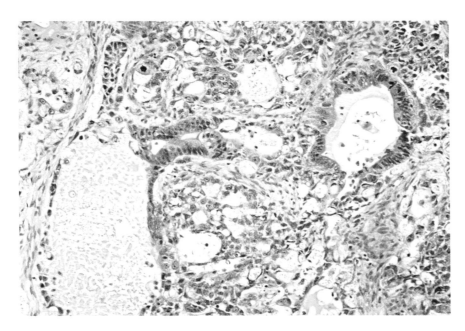

Figure 4-57

YOLK SAC TUMOR

Well-defined foci of columnar, glandular epithelium focally connect to a cystic (vesicle-like) space.

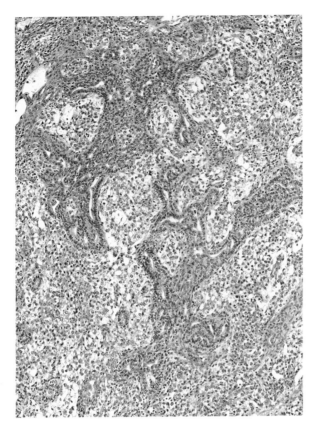

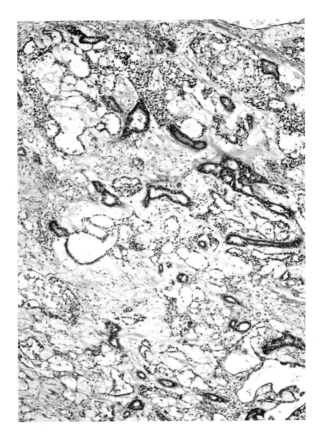

Figure 4-58

YOLK SAC TUMOR

The glandular component in this tumor is prominent, complex, and anastomosing.

Figure 4-59

YOLK SAC TUMOR

Numerous tubular glands are present in this tumor, which also has microcystic and macrocystic patterns.

Figure 4-60

YOLK SAC TUMOR

The glands are of simple tubular type and admixed with a microcystic pattern.

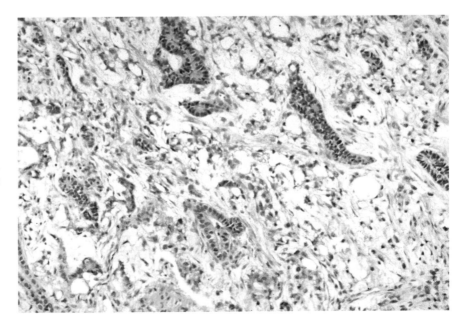

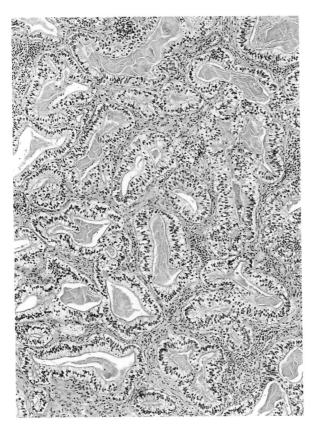

Figure 4-61

YOLK SAC TUMOR

This purely glandular tumor is composed of glands resembling secretory endometrium, with clear supranuclear and subnuclear cytoplasm.

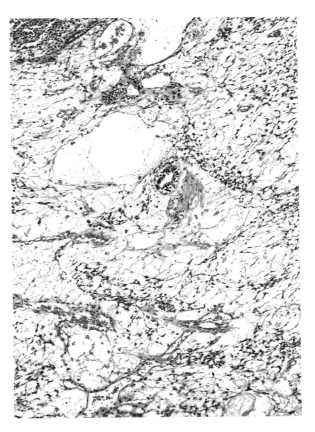

Figure 4-62

YOLK SAC TUMOR

Wispy strands of tumor cells are dispersed in a prominently myxoid stroma.

A myxoid component is common, particularly in association with a reticular pattern (figs. 4-40, 4-62, 4-63). The epithelial cells of the reticular pattern gradually disperse into a hyaluronic acid-rich, myxoid stroma and acquire stellate and spindled profiles, thereby constituting a *myxomatous pattern* (142). In addition to the spindled cells in a myxoid background, these foci have a prominent component of blood vessels, leading Teilum (122) to describe them as "angioblastic mesenchyme" analogous to extraembryonic mesenchyme (the "magma reticulare"). These elongated cells, while having a spindled, mesenchymal-like appearance, retain cytokeratin reactivity, supporting their derivation from the epithelial component of reticular yolk sac tumor (143). They are pluripotent, with the capacity to differentiate into skeletal muscle and cartilage (fig. 4-64) (143). The development of such differentiated somatic tissues creates semantic difficulties with respect to the classification of such cases as yolk sac tumor variants or teratomas. Our own approach is to accept scattered foci of somatic differentiation in an otherwise pure yolk sac tumor as yolk sac tumor, but to regard nodules of differentiated mesenchyme as teratomatous.

Rare yolk sac tumors have a cellular, neoplastic spindle cell component (fig. 4-65). Such foci develop in continuity with classic yolk sac tumor patterns, usually either reticular or myxomatous. These *sarcomatoid foci* retain reactivity for low molecular weight cytokeratins, supporting their derivation from epithelial yolk sac tumor elements and assisting in the distinction from tumors in the sex cord-stromal category that

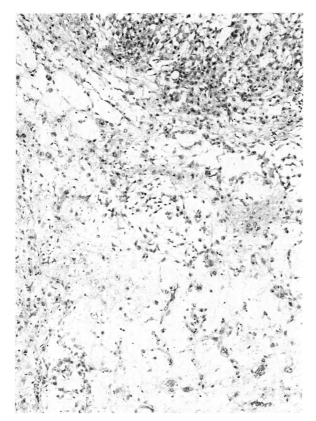

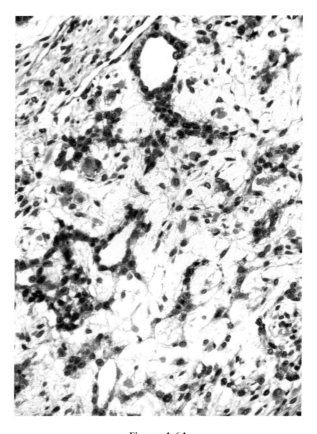

Figure 4-63

YOLK SAC TUMOR

A microcystic pattern (top) blends into a hypocellular, myxoid pattern, with stellate to spindle cells and frequent vessels. This pattern has been described as mesenchyme-like.

Figure 4-64

YOLK SAC TUMOR

Scattered rhabdomyoblasts are present in a myxoid zone.

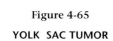

Figure 4-65

YOLK SAC TUMOR

A cellular, focally sarcomatoid pattern composed of oval and spindle cells is adjacent to a microcystic pattern.

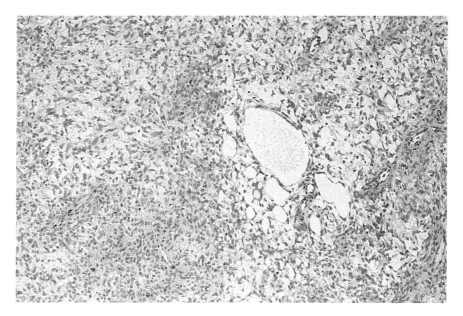

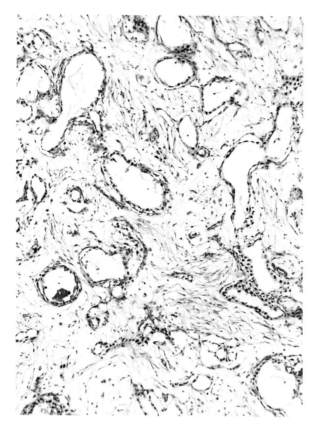

Figure 4-66

YOLK SAC TUMOR

In this polyvesicular vitelline pattern, vesicles, some with constrictions (upper left), are present in a loose, hypocellular stroma. The vesicles recapitulate the embryonic subdivision of the larger primary yolk sac into the smaller secondary yolk sac. (Fig. 3-19 from Young RH, Scully RE: Testicular tumors. Chicago: ASCP Press; 1990:57.)

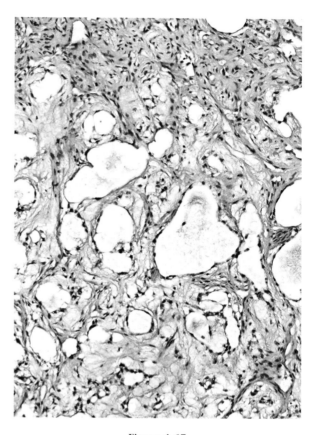

Figure 4-67

YOLK SAC TUMOR

Eccentrically constricted vesicles are set in a myxoid to fibrous stroma in this polyvesicular vitelline pattern.

may share some histologic features. Although some would regard these tumors as variants of myxomatous or reticular patterns, our preference is to categorize them as sarcomatoid to emphasize the need to consider yolk sac tumor in the differential diagnosis of a spindle cell tumor in a limited sample.

The *polyvesicular vitelline pattern* of yolk sac tumor consists of cysts scattered in a variably cellular mesenchyme that ranges from edematous (fig. 4-66) to fibrous and cellular (fig. 4-67). Some of the cysts show eccentric constriction (figs. 4-66–4-69), giving rise to a lopsided, figure-eight shape. These cysts are lined by a layer of flattened to columnar epithelium. Sometimes, a transition from flattened to cuboidal or columnar epithelium is identified within a cyst near the point of constriction (fig. 4-68). In the taller epithelial cells, basal or apical vacuolation of the cytoplasm may be seen. Sometimes the lining epithelium has a definite enteric appearance, with apical brush borders. In other cases, the lining is flat, with a deceptively bland appearance (fig. 4-69). Teilum (144) made an analogy between the constricted vesicles of this pattern and the embryonic subdivision of the primary yolk sac into the secondary yolk sac. The polyvesicular vitelline pattern is rare in testicular yolk sac tumors (about 8 percent of cases [75]), and it is almost always associated with other yolk sac tumor patterns. In our experience, it rarely predominates to the extent seen in occasional ovarian examples.

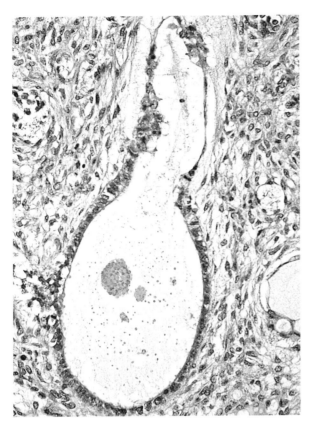

Figure 4-68

YOLK SAC TUMOR

A tumor with the polyvesicular vitelline pattern has a single vesicle with epithelium that varies from flat to columnar. Note the eccentric constriction of the vesicle.

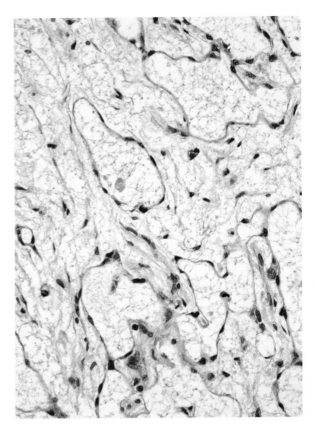

Figure 4-69

YOLK SAC TUMOR

Irregularly constricted vesicles are lined by flattened, bland-appearing tumor cells in this polyvesicular vitelline pattern.

The *hepatoid pattern* occurs in approximately 20 percent of yolk sac tumors (75,145), commonly as small clusters of liver-like cells arranged in nests (fig. 4-70), tubules, or trabeculae (fig. 4-71). In some unusual cases, there may be a predominant hepatoid pattern (fig. 4-72) and we have seen almost pure cases on rare occasion (fig. 4-73). The cells are polygonal and have abundant eosinophilic cytoplasm and a large nucleus with variably prominent nucleoli (figs. 4-74, 4-75). Bile canaliculi can be identified, but bile is only rarely seen (fig. 4-71). Hyaline globules occur commonly in hepatoid foci (fig. 4-74). The hepatoid foci are usually intensely reactive for AFP.

Parietal differentiation refers to the presence of eosinophilic bands of basement membrane material in the extracellular space between neoplastic cells (fig. 4-76). The basement membrane material is felt to represent a reiteration of the parietal layer of the embryonic yolk sac of the rodent that synthesizes a thick basement membrane (Reichert membrane) (75,144). It is a common but typically focal finding in yolk sac tumors: 92 percent of cases in a series of 50 yolk sac tumors (of which 36 were testicular in origin) contained such foci (75). Parietal differentiation may be identified in numerous yolk sac tumor patterns (figs. 4-77, 4-78), and its identification is helpful in recognizing yolk sac tumor in small biopsy specimens, especially at metastatic sites. Rarely, the basement membrane material becomes a predominant element, with neoplastic cells embedded within an eosinophilic matrix (figs. 4-79, 4-80). Patients with metastatic yolk sac tumor treated by chemotherapy may have recurrences with a pure parietal pattern.

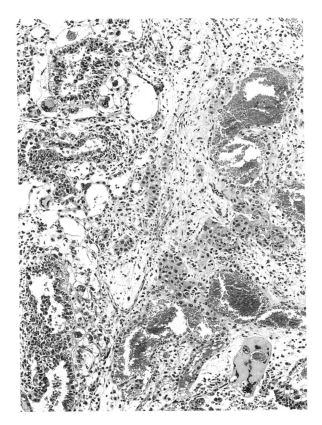

Figure 4-70

YOLK SAC TUMOR

Clusters of hepatoid cells with abundant eosinophilic cytoplasm are at the periphery of a nodule of a microcystic yolk sac tumor. Occasional syncytiotrophoblast cells are also present.

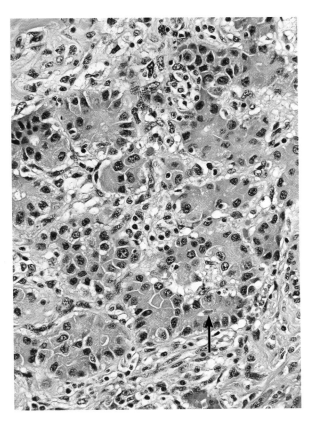

Figure 4-71

YOLK SAC TUMOR

Nests and thick trabeculae of hepatoid cells have occasional dilated canaliculi containing bile (arrow), a rare finding.

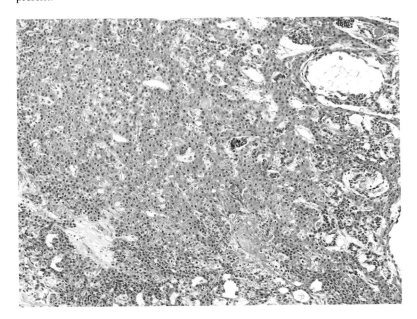

Figure 4-72

YOLK SAC TUMOR

This tumor has a predominant hepatoid pattern (left and center) that merges with microcystic foci.

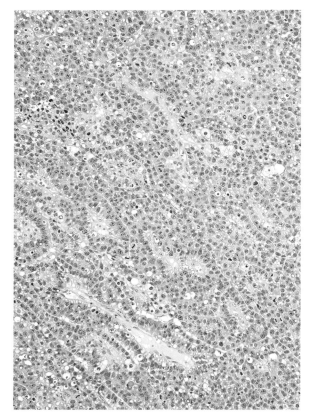

Figure 4-73

YOLK SAC TUMOR

A purely hepatoid yolk sac tumor forms thick trabeculae.

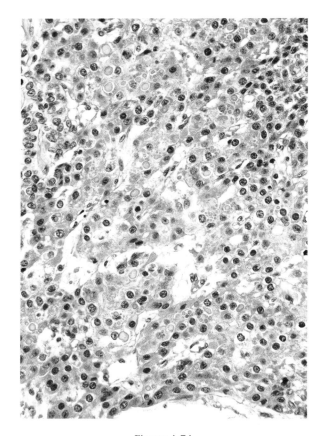

Figure 4-74

YOLK SAC TUMOR

A high-power view of a hepatoid area shows numerous intracytoplasmic hyaline globules.

Figure 4-75

YOLK SAC TUMOR

In this solid hepatoid focus, the tumor cells have prominent nucleoli.

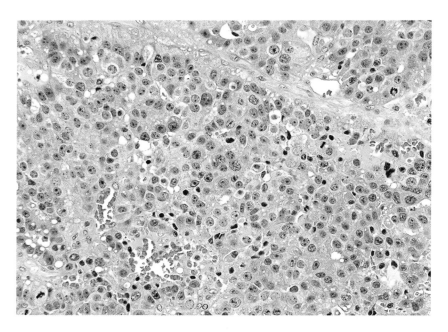

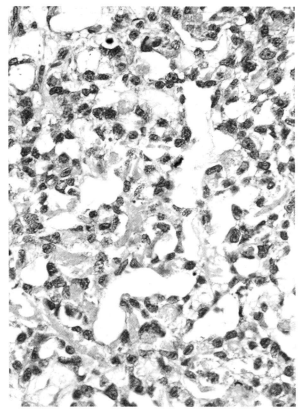

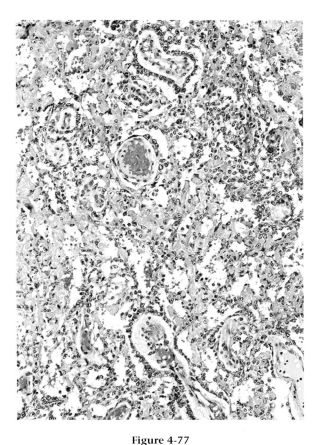

Figure 4-76

YOLK SAC TUMOR

Eosinophilic basement membrane material is deposited in the extracellular space in a reticular pattern.

Figure 4-77

YOLK SAC TUMOR

Abundant basement membrane deposits (parietal differentiation) are present in a tumor with endodermal sinus-like and microcystic patterns.

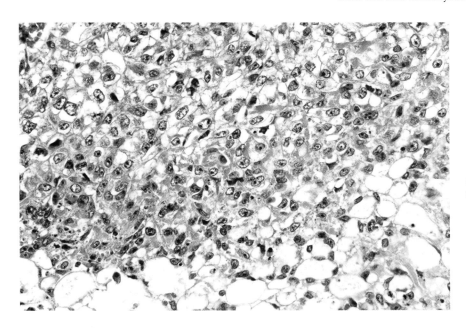

Figure 4-78

YOLK SAC TUMOR

There are solid and microcystic patterns with parietal differentiation.

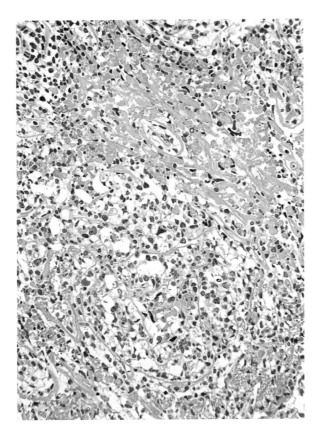

Figure 4-79

YOLK SAC TUMOR

This tumor has parietal and microcystic patterns.

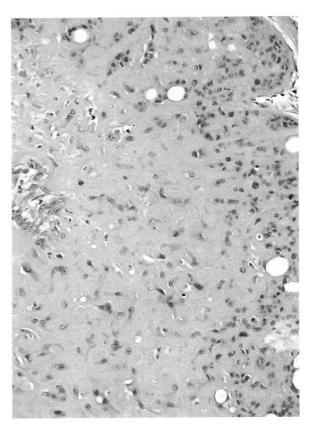

Figure 4-80

YOLK SAC TUMOR

Basement membrane-rich matrix contains scattered neoplastic cells in this parietal pattern tumor. Residual microcysts are also apparent.

Several series have addressed the frequency of various yolk sac tumor patterns, using a four-pattern classification system consisting of reticular, endodermal sinus, solid, and polyvesicular vitelline (18,75,146). Most agree that the reticular pattern is the most common, followed by solid and endodermal sinus patterns; the polyvesicular vitelline pattern is unusual (75,146). Macrocystic, papillary, and glandular-alveolar patterns appear to occur more prominently in children than in adults (136). In a series of 70 cases, a "vacuolated network" (91 percent) and microcystic patterns (67 percent) (we consider this in the reticular category) were the most common, followed by myxomatous (51 percent), macrocystic (44 percent), solid (27 percent), hepatoid (23 percent), "labyrinthine" (17 percent) (we consider this a variant of the endodermal sinus pattern), and endodermal sinus (9 percent) patterns (18). It is evident that although endodermal sinus

structures are a distinctive feature of yolk sac tumor, their presence cannot be relied upon to establish a diagnosis.

Another characteristic finding is the presence of hyaline eosinophilic globules in the cytoplasm of the neoplastic cells. These are not specific for yolk sac tumor but are observed in other malignant neoplasms as well; however, they are rarely identified in other forms of testicular germ cell tumor (75). The globules tend to occur in clusters and vary in size from 1 μm or less to more than 50 μm (figs. 4-74, 4-81). Sometimes they are confused with erythrocytes but they are more variable in size and are periodic acid–Schiff (PAS) positive and diastase resistant. Only occasional globules stain for AFP, although other serum proteins may be present. Many observers have felt that they occur both

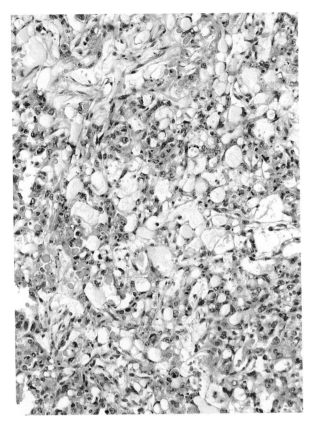

Figure 4-81

YOLK SAC TUMOR

Numerous round, eosinophilic hyaline globules in a microcystic yolk sac tumor.

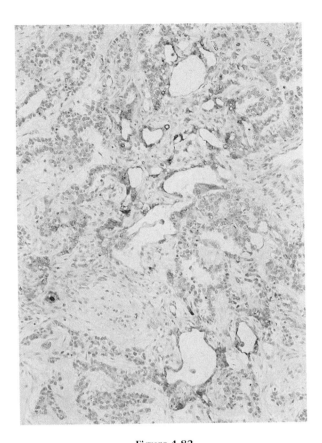

Figure 4-82

YOLK SAC TUMOR

There is patchy AFP positivity in a microcystic region.

extracellularly and intracellularly; electron micrographs of non-necrotic yolk sac tumor elements, however, verify that the globules are typically intracellular. It is possible that they appear to be extracellular by light microscopy as a consequence of necrosis and cytolysis, with extrusion into the extracellular space, or because the intact cytoplasm that surrounds them is too scant to be resolved by light microscopy.

Hematopoietic foci are identified in an occasional yolk sac tumor. Erythroblasts within the blood vessels or mesenchymal component of the tumor are the most common.

An interesting aspect of yolk sac tumors is an absence of IGCNU, unclassified type, in the childhood cases (147,148) in contrast to those of adults. As discussed in chapter 2, there is good evidence that the pediatric tumors form through a fundamentally different mechanism.

Immunohistochemical Findings. The frequency of AFP positivity in three series of yolk sac tumors varied from 74 to 100 percent (38,39,149), although childhood cases were more often negative in one study (39) but not in a second (9). Positivity occurs as a cytoplasmic blush that is often focal and patchy (figs. 4-82, 4-83). Hepatoid foci are often intensely reactive. The hyaline globules are usually AFP negative.

Reactivity for glypican 3 occurs in almost all yolk sac tumors and characteristically has a cytoplasmic and membranous distribution (fig. 4-84). This contrasts with negative staining in seminoma and uncommon (5 percent) positivity in embryonal carcinoma (76,77). In contrast to seminoma and embryonal carcinoma, OCT3/4 is negative in yolk sac tumor (24,150). CD30 is also absent (25,151,152), another difference with embryonal carcinoma.

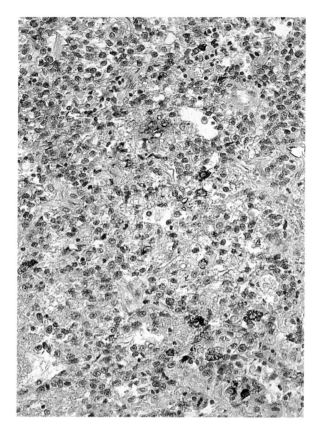

Figure 4-83

YOLK SAC TUMOR

Scattered AFP-positive tumor cells are seen in a yolk sac tumor with a solid pattern.

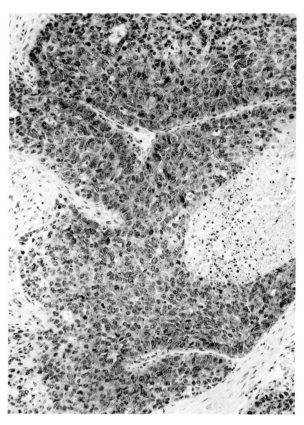

Figure 4-84

YOLK SAC TUMOR

An immunostain for glypican-3 highlights the cytoplasmic membranes in this tumor with a solid pattern.

Pancytokeratin marks almost all cases and is usually intensely positive (38,153); in contrast, CK7 is typically negative or only focally reactive (154). The nuclear transcription factor SALL4 is positive in yolk sac tumor as well as other testicular germ cell tumors (45). Alpha-1-antitrypsin positivity occurs in about 50 percent of yolk sac tumors (38,149). Reactivity to CEA has been reported in occasional cases: 4 of 32 cases (13 percent) in two series were positive (38,47) and the reactivity was localized to the enteric glands (47,75). Vimentin is routinely seen in the spindle cell component (153), which also reacts in many cases for pancytokeratin. EMA is usually negative (6 percent) (38) and therefore useful in helping to distinguish yolk sac tumor from somatic carcinomas in metastatic sites, as is CK7. PLAP reactivity varied from 1 to 85 percent in four studies (38,41,42,155). Laminin

is identifiable in the basement membrane component (75) and positivity for albumin, ferritin, neuron-specific enolase, and Leu-7 has been reported in some cases (38,47). Renal cell carcinoma antigen is highly expressed in yolk sac tumors (156) and p53 is heterogeneously positive (49). CD34 occurs in a minority of cases, which contrasts with its negativity in seminoma and embryonal carcinoma.

Ultrastructural Findings. Electron microscopic examination shows clusters of epithelial cells conjoined by tight junctional complexes and desmosomes (fig. 4-85) and occasionally forming extracellular lumens with apical microvilli. Abundant extracellular spaces frequently contain bands and irregularly shaped globular deposits of electron-dense basement membrane material (fig. 4-86) (75,157,158), with similar material in the dilated cisternae of the rough

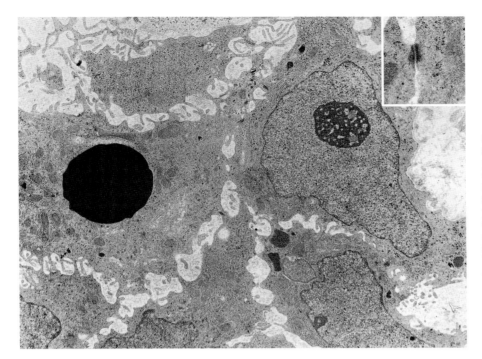

Figure 4-85

YOLK SAC TUMOR

Electron micrograph of a yolk sac tumor with a solid pattern. There are prominent cytoplasmic processes in the extracellular space, mitochondria often surrounded by rough endoplasmic reticulum, and a densely osmiophilic intracytoplasmic inclusion, representing a hyaline globule. Desmosomes connect adjacent cells (inset).

Figure 4-86

YOLK SAC TUMOR

Basement membrane material is present within dilated cisternae of the endoplasmic reticulum and also appears as osmiophilic, irregularly shaped deposits in the extracellular space. Glycogen particles are present in the cytoplasm.

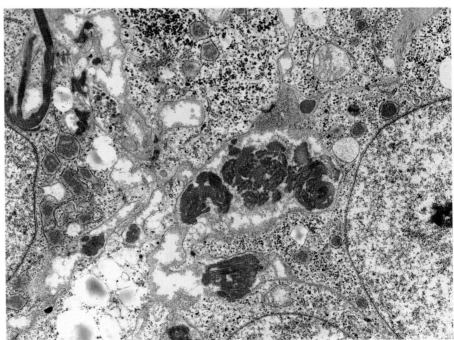

endoplastic reticulum of the adjacent cells (53). The deposits within the endoplasmic reticulum often have a central lucent zone, creating a doughnut-like appearance (53). In addition, some cells have nonmembrane-bound, densely osmiophilic, homogeneous, round cytoplasmic globules corresponding to the hyaline globules seen by light microscopy (fig. 4-85) (75,159). Glycogen may be conspicuous (157,160). The nuclei are usually irregular in shape and have a thread-like nucleolonema, as seen in seminoma. Enteric glands have microvilli with long anchoring rootlets (fig. 4-

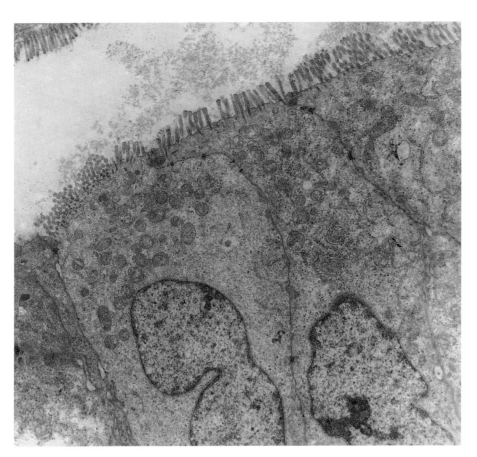

Figure 4-87

YOLK SAC TUMOR

A portion of a glandular pattern in a yolk sac tumor showing prominent apical microvilli with cytoplasmic rootlets.

87) and glycocalyx with glycocalyceal bodies, as seen in intestinal absorptive cells (75).

Cytologic Findings. In aspiration smears, yolk sac tumor often forms tight, rounded clusters of epithelial cells (fig. 4-88) (56,161). These cellular clusters are sometimes covered by a layer of flattened tumor cells (56). A characteristic feature is the association of these groups with a loosely cohesive spindle cell component (fig. 4-89). Such spindle to stellate cells may be seen in a metachromatic, myxomatous stroma (fig. 4-89). The branching capillary pattern seen in aspirations of embryonal carcinomas are not identified (56). Papillary and acinar arrangements are also characteristic (162,163). Hepatoid foci form sheets and trabeculae of polygonal cells with associated endothelial cells (164). The nuclei are often ovoid, with irregular nuclear membranes, coarse chromatin, and one or more nucleoli (fig. 4-90) (161).

Two cell types have been described, distinguished by their cytoplasmic appearances (161). One has distinct cell borders and solid cytoplasm with only small vacuoles. The other has indistinct cellular borders, tends to form syncytial clusters of cells, and has hypervacuolated or bubbly cytoplasm (fig. 4-91) (161,162). The background is often mucoid, with foamy histiocytes (muciphages) (161,162). In addition, intracytoplasmic hyaline globules and intercellular basement membrane material are identified in some cases (161,162,165). Seminoma, in contrast to yolk sac tumor, lacks the hypervacuolated cells (161). The distinctive Schiller-Duval bodies are not typically apparent in cytologic preparations, but when found, consist of tumor cells coating thin-walled, branching vessels that have occasional bulbous protrusions of attached epithelium (166). This causes an overall appearance that has been likened to a balloon animal (166).

Special Techniques. Karyotypic analysis of childhood yolk sac tumors fails to identify the i(12p) marker chromosome that is characteristic of postpubertal testicular germ cell tumors

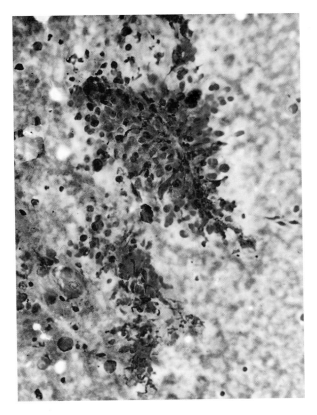

Figure 4-88

YOLK SAC TUMOR

A fine needle aspiration cytology specimen shows cohesive aggregates of tumor cells with occasional dispersed neoplastic spindle cells (Diff-Quik stain).

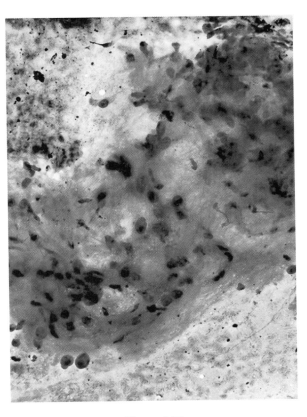

Figure 4-89

YOLK SAC TUMOR

Neoplastic spindle and polygonal cells are dispersed in a metachromatic, myxomatous stroma (Diff-Quik stain).

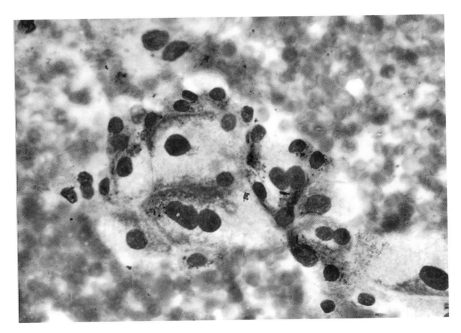

Figure 4-90

YOLK SAC TUMOR

The tumor cells have pleomorphic, ovoid nuclei with coarse chromatin and prominent nucleoli (Diff-Quik stain).

161

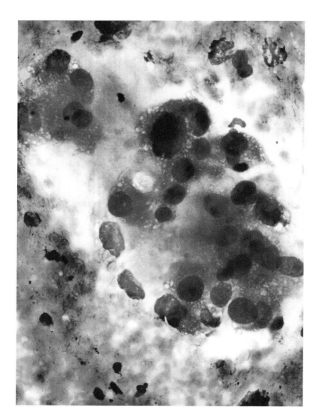

Figure 4-91

YOLK SAC TUMOR

The tumor cells have vacuolated to bubbly cytoplasm (Diff-Quik stain).

(167,168); instead, there are frequent anomalies of 1p, 6q, and 3q (168–170). The ploidy values are often either diploid or hypertriploid/peritetraploid (169,171), in contrast to the hyperdiploid/hypotriploid nature of adult nonseminomatous germ cell tumors, which are rarely diploid (171). Pediatric yolk sac tumors have more highly methylated DNA than adult germ cell tumors, in accord with the derivation of the latter from neoplastic germ cells with the characteristics of primordial germ cells having loss of genomic imprinting (172). There is a high frequency of inactivation of the adenomatous polyposis coli (*APC*) gene and the *RUNX3* gene in the yolk sac tumors of boys through a combination of promoter methylation and allelic loss (173,174). These observations, in conjunction with the usual absence of IGCNU in childhood yolk sac tumors (147,148), indicate a different formative pathway from the postpubertal tumors.

Some insight into the formation of yolk sac tumor has been gained by xenograft cultures. Cells from a mixed germ cell tumor that were grown in vitro produced tumors in nude mice that were initially composed of embryonal carcinoma and yolk sac tumor but that later had the appearance of yolk sac tumor with a peripheral rim of embryonal carcinoma, supporting the differentiation of embryonal carcinoma into yolk sac tumor (175). Additional work using in vitro germ cell lines derived from human tumors shows the potential for differentiation of some, but not all, embryonal carcinoma cells into yolk sac tumor (176). Xenograft studies suggest that seminoma may also differentiate to yolk sac tumor (177,178), as do tumors composed largely of seminoma with peripheral, multifocal rims of yolk sac tumor (179).

Differential Diagnosis. Juvenile granulosa cell tumor is a major consideration in the differential diagnosis of infants with yolk sac tumor (see chapter 6). Juvenile granulosa cell tumor presents, in most cases, prior to 6 months of age and many are congenital (180–184). This contrasts with yolk sac tumor, which uncommonly is encountered in patients less than 6 months old and has not been reported as a congenital tumor (123,124). The solid and cystic areas of juvenile granulosa cell tumor, the latter representing follicular differentiation (181,185), may be confused with the solid and reticular-cystic patterns of yolk sac tumor. A high mitotic rate may be seen in each tumor. The follicles of juvenile granulosa cell tumor, however, often are lined by several distinct layers of tumor cells and frequently are arranged in a lobular fashion with an intervening fibrous stroma, whereas the cysts in yolk sac tumor are, on average, smaller, more closely packed, and coalesce to a greater degree. An exception is the polyvesicular vitelline pattern of yolk sac tumor, but its association with typical yolk sac tumor will almost invariably aid in differentiation. The cells in most juvenile granulosa cell tumors are less primitive in appearance than those of yolk sac tumor. Cytoplasmic reactivity for AFP and negativity for alpha-inhibin contrast with the findings in juvenile granulosa cell tumor (52,183,186). Serum AFP levels in infants may not be of much use in differentiation since levels do not fall into the normal adult range until 8 months of age (187).

Rarely, Sertoli cell tumors have foci vaguely reminiscent of the reticular pattern of yolk sac tumor when edema, microcystic change, or combinations thereof are present. The nuclear characteristics in these foci are, however, generally not as primitive as in cases of yolk sac tumor, and the other patterns present, particularly the typical tubular morphology of Sertoli cell neoplasia, should facilitate the correct diagnosis. Of course, in the rare case in which it is deemed appropriate, immunohistochemical differences help in diagnosis.

Sarcomatous patterns of yolk sac tumor may simulate unclassified sex cord-stromal tumors. The latter may show foci of cystic change that further enhances this resemblance. An association with more distinctive yolk sac tumor patterns, as well as the typical presence, in the postpubertal yolk sac tumor, of IGCNU, resolves the issue. Stains for AFP, glypican 3, and alpha-inhibin are useful (see Tables 3-1 and 6-2), although in our experience, it is common for all of these to be negative in spindle cell tumors considered in this differential.

The differentiation of solid pattern yolk sac tumor and seminoma is discussed in chapter 3. From a clinical standpoint, this distinction is much more crucial than the differentiation of embryonal carcinoma from yolk sac tumor. The latter, however, may be important in determining the appropriateness of surveillance-only management since a yolk sac tumor component correlates with a decreased risk of relapse and embryonal carcinoma with a higher likelihood (90,188). Both embryonal carcinoma and yolk sac tumor may have glandular, solid, and papillary patterns; their distinction is discussed in the section on embryonal carcinoma earlier in this chapter. There remain occasional cases in which it is almost arbitrary whether a particular focus represents yolk sac tumor or embryonal carcinoma; in our experience with such cases, if the remainder of the neoplasm shows areas of both tumor types, such foci are probably transitional forms. Immunostains for CD30, OCT3/4, AFP, and glypican 3 (see Table 3-1) can help with the differential.

Rare pure glandular yolk sac tumors may be confused with teratoma (fig. 4-61). The enteric glands of yolk sac tumor lack a circumferential smooth muscle component, unlike many glands in teratomas (189). In addition, they often branch extensively, unlike the typically more simplified oval to round glands of teratoma. The presence of an admixture of teratomatous glands with other types of teratomatous tissues is also helpful. The glands of yolk sac tumor, in our experience, are frequently reactive for AFP and negative for EMA and CK7; teratomatous glands tend to have an opposite pattern of immunoreactivity, although some limited AFP reactivity can be seen.

Invasion of the rete testis by germ cell tumor elements may provoke a hyperplastic reaction of the epithelium, with the development of vacuoles and intracytoplasmic hyaline globules that may be misinterpreted as reticular yolk sac tumor (see chapter 8; fig. 8-79) (190). Differentiation depends on the scanning magnification observation of the characteristic branching pattern of the rete testis, and the high-power observation of the bland cytologic features of the hyperplastic rete epithelial cells (190). The rete epithelium, in contrast to yolk sac tumor, is strongly positive for CK7 and negative for AFP and glypican 3.

Treatment and Prognosis. The treatment of adults with yolk sac tumor (almost always as a component of a mixed germ cell tumor) does not differ from that outlined for nonseminomatous tumors in the section on embryonal carcinoma.

The approach to pediatric yolk sac tumors is often different. The current trend is conservative management of patients with clinical disease limited to the testis who lack postorchiectomy elevation of serum AFP. These patients receive close follow-up after radical orchiectomy rather than retroperitoneal lymph node dissection (191). Chemotherapy is given if relapse occurs (191,192). The rationale for this approach is based on the more frequent early stage status of pediatric yolk sac tumor compared to the postpubertal nonseminomatous tumors, with from 80 to more than 90 percent of neoplasms confined to the testis at diagnosis (131,132,193). Pediatric yolk sac tumors appear to behave less aggressively than adult nonseminomatous germ cell tumors (9,194) and the frequency of retroperitoneal metastases is low (4 to 14 percent) (132,195), with metastases more commonly developing by hematogenous routes to the lungs (125,132,196). Some, however, advocate staging lymph node dissection based on their belief that the nodal metastatic rate is higher than the usual quoted figures and that some yolk sac tumors are not associated with AFP elevation, making early diagnosis of relapse on surveillance-only protocols difficult (197). One study, for instance, failed to identify AFP elevations in 23 percent of prepubertal boys with yolk sac tumor at presentation (131).

Most studies do not discriminate between patients having nonseminomatous tumors with or without a yolk sac tumor component, making the relevance of a yolk sac tumor component hard to impossible to evaluate. There is, however, evidence that a yolk sac tumor component in a stage I mixed germ cell tumor of the testis may convey a somewhat better prognosis (95,167,198). In a study examining surveillance-only in the postorchiectomy follow-up of patients with clinical stage I nonseminomatous tumors, a multivariate analysis identified a yolk sac tumor component as a significant predictor for the absence of relapse (95). On the other hand, yolk sac tumor elements in patients with stage III testicular germ cell tumors are associated with a poor prognosis (199). This information does not contradict the other study but likely indicates that yolk sac tumor has both less metastatic potential and less chemosensitivity than embryonal carcinoma. Thus, its prognostic significance varies depending on whether or not it has disseminated. A study supporting this viewpoint documented a much higher frequency of yolk sac tumor elements during the chemotherapeutic era compared to the prechemotherapeutic era in autopsy cases (200).

Children with yolk sac tumor have a favorable prognosis, although there are some controversial aspects. In a literature review (antedating, for the most part, the revolution in the chemotherapeutic management of testicular germ cell tumors), there was a significant difference in mortality rates for children with yolk sac tumors who were less than 2 years of age (11 percent) compared to older children (77 percent) (125). More recent studies report overall survival rates in excess of 90 percent (131,191,201) and fail to identify a difference in survival with respect to age (131,201), and no difference in survival for different patterns of yolk sac tumor. It appears that the natural history of childhood yolk sac tumor is significantly different according to the

age of the patient but that advances in treatment have made this difference moot. Most (88 percent) children with yolk sac tumor present with clinical stage I disease, do not require post-orchiectomy treatment, and remain disease free. If relapse occurs (most commonly involving the lungs), almost all are effectively managed with cisplatin-based chemotherapy.

CHORIOCARCINOMA AND OTHER RARE FORMS OF TROPHOBLASTIC NEOPLASIA

Choriocarcinoma

Definition. *Choriocarcinoma* is a highly malignant tumor displaying trophoblastic differentiation. It is typically composed of an intimate admixture of multinucleated syncytiotrophoblast cells and mononucleated trophoblast cells.

General Features. Pure choriocarcinoma is rare, representing only 0.3 percent of 6,000 testis tumors in the files of the American Testicular Tumor Registry (4). Focal choriocarcinoma mixed with other germ cell tumor components is identified in about 8 percent of testicular germ cell tumors (2). There are no known distinct epidemiologic features.

Clinical Features. Unlike the other testicular germ cell tumors, patients with pure choriocarcinoma more commonly present with symptoms related to metastatic disease rather than a testicular mass. This is secondary to its frequent early and widespread dissemination prior to the development of a palpable lesion. Indeed, even after the establishment of a diagnosis of metastatic choriocarcinoma, a significant number of patients do not have palpable abnormalities in the testes. The typical presenting symptoms are hemoptysis secondary to pulmonary metastases, back pain due to retroperitoneal spread, gastrointestinal bleeding, and neurologic symptoms secondary to central nervous system involvement. Rare patients present with skin metastases (202). Most patients are in their second or third decades. No cases have been reported in prepubertal boys.

Pure tumors are often associated with marked elevations in serum levels of hCG, with values commonly greater than 100,000 IU/L. As a reflection of hormonal abnormalities associated with hCG elevations, about 10 percent of patients have clinical gynecomastia (122), which may be a presenting complaint (fig. 4-

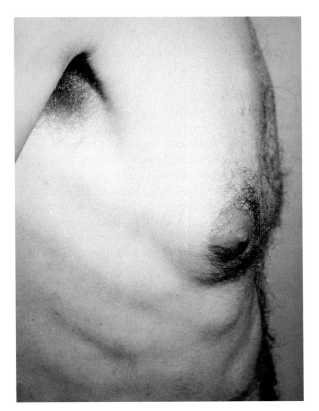

Figure 4-92

**GYNECOMASTIA IN A PATIENT
WITH CHORIOCARCINOMA**

(Courtesy of Dr. D. Gersell, St. Louis, MO.)

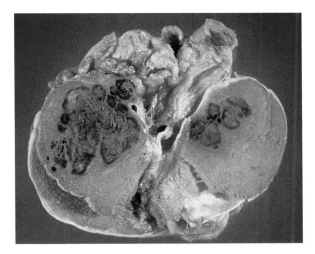

Figure 4-93

CHORIOCARCINOMA

An irregularly shaped, hemorrhagic area in the testis is the typical gross appearance.

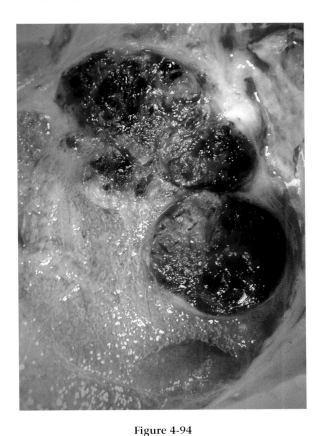

Figure 4-94

CHORIOCARCINOMA

Two distinct hemorrhagic and variegated nodules are seen.

92). A "choriocarcinoma syndrome" is caused by visceral hemorrhages due to metastases (203). Thyrotoxicosis may also occur in these patients secondary to the extreme hCG elevations and the fact that hCG has activity similar to thyroid-stimulating hormone (203,204).

Gross Findings. The external appearance of a testis with pure choriocarcinoma is often not distorted, reflecting the typically small size of these tumors. On cut section, a centrally necrotic and hemorrhagic nodule is often identified (fig. 4-93), sometimes with ill-defined, gray to tan tissue at the periphery. Two or more distinct nodules are present in some cases (fig. 4-94). In other cases, the entire testis may be hemorrhagic, often with some cystic change and separate nodules of clotted blood and tumor (fig. 4-95). Occasionally, only a hemosiderin-containing scar is identified in the testis, despite metastases (see chapter 5, Regressed Germ Cell Tumors).

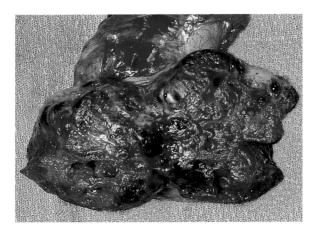

Figure 4-95

CHORIOCARCINOMA

This diffusely hemorrhagic tumor shows cystic change and distinct nodules of clotted blood and tumor.

Microscopic Findings. Most choriocarcinomas are extensively hemorrhagic and necrotic (fig. 4-96), often with little viable tumor. Diagnostic foci are typically identified at the periphery of the hemorrhagic/necrotic lesion, where there is usually an admixture of syncytiotrophoblast cells and mononuclear trophoblast cells (fig. 4-97), creating a "biphasic" pattern. In the best-differentiated examples, the cellular areas show well-defined syncytiotrophoblast cells that "cap" masses of proliferating mononucleated trophoblast cells in a pattern often described as villus-like, although stromal cores similar to those of placental villi are absent (figs. 4-98, 4-99). There is, however, one unique report of a metastatic testicular choriocarcinoma that reproduced villus-like structures with evident stromal cores (205). In other examples, the mixture

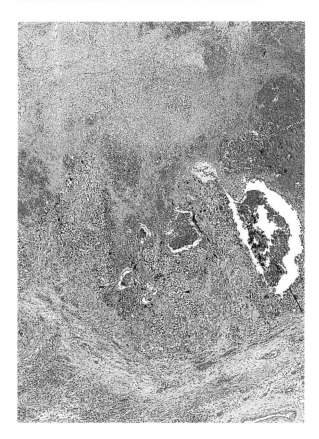

Figure 4-96

CHORIOCARCINOMA

There are large areas of hemorrhage and necrosis with a peripheral rim of viable tumor.

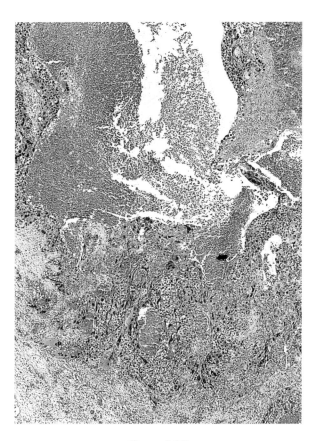

Figure 4-97

CHORIOCARCINOMA

This focus shows the diagnostic admixture of syncytiotrophoblast and mononucleated trophoblast cells at the periphery of a zone of hemorrhage and necrosis.

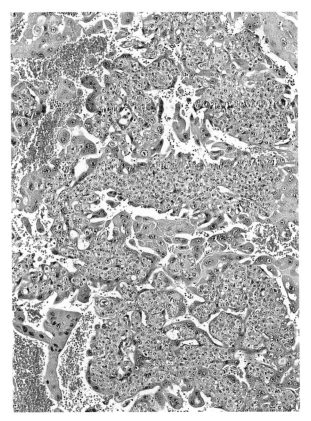

Figure 4-98

CHORIOCARCINOMA

The mononucleated trophoblast component consists of sheet-like collections of cells with pale cytoplasm and distinct borders that are "capped" by multinucleated cells (syncytiotrophoblasts) with dark, eosinophilic cytoplasm.

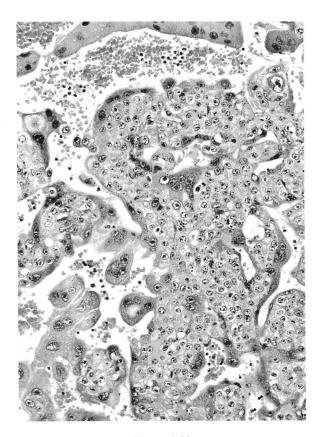

Figure 4-99

CHORIOCARCINOMA

A central collection of pale mononucleated trophoblast cells is surrounded by multinucleated syncytiotrophoblasts with eosinophilic cytoplasm and vesicular nuclei.

of syncytiotrophoblasts and mononucleated trophoblasts appears random (fig. 4-100). In some cases, the syncytiotrophoblast cells appear compressed and relatively inconspicuous (fig. 4-101). Uncommonly, syncytiotrophoblast cells are rare, creating a "monophasic" appearance (fig. 4-102). Occasionally, distinct areas of syncytiotrophoblast cells are seen; at other times, the distinction between syncytiotrophoblast and mononucleated trophoblast is indistinct, but there is a nodular proliferation of trophoblastic cells that range from small to large, mononucleated and occasional multinucleated forms (fig. 4-103). Many of the cells in these cases are similar to intermediate trophoblasts of gestational tissues, having large, single, or occasionally double nuclei and abundant, well-defined, eosinophilic cytoplasm, a resemblance further supported by immunostaining (206).

A distinctive feature in most cases is prominent blood vessel invasion; clumps of cohesive syncytiotrophoblasts and mononucleated trophoblasts are easily identified within the vessel lumens (fig. 4-104). In tumors with extensive necrosis, remnant syncytiotrophoblast cells are identifiable within the central necrotic coagulum (fig. 4-105), and such cells may be highlighted by immunostains for hCG (see below). It is necessary to have stringent criteria for the diagnosis of choriocarcinoma since it is common to see syncytiotrophoblast cells without associated mononucleated trophoblasts in other germ cell tumors, particularly embryonal carcinoma, seminoma, and mixed germ cell tumors with those components.

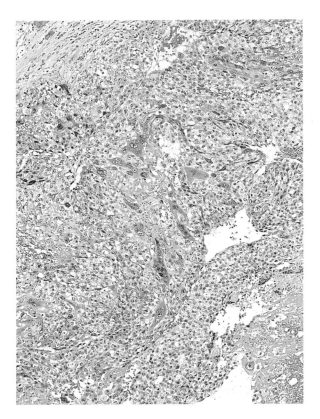

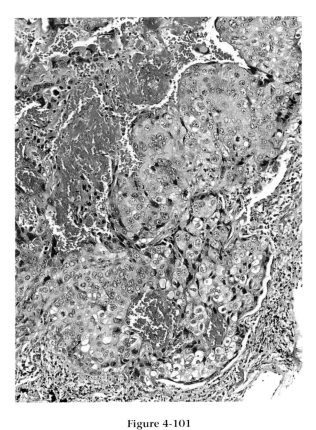

Figure 4-100

CHORIOCARCINOMA

This tumor shows a more or less random admixture of mononucleated trophoblast cells and larger, syncytiotrophoblast cells, with a subtle impression of the more "classic" mantling by the syncytiotrophoblast cells.

Figure 4-101

CHORIOCARCINOMA

The syncytiotrophoblast cells are less conspicuous and have a focal spindle cell configuration with darkly staining, smudged nuclei.

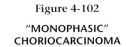

Figure 4-102

"MONOPHASIC" CHORIOCARCINOMA

There is a diffuse arrangement of mononucleated trophoblast cells with interspersed foci of necrosis and fibrin deposits.

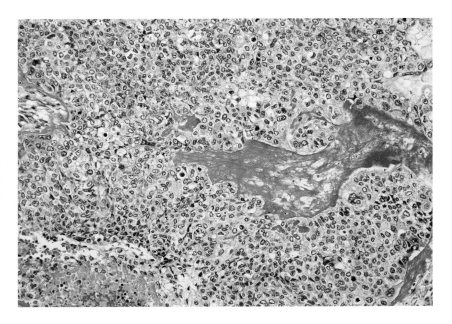

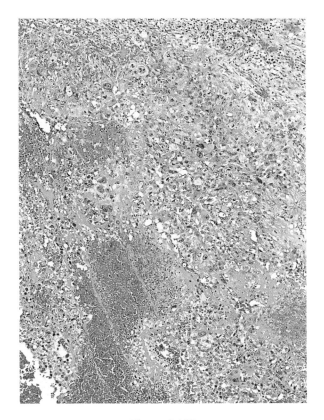

Figure 4-103

CHORIOCARCINOMA

There is a spectrum of malignant trophoblastic cells, from small to large mononucleated forms.

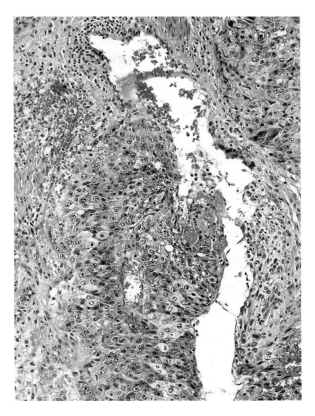

Figure 4-104

CHORIOCARCINOMA

A focus of tumor consisting mostly of mononucleated trophoblast cells invades the lumen of a blood vessel. Fibrin is seen on the tumor surface.

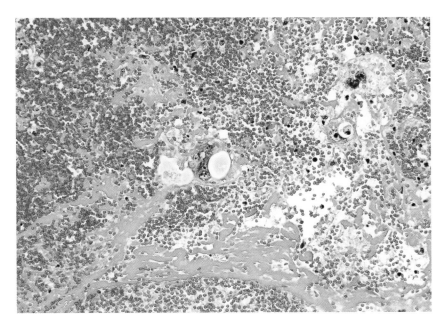

Figure 4-105

CHORIOCARCINOMA

Degenerate syncytiotrophoblast cells are recognizable within the central hemorrhagic zone of this tumor.

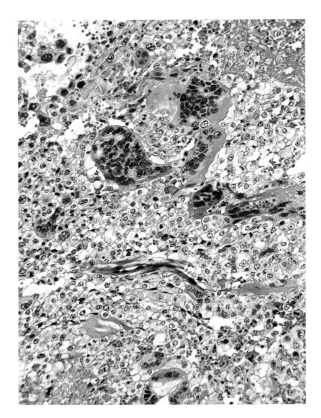

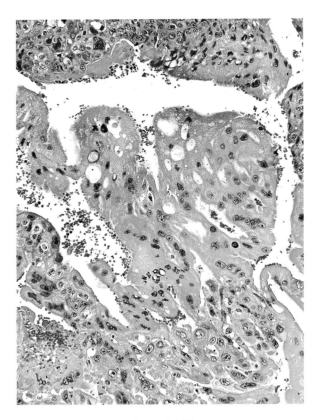

Figure 4-106

CHORIOCARCINOMA

Syncytiotrophoblast cells with numerous, often smudged nuclei are admixed with mononucleated trophoblast cells with clear cytoplasm and well-defined cytoplasmic membranes.

Figure 4-107

CHORIOCARCINOMA

Large syncytiotrophoblast cells have multiple cytoplasmic lacunae that occasionally contain eosinophilic material.

Syncytiotrophoblast cells in choriocarcinoma have a variable morphology. They are most easily recognized when they occur as large cells with eosinophilic to amphophilic cytoplasm; several to numerous vesicular to deeply chromatic, irregular, sometimes smudged nuclei (figs. 4-99, 4-106); and distinct cytoplasmic vacuoles or lacunae (fig. 4-107). Such vacuoles or lacunae may contain erythrocytes or an eosinophilic precipitate. Nucleoli may be prominent in cells with less dense nuclei (fig. 4-99). Less distinctive variants of syncytiotrophoblasts occur. In some instances, multinucleation is not prominent, although giant nuclei are seen (fig. 4-103). Cytoplasmic vacuoles are often not identified, and the syncytiotrophoblasts may be small and mainly distinguished from the associated mononucleated trophoblast cells by more deeply staining cytoplasm, smudged nuclei, and a syncytial appearance (fig. 4-104)

(19). Syncytiotrophoblasts are mitotically inactive and do not incorporate ³H-thymidine (207). They often abut thin-walled capillaries adjacent to foci of hemorrhage.

The mononucleated trophoblast cells usually have pale cytoplasm and mildly pleomorphic nuclei with prominent nucleoli (fig. 4-99). Discrete cell borders are usually apparent (fig. 4-106). In contrast to the nonproliferative syncytiotrophoblast cells, they often show conspicuous numbers of mitotic figures. Traditionally, mononucleated trophoblast cells have been considered to show cytotrophoblastic differentiation, but it is now clear that they may also resemble intermediate trophoblast cells (206,208), so we feel it is better to designate them descriptively as "mononucleated trophoblast" cells. Mononucleated trophoblast cell types typically have more densely eosinophilic cytoplasm and larger

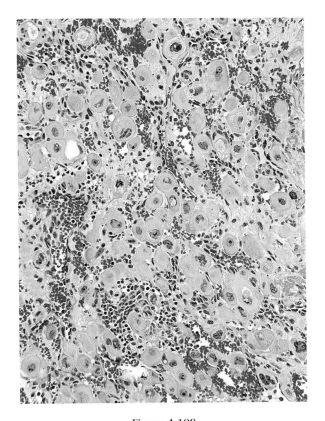

Figure 4-108

CHORIOCARCINOMA

This focus of pure intermediate-type trophoblast cells occurred in an otherwise typical choriocarcinoma. The dense, eosinophilic cytoplasm imparts a vaguely squamoid appearance.

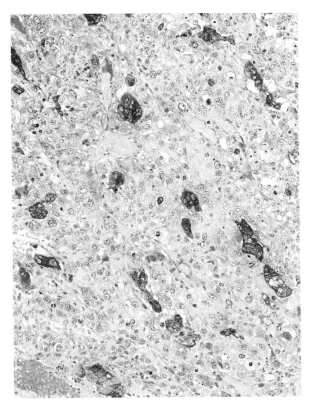

Figure 4-109

CHORIOCARCINOMA

The multinucleated syncytiotrophoblast cells stain intensely with anti-human chorionic gonadotropin (hCG) (anti-hCG immunostain).

nuclei than the classic cytotrophoblast cells (fig. 4-108); as a consequence, those tumors whose mononucleated component is skewed toward these variant trophoblastic morphologies tend to be less biphasic in appearance (figs. 4-102, 4-103) than those with a predominance of cytotrophoblastic differentiation.

Most choriocarcinomas do not generate a significant host inflammatory reaction. There is a report, however, of a rare case that had both an extensive lymphocytic infiltrate and a prominent granulomatous reaction (209).

Immunohistochemical Findings. hCG is the most valuable marker for choriocarcinoma and is positive in the syncytiotrophoblast component in essentially all cases (fig. 4-109). It is also positive within occasional large mononucleated trophoblast cells (38,149,206). The classic cytotrophoblast cells are generally

weakly positive or negative for hCG (figs. 4-109, 4-110). Pregnancy-specific beta-1-glycoprotein (SP1) and HPL are also positive within the syncytiotrophoblast cells and within trophoblastic cells of intermediate type (206). Inhibin is positive in syncytiotrophoblast cells (52,208), as is epidermal growth factor receptor (210,211) and glypican 3 (76,77). Patchy PLAP positivity occurs in 54 percent of choriocarcinomas (38); CEA is demonstrable in 25 percent of cases in both syncytiotrophoblast (212) and cytotrophoblast (38) cells. Cytokeratins occur in all cell types (19,38), usually cytokeratins 7, 8, 18, and 19 (213). Antibodies to CK7 mark a number of trophoblastic cells in choriocarcinoma, contrasting with the typically negative staining in seminoma, embryonal carcinoma, and yolk sac tumor (154). Nuclear reactivity for p63 is identified in the cytotrophoblastic component

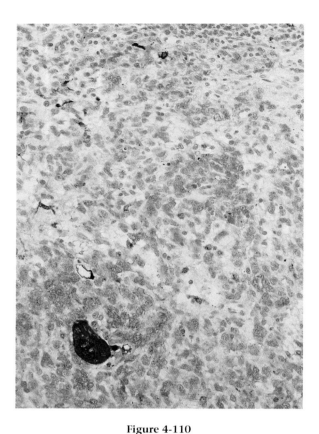

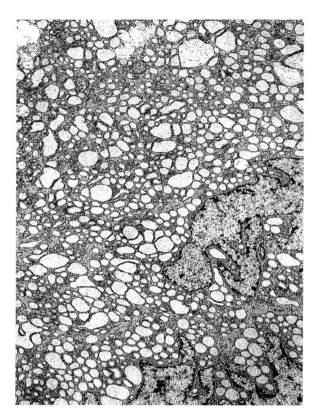

Figure 4-110

CHORIOCARCINOMA

There is weak but diffuse positivity for hCG in the predominant mononucleated trophoblasts, with strong reactivity in the rare syncytiotrophoblasts.

Figure 4-111

CHORIOCARCINOMA

An electron micrograph shows a syncytiotrophoblast cell with irregularly shaped nuclei in a shared cytoplasm. There are numerous dilated cisternae of rough endoplasmic reticulum producing a honeycomb-like pattern.

(214). Unlike seminoma, embryonal carcinoma, and yolk sac tumor, many choriocarcinomas (46 percent) react with antibodies directed against EMA, mainly in syncytiotrophoblast cells (38). A heterogeneous pattern of positivity for p53 has also been identified in choriocarcinomas (49).

Ultrastructural Findings. On ultrastructural examination, syncytiotrophoblast cells demonstrate several nuclei in a shared cytoplasm; there is also a strikingly prominent rough endoplasmic reticulum, with dilated cisternae frequently producing a honeycomb-like pattern (fig. 4-111) (215). The cisternae contain electron-dense, protein-like material that is also identifiable in the surrounding extracellular space (53). Desmosome-like attachments join adjacent cells, both syncytiotrophoblast and mononucleated trophoblast, and prominent interdigitating microvilli are present on the cell membranes

of the syncytiotrophoblasts. In contrast, the cytoplasm of mononucleated trophoblast cells contains only short profiles of tubular endoplasmic reticulum with numerous free cytoplasmic ribosomes (fig. 4-112). The nuclei of mononucleated trophoblast cells are more regular and round than those of embryonal carcinoma cells, although heterochromatin clumps and nucleoli remain prominent (53). Some cells have features intermediate between syncytiotrophoblasts and mononucleated trophoblasts (215), which, in conjunction with similar nuclear features (53), supports a derivation of syncytiotrophoblasts from mononucleated trophoblasts.

Cytologic Findings. The key diagnostic findings for choriocarcinoma are admixtures of malignant mononucleated cells with the more distinctive multinucleated syncytiotrophoblastic

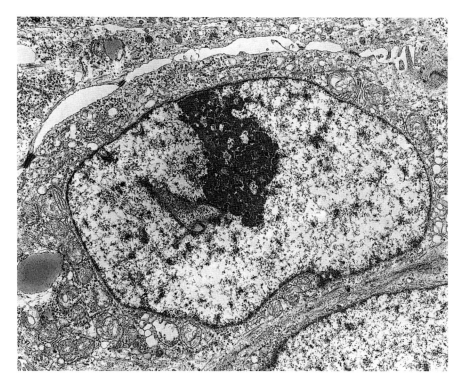

Figure 4-112

CHORIOCARCINOMA

An electron micrograph shows a cytotrophoblast cell with simple-appearing cytoplasm that contains scattered cisternae of rough endoplasmic reticulum, mitochondria, and a lipid droplet. The nucleus is round with a prominent nucleolus. Well-developed desmosomes (upper left) join the cell to an adjacent one.

giant cells, usually in a background of necrotic debris, fibrin, and hemorrhage (fig. 4-113). The mononucleated trophoblasts, by themselves, are not easily recognized as derived from choriocarcinoma. They typically occur in small clusters of irregular to oval-shaped cells with pale to clear, granular to vacuolated cytoplasm; large nuclei with dispersed chromatin; and a single prominent nucleolus (fig. 4-114). The syncytiotrophoblast cells vary from scant to numerous and may "cap" the mononucleated cells (fig. 4-113) or be randomly dispersed with them. The cytoplasm is usually dense and granular but may have fine vacuoles. The multiple nuclei vary from a few to numerous, and often have condensed chromatin with a variably prominent nucleolus (216).

Differential Diagnosis. Choriocarcinoma with extensive hemorrhagic necrosis must be distinguished from hemorrhagic testicular infarction due to torsion, trauma, thromboembolic disease, or hypercoagulable states. Most patients with testicular infarction have painful, diffuse testicular enlargement, in contrast to most patients with choriocarcinoma. Furthermore, the testis, at least in the earlier stages of hemorrhagic infarction, is edematous, and residual outlines

of seminiferous tubules can usually be identified within the infarcted area (see chapter 8, fig. 8-22); such outlines are not identified within the cystic/hemorrhagic portions of extensively necrotic choriocarcinomas. Generous sampling and sections from the periphery of the lesion are more apt to identify recognizable tumor cells. Sections of nontumorous testis may permit identification of IGCNU within intact seminiferous tubules. Stains for hCG may identify trophoblastic cells, but the necrotic background often causes a high level of nonspecific staining, which makes interpretation difficult.

Choriocarcinoma must be distinguished from other testicular germ cell tumors with intermingled syncytiotrophoblast cells. The syncytiotrophoblast cells that occur in seminoma are dispersed as individual cells and small clusters, with the surrounding neoplasm having the typical morphology of seminoma, including the characteristic lymphoid infiltrate and fibrous septa. In choriocarcinoma, the cells associated with the syncytiotrophoblasts are mononucleated trophoblasts, the tumor usually has a greater hemorrhagic and necrotic background, and there are no stromal (fibrous septa) and lymphoid components.

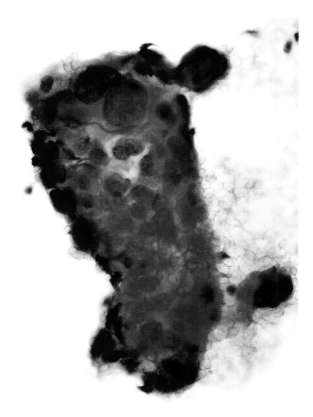

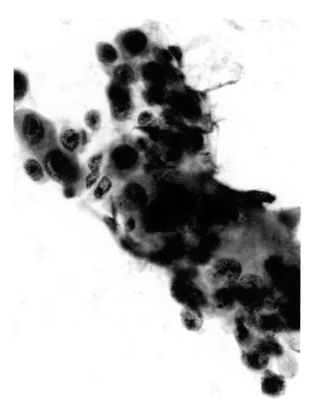

Figure 4-113

CHORIOCARCINOMA

A fine needle aspiration specimen of metastatic choriocarcinoma shows a cluster of cohesive malignant cells with marked variation in nuclear size. The syncytiotrophoblast cells have very large nuclei and are peripherally located, "capping" the mononucleated trophoblast cells. The background is hemorrhagic (Papanicolau stain).

Figure 4-114

CHORIOCARCINOMA

A fine needle aspiration specimen of metastatic choriocarcinoma shows a cluster of cohesive, malignant, mononucleated trophoblast cells with lightly staining cytoplasm. Some of the nuclei have very large nucleoli.

Most embryonal carcinomas with syncytiotrophoblasts are readily distinguished from choriocarcinoma. A problem arises with embryonal carcinomas with the "appliqué" pattern in which there are dark, smudged cells resembling syncytiotrophoblasts admixed with embryonal carcinoma cells, creating a biphasic appearance mimicking choriocarcinoma. A lack of hemorrhage in such a case favors embryonal carcinoma. In difficult cases, the diagnosis is made with immunostains against hCG, CD30, and OCT3/4: the former is negative and the latter two positive in embryonal carcinoma in contrast to choriocarcinoma. We have seen some cases that have hybrid features of these two tumors and may represent "transitional" forms, as illustrated by Friedman and Moore (3) and Dixon and Moore (17).

Spread and Metastasis. Choriocarcinoma may metastasize hematogenously in the absence of lymph node involvement (217). In autopsy studies, not only was there involvement of the usual metastatic sites of testicular germ cell tumors, but also of the lungs (100 percent), liver (86 percent), gastrointestinal tract (71 percent), and spleen, brain, and adrenal gland (56 percent) (4). A disproportionate number of brain metastases at autopsy in patients with metastatic testicular germ cell tumors are choriocarcinomas (218).

Treatment and Prognosis. Because of its tendency to disseminate widely by hematogenous routes prior to diagnosis, pure choriocarcinoma carries a worse prognosis than other testicular germ cell tumors. Also, a greater amount of choriocarcinoma in mixed germ cell tumors has

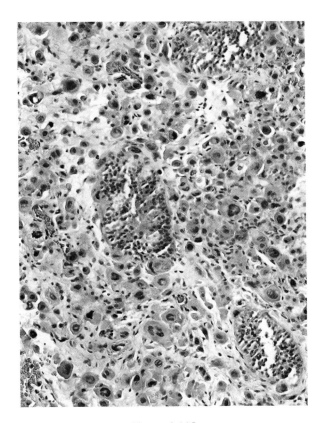

Figure 4-115

PLACENTAL SITE TROPHOBLASTIC TUMOR

Atypical, mostly mononucleated intermediate trophoblast cells invade the interstitium. Residual seminiferous tubules are visible.

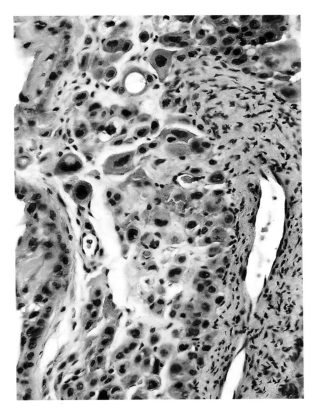

Figure 4-116

PLACENTAL SITE TROPHOBLASTIC TUMOR

Mononucleated trophoblast cells invade the wall of a thick blood vessel.

an adverse impact on prognosis (17,219-221). It remains unclear whether there is a threshold amount of choriocarcinoma below which deterioration in prognosis does not occur. Multivariate analyses of clinical prognostic factors in patients with metastatic nonseminomatous germ cell tumors have shown a worse prognosis associated with increased levels of serum hCG (203,222,223) and with the identification of choriocarcinomatous or trophoblastic elements in the primary tumor (203,222,224,225). A high mortality rate is associated with a "choriocarcinoma syndrome" where patients have hemorrhagic visceral metastases, including in the brain (203). Despite these findings, some patients with metastatic testicular choriocarcinoma are cured by chemotherapy (203,226). Four of seven patients (57 percent) with metastatic choriocarcinoma, with or without embryonal

carcinoma, were disease-free on follow-up in one study (203).

Placental Site Trophoblastic Tumor

There are two documented testicular cases of a neoplasm resembling the *placental site trophoblastic tumor* of the uterus (PSTT) (227–229). One (228) occurred in a 16-month-old boy and consisted of mostly mononucleated trophoblastic cells in a fibrous to edematous stroma. The cells had a moderate amount of dense, eosinophilic to amphophilic cytoplasm and hyperchromatic, smudged nuclei with occasional binucleated forms (fig. 4-115). Distinct populations of syncytiotrophoblastic and cytotrophoblastic cells were absent. Small zones of hemorrhage occurred and the tumor cells invaded the vessel walls (fig. 4-116). There was strong and diffuse immunohistochemical reactivity for HPL (fig. 4-117),

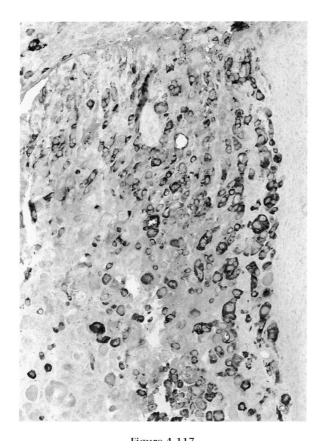

Figure 4-117

PLACENTAL SITE TROPHOBLASTIC TUMOR

Strong positivity for human placental lactogen (HPL) is present (anti-HPL immunostain).

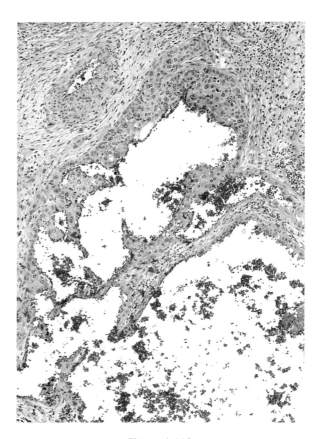

Figure 4-118

CYSTIC TROPHOBLASTIC TUMOR

This cystic space contains blood and is lined by squamoid-appearing, non-necrotic trophoblastic cells.

with only focal reactivity for hCG. The patient was well 8 years after orchiectomy, without adjuvant therapy. A second case (229) occurred in the testis of a 24-year-old man in association with teratoma and was morphologically similar to the first case. The patient was alive and well 3 years after orchiectomy without additional treatment. Another case of PSTT was reported in a retroperitoneal metastasis of a patient whose testicular tumor had small foci of intermediate trophoblast cells (230). Because choriocarcinomas may have foci with a predominance of intermediate trophoblast cells (fig. 4-108), it is important that the entire tumor is composed of intermediate-type trophoblasts and that the usual patterns of choriocarcinoma are absent. We have also seen partially regressed choriocarcinomas where the residual neoplastic cells have almost entirely consisted of intermediate trophoblasts, although in a background

of fibrosis and siderophages. Evidence of such regression is helpful in the distinction from placental site trophoblastic tumor.

Cystic Trophoblastic Tumor

This distinctive form of trophoblastic neoplasm is mostly seen in metastatic sites following chemotherapy for germ cell tumors that may or may not have had an identifiable choriocarcinoma component (231). We have seen occasional cases as well in primary, untreated testicular germ cell tumors of mixed type that lacked a choriocarcinoma component. They consisted of cysts lined by one or multiple layers of mostly mononucleated, often squamoid trophoblast cells with eosinophilic to pale cytoplasm, sometimes having distinct vacuoles (fig. 4-118). The cyst may be either empty or contain small amounts of blood. Stains for hCG are typically only focally positive in the epithelium. These lesions are invariably associated with other forms of germ cell tumor, making assessment of their biologic behavior impossible. When seen at metastatic sites after chemotherapy, they have had a clinical course similar to that of teratoma (231).

TERATOMA

Definition. *Teratoma* is a neoplasm of germ cell origin that differentiates to form somatic-type tissues typical of either adult or embryonic development. The *dermoid cyst* is recognized as a specific subcategory of teratoma. The nosologic position of epidermoid cyst is debatable, and it is considered separately.

General Features. Pure teratomas account for 3 to 4 percent of testicular germ cell tumors (2,232). They occur in two distinct age groups, and the prognosis of the lesion differs accordingly. Teratomas are the second most common germ cell tumor of infancy and childhood, representing 29 percent of cases in two combined prepubertal testicular tumor registries (123,124) and occurring at a median age of 13 months (124). Most occur prior to 4 years of age (123,124). In this group, teratomas are almost always pure. The second age group prone to develop teratoma is young adults, with the typical age distribution as seen for other germ cell tumors. These teratomas are most commonly admixed with other types of germ cell tumor (i.e., mixed germ cell tumors, see chapter 5), rather than pure; about 50 percent of mixed germ cell tumors have a teratoma component (2,232).

Associated congenital anomalies have been described in patients with childhood germ cell tumors, including teratomas: inguinal hernia (7 percent), testicular malformation or maldescent (5 percent), other genitourinary tract anomalies (2.5 percent), Down syndrome (2 percent), Klinefelter syndrome (1.5 percent), xeroderma pigmentosa (0.5 percent), ataxia (0.5 percent), hemihypertrophy (0.5 percent), spina bifida (0.5 percent), hemophilia (0.5 percent), umbilical hernia (0.5 percent), and retrocaval ureter (0.5 percent) (233). In postpubertal patients, the general epidemiologic features of germ cell tumors apply (see chapter 1).

It is not unusual for postpubertal patients with pure testicular teratomas to develop metastases that contain nonteratomatous germ cell tumor elements (221,234–236). Our explanation for this phenomenon is that teratoma of the postpubertal testis almost always develops from a malignant nonteratomatous germ cell tumor precursor. This precursor may metastasize but also differentiate in the testis to form teratoma. The malignant potential of postpubertal teratoma contrasts with the benign behavior of prepubertal teratoma, with a rare possible exception (237). The difference in biologic behavior of pure teratoma in prepubertal and postpubertal patients reflects a fundamentally different pathogenesis in these two groups, and this is reflected by the absence of IGCNU in the former and its presence in the latter (238), as well as genetic differences (see chapter 2).

Although a distinction has been made between mature and immature teratoma in the past, the current World Health Organization (WHO) classification no longer recognizes these subsets. The rationale for this approach is the lack of any known differences in behavior or management implications for "mature" versus "immature" teratoma.

Clinical Features. Most patients seek medical consultation because of testicular enlargement. Postpubertal patients, in addition, may have symptoms due to metastatic involvement. In three series, the metastatic frequency in postpubertal patients with pure teratomas ranged from 20 to 46 percent (234,236,239), figures that are likely falsely elevated because they derive from referral centers that have selection bias. In patients with pure teratomas, the usual serum markers are negative, although some adult patients may have marker elevations due to discordant histologies in the testis compared to metastases. In addition, several studies have documented endodermal derivatives in teratomas that immunostain for AFP (47,149,240), so some degree of serum AFP elevation is theoretically compatible with a diagnosis of pure teratoma, although we are not aware of any such testicular cases. Children less than 8 months old may have physiologically "elevated" AFP levels unrelated to the tumor (241).

Gross Findings. Pure teratomas are usually nodular and distort the tunica albuginea. Extratesticular extension is rare (17). The cut surface is usually cystic and solid, with the cysts

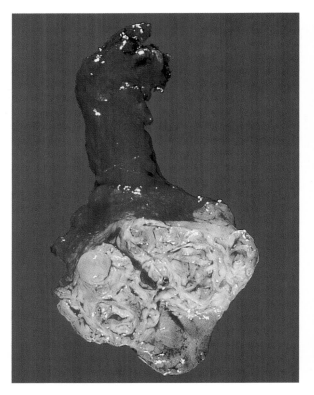

Figure 4-119

TERATOMA

The typical cut surface of a teratoma composed of "mature" elements shows multiple cysts that contain serous to mucoid fluid.

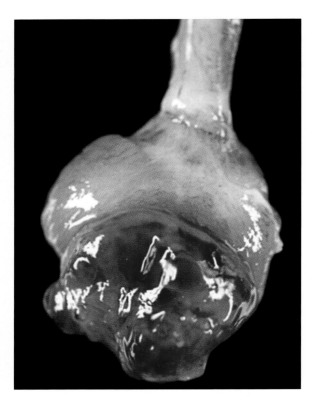

Figure 4-120

TERATOMA

This teratoma from a child is extensively mucoid.

filled with mucoid, keratinous, or serous-type fluid (figs. 4-119). The solid areas may contain translucent, gray-white nodules. Occasional tumors, more commonly those in children in our experience, are myxoid (fig. 4-120). Small, white to yellow nodular excrescences represent keratin protruding from the center of squamous epithelial-lined nests (fig. 4-121). Hair is rarely identified except in dermoid cysts. Small patches of black pigment may be seen (corresponding to melanin-containing choroidal epithelium). Immature tissues are most frequently solid and have an encephaloid, hemorrhagic, or necrotic appearance (fig. 4-122). Dermoid cysts are rare and have a similar appearance to their much more common ovarian counterpart; they are usually unilocular and filled with grumous, keratinous material and hair, with protruding nodules in the cyst wall (fig. 4-123). Particularly large teratomas may be seen in intra-abdominal

testes since they do not come to clinical attention as quickly as those in the scrotum (fig. 4-124). Small teratomas in adults are sometimes associated with massive retroperitoneal metastases of nonteratomatous germ cell tumors (fig. 4-125)

Microscopic Findings. Because of important morphologic differences, postpubertal and prepubertal teratomas are considered separately.

Postpubertal Teratoma. Various elements, commonly but not invariably deriving from the three germ layers, are identified. Nests of squamous epithelium within a fibrous stroma, some centrally cystic and containing keratin, are frequent (fig. 4-126). Many cysts are lined by glandular epithelium of enteric type, showing both absorptive and goblet cells (fig. 4-127); some contain only mucinous cells. Other glands are lined by ciliated respiratory-type epithelium. Some glands may be architecturally complex,

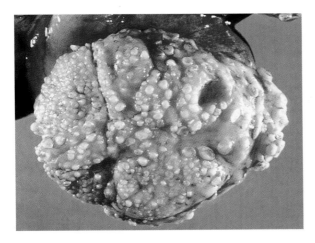

Figure 4-121

TERATOMA

There are multiple nodular excrescences of keratin protruding from small, squamous epithelial-lined cysts. (Fig. 3.38 from Young RH, Scully RE. Testicular tumors. Chicago: ASCP Press; 1990:66.)

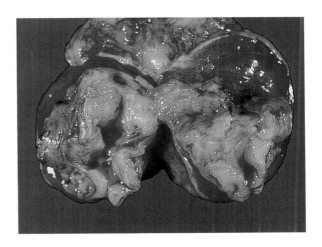

Figure 4-122

TERATOMA

The cut surface of a teratoma with an abundant amount of immature neuroectodermal tissue is predominantly solid and encephaloid.

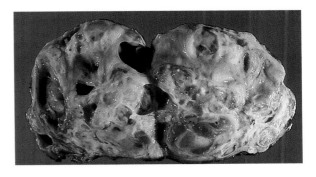

Figure 4-124

TERATOMA

This large neoplasm replaced an intra-abdominal testis.

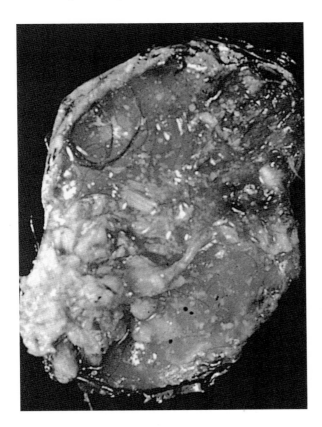

Figure 4-123

DERMOID CYST

A hair-containing cyst has central keratinous material.

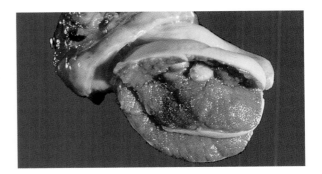

Figure 4-125

TERATOMA

The patient with this small tumor presented with a retroperitoneal metastasis that contained yolk sac tumor.

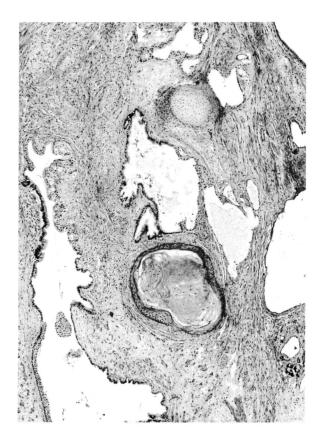

Figure 4-126

TERATOMA

This tumor has a squamous epithelial-lined cyst, a nodule of cartilage, and cysts lined by simple, columnar and cuboidal epithelium. At the lower left, the large cyst is partially lined by transitional epithelium.

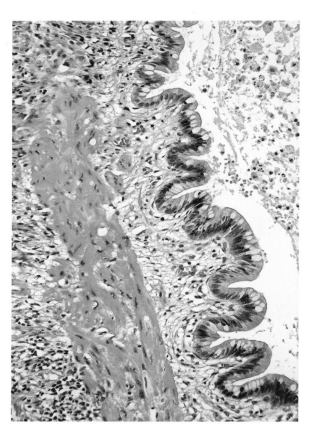

Figure 4-127

TERATOMA

This cyst is lined by enteric-type epithelium having absorptive and goblet cells. There is a subepithelial layer of smooth muscle.

with frequent outpouchings or a cribriform arrangement (fig. 4-128). Nests of transitional epithelium are common. Pigmented, retinal-type epithelium is present in occasional cases (fig. 4-129). Epithelium typical of kidney, liver, prostate gland (242,243), pancreas, thyroid gland (fig. 4-130), or choroid plexus is unusual, with a rare report of "struma testis" (244). A focal surface covering of meninges with neuroglia may rarely be seen (3), and we have seen one case in which meninges were prominent (fig. 4-131). Rarely, foci resembling pleomorphic adenoma of the salivary gland are seen (3). Perforation of keratin-containing squamous cysts often induces an inflammatory reaction with foreign body giant cells.

Incomplete organoid differentiation may be seen, most commonly in the form of smooth

muscle cells encircling enteric and respiratory epithelial-lined glands, and mimicking intestine and bronchus, respectively (fig. 4-132). In addition to smooth muscle, other frequently found stromal tissues include hypocellular fibrous tissue, hyaline cartilage (fig. 4-133), and, less commonly, adipose tissue. Rarely, a tumor consists almost exclusively of cartilage (fig. 4-134). Foci of neuroglia, sometimes with ependymal differentiation, are common. Bone is less frequent but may contain hematopoietic marrow.

Significant cytologic atypia of various elements may be encountered in postpubertal teratomas, regardless of their "mature" or "immature" nature. Thus, certain tissues show nuclear enlargement and hyperchromasia, and occasional mitotic figures, both within mesenchymal and epithelial types (figs. 4-133,

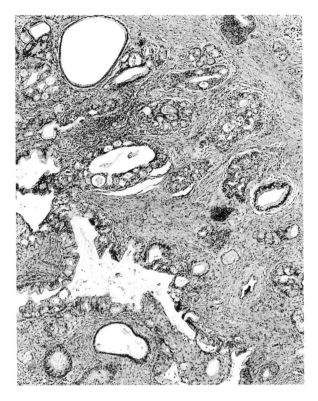

Figure 4-128

TERATOMA

There are complex glands, some with a cribriform pattern.

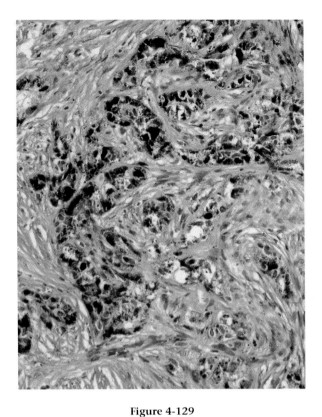

Figure 4-129

TERATOMA

This tumor contains pigmented retinal-type epithelium.

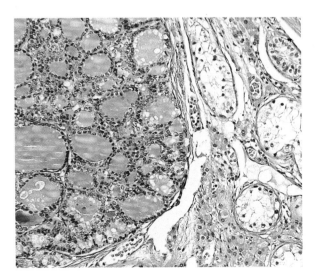

Figure 4-130

TERATOMA

Thyroid tissue is present.

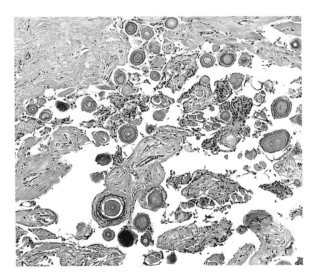

Figure 4-131

TERATOMA

Prominent meningeal tissue with numerous psammoma bodies is formed.

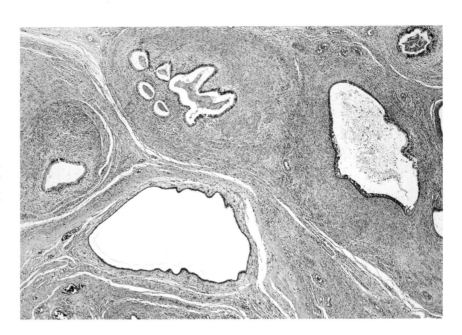

Figure 4-132

TERATOMA

This teratoma shows gut-like structures lined by enteric epithelium with absorptive and goblet cells and encircled by smooth muscle.

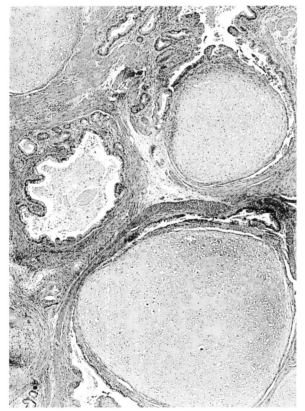

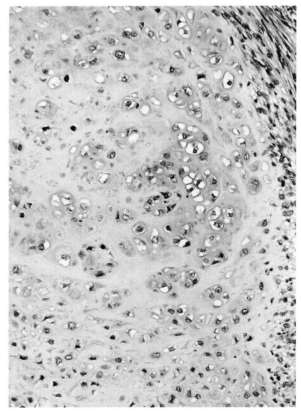

Figure 4-133

TERATOMA

Left: There are nodules of cartilage, glands lined by enteric-type epithelium, and fibromuscular stroma.
Right: The cartilage is cellular and cytologically atypical.

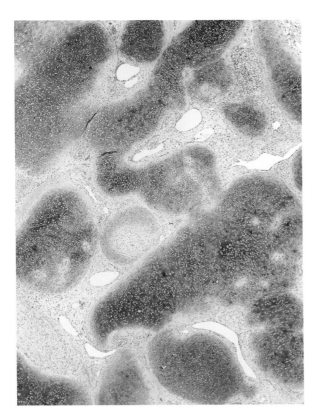

Figure 4-134

TERATOMA

Cartilage is predominant in this case.

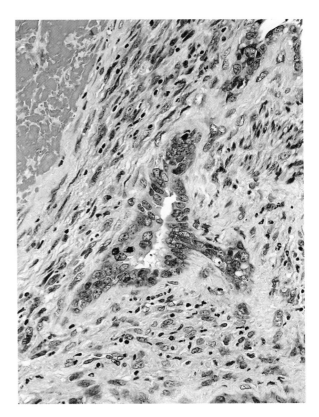

Figure 4-135

TERATOMA

There is significant atypia of the glandular epithelium and the surrounding stroma. Atypical glands such as this may be confused with embryonal carcinoma.

4-135). In some cases, the appearance of atypical teratomatous epithelium overlaps to a degree with that of embryonal carcinoma (fig. 4-135), although the nuclei are less pleomorphic and immunohistochemical differences remain.

Embryonic-like immature tissues are usually of neuroectodermal type and less commonly have a nephroblastic appearance. Neuroectoderm often consists of cells arranged in tubules (fig. 4-136) and rosettes (fig. 4-137), with foci of more diffuse growth (fig. 4-138). Primitive neural-type tubules may be formed, consisting of columnar, stratified tumor cells with apical mitotic figures arranged in a radial fashion around a central lumen and separated from the surrounding stroma by an investing basement membrane (fig. 4-136). Ependymoblastic-type rosettes are also seen; these usually consist of a radial arrangement of tumor cells around a small luminal space with a nuclear free zone of

fibrillary eosinophilic cytoplasm in the immediately subluminal zone (fig. 4-139). Such rosettes tend to blend with the surrounding cells, lacking the investing basement membrane of the neural-type tubules. Blastema-like foci consist of oval to spindle cells with scant cytoplasm in generally nodular arrays; the frequent admixture with primitive-appearing tubules lined by cuboidal to columnar cells with scant cytoplasm and high nuclear to cytoplasmic ratios creates an appearance similar to nephroblastoma (fig. 4-140). Sometimes primitive-appearing tubules occur in the absence of blastema (figs. 4-141, 4-142). Embryonic rhabdomyoblastic tissue is sometimes identified (fig. 4-143), as well as more mature-appearing, fetal-type skeletal muscle (fig. 4-144). In contrast to teratoma with a secondary malignant component (described separately), these highly immature elements

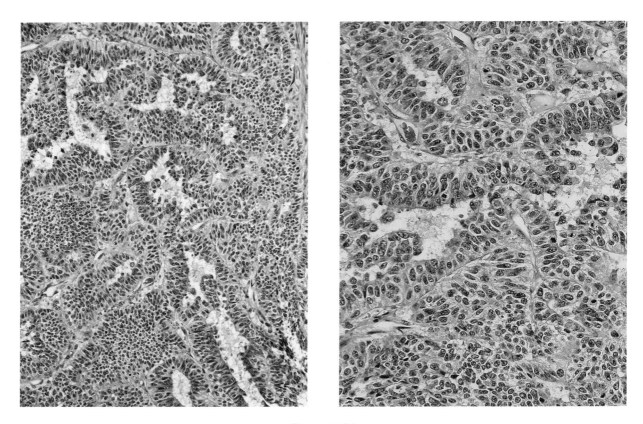

Figure 4-136

TERATOMA

Left: Multiple embryonic-type neural tubules are lined by stratified columnar cells with frequent mitotic figures.

Right: The tubules are lined by stratified, atypical columnar cells with occasional mitotic figures along the luminal edge.

Figure 4-137

TERATOMA

This focus of immature neuro-ectoderm forms multiple true rosettes.

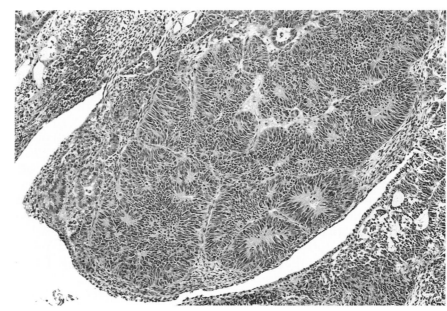

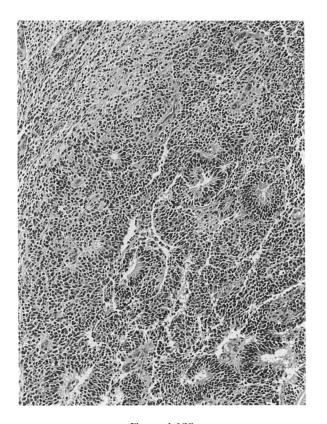

Figure 4-138

TERATOMA

The tumor cell are arranged in tubules and rosettes but also more diffusely.

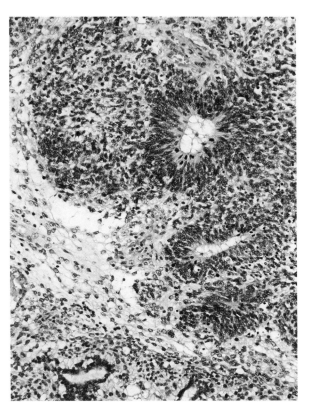

Figure 4-139

TERATOMA

Ependymoblastic rosettes are present.

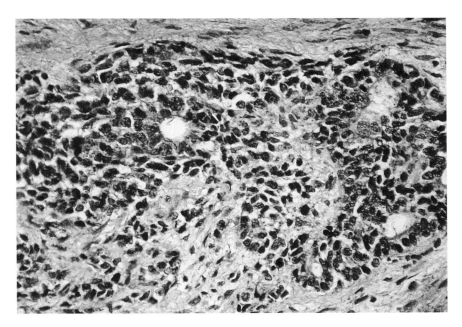

Figure 4-140

TERATOMA

This focus shows blastema with occasional primitive-appearing tubules.

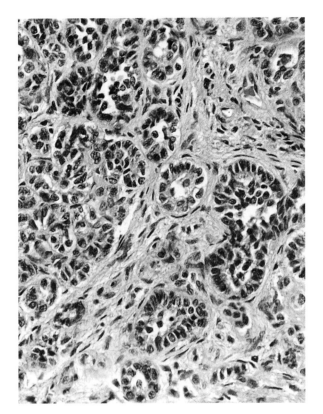

Figure 4-141

TERATOMA

There are foci of embryonal tubules.

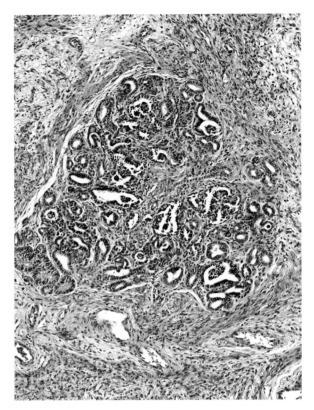

Figure 4-142

TERATOMA

A small, circumscribed focus of primitive tubules, some showing glomeruloid features, is seen.

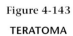

Figure 4-143

TERATOMA

This large focus of embryonic rhabdomyoblastic tissue adjacent to glandular epithelium (top) is distinguished from embryonal rhabdomyosarcoma on the basis of size.

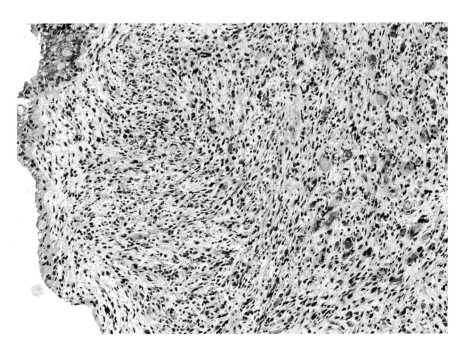

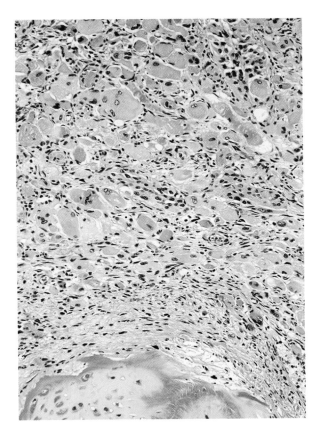

Figure 4-144

TERATOMA

Fetal-type muscle fibers are adjacent to a nodule of cartilage.

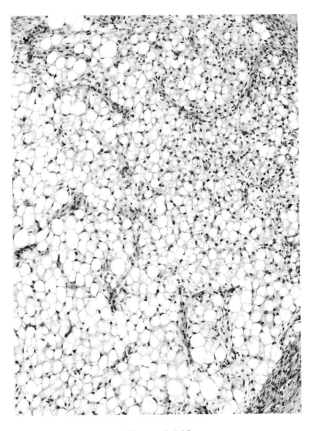

Figure 4-145

TERATOMA

This focus of adipose tissue has a fetal-type appearance, with small adipocytes and prominent vascularity.

do not show significant stromal overgrowth but characteristically interweave with other teratomatous structures.

Less immature, fetal-type tissues may also be seen, including: cellular islands of cartilage (fig. 4-134); adipose tissue, often with a prominent vascular pattern (fig. 4-145); and a nonspecific, spindle cell stroma that sometimes encircles glands or epithelial islands in an apparent reiteration of developing gastrointestinal tract, respiratory tract, tooth buds, or hair follicles (figs. 4-146, 4-147).

IGCNU is present in the seminiferous tubules peripheral to postpubertal teratomas in about 90 percent of the cases. The background testis is frequently atrophic, showing spermatogenic cell loss, peritubular and tubular sclerosis, and sometimes tubular microliths.

Prepubertal Teratoma. In contrast to postpubertal tumors, prepubertal teratomas have well-defined, organoid morphologies. Some show perfectly formed gastrointestinal structures with the normal tissue compartments arranged in the characteristic fashion (fig. 4-148). The pancreas may show lobular arrangements of acinar cells with intervening ducts and scattered islets of Langerhans (fig. 4-149). Other organ-like structures may be encountered, but a more random admixture of various elements is also seen. Immature, embryonic-type tissue is less commonly encountered than in the postpubertal tumors. The cytologic atypia that is frequent in the postpubertal cases is not seen, nor are mitotic figures as frequent, although they may be identified in foci that correspond to the normal proliferative compartments of "organs" that are mimicked by the teratoma.

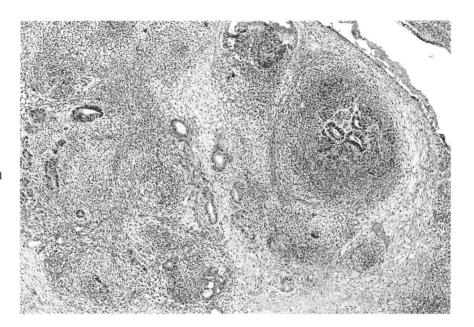

Figure 4-146

TERATOMA

The cellular, spindle cell stroma encircles small glands.

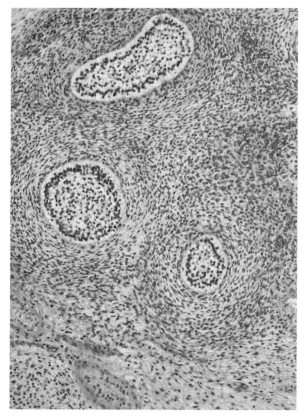

Figure 4-147

TERATOMA

The mildly hypercellular, spindle cell stroma forms concentric arrays around nests of squamous epithelium.

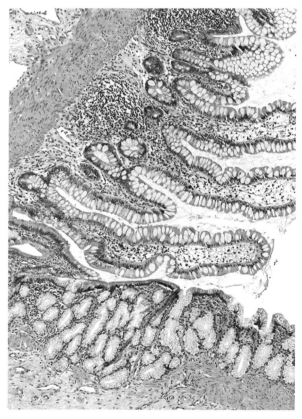

Figure 4-148

TERATOMA

This prepubertal case reiterates small intestinal and gastric pyloric mucosa.

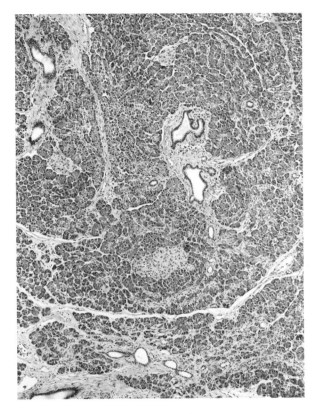

Figure 4-149

TERATOMA

In this case from a prepubertal boy, lobules of pancreatic parenchyma are formed consisting of acinar tissue, ducts, and islets of Langerhans.

Unlike the postpubertal teratomas, there is absence of IGCNU, although some abnormalities in the germ cell population may be appreciable in some cases, including nuclear enlargement and multinucleation (see chapter 2). Such cells, however, lack the seminoma-like features of IGCNU.

Immunohistochemical Findings. The immunohistochemical findings in teratomas reflect those normally found in the components that it reproduces (153,245,246), and only those of differential diagnostic importance are mentioned here. AFP is demonstrable in either glands of enteric or respiratory type or in cells showing hepatic differentiation (240); it is seen in 19 to 36 percent of teratomas (47,149,240). Alpha-1-antitrypsin is identified in teratomatous epithelium in 57 percent of cases and CEA and ferritin in about half of the cases (47). PLAP posi-

tivity occurs in the glandular component of 4 to 27 percent of teratomas (41,42,247); glypican 3 reactivity is present in immature elements of 38 percent (76); SOX2 positivity occurs in the immature neuroectodermal elements of 80 percent (34,35), and SOX17 reactivity is seen in about 40 percent (35). Focal SALL4 reactivity occurs in 80 percent of teratomas (45). p53 expression is identified in teratomatous epithelium (49) whereas OCT3/4 stains are negative (23,24).

Special Techniques. Cytogenetic study of postpubertal teratomas shows complex abnormalities with the frequent formation of i(12p) and nonrandom rearrangements involving 1p32-36 and 7q11.2 (248). These tumors are aneuploid, with DNA values in the hypotriploid range (249,250). In contrast, prepubertal teratomas are diploid and have normal cytogenetic findings (251) with interphase cytogenetic analysis (252) and comparative genomic hybridization (253).

The residual teratomatous lesions seen in postpubertal patients following chemotherapy have an aneuploid DNA index (249,250,254), with some cases showing further evolution of clones of cells with different aneuploid peaks from the primary tumor (249,250). The presence of fewer chromosomes in such metastases compared to the primary tumors argues that chemotherapy selects for a component with a capacity for differentiation (255).

Differential Diagnosis. The lesions that are most apt to be confused with postpubertal teratoma are dermoid cyst and epidermoid cyst. The mostly cystic nature of dermoid cyst contrasts with the usual solid and cystic pattern of teratoma. Dermoid cyst, by definition, has a skin-like surface with the usual adnexal structures (hair follicles with sebaceous glands, sweat glands) lining a cavity, whereas this organoid reiteration of skin is rarely identified in usual teratomas. Additionally, dermoid cysts lack immature elements, in contrast to many teratomas. The absence of IGCNU and the presence of intact spermatogenesis contrast with the usual presence of IGCNU and frequent impaired spermatogenesis with atrophic change of usual teratoma. A lipogranulomatous reaction in the parenchyma adjacent to the lesion favors dermoid cyst over teratoma. The demonstration of 12p amplification is diagnostic of teratoma as opposed to dermoid cyst.

Epidermoid cysts are grossly distinct from teratomas. They are a single cyst containing abundant amounts of keratin arranged in parallel laminae resulting in a characteristic targetoid appearance. This contrasts with the more complex, typically solid, cystic, and variegated cut surface of most teratomas. Microscopically, epidermoid cysts lack any component other than a cyst lined by keratinizing squamous epithelium (see chapter 8). No teratomatous or adnexal structures are present. Unlike postpubertal teratomas, they are not associated with IGCNU (238,256) and show no cytologic atypia. They are uniformly benign (257,258).

Spread and Metastasis. One study found local spread beyond the testis in 6 percent of postpubertal teratomas and metastases at presentation in 24 percent, although some were not pure teratomas but had seminoma components (259). In three referral centers, 20 to 46 percent of pure postpubertal teratomas had metastases (234,236,239). The pattern of metastasis is similar to that of other germ cell tumors, with initial involvement of retroperitoneal lymph nodes. In autopsy studies of patients with metastatic testicular teratoma, 100 percent had involvement of para-aortic and iliac lymph nodes; 83 percent, liver; 72 percent, bilateral lung; 36 percent, bone; 35 percent, pleura; and 25 percent, intestine (17).

It is common to find pure teratomatous metastases following the chemotherapeutic treatment of nonseminomatous germ cell tumors (260,261). This situation is highly associated with the presence of teratomatous elements in the testis (262–267), with the implication that either: 1) such teratomatous elements metastasized and were selected for by chemotherapy or 2) a nonteratomatous germ cell tumor metastasized but differentiated, because of an inherent tendency as evidenced by the testicular lesion, to teratoma, which was selected for by chemotherapy.

Treatment and Prognosis. Pure testicular teratomas in prepubertal boys are benign and are managed by orchiectomy alone (221,268). Pure testicular teratomas in postpubertal patients are uncommon, so treatment data are limited. In Dixon and Moore's studies (259), testicular teratomas, with or without seminoma, were associated with a 30 percent 5-year mortality rate. In another study (269), 18 patients

with teratomas (some of whom also had a seminoma component) had orchiectomy followed by retroperitoneal lymph node dissection and achieved a 5-year survival rate of 100 percent. In another study (236), 41 adult patients with pure teratoma were treated with retroperitoneal lymphadenectomy and, in some cases, chemotherapy; 6 patients developed recurrences, 3 of whom were successfully treated, while 1 patient died of progressive tumor, another from treatment-related angiosarcoma, and a third had persistent tumor at last follow-up. In the experience of the British Testicular Tumor Panel (221), 2 of 12 adult patients with pure testicular teratoma died of tumor. Both had metastases of nonteratomatous type (embryonal carcinoma and choriocarcinoma). The presence of mature teratomatous elements in the testicular tumors of patients with clinical disease limited to the testis correlates with a decreased likelihood of occult metastases (88,91,96,98).

When pure teratomas are found in metastatic sites after chemotherapy (usually for patients who had mixed germ cell tumors of the testis), the outcome is favorable (260,261), except in those rare instances in which a secondary malignant component has occurred (270–272). Disease-free survival rates of 87 to 94 percent are reported on follow-up of patients with completely resected, pure teratomatous metastases (272–274). Surgical excision of such lesions is indicated because they are genotypically abnormal (249,250,254) and are susceptible to transform into aggressively behaving neoplasms (249). Additionally, teratomatous lesions, even in the absence of such transformation, may progressively enlarge and ultimately cause lethal complications due to their local effects, the "growing teratoma syndrome" (275,276).

Dermoid Cyst

Dermoid cysts are rare, specialized forms of mature teratoma analogous to the more commonly occurring ovarian lesions. They consist of central keratinous material, often containing hairs (see fig. 4-123), surrounded by a cyst wall composed of keratinizing squamous epithelium with skin appendages, including hair follicles and sebaceous glands (fig. 4-150) (277–283). Ciliated (fig. 4-151) and goblet cell-containing epithelium are seen in some cases, as is cartilage, fibrous tissue, and neuroglia. In one case, there

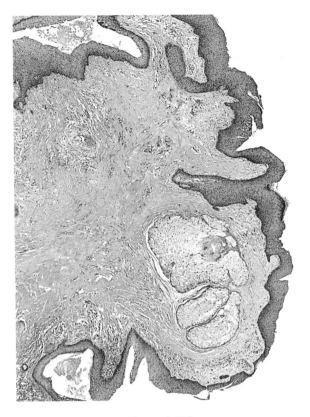

Figure 4-150

DERMOID CYST

The wall of a dermoid cyst consists of a squamous epithelial lining, sebaceous glands, and fibrous stroma.

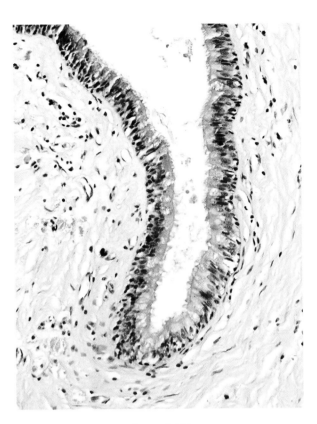

Figure 4-151

DERMOID CYST

This cyst from a portion of a dermoid cyst is lined by ciliated epithelium.

was well-formed intestinal mucosa (fig. 4-152). There is often an associated lipogranulomatous reaction in the adjacent testicular parenchyma (fig. 4-153) because of leakage of oily sebum from the cyst. Some cases have an appearance resembling pilomatrixoma, with the characteristic "shadow" cells (283), although such cells are not specific for dermoid cysts but may also be seen in usual teratomas (284). The seminiferous tubules surrounding dermoid cysts do not contain IGCNU and lack the diffuse atrophy so often seen with usual adult teratomas. Dermoid cysts, even in postpubertal patients, lack the amplification of chromosome 12p characteristic of usual teratomas (unpublished observation, 2012).

Teratoma with a Secondary Malignant Component

Teratoma with a secondary malignant component results from the independent growth of an atypical teratomatous element and has only been encountered in postpubertal cases. It is preferable to use this term rather than "teratoma with malignant transformation" because the latter implies that teratomas lacking this change are benign, which is not the case. Most of these tumors represent excessive proliferations of embryonic-type atypical elements, forming neoplasms resembling primitive neuroectodermal tumors (fig. 4-154; see following section, Monodermal and Highly Specialized Teratomas), nephroblastomas (fig. 4-155) or other blastomatous type neoplasms, and embryonal and alveolar rhabdomyosarcomas (fig. 4-156). Our guideline for distinguishing between such tumors and teratomas with large amounts of immature elements is overgrowth by a pure population of the atypical element such that it occupies a single, low-power (4X objective) microscopic field (270), as has been employed in recognizing malignant change in phyllodes

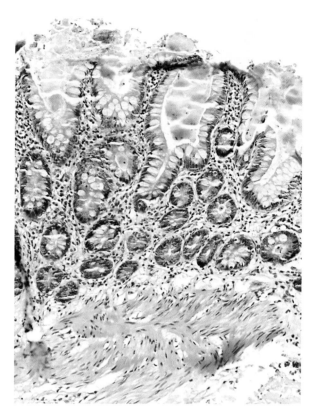

Figure 4-152

DERMOID CYST

Intestinal mucosa is formed.

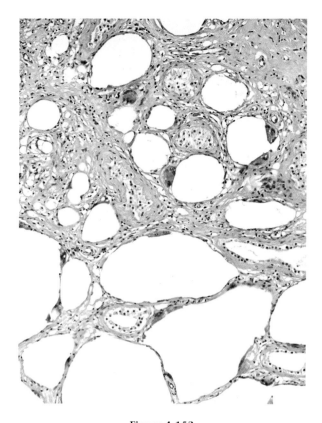

Figure 4-153

**LIPOGRANULOMATOUS REACTION
ADJACENT TO DERMOID CYST**

Figure 4-154

**PRIMITIVE
NEUROECTODERMAL
TUMOR IN TERATOMA**

Primitive neural tubules and
true rosettes are formed.

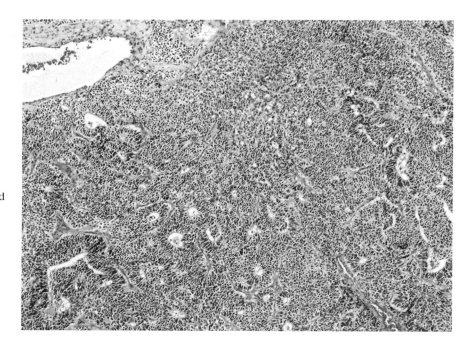

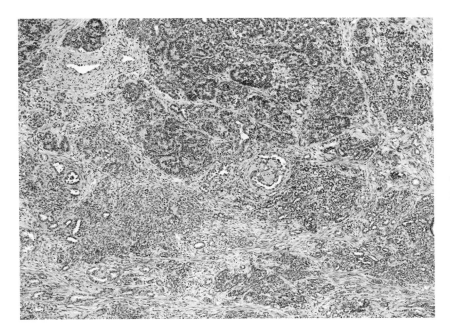

Figure 4-155

NEPHROBLASTOMA IN TERATOMA

There is a triphasic proliferation of primitive tubules, sometimes forming glomeruloid structures, blastema, and stroma.

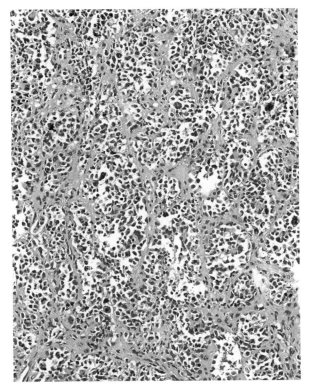
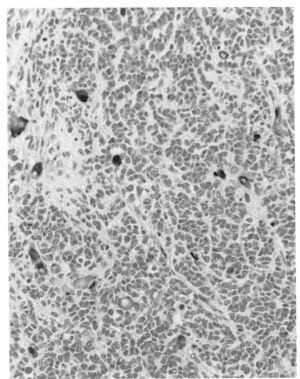

Figure 4-156

RHABDOMYOSARCOMA IN TERATOMA

Left: Primitive rhabdomyoblasts with discohesion and scattered giant tumor cells create an overall pattern of alveolar rhabdomyosarcoma.

Right: A focus of embryonal rhabdomyosarcoma from a different case consists of small, hyperchromatic, primitive skeletal muscle cells arranged in cords and nests. Scattered cells are reactive for desmin (immunoperoxidase stain with antidesmin).

tumors of the breast (285). Rarely, somatic-type carcinomas develop from teratomatous epithelium, for instance, adenocarcinomas derived from enteric-type glandular structures. Such carcinomas are recognizable by their pattern of stromal invasion, usually with associated desmoplasia.

The significance of a secondary malignant component in teratoma remains unclear. In two studies, testicular teratomas with secondary malignant components did not confer a worse outcome than those lacking such a component (271,286). This perhaps indicates that the criterion for their diagnosis (see above) is at too low a threshold. This is an area that requires additional study. Nonetheless, it is clear that secondary teratomatous malignancies have a poor outcome when they are found at metastatic sites, usually after the patient has received chemotherapy (270,287–291).

MONODERMAL AND HIGHLY SPECIALIZED TERATOMAS

Carcinoid Tumor

General and Clinical Features. Primary *carcinoid tumors* occur either as a pure testicular neoplasm (about 75 percent of the cases) or in association with a testicular teratoma (about 25 percent) (292–294). These tumors are rare: only 12 cases were found among the files of testicular tumors at the Armed Forces Institute of Pathology (AFIP), a frequency of 0.17 percent (293).

Carcinoid tumors tend to occur in older patients than most other types of testicular germ cell tumor, with a mean and median age of 46 years (293,294) and a range of 10 to 83 years (292,294,295). One carcinoid tumor occurred in a cryptorchid testis (296), but this may be a coincidence. Most patients present with testicular enlargement that may or may not be associated with pain. Often the clinical history of a mass is long, with a mean of 38 months (294). Rarely, the presentation is related to a metastasis (297). Although metastases develop in only a minority of cases (see below), most tumors that do metastasize have already spread at presentation (297). Hydroceles are described in about 10 percent of patients (294). The carcinoid syndrome is unusual, occurring in about 12 percent of cases (294), but serotonin or its metabolites are abnormally high in a greater

number of patients (294). On the other hand, serotonin metabolites may be negative, even when serotonin is subsequently identified in the tumor by immunohistochemistry (298). A metastatic primary testicular carcinoid was associated with very high levels of 5-hydroxyindole acetic acid in the urine (299). The presence of the carcinoid syndrome correlates with malignant behavior. This suggests that many tumors synthesize serotonin but in insufficient quantities to produce a carcinoid syndrome unless disseminated.

Gross Findings. Pure carcinoid tumors are usually solid, well-circumscribed, pale yellow to brown neoplasms (fig. 4-157). The reported size range is 0.5 to 11.0 cm, with a mean of 3.5 cm (294). Pure carcinoid tumors tend to be larger than those associated with a teratoma (294), which they outnumber by a 3-4 to 1 ratio (297). They do not invade surrounding structures.

Microscopic Findings. An insular pattern is usual, with small nests and acini separated by a fibrous to hyalinized stroma (fig. 4-158). The cells have moderate to abundant eosinophilic cytoplasm, often with distinct granularity, and round nuclei with coarse ("salt and pepper") chromatin granules (fig. 4-159). Both argyrophil and argentaffin stains are positive; faint mucin staining may occur in glandular lumens. There is one report of a primary testicular carcinoid tumor with extensive cutaneous metastases that had the trabecular growth pattern often seen in foregut carcinoid tumors (295). For the few cases associated with teratoma, there may be close juxtaposition of the carcinoid tumor with enteric or respiratory elements (293,300,301). In our experience, mostly with pure carcinoid tumors, and that of others (302), there is absence of IGCNU, although two testicular carcinoids, one pure and the other with teratoma, had adjacent IGCNU (303,304). These observations raise the possibility that most testicular carcinoids develop by a mechanism different from the majority of postpubertal teratomas.

Immunohistochemical Findings and Special Techniques. Immunohistochemical studies are positive for chromogranin, synaptophysin, neuron-specific enolase, serotonin, and cytokeratin (294,303,305,306), with some cases also positive for beta-catenin (nuclear and cytoplasmic), gastrin, gastrin-releasing peptide,

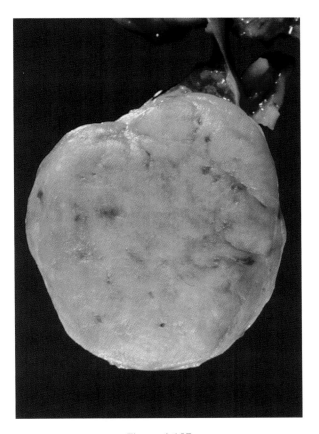

Figure 4-157

CARCINOID TUMOR

This tumor has a solid, tan to yellow cut surface.

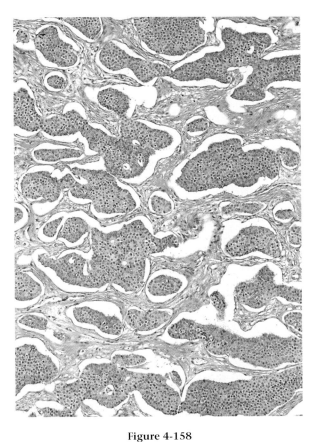

Figure 4-158

CARCINOID TUMOR

There are well-defined acini and solid islands of cells separated by a fibrous stroma.

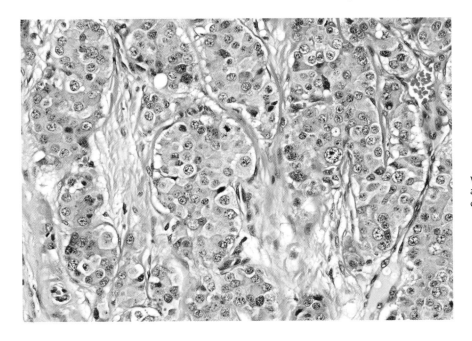

Figure 4-159

CARCINOID TUMOR

The cells have round nuclei with granular chromatin and abundant, lightly eosinophilic cytoplasm.

neurofilament, substance P, and vasoactive intestinal polypeptide (294,298,303,306). On ultrastructural examination, the pleomorphic neurosecretory granules characteristic of mid-gut-type carcinoid tumors are usually seen (292,294,298,306), although some tumors have more regular round to oval granules (294).

Flow cytometric study of three cases demonstrated near-diploid, aneuploid peaks and low S-phase values (less than 5 percent), consistent with indolent, malignant tumors (294). One study, using a fluorescence in situ hybridization (FISH) method, identified i(12p) in four testicular carcinoid tumors that were associated with "mature" teratomas (303), suggesting a pathogenesis similar to usual teratoma of the adult testis. On the other hand, three pure carcinoid tumors lacked numerical abnormalities of the X chromosome, in contrast to many usual teratomas and implicating a different pathogenesis (306).

Differential Diagnosis. The major entity in the differential is metastatic carcinoid. The presence of associated teratomatous elements indicates a primary nature, as does IGCNU, but both of these findings are usually absent. Bilaterality, multifocal involvement, and lymphatic/vascular invasion all favor metastasis. Clinical evidence of extratesticular involvement is also important in making this determination. The ileum is a favored site of origin for carcinoid tumors metastatic to the testis (297).

Sertoli cell tumors may be mistaken for carcinoid tumors because they grow in cords, trabeculae, and nests. Furthermore, they typically have abundant eosinophilic cytoplasm and infrequent mitotic figures, features that are shared by carcinoid tumors. The cytoplasmic granularity, coarse chromatin, and absence of tubules in carcinoid tumor, however, contrast with Sertoli cell tumor. Additionally, Sertoli cell tumors often have prominent stromal fibrosis and hyalinization with thick-walled blood vessels and hemosiderin deposits, whereas such features are not conspicuous in most carcinoid tumors. Immunoreactivity for alpha-inhibin occurs in some Sertoli cell tumors (52,307,308) but is not expected in testicular carcinoids based on the experience with the ovarian counterpart (309), although this has not been specifically studied. A potential pitfall in this differential diagnosis is the frequent reactivity of Sertoli cell tumors for neuroendocrine markers, including chromogranin and synaptophysin (308,310), possibly contributing to misinterpretation.

Treatment and Prognosis. Overall, patients with primary carcinoid tumors have a favorable prognosis, although metastases occasionally develop. Fatal metastatic disease developed in 1 of the 12 patients in the AFIP series (293), while a second had a clinical diagnosis of metastatic involvement. A literature review identified a 13 percent metastatic rate (297), but the figure may potentially be higher since late metastases, 15 years or more after orchiectomy, occur (299). It is also likely that metastatic cases are disproportionately reported, and most primary testicular carcinoid tumors are cured by orchiectomy, which, with clinical follow-up, is the usual form of therapy. For this reason we prefer the traditional nomenclature of "carcinoid tumor" for this low-grade, indolent tumor rather than "low-grade neuroendocrine carcinoma," as has been advocated by some, because the latter connotes a more aggressive neoplasm. Larger tumors are more apt to metastasize (median size of metastasizing tumors, 7.0 cm versus 3.6 cm for nonmetastasizing [297]), as are those associated with a clinical carcinoid syndrome (294). In one study, necrosis, mitotic rate, and vascular invasion did not correlate with malignancy (294). Small tumor size and an association with teratomatous elements are favorable factors (294,297).

Primitive Neuroectodermal Tumor

Primitive neuroectodermal tumors (PNETs) of the testis represent overgrowth of embryonic-appearing, neuroectodermal tissue (21,291,311–313). Some are pure PNETs (311–313), but most have a small component of a mixed germ cell tumor (21,291). In the latter case, distinction from teratoma with immature neural elements is based on the size of the primitive neuroectodermal component.

These tumors occur in young adults and, when large, are typically gray/white to tan, hemorrhagic, and partially necrotic (fig. 4-160) (311,313). Microscopically, there are areas of small, poorly differentiated malignant cells (311,313). Most tumors have foci of overt neuroectodermal differentiation in the form of

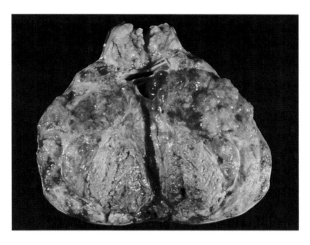

Figure 4-160

PRIMITIVE NEUROECTODERMAL TUMOR

The highly malignant nature of this tumor is suggested by the necrosis and hemorrhage within this large mass that replaced the testis. (Fig. 3.46 from Young RH, Scully RE. Testicular tumors. Chicago: ASCP Press; 1990:70.)

primitive neural-type tubules lined by stratified epithelium (fig. 4-161), ependymal-type rosettes (fig. 4-162), neuroblastic cells in an eosinophilic, fibrillary neuropil (fig. 4-163), or cellular atypical glia (291,311). They, therefore, resemble the PNETs of the central nervous system that typically occur in the posterior fossa of children (314), with a disproportionate number (compared to the brain tumors) having the features of medulloepithelioma (291,315). A rare melanotic variant closely resembled the paratesticular retinal anlage tumor but was considered to be of germ cell derivation given its testicular origin (316). Ultrastructural examination showed neurosecretory granules in one PNET (313). Unlike peripheral PNETs, these tumors are not associated with chromosome 22 translocations (315).

In the absence of light microscopic evidence of neural differentiation, confusion may occur with other small cell tumors of the testis such

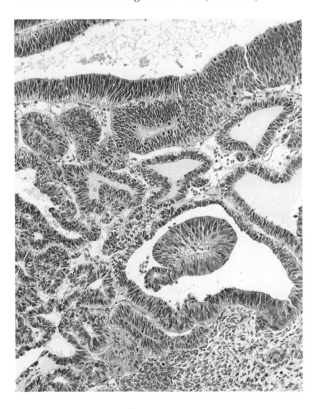

Figure 4-161

PRIMITIVE NEUROECTODERMAL TUMOR

Primitive neural tubules are lined by stratified atypical neuroepithelium in a pattern similar to medulloepithelioma.

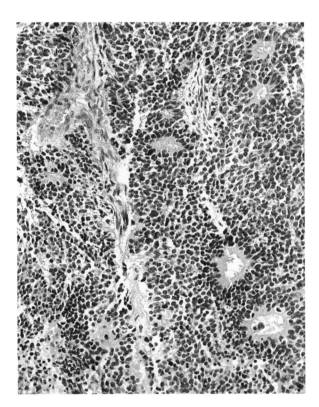

Figure 4-162

PRIMITIVE NEUROECTODERMAL TUMOR

Ependymal-type true rosettes are formed in an otherwise solid area.

197

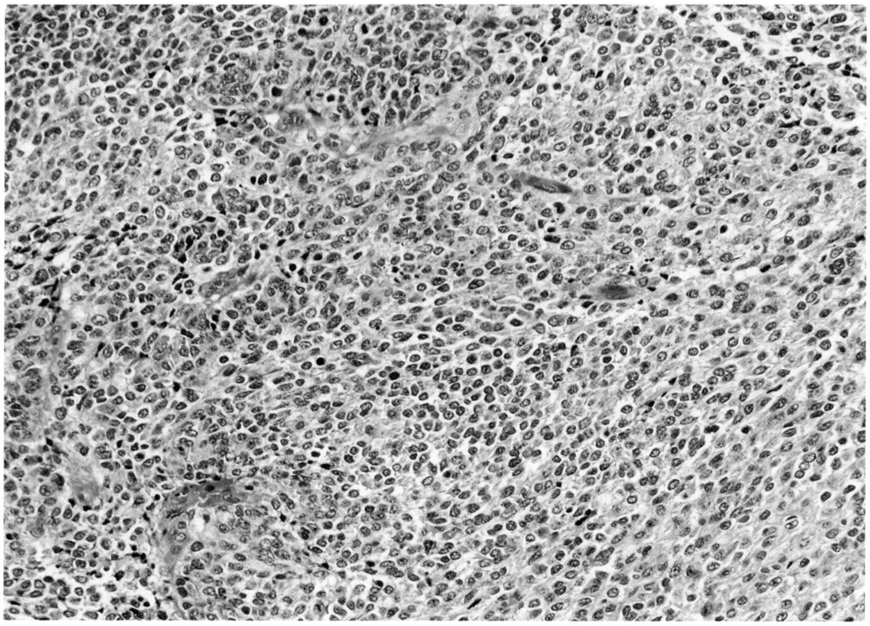

Figure 4-163

PRIMITIVE NEUROECTODERMAL TUMOR

Primitive neural cells are present in a neurofibrillary matrix.

as lymphoma, embryonal rhabdomyosarcoma, or metastatic small cell carcinoma (313). This differential diagnosis is aided by immunohistochemical markers directed against neural and neuroendocrine markers as well as lymphoid and muscle markers (317,318). Electron microscopy may be of additional help (317). Desmoplastic small round cell tumor may rarely demonstrate tubules and rosettes, but it is based in the paratestis and shows the characteristic polyimmunophenotype (319).

Overgrowth of embryonic-type renal tissue, thereby resembling nephroblastoma, may be confused with PNET. Glomeruloid-like epithelial structures, lack of neurofibrillary matrix, absence of distinct rosettes or pseudorosettes, and diffuse cytokeratin reactivity and nuclear WT-1 positivity support nephroblastoma over PNET.

In one series, when focal PNETs were found in the testis, there was no effect on prognosis (291). On the other hand, there was a high mortality rate when PNETs occurred in metastatic sites, always in patients previously treated with chemotherapy (291).

REFERENCES

1. Mostofi FK, Sesterhenn IA, Davis CJ Jr. Developments in histopathology of testicular germ cell tumors. Semin Urol 1988;6:171-88.
2. Jacobsen GK, Barlebo H, Olsen J, et al. Testicular germ cell tumours in Denmark 1976-1980: pathology of 1058 consecutive cases. Acta Radiol Oncol 1984;23:239-47.
3. Friedman NB, Moore RA. Tumors of the testis: a report on 922 cases. Milit Surgeon 1946;99:573-93.
4. Mostofi FK, Price EB Jr. Tumors of the male genital system. Atlas of Tumor Pathology, 2nd Series, Fascicle 8. Washington D.C.: Armed Forces Institute of Pathology; 1973.
5. Mostofi FK, Sobin LH. Histological typing of testicular tumors (international histological classification of tumors, No. 16). Geneva: World Health Organization; 1977.
6. Shah VI, Amin MB, Linden MD, Zarbo RJ. Immunohistologic profile of spindle cell elements in non-seminomatous germ cell tumors (NS-GCT): histogenetic implications. Mod Pathol 1998;11:96A.
7. Pugh RC. Testicular tumours—introduction. In: Pugh RC, ed. Pathology of the testis. Oxford: Blackwell Scientific; 1976:139-59.
8. Steyerberg EW, Keizer HJ, Fossa SD, et al. Prediction of residual retroperitoneal mass histology after chemotherapy for metastatic nonseminomatous germ cell tumor: multivariate analysis of individual patient data from six study groups. J Clin Oncol 1995;13:1177-87.
9. Visfeldt J, Jorgensen N, Muller J, Moller H, Skakkebaek NE. Testicular germ cell tumours of childhood in Denmark, 1943-1989: incidence and evaluation of histology using immunohistochemical techniques. J Pathol 1994;174:39-47.
10. Terenziani M, Piva L, Spreafico F, et al. Clinical stage I nonseminomatous germ cell tumors of the testis in childhood and adolescence: an analysis of 31 cases. J Pediatr Hematol Oncol 2002;24:454-8.
11. Saukko P, Lignitz E. [Sudden death caused by malignant testicular tumors.] Z Rechtsmed 1990;103:529-36. [German]
12. Aronsohn RS, Nishiyama RH. Embryonal carcinoma. An unexpected cause of sudden death in a young adult. JAMA 1974;229:1093-4.
13. Williams SD, Einhorn LH. Neoplasms of the testis. In: Calabresi P, Schein PS, Rosenberg SA, eds. Medical oncology: basic principles and clinical management of cancer. New York: Macmillan; 1985:1077-88.
14. Rodriguez PN, Hafez GR, Messing EM. Nonseminomatous germ cell tumor of the testicle: does extensive staging of the primary tumor predict the likelihood of metastatic disease? J Urol 1986;136:604-8.
15. Javadpour N. The role of biologic tumor markers in testicular cancer. Cancer 1980;45:1755-61.
16. Bosl GJ, Lange PH, Nochomovitz LE, et al. Tumor markers in advanced non-seminomatous testicular cancer. Cancer 1981;47:572-6.
17. Dixon FJ, Moore RA. Tumors of the male sex organs. Atlas of Tumor Pathology, 1st series, Fascicles 31b & 32. Washington, D.C.: Armed Forces Institute of Pathology; 1952.
18. Jacobsen GK. Histogenetic considerations concerning germ cell tumours. Morphological and immunohistochemical comparative investigation of the human embryo and testicular germ cell tumours. Virchows Arch [A] 1986;408:509-25.
19. Jacobsen GK, Talerman A. Atlas of germ cell tumours. Copenhagen: Munksgaard; 1989.
20. Moriyama N, Daly JJ, Keating MA, Lin CW, Prout GR Jr. Vascular invasion as a prognosticator of metastatic disease in nonseminomatous germ cell tumors of the testis. Importance in "surveillance only" protocols. Cancer 1985;56:2492-8.
21. Young RH, Scully RE. Testicular tumors. Chicago: ASCP Press; 1990.
22. Nazeer T, Ro JY, Kee KH, Ayala AG. Spermatic cord contamination in testicular cancer. Mod Pathol 1996;9:762-6.
23. Looijenga LH, Stoop H, de Leeuw HP, et al. POU5F1 (OCT3/4) identifies cells with pluripotent potential in human germ cell tumors. Cancer Res 2003;63:2244-50.
24. Jones TD, Ulbright TM, Eble JN, Cheng L. OCT4 staining in testicular tumors: a sensitive and specific marker for seminoma and embryonal carcinoma. Am J Surg Pathol 2004;28:935-40.
25. Ferreiro JA. Ber-H2 expression in testicular germ cell tumors. Hum Pathol 1994;25:522-4.
26. Lau SK, Weiss LM, Chu PG. Association of intratubular seminoma and intratubular embryonal carcinoma with invasive testicular germ cell tumors. Am J Surg Pathol 2007;31:1045-9.
27. Leroy X, Augusto D, Leteurtre E, Gosselin B. CD30 and CD117 (c-kit) used in combination are useful for distinguishing embryonal carcinoma from seminoma. J Histochem Cytochem 2002;50:283-5.

28. Cheville JC, Rao S, Iczkowski KA, Lohse CM, Pankratz VS. Cytokeratin expression in seminoma of the human testis. Am J Clin Pathol 2000;113:583-8.

29. Kneile JR, Tan G, Suster S, Wakely PE Jr. Expression of CD30 (Ber-H2) in nasopharyngeal carcinoma, undifferentiated type and lymphoepithelioma-like carcinoma. A comparison study with anaplastic large cell lymphoma. Histopathology 2006;48:855-61.

30. Mechtersheimer G, Moller P. Expression of Ki-1 antigen (CD30) in mesenchymal tumors. Cancer 1990;66:1732-7.

31. Kahle PJ. Retroperitoneal seminoma (germinoma): report of a case; histogenetic and diagnostic considerations. Am Surg 1954;20:538-48.

32. Schwarting R, Gerdes J, Durkop H, Falini B, Pileri S, Stein H. BER-H2: a new anti-Ki-1 (CD30) monoclonal antibody directed at a formol-resistant epitope. Blood 1989;74:1678-89.

33. Santagata S, Ligon KL, Hornick JL. Embryonic stem cell transcription factor signatures in the diagnosis of primary and metastatic germ cell tumors. Am J Surg Pathol 2007;31:836-45.

34. Gopalan A, Dhall D, Olgac S, et al. Testicular mixed germ cell tumors: a morphological and immunohistochemical study using stem cell markers, OCT3/4, SOX2 and GDF3, with emphasis on morphologically difficult-to-classify areas. Mod Pathol 2009;22:1066-74.

35. Nonaka D. Differential expression of SOX2 and SOX17 in testicular germ cell tumors. Am J Clin Pathol 2009;131:731-6.

36. Boseman FT, Giard RW, Kruseman AC, Knijenenburg G, Spaander PJ. Human chorionic gonadothropin and alpha-fetoprotein in testicular germ cell tumors: a retrospective immunohistochemical study. Histopathology 1980;4:673-84.

37. Stiller D, Bahn H, Pressler H. Immunohistochemical demonstration of alpha-fetoprotein in testicular germ cell tumors. Acta Histochem Suppl (Jena) 1986;33:225-31.

38. Niehans GA, Manivel JC, Copland GT, Scheithauer BW, Wick MR. Immunohistochemistry of germ cell and trophoblastic neoplasms. Cancer 1988;62:1113-23.

39. Mostofi FK, Sesterhenn IA, Davis CJ Jr. Immunopathology of germ cell tumors of the testis. Semin Diagn Pathol 1987;4:320-41.

40. Wittekind C, Wichmann T, Von Kleist S. Immunohistological localization of AFP and HCG in uniformly classified testis tumors. Anticancer Res 1983;3:327-30.

41. Manivel JC, Jessurun J, Wick MR, Dehner LP. Placental alkaline phosphatase immunoreactivity in testicular germ cell tumors. Am J Surg Pathol 1987;11:21-9.

42. Burke AP, Mostofi FK. Placental alkaline phosphatase immunohistochemistry of intratubular malignant germ cells and associated testicular germ cell tumors. Hum Pathol 1988;19:663-70.

43. Lifschitz-Mercer B, Fogel M, Moll R, et al. Intermediate filament protein profiles of human testicular non-seminomatous germ cell tumors: correlation of cytokeratin synthesis to cell differentiation. Differentiation 1991;48:191-8.

44. Battifora H, Sheibani K, Tubbs RR, Kopinski MI, Sun TT. Antikeratin antibodies in tumor diagnosis: distinction between seminoma and embryonal carcinoma. Cancer 1984;54:843-8.

45. Cao D, Li J, Guo CC, Allan RW, Humphrey PA. SALL4 is a novel diagnostic marker for testicular germ cell tumors. Am J Surg Pathol 2009;33:1065-77.

46. Murakami SS, Said JW. Immunohistochemical localization of lactate dehydrogenase isoenzyme 1 in germ cell tumors of the testis. Am J Clin Pathol 1984;81:293-6.

47. Jacobsen GK, Jacobsen M, Clausen PP. Distribution of tumor-associated antigens in the various histologic components of germ cell tumors of the testis. Am J Surg Pathol 1981;5:257-66.

48. Visfeldt J, Giwercman A, Skakkebaek NE. Monoclonal antibody 43-9F: an immunohistochemical marker of embryonal carcinoma of the testis. APMIS 1992;100:63-70.

49. Bartkova J, Bartek J, Lukas J, et al. p53 protein alterations in human testicular cancer including pre-invasive intratubular germ-cell neoplasia. Int J Cancer 1991;49:196-202.

50. Ulbright TM, Orazi A, de Riese W, et al. The correlation of P53 protein expression with proliferative activity and occult metastases in clinical stage I non-seminomatous germ cell tumors of the testis. Mod Pathol 1994;7:64-8.

51. McCluggage WG, Ashe P, McBride H, Maxwell P, Sloan JM. Localization of the cellular expression of inhibin in trophoblastic tissue. Histopathology 1998;32:252-6.

52. Kommoss F, Oliva E, Bittinger F, et al. Inhibin-alpha CD99, HEA125, PLAP, and chromogranin immunoreactivity in testicular neoplasms and the androgen insensitivity syndrome. Hum Pathol 2000;31:1055-61.

53. Srigley JR, Mackay B, Toth P, Ayala A. The ultrastructure and histogenesis of male germ neoplasia with emphasis on seminoma with early carcinomatous features. Ultrastruc Pathol 1988;12:67-86.

54. Roth LM, Gillespie JJ. Ultrastructure of testicular tumors. In: Talerman A, Roth LM, eds. Pathology of the testis and its adnexa. New York: Churchill-Livingstone; 1986:155-68.

55. Ulbright TM, Goheen MP, Roth LM, Gillespie JJ. The differentiation of carcinomas of teratomatous origin from embryonal carcinoma. A light and electron microscopic study. Cancer 1986;57:257-63.

56. Baslev E, Francis D, Jacobsen GK. Testicular germ cell tumors: classification based on fine needle aspiration biopsy. Acta Cytol 1990;34:690-4.

57. Highman WJ, Oliver RT. Diagnosis of metastases from testicular germ cell tumours using fine needle aspiration cytology. J Clin Pathol 1987;40:1324-33.

58. Koss LG, Zajicek J. Aspiration biopsy. In: Koss LG, ed. Diagnostic cytology and its histopathologic basis, 4th ed. Philadelphia: JB Lippincott; 1992:1234-402.

59. Fossä SD, Nesland JM, Waehre H, Amellem O, Pettersen EO. DNA ploidy in the primary tumor from patients with nonseminomatous testicular germ cell tumors clinical stage I. Cancer 1991;67:1874-7.

60. Oosterhuis JW, Castedo SM, de Jong B, et al. Ploidy of primary germ cell tumors of the testis. Pathogenetic and clinical relevance. Lab Invest 1989;60:14-21.

61. Delozier-Blanchet CD, Walt H, Engel E, Vuagnat P. Cytogenetic studies of human testicular germ cell tumours. Int J Androl 1987;10:69-77.

62. Castedo SM, de Jong B, Oosterhuis JW, et al. i(12p)-negative testicular germ cell tumors. A different group? Cancer Genet Cytogenet 1988;35:171-8.

63. Blough RI, Heerema NA, Albers P, Foster RS. Fluorescence in situ hybridization on nuclei from paraffin-embedded tissue in low stage pure embryonal carcinoma of the testis. J Urol 1998;159:240-4.

64. Motzer RJ, Rodriguez E, Reuter VE, et al. Genetic analysis as an aid in diagnosis for patients with midline carcinomas of uncertain histologies. J Natl Cancer Inst 1991;83:341-6.

65. Korkola JE, Houldsworth J, Chadalavada RS, et al. Down-regulation of stem cell genes, including those in a 200-kb gene cluster at 12p13.31, is associated with in vivo differentiation of human male germ cell tumors. Cancer Res 2006;66:820-7.

66. Hart AH, Hartley L, Parker K, et al. The pluripotency homeobox gene NANOG is expressed in human germ cell tumors. Cancer 2005;104:2092-8.

67. Skotheim RI, Autio R, Lind GE, et al. Novel genomic aberrations in testicular germ cell tumors by array-CGH, and associated gene expression changes. Cell Oncol 2006;28:315-26.

68. Skotheim RI, Lind GE, Monni O, et al. Differentiation of human embryonal carcinomas in vitro and in vivo reveals expression profiles relevant to normal development. Cancer Res 2005;65:5588-98.

69. Faulkner SW, Leigh DA, Oosterhuis JW, Roelofs H, Looijenga LH, Friedlander ML. Allelic losses in carcinoma in situ and testicular germ cell tumours of adolescents and adults: evidence suggestive of the linear progression model. Br J Cancer 2000;83:729-36.

70. Lind GE, Skotheim RI, Fraga MF, Abeler VM, Esteller M, Lothe RA. Novel epigenetically deregulated genes in testicular cancer include homeobox genes and SCGB3A1 (HIN-1). J Pathol 2006;210:441-9.

71. Sperger JM, Chen X, Draper JS, et al. Gene expression patterns in human embryonic stem cells and human pluripotent germ cell tumors. Proc Nat Acad Sci USA 2003;100:13350-5.

72. Damjanov I, Fox N, Knowles BB, Solter D, Lange PH, Fraley EE. Immunohistochemical localization of stage-specific embryonic antigens in human testicular germ cell tumors. Am J Pathol 1982;108:225-30.

73. Damjanov I, Andrews PW. Ultrastructural differentiation of a clonal human embryonal carcinoma cell line in vitro. Cancer Res 1983;43:2190-8.

74. Damjanov I, Clark RK, Andrews PW. Cytoskeleton of human embryonal carcinoma cells. Cell Differ 1984;15:133-9.

75. Ulbright TM, Roth LM, Brodhecker CA. Yolk sac differentiation in germ cell tumors. A morphologic study of 50 cases with emphasis on hepatic, enteric and parietal yolk sac features. Am J Surg Pathol 1986;10:151-64.

76. Zynger DL, Dimov ND, Luan C, Teh BT, Yang XJ. Glypican 3: a novel marker in testicular germ cell tumors. Am J Surg Pathol 2006;30:1570-5.

77. Ota S, Hishinuma M, Yamauchi N, et al. Oncofetal protein glypican-3 in testicular germ-cell tumor. Virchows Arch 2006;449:308-14.

78. Ferry JA, Ulbright TM, Young RH. Anaplastic large cell lymphoma presenting in the testis. J Urol Pathol 1997;5:139-47.

79. Ulbright TM, Young RH. Metastatic carcinoma to the testis: a clinicopathologic analysis of 26 non-incidental cases with emphasis on deceptive features. Am J Surg Pathol 2008;32:1683-93.

80. de Bruin MJ, Oosterhof GO, Debruyne FM. Nerve-sparing retroperitoneal lymphadenectomy for low stage testicular cancer. Br J Urol 1993;71:336-9.

81. Spermon JR, Roeleveld TA, van der Poel HG, et al. Comparison of surveillance and retroperitoneal lymph node dissection in Stage I nonseminomatous germ cell tumors. Urology 2002;59:923-9.

82. Rowland RG, Donohue JP. Scrotum and testis. In: Gillenwater JY, Grayhack JT, Howards SS, Duckett JW, eds. Adult and pediatric urology, 2nd ed. St. Louis: Mosby Year Book; 1991:1565-98.

83. Stephenson AJ, Bosl GJ, Bajorin DF, Stasi J, Motzer RJ, Sheinfeld J. Retroperitoneal lymph node dissection in patients with low stage testicular cancer with embryonal carcinoma predominance and/or lymphovascular invasion. J Urol 2005;174:557-60.

84. Richie JP, Kantoff PW. Is adjuvant chemotherapy necessary for patients with stage B1 testicular cancer? J Clin Oncol 1991;9:1393-6.

85. Sturgeon JF, Jewett MA, Alison RE, et al. Surveillance after orchidectomy for patients with clinical stage I nonseminomatous testis tumors. J Clin Oncol 1992;10:564-8.

86. Sogani PC, Fair WR. Surveillance alone in the treatment of clinical stage I nonseminomatous germ cell tumor of the testis (NSGCT). Semin Urol 1988;6:53-6.

87. Divrik RT, Akdoan B, Ozen H, Zorlu F. Outcomes of surveillance protocol of clinical stage I nonseminomatous germ cell tumors—is shift to risk adapted policy justified? J Urol 2006;176:1424-9.

88. Fung CY, Kalish LA, Brodsky GL, Richie JP, Garnick MB. Stage I nonseminomatous germ cell testicular tumor: prediction of metastatic potential by primary histopathology. J Clin Oncol 1988;6:1467-73.

89. Dunphy CH, Ayala AG, Swanson DA, Ro JY, Logothetis C. Clinical stage I nonseminomatous and mixed germ cell tumors of the testis. A clinicopathologic study of 93 patients on a surveillance protocol after orchiectomy alone. Cancer 1988;62:1202-6.

90. Jacobsen GK, Rorth M, Osterlind K, et al. Histopathological features in stage I non-seminomatous testicular germ cell tumours correlated to relapse. Danish Testicular Cancer Study Group. APMIS 1990;98:377-82.

91. Wishnow KI, Johnson DE, Swanson DA, et al. Identifying patients with low-risk clinical stage I nonseminomatous testicular tumors who should be treated by surveillance. Urology 1989;34:339-43.

92. Javadpour N, Canning DA, O'Connell KJ, Young JD. Predictors of recurrent clinical stage I nonseminomatous testicular cancer. A prospective clinicopathologic study. Urology 1986;27:508-11.

93. Costello AJ, Mortensen PH, Stillwell RG. Prognostic indicators for failure of surveillance management of stage I non-seminomatous germ cell tumours. Aust N Z J Surg 1989;59:119-22.

94. Fossä SD, Aass N, Kaalhus O. Testicular cancer in young Norwegians. J Surg Oncol 1988;39:43-63.

95. Freedman LS, Parkinson MC, Jones WG, et al. Histopathology in the prediction of relapse of patients with stage I testicular teratoma treated by orchidectomy alone. Lancet 1987;2:294-8.

96. Moul JW, McCarthy WF, Fernandez EB, Sesterhenn IA. Percentage of embryonal carcinoma and of vascular invasion predicts pathological stage in clinical stage I nonseminomatous testicular cancer. Cancer Res 1994;54:362-4.

97. Fernandez EB, Sesterhenn IA, McCarthy WF, Mostofi FK, Moul JW. Proliferating cell nuclear antigen expression to predict occult disease in clinical stage I nonseminomatous testicular germ cell tumors. J Urol 1994;152:1133-8.

98. Gels ME, Hoekstra HJ, Sleijfer DT, et al. Detection of recurrence in patients with clinical stage I nonseminomatous testicular germ cell tumors and consequences for further follow-up: a single-center 10-year experience. J Clin Oncol 1995;13:1188-94.

99. Raghavan D, Vogelzang NJ, Bosl GJ, et al. Tumor classification and size in germ-cell testicular cancer: influence on the occurrence of metastases. Cancer 1982;50:1591-5.

100. Nicolai N, Pizzocaro G. A surveillance study of clinical stage I nonseminomatous germ cell tumors of the testis: 10-year followup. J Urol 1995;154:1045-9.

101. de Riese WT, Albers P, Walker EB, et al. Predictive parameters of biologic behavior of early stage nonseminomatous testicular germ cell tumors. Cancer 1994;74:1335-41.

102. Moul JW, Foley JP, Hitchcock CL, et al. Flow cytometric and quantitative histological parameters to predict occult disease in clinical stage I nonseminomatous testicular germ cell tumors. J Urol 1993;150:879-83.

103. Albers P, Miller GA, Orazi A, et al. Immunohistochemical assessment of tumor proliferation and volume of embryonal carcinoma identify patients with clinical stage A nonseminomatous testicular germ cell tumor at low risk for occult metastasis. Cancer 1995;75:844-50.

104. Albers P, Ulbright TM, Albers J, et al. Tumor proliferative activity is predictive of pathological stage in clinical stage A nonseminomatous testicular germ cell tumors. J Urol 1996;155:579-86.

105. de Riese WT, de Riese C, Ulbright TM, et al. Flow-cytometric and quantitative histologic parameters as prognostic indicators for occult retroperitoneal disease in clinical-stage-I nonseminomatous testicular germ-cell tumors. Int J Cancer 1994;57:628-33.

106. Allhoff EP, Liedkes S, Wittekind C, et al. DNA content in NSGCT/CSI: a new prognosticator for biologic behaviour. J Cancer Res Clin Oncol 1990;1(Suppl):592.

107. de Graaff WE, Sleijfer DT, de Jong B, Dam A, Koops HS, Oosterhuis JW. Significance of aneuploid stemlines in testicular nonseminomatous germ cell tumors. Cancer 1993;72:1300-4.

108. Kondagunta GV, Sheinfeld J, Mazumdar M, et al. Relapse-free and overall survival in patients with pathologic stage II nonseminomatous germ cell cancer treated with etoposide and cisplatin adjuvant chemotherapy. J Clin Oncol 2004;22:464-7.

109. Morse MJ, Whitmore WF. Neoplasms of the testis. In: Walsh PC, Gittes RF, Perlmutter AD, Stamey TA, eds. Campbell's urology. Philadelphia: W.B. Saunders; 1986:1535-82.

110. Einhorn LH. Chemotherapy of disseminated testicular cancer. In: Skinner DG, Lieskovsky G, eds. Diagnosis and management of genitourinary cancer. Philadelphia: W.B. Saunders; 1988:526-31.

111. Ulbright TM, Roth LM. A pathologic analysis of lesions following modern chemotherapy for metastatic germ cell tumors. Pathol Ann 1990;25(Pt 1):313-40.

112. Geller NL, Bosl GJ, Chan EY. Prognostic factors for relapse after complete response in patients with metastatic germ cell tumors. Cancer 1989;63:440-5.

113. Mead GM, Stenning SP, Parkinson MC, et al. The Second Medical Research Council study of prognostic factors in nonseminomatous germ cell tumors. Medical Research Council Testicular Tumour Working Party. J Clin Oncol 1992;10:85-94.

114. Vogelzang NJ. Prognostic factors in metastatic testicular cancer. Int J Androl 1987;10:225-37.

115. Stoter G, Sylvester R, Sleijfer DT, et al. Multivariate analysis of prognostic variables in patients with disseminated non-seminomatous testicular cancer: results from an EORTC multi-institutional phase III study. Int J Androl 1987;10:239-46.

116. Peckham M. Testicular cancer. Acta Oncol 1988;27:439-53.

117. Einhorn LH. Cancer of the testis: a new paradigm. Hosp Pract 1986;April 15:165-78.

118. Marrett LD, Weir HK, Clarke EA, Magee CJ. Rates of death from testicular cancer in Ontario from 1964-82: analysis by major histologic subgroups. Can Med Assoc J 1986;135:999-1002.

119. Teilum G. "Mesonephroma ovarii" (Schiller)—an extra-embryonic mesoblastoma of germ cell origin in the ovary and the testis. Acta Pathol Microbiol Scand 1950;27:249-61.

120. Teilum G. Endodermal sinus tumors of the ovary and testis: comparative morphogenesis of the so-called mesonephroma ovarii (Schiller) and extraembryonic (yolk sac-allantoic) structures of the rat's placenta. Cancer 1959;12:1092-105.

121. Teilum G. Gonocytoma: homologous ovarian and testicular tumors I: with discussion of "mesonephroma ovarii" (Schiller: Am J Cancer 1939). Acta Pathol Microbiol Scand 1946;23:242-51.

122. Teilum G. Special tumors of ovary and testis and related extragonadal lesions. Philadelphia: J. B. Lippincott; 1976.

123. Lee SD, Korean Society of Pediatric Urology. Epidemiological and clinical behavior of prepubertal testicular tumors in Korea. J Urol 2004;172:674-8.

124. Ross JH, Rybicki L, Kay R. Clinical behavior and a contemporary management algorithm for prepubertal testis tumors: a summary of the Prepubertal Testis Tumor Registry. J Urol 2002;168:1675-8.

125. Brosman SA. Testicular tumors in prepubertal children. Urology 1979;13:581-8.

126. Pierce GB, Bullock WK, Huntington RW. Yolk sac tumors of the testis. Cancer 1970;25:644-58.

127. Steinbronn DV, Hicks TH, Carrel WH. Mixed germ cell testis tumor in an 86-year-old man. J Urol 1999;162:161.

128. Talerman A. Endodermal sinus (yolk sac) tumor elements in testicular germ-cell tumors in adults: comparison of prospective and retrospective studies. Cancer 1980;46:1213-7.

129. Brown LM, Pottern LM, Hoover RN, Devesa SS, Aselton P, Flannery JT. Testicular cancer in the United States: trends in incidence and mortality. Int J Epidemiol 1986;15:164-70.

130. Bradfield JS, Hagen RO, Ytredal DO. Carcinoma of the testis: an analysis of 104 patients with germinal tumors of the testis other than seminoma. Cancer 1973;31:633-40.

131. Kaplan GW, Cromie WC, Kelalis PP, Silber I, Tank ES Jr. Prepubertal yolk sac testicular tumors—report of the testicular tumor registry. J Urol 1988;140:1109-12.

132. Grady RW, Ross JH, Kay R. Patterns of metastatic spread in prepubertal yolk sac tumor of the testis. J Urol 1995;153:1259-61.

133. Talerman A, Haije WG, Baggerman L. Serum alphafetoprotein (AFP) in patients with germ cell tumors of the gonads and extragonadal sites: correlation between endodermal sinus (yolk sac) tumor and raised serum AFP. Cancer 1980;46:380-5.

134. Jacobsen GK. Alpha-fetoprotein (AFP) and human chorionic gonadotropin (HCG) in testicular germ cell tumours. Acta Pathol Microbiol Immunol Scand [A] 1983;91:183-90.

135. Brown NJ. Yolk-sac tumour ("orchioblastoma") and other testicular tumours of childhood. In: Pugh RC, ed. Pathology of the testis. Oxford: Blackwell Scientific; 1976:356-70.

136. Talerman A. Germ cell tumors. In: Talerman A, Roth LM, eds. Pathology of the testis and its adnexa. New York: Churchill Livingstone; 1986:29-65.

137. Clement PB, Young RH, Scully RE. Endometrioid-like variant of ovarian yolk sac tumor. A clinicopathological analysis of eight cases. Am J Surg Pathol 1987;11:767-78.

138. Cohen MB, Friend DS, Molnar JJ, Talerman A. Gonadal endodermal sinus (yolk sac) tumor with pure intestinal differentiation: a new histologic type. Pathol Res Pract 1987;182:609-16.

139. Moran CA, Suster S. Yolk sac tumors of the mediastinum with prominent spindle cell features: a clinicopathologic study of three cases. Am J Surg Pathol 1997;21:1173-7.

140. Prat J, Bhan AK, Dickersin GR, Robboy S, Scully RE. Hepatoid yolk sac tumor of the ovary (endodermal sinus tumor with hepatoid differentiation): a light microscopic, ultrastructural, and immunohistochemical study of seven cases. Cancer 1982;50:2355-68.

141. Horie Y, Kato M. Hepatoid variant of yolk sac tumor of the testis. Pathol Int 2000;50:754-8.

142. Pugh RC, Parkinson C. The origin and classification of testicular germ cell tumours. Int J Androl 1981;4(Suppl):15-25.

143. Michael H, Ulbright TM, Brodhecker CA. The pluripotential nature of the mesenchyme-like component of yolk sac tumor. Arch Pathol Lab Med 1989;113:1115-9.

144. Teilum G. Classification of endodermal sinus tumor (mesoblastoma vitellinum) and so-called "embryonal carcinoma" of the ovary. Acta Pathol Microbiol Scand 1965;64:407-29.

145. Jacobsen GK, Jacobsen M. Possible liver cell differentiation in testicular germ cell tumours. Histopathology 1983;7:537-48.

146. Fujimoto J, Hata J, Ishii E, et al. Differentiation antigens defined by mouse monoclonal antibodies against human germ cell tumors. Lab Invest 1987;57:350-8.

147. Manivel JC, Simonton S, Wold SE, Dehner LP. Absence of intratubular germ cell neoplasia in testicular yolk sac tumors in children. Arch Pathol Lab Med 1988;112:641-5.

148. Koide O, Iwai S, Baba K, Iri H. Identification of testicular atypical germ cells by an immunohistochemical technique for placental alkaline phosphatase. Cancer 1987;60:1325-30.

149. Jacobsen GK, Jacobsen M. Alpha-fetoprotein (AFP) and human chorionic gonadotropin in testicular germ cell tumours: a prospective immunohistochemical study. Acta Pathol Microbiol Scand A 1983;91:165-76.

150. Willmore-Payne C, Holden JA, Chadwick BE, Layfield LJ. Detection of c-kit exons 11- and 17-activating mutations in testicular seminomas by high-resolution melting amplicon analysis. Mod Pathol 2006;19:1164-9.

151. de Peralta-Venturina MN, Ro JY, Ordonez NG, Ayala AG. Diffuse embryoma of the testis. An immunohistochemical study of two cases. Am J Clin Pathol 1994;102:402-5.

152. Pallesen G, Hamilton-Dutoit SJ. Ki-1 (CD30) antigen is regularly expressed in tumor cells of embryonal carcinoma. Am J Pathol 1988;133:446-50.

153. Miettinen M, Virtanen I, Talerman A. Intermediate filament proteins in human testis and testicular germ-cell tumors. Am J Pathol 1985;120:402-10.

154. Damjanov I, Osborn M, Miettinen M. Keratin 7 is a marker for a subset of trophoblastic cells in human germ cell tumors. Arch Pathol Lab Med 1990;114:81-3.

155. Shah VI, Amin MB, Linden MD, Zarbo RJ. Utility of a selective immunohistochemical (IHC) panel in the detection of components of mixed germ cell tumors (GCT) of testis. Mod Pathol 1998;11:95A.

156. Yan M, Ghorab Z, Nadji M. Renal cell carcinoma antigen is expressed by yolk sac tumors and yolk sac elements of embryonal carcinomas. Appl Immunohistochem Molecul Morphol 2003;11:113-5.

157. Gonzalez-Crussi F, Roth LM. The human yolk sac and yolk sac carcinoma: an ultrastructural study. Hum Pathol 1976;7:675-91.

158. Nogales-Fernandez F, Silverberg SG, Bloustein PA, Martinez-Hernandez A, Pierce GB. Yolk sac carcinoma (endodermal sinus tumor): ultrastructure and histogenesis of gonadal and extragonadal tumors in comparison with normal human yolk sac. Cancer 1977;39:1462-74.

159. Nakanishi I, Kawahara E, Kajikawa K, Miwa A, Terahata S. Hyaline globules in yolk sac tumor. Histochemical, immunohistochemical and electron microscopic studies. Acta Pathol Jap 1982;32:733-9.

160. Roth LM, Gillespie JJ. Pathology and ultrastructure of germinal neoplasia of the testis. In: Einhorn LH, ed. Testicular tumors: management and treatment. New York: Masson; 1980:1-28.

161. Akhtar M, Ali MA, Sackey K, Jackson D, Bakry M. Fine-needle aspiration biopsy diagnosis of endodermal sinus tumor: histologic and ultrastructural correlations. Diagn Cytopathol 1990;6:184-92.

162. Dominguez-Franjo P, Vargas J, Rodriguez-Peralto JL, et al. Fine needle aspiration biopsy findings in endodermal sinus tumors. A report of four cases with cytologic, immunocytochemical and ultrastructural findings. Acta Cytol 1993;37:209-15.

163. Afroz N, Khan N, Chana RS. Cytodiagnosis of yolk sac tumor. Indian J Pediatr 2004;71:939-42.

164. Ceyhan K, Utkan G, Dincol D, Erdogan N, Erekul S, Umudum H. Fine needle aspiration biopsy features with histologic correlation in mediastinal hepatoid yolk sac tumor presenting with sternum metastasis: a case report. Acta Cytol 2007;51:610-5.

165. Chhieng DC, Lin O, Moran CA, et al. Fine-needle aspiration biopsy of nonteratomatous germ cell tumors of the mediastinum. Am J Clin Pathol 2002;118:418-24.

166. Yang GC. Fine-needle aspiration cytology of Schiller-Duval bodies of yolk-sac tumor. Diagn Cytopathol 2000;23:228-32.

167. Oosterhuis JW, Castedo SM, de Jong B, et al. Karyotyping and DNA flow cytometry of an orchidoblastoma. Cancer Genet Cytogenet 1988;36:7-11.

168. Perlman EJ, Cushing B, Hawkins E, Griffin CA. Cytogenetic analysis of childhood endodermal sinus tumors: a Pediatric Oncology Group study. Pediatr Pathol 1994;14:695-708.

169. van Echten J, Timmer A, van der Veen AY, Molenaar WM, de Jong B. Infantile and adult testicular germ cell tumors. a different pathogenesis? Cancer Genet Cytogenet 2002;135:57-62.

170. Perlman EJ, Hu J, Ho D, Cushing B, Lauer S, Castleberry RP. Genetic analysis of childhood endodermal sinus tumors by comparative genomic hybridization. J Pediatr Hematol Oncol 2000;22:100-5.

171. de Jong B, Oosterhuis JW, Castedo SM, Vos A, te Meerman GJ. Pathogenesis of adult testicular germ cell tumors. A cytogenetic model. Cancer Genet Cytogenet 1990;48:143-67.

172. Sievers S, Alemazkour K, Zahn S, et al. IGF2/H19 imprinting analysis of human germ cell tumors (GCTs) using the methylation-sensitive single-nucleotide primer extension method reflects the origin of GCTs in different stages of primordial germ cell development. Genes Chromosomes Cancer 2005;44:256-64.

173. Kato N, Shibuya H, Fukase M, Tamura G, Motoyama T. Involvement of adenomatous polyposis coli (APC) gene in testicular yolk sac tumor of infants. Hum Pathol 2006;37:48-53.

174. Kato N, Tamura G, Fukase M, Shibuya H, Motoyama T. Hypermethylation of the RUNX3 gene promoter in testicular yolk sac tumor of infants. Am J Pathol 2003;163:387-91.

175. Vogelzang NJ, Bronson D, Savino D, Vessella RL, Fraley EF. A human embryonal-yolk sac carcinoma model system in athymic mice. Cancer 1985;55:2584-93.

176. Motoyama T, Watanabe H, Yamamoto T, Sekiguchi M. Human testicular germ cell tumors in vitro and in athymic nude mice. Acta Pathol Jap 1987;37:431-48.

177. Raghavan D, Heyderman E, Monaghan P, et al. Hypothesis: when is a seminoma not a seminoma? J Clin Pathol 1981;34:123-8.

178. Monaghan P, Raghavan D, Neville M. Ultrastructure of xenografted human germ cell tumors. Cancer 1982;49:683-97.

179. Czaja JT, Ulbright TM. Evidence for the transformation of seminoma to yolk sac tumor, with histogenetic considerations. Am J Clin Pathol 1992;97:468-77.

180. Harms D, Kock LR. Testicular juvenile granulosa cell and Sertoli cell tumours: a clinicopathological study of 29 cases from the Kiel Paediatric Tumour Registry. Virchows Arch 1997;430:301-9.

181. Lawrence WD, Young RH, Scully RE. Juvenile granulosa cell tumor of the infantile testis. A report of 14 cases. Am J Surg Pathol 1985;9:87-94.

182. Lawrence WD, Young RH, Scully RE. Sex cord-stromal tumors. In: Talerman A, Roth LM, eds. Pathology of the testis and its adnexa. New York: Churchill Livingstone; 1986:67-92.

183. Shukla AR, Huff DS, Canning DA, et al. Juvenile granulosa cell tumor of the testis: contemporary clinical management and pathological diagnosis. J Urol 2004;171:1900-2.

184. Thomas JC, Ross JH, Kay R. Stromal testis tumors in children: a report from the prepubertal testis tumor registry. J Urol 2001;166:2338-40.

185. Chan JK, Chan VS, Mak KL. Congenital juvenile granulosa cell tumour of the testis: report of a case showing extensive degenerative changes. Histopathology 1990;17:75-80.

186. Goswitz JJ, Pettinato G, Manivel JC. Testicular sex cord-stromal tumors in children: clinicopathologic study of sixteen children with review of the literature. Pediatr Pathol Lab Med 1996;16:451-70.

187. Wu JT, Book L, Sudar K. Serum alpha fetoprotein (AFP) levels in normal infants. Pediatr Res 1981;15:50-2.

188. Loehrer PJ Sr, Williams SD, Einhorn LH. Testicular cancer: the quest continues. J Natl Cancer Inst 1988;80:1373-82.

189. Martinazzi M, Crivelli F, Zampatti C. Immunohistochemical study of hepatic and enteric structures in testicular endodermal sinus tumors. Bas Appl Histochem 1988;32:239-45.

190. Ulbright TM, Gersell DJ. Rete testis hyperplasia with hyaline globule formation. A lesion simulating yolk sac tumor. Am J Surg Pathol 1991;15:66-74.

191. Mann JR, Raafat F, Robinson K, et al. The United Kingdom Children's Cancer Study Group's second germ cell tumor study: carboplatin, etoposide, and bleomycin are effective treatment for children with malignant extracranial germ cell tumors, with acceptable toxicity. J Clin Oncol 2000;18:3809-18.

192. Carroll WL, Kempson RL, Govan DE, Freiha FS, Shochat SJ, Link MP. Conservative management of testicular endodermal sinus tumor in childhood. J Urol 1985;13:1011-4.

193. Sabio H, Burgert EO Jr, Farrow GM, Kelalis PP. Embryonal carcinoma of the testis in childhood. Cancer 1974;34:2118-21.

194. Marshall S, Lyon RP, Scott MP. A conservative approach to testicular tumors in children: 12 cases and their management. J Urol 1983;129:350-1.

195. Kramer SA. Pediatric urologic oncology. Urol Clin North Am 1985;12:31-42.

196. Drago JR, Nelson RP, Palmer JM. Childhood embryonal carcinoma of testes. Urology 1978;12:499-504.

197. Kaplan WE, Firlit CF. Treatment of testicular yolk sac carcinoma in the young child. J Urol 1981;126:663-4.

198. Sweetenham JW, Whitehouse JM, Williams CJ, Mead GM. Involvement of the gastrointestinal tract by metastases from germ cell tumors of the testis. Cancer 1988;61:2566-70.

199. Logothetis CJ, Samuels ML, Trindade A, Grant C, Gomez L, Ayala A. The prognostic significance of endodermal sinus tumor histology among patients treated for stage III nonseminomatous germ cell tumors of the testes. Cancer 1984;53:122-8.

200. Nseyo UO, Englander LS, Wajsman Z, Huben RP, Pontes JE. Histological patterns of treatment failures in testicular germ cell neoplasms. J Urol 1985;133:219-20.

201. Hawkins EP, Finegold MJ, Hawkins HK, Krischer JP, Starling KA, Weinberg A. Nongerminomatous malignant germ cell tumors in children: a review of 89 cases from the Pediatric Oncology Group, 1971-1984. Cancer 1986;58:2579-84.

202. Chhieng DC, Jennings TA, Slominski A, Mihm MC Jr. Choriocarcinoma presenting as a cutaneous metastasis. J Cutan Pathol 1995;22:374-7.

203. Logothetis CJ, Samuels ML, Selig DE, et al. Cyclic chemotherapy with cyclophosphamide, doxorubicin, and cisplatin plus vinblastine and bleomycin in advanced germ cell tumors: results with 100 patients. Am J Med 1986;81:219-28.

204. Giralt S, Dexeus F, Amato R, Sella A, Logothetis C. Hyperthyroidism in men with germ cell tumors and high levels of beta-human chorionic gonadotropin. Cancer 1992;69:1286-90.

205. Silva EG. Chorionic villous-like structures in metastatic testicular choriocarcinoma. Cancer 1987;60:207-10.

206. Manivel JC, Niehans G, Wick MR, Dehner LP. Intermediate trophoblast in germ cell neoplasms. Am J Surg Pathol 1987;11:693-701.

207. Rabes HM. Proliferation of human testicular tumours. Int J Androl 1987;10:127-37.

208. Pelkey TJ, Frierson HF Jr, Mills SE, Stoler MH. Detection of the alpha-subunit of inhibin in trophoblastic neoplasia. Hum Pathol 1999;30:26-31.

209. Go JH. Pure choriocarcinoma of testis with tumor-infiltrating lymphocytes and granulomas. Yonsei Med J 2006;47:887-91.

210. Hechelhammer L, Storkel S, Odermatt B, Heitz PU, Jochum W. Epidermal growth factor receptor is a marker for syncytiotrophoblastic cells in testicular germ cell tumors. Virchows Arch 2003;443:28-31.

211. Moroni M, Veronese S, Schiavo R, et al. Epidermal growth factor receptor expression and activation in nonseminomatous germ cell tumors. Clinical Cancer Research 2001;7:2770-5.

212. Lind HM, Haghighi P. Carcinoembryonic antigen staining in choriocarcinoma. Am J Clin Pathol 1986;86:538-40.

213. Clark RK, Damjanov I. Intermediate filaments of human trophoblast and choriocarcinoma cell lines. Virchows Arch [A] 1985;407:203-8.

214. Emanuel PO, Unger PD, Burstein DE. Immunohistochemical detection of p63 in testicular germ cell neoplasia. Ann Diagn Pathol 2006;10:269-73.

215. Pierce GB Jr, Midgley AR Jr. The origin and function of human syncytiotrophoblastic giant cells. Am J Pathol 1963;43:153-73.

216. Akhtar M, al Davel F. Is it feasible to diagnose germ-cell tumors by fine-needle aspiration biopsy? Diagn Cytopathol 1997;16:72-7.

217. Barsky SH. Germ cell tumors of the testis. In: Javadpour N, Barsky SH, eds. Surgical pathology of urologic diseases. Baltimore: Williams & Wilkins; 1987:224-46.

218. Bredael JJ, Vugrin D, Whitmore WF Jr. Autopsy findings in 154 patients with germ cell tumors of the testis. Cancer 1982;50:548-51.

219. Mostofi FK, Spaander P, Grigor K, Parkinson CM, Shakkebaek NE, Oliver RT. Consensus on pathological classifications of testicular tumours. Prog Clin Biol Res 1990;357:267-76.

220. Damjanov I. Tumors of the testis and epididymis. In: Murphy WM, ed. Urological pathology. Philadelphia: W.B.Saunders; 1989:314-79.

221. Pugh RC, Cameron KM. Teratoma. In: Pugh RC, ed. Pathology of the testis. Oxford: Blackwell Scientific; 1976:199-244.

222. Vaeth M, Schultz HP, von der Maase H, et al. Prognostic factors in testicular germ cell tumours: experiences with 1058 consecutive cases. Acta Radiol Oncol 1984;23:271-85.

223. Bosl GJ, Geller NL, Cirrincione C, et al. Multivariate analysis of prognostic variables in patients with metastatic testicular cancer. Cancer Res 1983;43:3403-7.

224. Stoter G, Sylvester R, Sleijfer DT, et al. A multivariate analysis of prognostic factors in disseminated non-seminomatous testicular cancer. Prog Clin Biol Res 1988;269:381-93.

225. Seguchi T, Iwasaki A, Sugao H, Nakano E, Matsuda M, Sonoda T. [Clinical statistics of germinal testicular cancer.] Nippon Hinyokika Gakkai Zasshi 1990;81:889-94. [Japanese]

226. Brigden ML, Sullivan LD, Comisarow RH. Stage C pure choriocarcinoma of the testis: a potentially curable lesion. CA Cancer J Clin 1982;32:82-4.

227. Young RH, Kurman RJ, Scully RE. Proliferations and tumors of intermediate trophoblast of the placental site. Semin Diagn Pathol 1988;5:223-37.

228. Ulbright TM, Young RH, Scully RE. Trophoblastic tumors of the testis other than classic choriocarcinoma: "monophasic" choriocarcinoma and placental site trophoblastic tumor: a report of two cases. Am J Surg Pathol 1997;21:282-8.

229. Petersson F, Grossmann P, Vanecek T, et al. Testicular germ cell tumor composed of placental site trophoblastic tumor and teratoma. Hum Pathol 2010;41:1046-50.

230. Suurmeijer AJ, Gietema JA, Hoekstra HJ. Placental site trophoblastic tumor in a late recurrence of a nonseminomatous germ cell tumor of the testis. Am J Surg Pathol 2004;28:830-3.

231. Ulbright TM, Henley JD, Cummings OW, Foster RS, Cheng L. Cystic trophoblastic tumor: a nonaggressive lesion in postchemotherapy resections of patients with testicular germ cell tumors. Am J Surg Pathol 2004;28:1212-6.

232. von Hochstetter AR, Hedinger CE. The differential diagnosis of testicular germ cell tumors in theory and practice: a critical analysis of two major systems of classification and review of 389 cases. Virchows Arch A Pathol Anat Histol 1982;396:247-77.

233. Gilman PA. The epidemiology of human teratomas. In: Damjanov I, Knowles BB, Solter D, eds. The human teratomas: experimental and clinical biology. Clinton, NJ: Humana Press; 1983:81-104.

234. Simmonds PD, Lee AH, Theaker JM, Tung K, Smart CJ, Mead GM. Primary pure teratoma of the testis. J Urol 1996;155:939-42.

235. Stevens MJ, Norman AR, Fisher C, Hendry WF, Dearnaley DP, Horwich A. Prognosis of testicular teratoma differentiated. Br J Urol 1994;73:701-6.

236. Leibovitch I, Foster RS, Ulbright TM, Donohue JP. Adult primary pure teratoma of the testis. The Indiana experience. Cancer 1995;75:2244-50.

237. Hasegawa T, Maeda K, Kamata N, Okita Y. A case of immature teratoma originating in intra-abdominal undescended testis in a 3-month-old infant. Pediatr Surg Int 2006;22:570-2.

238. Manivel JC, Reinberg Y, Niehans GA, Fraley EE. Intratubular germ cell neoplasia in testicular teratomas and epidermoid cysts. Correlation with prognosis and possible biologic significance. Cancer 1989;64:715-20.

239. Sesterhenn IA, Mesonero C, Davis CJ, Mostofi FK. Testicular teratomas in adults. Histopathology 2002;41 (suppl 1):24.

240. Mostofi FK, Sesterhenn IA. Pathology of germ cell tumors of testes. Prog Clin Biol Res 1985;203:1-34.

241. Grady RW, Ross JH, Kay R. Epidemiological features of testicular teratoma in a prepubertal population. J Urol 1997;158:1191-2.

242. Unger PD, Cohen EL, Talerman A. Mixed germ cell tumor of the testis: a unique combination of seminoma and teratoma composed predominantly of prostatic tissue. J Urol Pathol 1998;9:257-63.

243. Woods CG, O'Brien BA, Cohen RJ. Benign prostatic glands as a tissue component of testicular teratoma: an uncommon histological finding. Pathology 2011;43:168-9.

244. Waxman M, Vuletin JC, Pertschuk LP, Bellamy J, Enu K. Pleomorphic atypical thyroid adenoma arising in struma testis: light microscopic, ultrastructural and immunofluorescent studies. Mt Sinai J Med 1982;49:13-7.

245. Brodner OG, Grube D, Helmstaedter V, Kreienbrink V, Wurster K, Forssmann WG. Endocrine GEP-cells in primary testicular teratoma. Virchows Arch A Pathol Anat Histol 1980;388:251-62.

246. Trojanowski JQ, Hickey WF. Human teratomas express differentiated neural antigens: an immunohistochemical study with anti-neurofilament, anti-glial filament, and anti-myelin basic protein monoclonal antibodies. Am J Pathol 1984;115:383-9.

247. Uchida T, Shimoda T, Miyata H, et al. Immunoperoxidase study of alkaline phosphatase in testicular tumor. Cancer 1981;48:1455-62.

248. Rodriguez E, Mathew S, Reuter V, Ilson DH, Bosl GJ, Chaganti RS. Cytogenetic analysis of 124 prospectively ascertained male germ cell tumors. Cancer Res 1992;52:2285-91.

249. Oosterhuis JW, de Jong B, Cornelisse CJ, et al. Karyotyping and DNA flow cytometry of mature residual teratoma after intensive chemotherapy of disseminated nonseminomatous germ cell tumor of the testis: a report of two cases. Cancer Genet Cytogenet 1986;22:149-57.

250. Molenaar WM, Oosterhuis JW, Meiring A, Sleyfer DT, Koops HS, Cornelisse CJ. Histology and DNA contents of a secondary malignancy arising in a mature residual lesion six years after chemotherapy for a disseminanted nonseminomatous testicular tumor. Cancer 1986;58:264-8.

251. Bussey KJ, Lawce HJ, Olson SB, et al. Chromosome abnormalities of eighty-one pediatric germ cell tumors: sex-, age-, site-, and histopathology-related differences—a Children's Cancer Group study. Genes Chromosomes Cancer 1999;25:134-46.

252. Stock C, Ambros IM, Lion T, et al. Detection of numerical and structural chromosome abnormalities in pediatric germ cell tumors by means of interphase cytogenetics. Genes Chromosomes Cancer 1994;11:40-50.

253. Mostert M, Rosenberg C, Stoop H, et al. Comparative genomic and in situ hybridization of germ cell tumors of the infantile testis. Lab Invest 2000;80:1055-64.

254. Sella A, el-Naggar A, Ro JY, et al. Evidence of malignant features in histologically mature teratoma. J Urol 1991;146:1025-8.

255. Castedo SM, Oosterhuis JW, de Jong B, et al. A residual mature teratoma with a more balanced karyotype than the primary testicular nonseminoma? Cancer Genet Cytogenet 1988;32:51-7.

256. Dieckmann KP, Loy V. Epidermoid cyst of the testis: a review of clinical and histogenetic considerations. Br J Urol 1994;73:436-41.

257. Shah KH, Maxted WC, Chun B. Epidermoid cysts of the testis: a report of three cases and an analysis of 141 cases from the world literature. Cancer 1981;47:577-82.

258. Price EB Jr. Epidermoid cysts of the testis: a clinical and pathologic analysis of 69 cases from the testicular tumor registry. J Urol 1969;102:708-13.

259. Dixon FJ, Moore RA. Testicular tumors: a clinicopathologic study. Cancer 1953;6:427-54.

260. Donohue JP, Roth LM, Zachary JM, Rowland RG, Einhorn LH, Williams SD. Cytoreductive surgery for metastatic testis cancer: tissue analysis of retroperitoneal masses after chemotherapy. J Urol 1982;127:1111-4.

261. Einhorn LH, Williams SD, Mandelbaum I, Donohue JP. Surgical resection in disseminated testicular cancer following chemotherapeutic cytoreduction. Cancer 1981;48:904-8.

262. Oosterhuis JW, Suurmeyer AJ, Sleyfer DT, Koops HS, Oldhoff J, Fleuren G. Effects of multiple-drug chemotherapy (cis-diammine-dichloroplatinum, bleomycin and vinblastine) on the maturation of retroperitoneal lymph node metastases of nonseminomatous germ cell tumors of the testis: no evidence for de novo induction of differentiation. Cancer 1983;51:408-16.

263. Steyerberg EW, Keizer HJ, Stoter G, Habbema JD. Predictors of residual mass histology following chemotherapy for metastatic non-seminomatous testicular cancer: a quantitative overview of 996 resections. Eur J Cancer 1994;30A:1231-9.

264. Jaeger N, Weissbach L, Bussar-Maatz R. Size and status of metastases after inductive chemotherapy of germ-cell tumors. Indication for salvage operation. World J Urol 1994;12:196-9.

265. Foster RS, Baniel J, Leibovitch I, et al. Teratoma in the orchiectomy specimen and volume of metastasis are predictors of retroperitoneal teratoma in low stage nonseminomatous testis cancer. J Urol 1996;155:1943-5.

266. Rabbani F, Gleave ME, Coppin CM, Murray N, Sullivan LD. Teratoma in primary testis tumor reduces complete response rates in the retroperitoneum after primary chemotherapy. The case for primary retroperitoneal lymph node dissection of stage IIb germ cell tumors with teratomatous elements. Cancer 1996;78:480-6.

267. Beck SD, Foster RS, Bihrle R, et al. Teratoma in the orchiectomy specimen and volume of metastasis are predictors of retroperitoneal teratoma in post-chemotherapy nonseminomatous testis cancer. J Urol 2002;168:1402-4.

268. Kooijman CD. Immature teratomas in children. Histopathology 1988;12:491-502.

269. Johnson DE, Bracken RB, Blight EM. Prognosis for pathologic stage I non-seminomatous germ cell tumors of the testis managed by retroperitoneal lymphadenectomy. J Urol 1976;116:63-8.

270. Ulbright TM, Loehrer PJ, Roth LM, Einhorn LH, Williams SD, Clark SA. The development of non-germ cell malignancies within germ cell tumors. A clinicopathologic study of 11 cases. Cancer 1984;54:1824-33.

271. Ahmed T, Bosl GJ, Hajdu SI. Teratoma with malignant transformation in germ cell tumors in men. Cancer 1985;56:860-3.

272. Loehrer PJ, Hui S, Clark S, et al. Teratoma following cisplatin-based combination chemotherapy for nonseminomatous germ cell tumors: a clinicopathological correlation. J Urol 1986;135:1183-9.

273. Zuk RJ, Jenkins BJ, Martin JE, Oliver RT, Baithun SI. Findings in lymph nodes of patients with germ cell tumours after chemotherapy and their relation to prognosis. J Clin Pathol 1989;42:1049-54.

274. Fossä SD, Aass N, Ous S, et al. Histology of tumor residuals following chemotherapy in patients with advanced nonseminomatous testicular cancer. J Urol 1989;142:1239-42.

275. Logothetis CJ, Samuels ML, Trindade A. The growing teratoma syndrome. Cancer 1982;50:1629-35.

276. Tongaonkar HB, Deshmane VH, Dalal AV, Kulkarni JN, Kamat MR. Growing teratoma syndrome. J Surg Oncol 1994;55:56-60.

277. Burt AD, Cooper G, MacKay C, Boyd JF. Dermoid cyst of the testis. Scott Med J 1987;32:146-8.

278. Broggi G, Appetito C, di Leone L, et al. Dermoid cyst in undescended testis in a 9-year-old boy. Urol Int 1991;47:110-2.

279. Gupta AK, Gupta MK, Gupta K. Dermoid cyst of the testis (a case report). Indian J Cancer 1986;23:21-3.

280. Assaf G, Mosbah A, Homsy Y, Michaud J. Dermoid cyst of testis in five-year-old-child. Urology 1983;22:432-4.

281. Dockerty MB, Priestly JT. Dermoid cysts of the testis. J Urol 1942;48:392-400.

282. Wegner HE, Herbst H, Loy V, Dieckmann KP. Testicular dermoid cyst in a 10-year-old child: case report and discussion of etiopathogenesis, diagnosis, and treatment. Urol Int 1995;54:109-11.

283. Ulbright TM, Srigley JR. Dermoid cyst of the testis: a study of five postpubertal cases, including a pilomatrixoma-like variant, with evidence supporting its separate classification from mature testicular teratoma. Am J Surg Pathol 2001;25:788-93.

284. Zamecnik M, Mukensnabl P, Curik R, Michal M. Shadow cell differentiation in testicular teratomas. A report of two cases. Cesk Patol 2005;41:102-6.

285. Ward RM, Evans HL. Cystosarcoma phyllodes. A clinicopathologic study of 26 cases. Cancer 1986;58:2282-9.

286. Guo CC, Punar M, Contreras AL, et al. Testicular germ cell tumors with sarcomatous components: an analysis of 33 cases. Am J Surg Pathol 2009;33:1173-8.

287. Comiter CV, Kibel AS, Richie JP, Nucci MR, Renshaw AA. Prognostic features of teratomas with malignant transformation: a clinicopathological study of 21 cases. J Urol 1998;159:859-63.

288. Lutke Holzik MF, Hoekstra HJ, Mulder NH, Suurmeijer AJ, Sleijfer DT, Gietema JA. Non-germ cell malignancy in residual or recurrent mass after chemotherapy for nonseminomatous testicular germ cell tumor. Ann Surg Oncol 2003;10:131-5.

289. Malagon HD, Valdez AM, Moran CA, Suster S. Germ cell tumors with sarcomatous components: a clinicopathologic and immunohisto-

chemical study of 46 cases. Am J Surg Pathol 2007;31:1356-62.

290. Motzer RJ, Amsterdam A, Prieto V, et al. Teratoma with malignant transformation: diverse malignant histologies arising in men with germ cell tumors. J Urol 1998;159:133-8.

291. Michael H, Hull MT, Ulbright TM, Foster RS, Miller KD. Primitive neuroectodermal tumors arising in testicular germ cell neoplasms. Am J Surg Pathol 1997;21:896-904.

292. Talerman A, Gratama S, Miranda S, Okagaki T. Primary carcinoid tumor of the testis: case report, ultrastructure and review of the literature. Cancer 1978;42:2696-706.

293. Berdjis CC, Mostofi FK. Carcinoid tumors of the testis. J Urol 1977;118:777-82.

294. Zavala-Pompa A, Ro JY, El-Naggar A, et al. Primary carcinoid tumor of testis. Immunohistochemical, ultrastructural, and DNA flow cytometric study of three cases with a review of the literature. Cancer 1993;72:1726-32.

295. Sullivan JL, Packer JT, Bryant M. Primary malignant carcinoid of the testis. Arch Pathol Lab Med 1981;105:515-7.

296. Finci R, Gunhan O, Celasun B, Gungor S. Carcinoid tumor of undescended testis. J Urol 1987;137:301-2.

297. Stroosma OB, Delaere KP. Carcinoid tumours of the testis. BJU Int 2008;101:1101-5.

298. Ordonez NG, Ayala AG, Sneige N, Mackay B. Immunohistochemical demonstration of multiple neurohormonal polypeptides in a case of pure testicular carcinoid. Am J Clin Pathol 1982;78:860-4.

299. Hosking DH, Bowman DM, McMorris SL, Ramsey EW. Primary carcinoid of the testis with metastases. J Urol 1981;125:255-6.

300. Berkheiser SW. Carcinoid tumor of the testis occurring in a cystic teratoma of the testis. J Urol 1959;82:352-5.

301. Simon HB, McDonald JR, Culp OS. Argentaffin tumor (carcinoid) occurring in a benign cystic teratoma of the testicle. J Urol 1954;72:892-4.

302. Reyes A, Moran CA, Suster S, Michal M, Dominguez H. Neuroendocrine carcinomas (carcinoid tumor) of the testis. A clinicopathologic and immunohistochemical study of ten cases. Am J Clin Pathol 2003;120:182-7.

303. Abbosh PH, Zhang S, MacLennan GT, et al. Germ cell origin of testicular carcinoid tumors. Clinical Cancer Res 2008;14:1393-6.

304. Merino J, Zuluaga A, Gutierrez-Tejero F, Del Mar Serrano M, Ciani S, Nogales FF. Pure testicular carcinoid associated with intratubular germ cell neoplasia. J Clin Pathol 2005;58:1331-3.

305. Ogawa A, Sugihara S, Nakazawa Y. A case of primary carcinoid tumor of the testis. Gan No Rinsho 1988;34:1629-34.

306. Kato N, Motoyama T, Kameda N, et al. Primary carcinoid tumor of the testis: Immunohistochemical, ultrastructural and FISH analysis with review of the literature. Pathol Int 2003;53:680-5.

307. McCluggage WG, Shanks JH, Whiteside C, Maxwell P, Banerjee SS, Biggart JD. Immunohistochemical study of testicular sex cord-stromal tumors, including staining with anti-inhibin antibody. Am J Surg Pathol 1998;22:615-9.

308. Iczkowski KA, Bostwick DG, Roche PC, Cheville JC. Inhibin A is a sensitive and specific marker for testicular sex cord-stromal tumors. Mod Pathol 1998;11:774-9.

309. Zhao C, Bratthauer GL, Barner R, Vang R. Comparative analysis of alternative and traditional immunohistochemical markers for the distinction of ovarian sertoli cell tumor from endometrioid tumors and carcinoid tumor: A study of 160 cases. Am J Surg Pathol 2007;31:255-66.

310. Kuroda N, Senzaki T, Yamasaki Y, et al. Sertoli cell tumor of the testis (not otherwise specified) with the expression of neuroendocrine markers and without the expression of inhibin-alpha. Pathol Int 2004;54:719-24.

311. Aguirre P, Scully RE. Primitive neuroectodermal tumor of the testis. Report of a case. Arch Pathol Lab Med 1983;107:643-5.

312. Nocks BN, Dann JA. Primitive neuroectodermal tumor (immature teratoma) of testis. Urology 1983;22:543-4.

313. Nistal M, Paniagua R. Primary neuroectodermal tumour of the testis. Histopathology 1985;9:1351-9.

314. Kleihues P, Cavenee WK, eds. Pathology and genetics of tumours of the nervous system. Lyon: IARC Press; 2000.

315. Ulbright TM, Hattab EM, Zhang S, et al. Primitive neuroectodermal tumors in patients with testicular germ cell tumors usually resemble pediatric-type central nervous system embryonal neoplasms and lack chromosome 22 rearrangements. Mod Pathol 2010;23:972-80.

316. Anagnostaki L, Jacobsen GK, Horn T, Sengelov L, Braendstrup O. Melanotic neuroectodermal tumour as a predominant component of an immature testicular teratoma. Case report with immunohistochemical investigations. APMIS 1992;100:809-16.

317. Schmidt D, Harms D, Pilon VA. Small-cell pediatric tumors: histology, immunohistochemistry, and electron microscopy. Clin Lab Med 1987;7:63-89.

318. Parham DM, Webber B, Holt H, Williams WK, Maurer H. Immunohistochemical Study of childhood rhabdomyosarcomas and related neoplasms. Results of an Intergroup Rhabdomyosarcoma Study Project. Cancer 1991;67:3072-80.

319. Cummings OW, Ulbright TM, Young RH, Dei Tos AP, Fletcher CDM, Hull MT. Desmoplastic small round cell tumors of the para-testicular region: a report of six cases. Am J Surg Pathol 1997;21:219-25.

5 MIXED GERM CELL TUMORS, REGRESSED GERM CELL TUMORS, AND GERM CELL-SEX CORD-STROMAL TUMORS

MIXED GERM CELL TUMORS

Definition. *Mixed germ cell tumors* contain more than one germ cell component. Seminoma with syncytiotrophoblast cells are, by convention, excluded from this category.

General Features. In a registry-based series of 1,053 consecutive testicular germ cell tumors, mixed tumors represented 69 percent of all nonseminomatous tumors and 32 percent of all cases (1). In a referral-based series of 513 testicular germ cell tumors, mixed tumors accounted for 91 percent of the nonseminomatous cases and 60 percent of all neoplasms, although this study included seminomas with syncytiotrophoblast giant cells in the mixed category (2). The more common combinations are listed in order of frequency in Table 5-1; the most frequent is embryonal carcinoma with one or more of teratoma, seminoma, or yolk sac tumor. The only germ cell tumor never seen as a component of a mixed germ cell tumor is spermatocytic seminoma.

For diagnosis, these tumors should be termed "mixed germ cell tumor, composed of ...," followed by a tabulation of the components, with an estimate of their percentage; for example: "mixed germ cell tumor composed of embryonal carcinoma (60 percent), yolk sac tumor (25 percent), seminoma (15 percent), and rare syncytiotrophoblast cells." The combination of embryonal carcinoma and teratoma has been termed *teratocarcinoma*, but it is preferable to list the components separately.

Clinical Features. Patients with mixed germ cell tumors generally present with testicular enlargement, sometimes associated with pain. The tumors occur at an average age of 30 years: patients with a predominance of embryonal carcinoma average 28 years and those with a predominance of seminoma, 33 years (3). Prepubertal patients rarely develop mixed germ cell tumors. Serum marker elevations are common and reflect the components of the tumors: alpha-fetoprotein (AFP) elevation is present at diagnosis in 45 percent of those whose tumors are limited to the testis and human chorionic gonadotropin (hCG) elevation in 33 percent; for patients with metastatic disease, high levels occur in about 60 percent and 55 percent of patients, respectively (4,5).

Gross Findings. The tumors are variegated (fig. 5-1). Solid white to gray areas may reflect a seminomatous component (fig. 5-2) whereas nonseminomatous elements more frequently are associated with areas of necrosis, hemorrhage, and cystic change (fig. 5-1A,B). Nondegenerative

Table 5-1

COMBINATIONS OF NEOPLASTIC GERM CELL TUMOR TYPES IN 352 MIXED GERM CELL TUMORS[a]

Tumor Types	Number (%)
EC[b] + T	90 (26%)
EC + S	55 (16%)
EC + YST + T	39 (11%)
EC + T + CC	26 (7%)
EC + T + S	22 (6%)
T + S	20 (6%)
EC + YST	15 (4%)
EC + YST + T + CC	15 (4%)
EC + CC	13 (4%)
EC + YST + T	12 (3%)
EC + YST + S	9 (3%)
Other combinations	36 (10%)

[a]Adapted from Jacobsen GK, Barlebo H, Olsen J, et al. Testicular germ cell tumours in Denmark 1976-1980: pathology of 1058 consecutive cases. Acta Radiol Oncol 1984;23:239-47.
[b]EC = embryonal carcinoma; T = teratoma; S = seminoma; YST = yolk sac tumor; CC = choriocarcinoma.

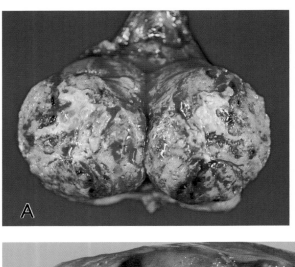

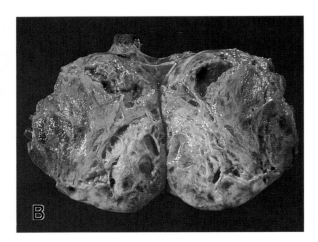

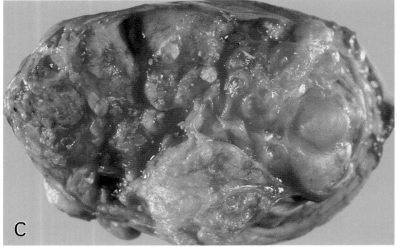

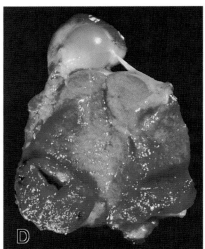

Figure 5-1

MIXED GERM CELL TUMORS

A: The cut surface has the usual variegated appearance, with areas of necrosis. This tumor had components of teratoma with immature elements, yolk sac tumor, and embryonal carcinoma. (Courtesy of Dr. P. R. Faught, Indianapolis, IN.)

B: There is prominent cystic degeneration in a tumor consisting of yolk sac tumor and embryonal carcinoma.

C: Cysts corresponding to a teratomatous component are present in a neoplasm that also contained embryonal carcinoma.

D: Beefy red areas are conspicuous in this tumor that had a prominent choriocarcinoma component as well as embryonal carcinoma.

cysts often correspond to dilated teratomatous glands (figs. 5-1C, 5-3).

Microscopic Findings. The individual components are identical to those seen in pure form (fig. 5-4). Closely associated components of embryonal carcinoma and yolk sac tumor (fig. 5-5) are especially frequent, the latter often being overlooked (fig. 5-6). Close inspection of such cases often discloses a less dense grouping of flattened or stellate cells directly adjacent to

a surface lining of more deeply staining embryonal carcinoma cells (fig. 5-6D). Seminoma may have subtle admixed foci of embryonal carcinoma (fig. 5-7), yolk sac tumor (fig. 5-8) or, rarely, choriocarcinoma (fig. 5-9). In choriocarcinoma, it is important to distinguish the mononucleated trophoblasts that admix with syncytiotrophoblasts from seminoma cells because of the different treatment and prognosis of patients with seminoma with

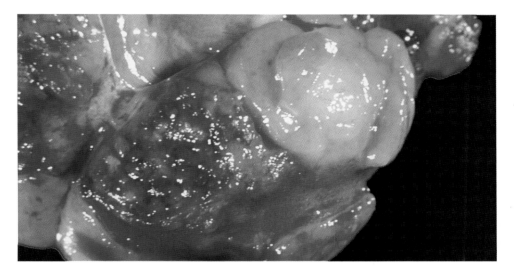

Figure 5-2

MIXED GERM CELL TUMOR

Two distinct components, embryonal carcinoma (lower left) and seminoma (upper right), were present, as could be suspected from the gross appearance.

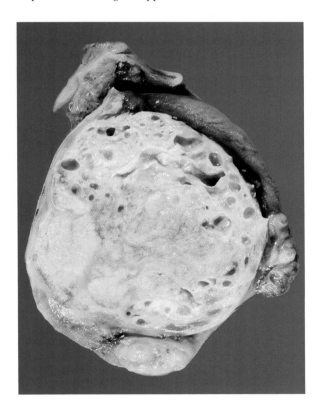

Figure 5-3

MIXED GERM CELL TUMOR

The teratomatous component in this tumor is evident as multiple cystically dilated glands.

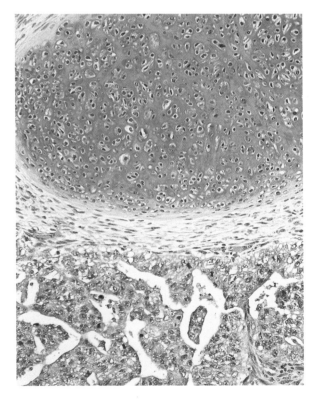

Figure 5-4

MIXED GERM CELL TUMOR

There is an admixture of embryonal carcinoma and teratomatous cartilage.

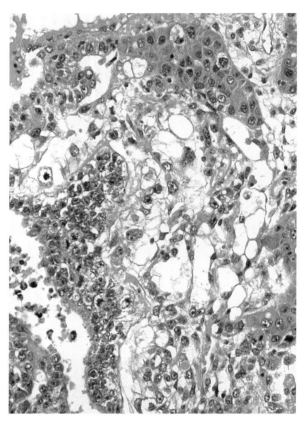
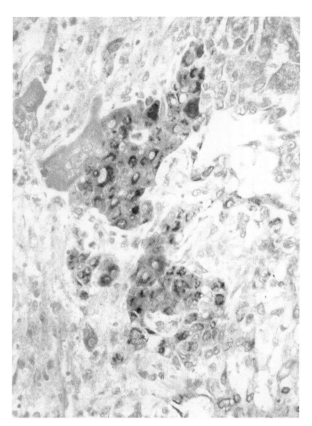

Figure 5-5

MIXED GERM CELL TUMOR

Left: There is admixture of embryonal carcinoma (lower left) with yolk sac tumor showing both reticular and hepatoid features (top).

Right: The liver-like cells are highlighted by an immunostain against alpha-fetoprotein (AFP).

syncytiotrophoblast cells as opposed to those with seminoma with choriocarcinoma. This is facilitated by using immunostains for OCT3/4, which are negative in trophoblasts and positive in seminoma cells. The yolk sac tumor foci are often readily appreciated when appropriate immunostains are employed (fig. 5-8). The usually clear cytoplasm of seminoma cells that contrasts with the denser cytoplasm and greater pleomorphism of embryonal carcinoma cells generally allows the distinction of these two components at scanning magnification, but in occasional cases (fig. 5-7B,C), the types merge imperceptibly. Appropriate immunostains may clarify their distinction. We have seen a single case of seminoma that had multiple microscopic foci of admixed squamous epithelial cells; this unique tumor was interpreted as seminoma and teratoma.

Two patterns of mixed germ cell tumor are sufficiently distinctive that they are separately subcategorized: polyembryoma and diffuse embryoma.

Polyembryoma. This distinctive mixed germ cell tumor is composed of embryonal carcinoma and yolk sac tumor, often with teratomatous components. The first two components are predominantly arranged in a pattern resembling the presomatic embryo prior to day 18 of development (6,7). For that reason, some authorities have considered it the most immature of teratomas. But because it behaves and is treated like a mixed germ cell tumor with embryonal carcinoma and yolk sac tumor components (8), we have categorized it as a unique form of mixed germ cell tumor, in accord with the classification of the World Health Organization (WHO) (9).

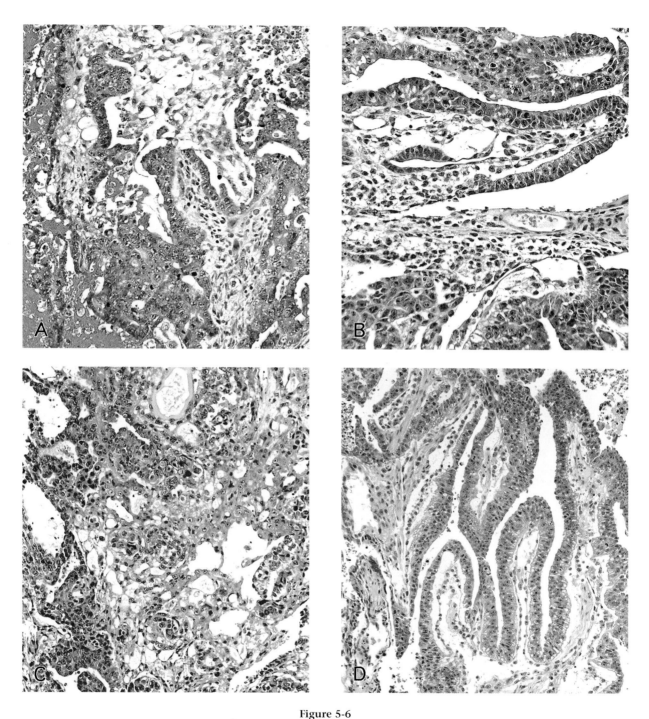

Figure 5-6

MIXED GERM CELL TUMORS

A: The loosely arranged, focally vacuolated cells represent yolk sac tumor that is associated with embryonal carcinoma.

B: Embryonal carcinoma cells with columnar profiles line villus-like processes. These processes contain cores of smaller, vacuolated to flattened yolk sac tumor cells.

C: In this area, the yolk sac tumor and embryonal carcinoma components do not contrast as much as they do in A and B, although they are still distinguishable.

D: A subtle, thin layer of yolk sac tumor cells parallels the more conspicuous embryonal carcinoma component.

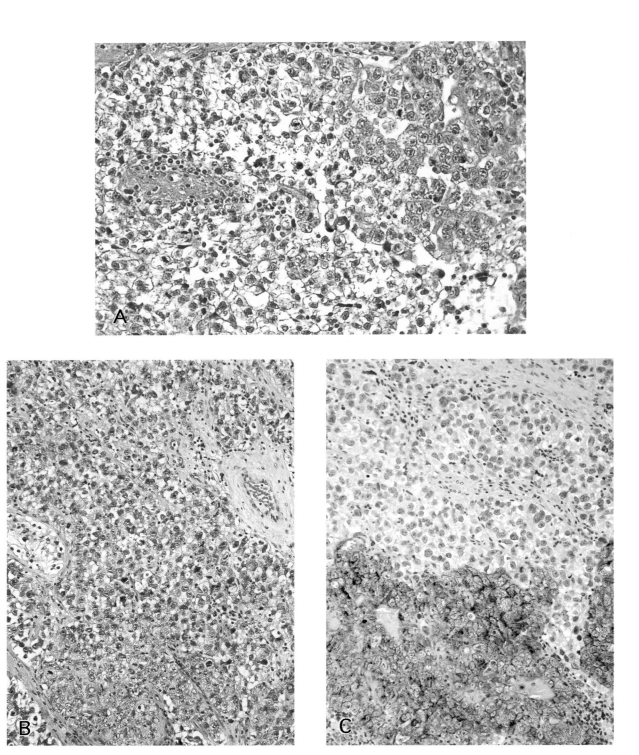

Figure 5-7

MIXED GERM CELL TUMORS

A: Seminoma (top) merges with embryonal carcinoma (bottom right).

B: In this tumor, the seminoma (top) is more difficult to distinguish from the embryonal carcinoma (bottom) than in A.

C: An immunostain for CD30 selectively highlights the embryonal carcinoma component in the tumor illustrated in B.

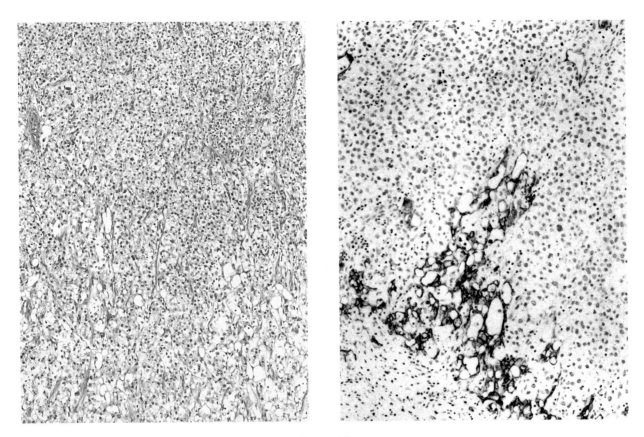

Figure 5-8

MIXED GERM CELL TUMOR

Left: There is a subtle blending of seminoma (top) with yolk sac tumor (bottom).
Right: The yolk sac tumor component is selectively highlighted by a cytokeratin immunostain.

In support of this approach, polyembryomatous foci always comprise a portion of a mixed germ cell tumor and have not been reported in pure form in the testis to our knowledge. The age range of patients is the same as for those with nonseminomatous germ cell tumors (6,8). Substantial AFP elevations occur (8).

The tumors are solid and cystic, the latter reflecting the frequently associated teratoma component. Foci of hemorrhage and necrosis are present (8).

On microscopic examination, there are numerous scattered embryo-like bodies ("embryoid bodies") (fig. 5-10). These bodies consist of a central plate of cuboidal to columnar embryonal carcinoma cells of one to four layers thickness, a "dorsal" amnion-like cavity typically lined by flattened epithelium, and a "ventral" yolk sac-like vesicle composed of reticular and myxo-matous yolk sac tumor (fig. 5-11). These bodies are from 0.2 to 0.7 mm in greatest dimension and are surrounded by myxoid, embryonic-type mesenchyme (fig. 5-10). They are often evenly spaced from one another, resulting in a distinctive picture. The "amnion" is usually composed of flattened cells, but both intestinal and squamous differentiation of the "amniotic epithelium" has been described (8). Argyrophilic cells may be identified in the intestinal component (8). Microscopic foci of yolk sac tumor often emanate from the yolk sac epithelium of the embryonic disc, and this is generally associated with breakdown of the classic organization of the embryoid body. Elements of yolk sac tumor and embryonal carcinoma are randomly arranged but still retain a vaguely zonal distribution (fig. 5-12). Hepatic differentiation may develop in these foci (8). Sometimes, the

217

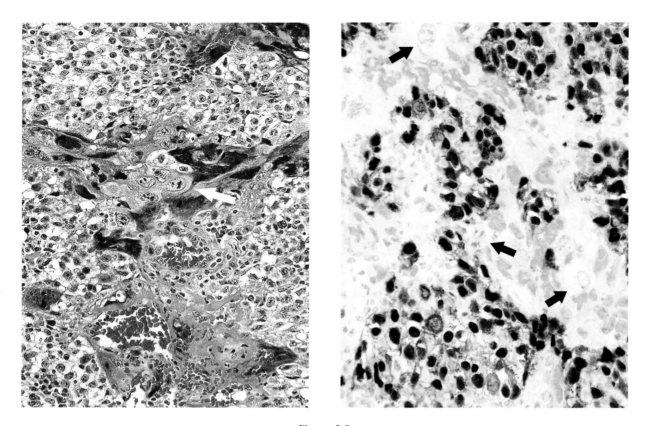

Figure 5-9

MIXED GERM CELL TUMOR

Left: A minor choriocarcinoma component is seen with seminoma. Syncytiotrophoblasts with multiple smudgy nuclei are mixed with large mononucleated trophoblast cells (arrow) that contrast with the smaller, surrounding seminoma cells.

Right: Neither the mononucleated trophoblast cells (cells at arrows with open chromatin) nor the syncytiotrophoblast cells (cells with multiple smudged nuclei) show nuclear staining for OCT3/4, in contrast to the seminoma cells.

Figure 5-10

POLYEMBRYOMA

Embryoid bodies are scattered in a loose mesenchyme analogous to extraembryonic mesenchyme.

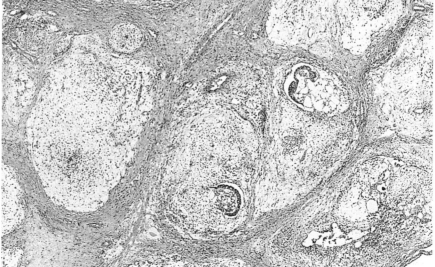

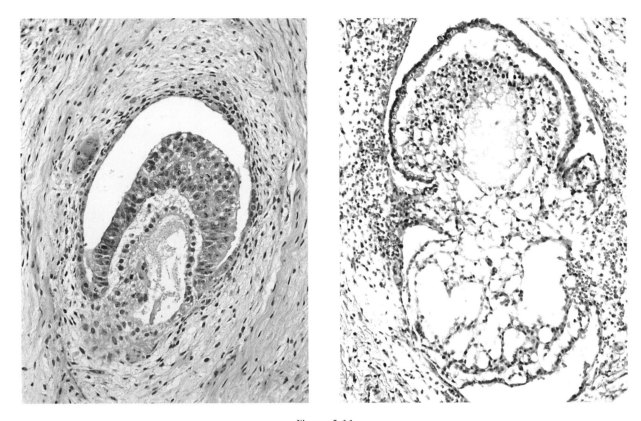

Figure 5-11

POLYEMBRYOMA

Left: High magnification of an embryoid body shows a central core of embryonal carcinoma mimicking the embryonic plate, with a "dorsal" amnion-like cavity and a "ventral" yolk sac-like structure. A syncytiotrophoblastic cell is also apparent close to the "amnion."

Right: Two embryoid bodies are fused and there is a central aggregate of yolk sac tumor epithelium. Invasion of the yolk sac epithelium beyond the embryoid body has not occurred.

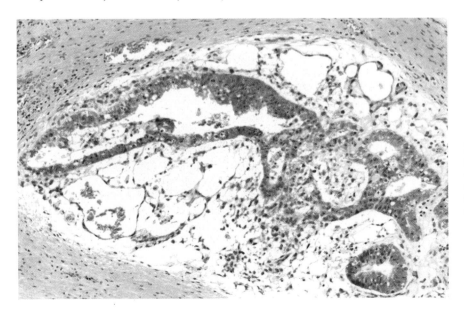

Figure 5-12

MIXED GERM CELL TUMOR

This mixed germ cell tumor has a poorly formed embryoid body with a central core of embryonal carcinoma around which is a haphazard arrangement of yolk sac tumor epithelium.

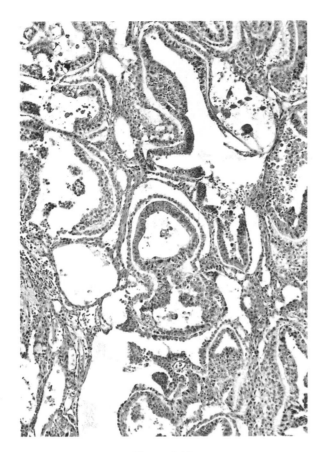

Figure 5-13

DIFFUSE EMBRYOMA

Embryonal carcinoma and yolk sac tumor are admixed in diffuse orderly ribbons and circular patterns.

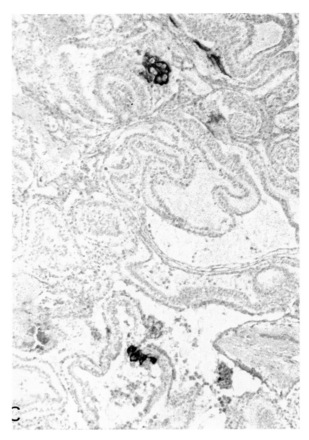

Figure 5-14

DIFFUSE EMBRYOMA

Syncytiotrophoblast cells are highlighted by an immunostain for human chorionic gonadotropin (hCG). The orderly arrangement is still perceptible. (Fig. 3.63 from Young RH, Scully RE. Testicular tumors. Chicago, ASCP Press; 1990:79.)

microscopic foci of yolk sac tumor elements in the embryoid bodies proliferate enough to justify a separate diagnosis of yolk sac tumor (*polyembryoma and yolk sac tumor*). Similarly, growth of the embryonal carcinoma component can lead to larger, circumscribed foci of ribbons and glands of embryonal carcinoma, often with admixed yolk sac tumor (fig. 5-12). Syncytiotrophoblast cells may be identified in close proximity to the "amnion" and "yolk sac" (6). Immunohistochemically, the yolk sac-like areas stain for AFP (8).

Diffuse Embryoma. This tumor is characterized by an intimate admixture of orderly arranged embryonal carcinoma and yolk sac tumor components in roughly equal proportions (fig. 5-13) (10,11). Minor trophoblastic (fig. 5-14) or teratomatous elements may also

occur, as well as liver-like cells. The yolk sac tumor elements may "garland" foci of embryonal carcinoma as a parallel layer of flattened epithelium, a pattern that has been described as "necklace-like" or "ribbon-like." This pattern is similar to that described as the "double-layered" pattern of embryonal carcinoma (fig. 5-15) (12,13), said to occur in 7 percent of embryonal carcinomas (12) and which we regard as diffuse embryoma and a form of mixed germ cell tumor. The flattened cell layer in such cases generally stains for AFP, supporting its yolk sac tumor nature (fig. 5-16).

Treatment and Prognosis. The treatment of mixed germ cell tumors is similar to that for other nonseminomatous tumors. The presence

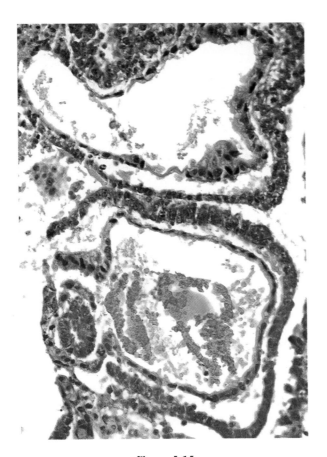

Figure 5-15

DIFFUSE EMBRYOMA

A higher magnification of the tumor seen in figure 5-13 shows an equal proportion of embryonal carcinoma and yolk sac tumor in a necklace-like arrangement.

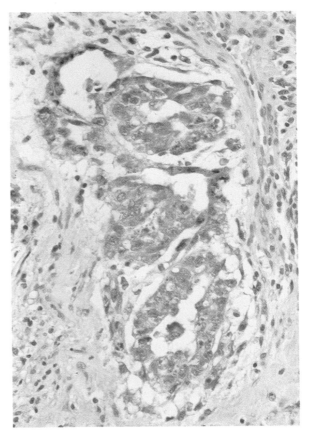

Figure 5-16

MIXED GERM CELL TUMOR

AFP is positive in the flattened cells representing the yolk sac tumor component, intermingled with embryonal carcinoma cells, which are negative (anti-AFP immunostain).

of some elements appears to modify the behavior of other components: embryonal carcinoma with teratoma has a lower metastatic rate than a pure embryonal carcinoma of the same size as the embryonal carcinoma component of the mixed tumor (14). This fact, in conjunction with the occurrence of different potentials for differentiation in human embryonal carcinoma cell lines (15–17), implies that embryonal carcinomas associated with teratoma have a greater inherent ability to differentiate than pure embryonal carcinomas and are therefore intrinsically less aggressive (18–21). The presence of yolk sac tumor elements is also associated with a lesser tendency to metastasize, and may also reflect a greater inherent tendency of the neoplasm to differentiate (22).

REGRESSED GERM CELL TUMORS

General and Clinical Features. In some patients who present with extragonadal germ cell tumors, careful clinical evaluation fails to reveal evidence of a conventional testicular primary neoplasm (23–26). Some of these patients may have primary neoplasms of extragonadal origin, presumably developing from misplaced germ cells. There is convincing evidence, however, that many of these patients have primary testicular neoplasms that have partially or completely regressed. Indeed, some patients only develop a clinically evident testicular tumor after metastatic disease is present (27). An occult testicular origin is most likely for those patients with retroperitoneal tumors (26,28). With isolated mediastinal or pineal involvement, there

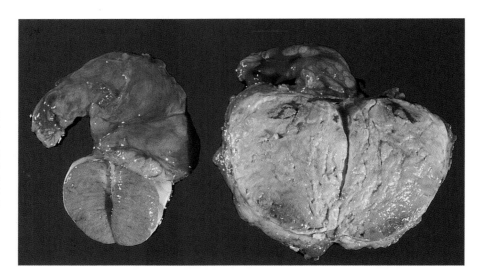

Figure 5-17

REGRESSED GERM CELL TUMOR

The patient presented with a large, mostly necrotic retroperitoneal tumor composed of seminoma and mature teratoma (right). The grossly normal testis (left) contained a microscopic area of scarring and mature teratoma.

is a higher probability of true extragonadal origin (28,29). In one series of 15 patients with retroperitoneal germ cell tumors who lacked clinical evidence of a primary testicular tumor, 53 percent had intratubular germ cell neoplasia, unclassified type (IGCNU) on testicular biopsies (28,30), suggesting the retroperitoneal tumors were metastases from regressed testicular primaries (31). This is not the case in patients with mediastinal germ cell tumors (28), although there are rare exceptions (32). Although a "field effect" causing independent neoplasia in both the testis and retroperitoneum has been suggested, this seems unlikely given the high rate of detection of IGCNU in this situation and the low rate of IGCNU in the contralateral testis of patients with testicular germ cell tumors (approximately 5 percent). A field effect also fails to explain why a comparable rate of IGCNU is not identified in association with mediastinal germ cell tumors.

The initial concept of spontaneous regression in testicular germ cell tumors was based on studies of patients who died of metastatic germ cell tumors and were found only at autopsy to have testicular abnormalities (33). In an autopsy series of 61 cases, "burnt-out" testicular primaries were found in 6 (10 percent) patients (34). Subsequently, several large series of regressed tumors, mostly in patients who presented with metastatic disease, were reported (35,36).

All forms of germ cell tumor may regress. Not unexpectedly, the single largest number of cases is attributable to regression of seminoma (36), which is the most common tumor type. A high proportion of choriocarcinomas regress (37), which is partly responsible for the frequent presentation of choriocarcinoma with metastatic disease rather than a testicular mass. Teratoma is more likely to persist than the other germ cell tumor types. Because a testicular primary may regress at the same time as metastases grow, huge metastatic deposits may occur with only microscopic testicular lesions (fig. 5-17).

Histologic discrepancies between the metastatic tumor and the residual, partially regressed testicular neoplasm are common (34). For instance, patients may present with metastatic embryonal carcinoma and only have microscopic foci of seminoma and scarring in the testis (24). Such cases may well represent mixed germ cell tumors in which the disseminated element regressed in the testis, while other components persisted. Another explanation for discrepancy between the morphology of the testicular tumor and the metastasis is transformation of tumor types (38).

Gross Findings. Gross examination may reveal only one or more, poorly demarcated (fig. 5-18) to circumscribed (fig. 5-19) zones of firm, white scar tissue. A scar surrounded by hemorrhage may represent a regressed choriocarcinoma. In cases that are not entirely regressed, cysts corresponding to dilated teratomatous glands, small firm nodules of cartilage, or necrotic foci (fig. 5-19) may be identified, as may foci grossly consistent with residual seminoma or embryonal carcinoma.

Microscopic Findings. On microscopic examination, the scarred zones are most frequently circumscribed areas of dense collagen (fig. 5-20), but they also may be irregular, stellate-shaped, sclerotic foci that dissect between seminiferous tubules (fig. 5-21). Within the scar, hyalinized

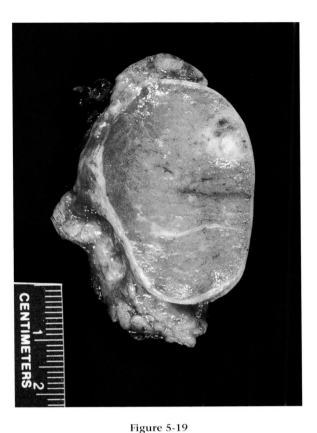

Figure 5-19

REGRESSED GERM CELL TUMOR

There is a small circumscribed zone of scarring that contains some necrotic foci.

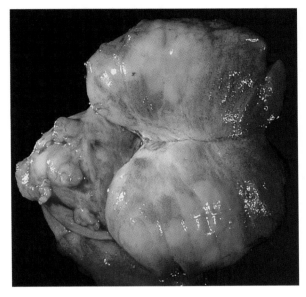

Figure 5-18

REGRESSED GERM CELL TUMOR

An irregularly outlined, firm, white zone of scarring is seen in the testis of a patient with extensive retroperitoneal seminoma.

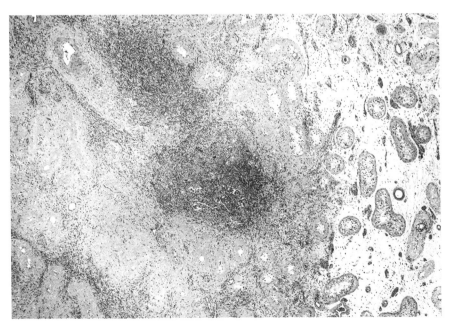

Figure 5-20

REGRESSED GERM CELL TUMOR

A circumscribed scar contains a patchy, dense lymphocytic infiltrate. Small foci of residual embryonal carcinoma were present in the center of the lymphoid aggregates (not visible at this magnification).

223

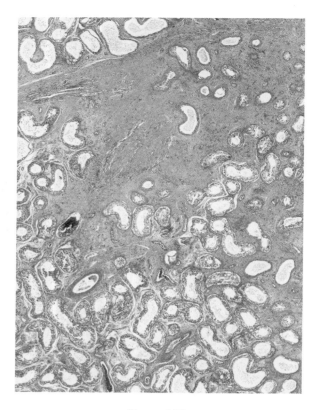

Figure 5-21

REGRESSED GERM CELL TUMOR

This scar has an irregular, dissecting configuration.

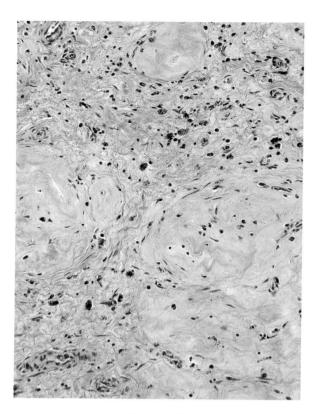

Figure 5-22

REGRESSED GERM CELL TUMOR

Hyalinized remnants of seminiferous tubules and scattered hemosiderin-containing macrophages are apparent in the center of a scar.

remnants of seminiferous tubules are identifiable in the majority of cases (fig. 5-22), as is a variably prominent lymphoplasmacytic infiltrate (fig. 5-23). Less common are hemosiderin-containing macrophages (fig. 5-22). For those tumors that have partially regressed, foci of any number of germ cell tumor types may be encountered (fig. 5-24). In about 15 percent of the cases, coarse intratubular calcifications are seen (fig. 5-25), representing the residue of the dystrophic calcification that occurs in the comedonecrosis of regressed intratubular embryonal carcinoma. Because intratubular embryonal carcinoma expands the seminiferous tubules, these calcifications are larger than the diameter of residual tubules, in contrast to most microliths.

Peripheral to the scar, the testicular parenchyma reflects the common background upon which germ cell tumors develop. There is almost always evidence of testicular atrophy, with many shrunken, partially hyalinized to com-

pletely sclerotic seminiferous tubules (fig. 5-26). In tubules that are more preserved, many have readily apparent thickening of the peritubular basement membrane and impaired spermatogenesis (fig. 5-26). A "Sertoli cell only" pattern is often present in at least some of the tubules. Intratubular microliths (psammoma body-like calcifications) (fig. 5-27), may be seen in about 25 percent of the cases. Intratubular granulomas are uncommon (fig. 5-28). IGCNU is identified in roughly half of the cases (fig. 5-27).

Findings that we consider pathognomonic of a regressed germ cell tumor include either a scar containing coarse intratubular calcifications that exceed the diameter of the peripheral non-atrophic, seminiferous tubules, or a scar with peripheral IGCNU. A scar associated with the other features mentioned above is supportive of a regressed germ cell tumor but not entirely diagnostic of that entity.

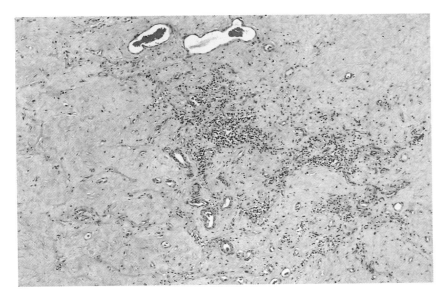

Figure 5-23

REGRESSED GERM CELL TUMOR

The central portion of a scar contains a lymphoplasmacytic infiltrate and prominent blood vessels, including thick-walled ones and some thin, arcuate ones.

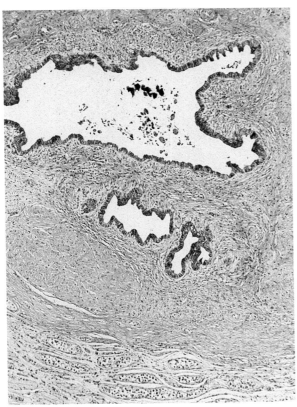

Figure 5-24

REGRESSED GERM CELL TUMOR

Teratomatous glands and cysts are present within the scarred zones.

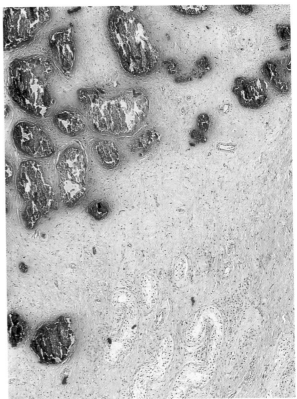

Figure 5-25

REGRESSED GERM CELL TUMOR

A scarred zone contains numerous round foci of dystrophic calcification with central necrotic debris in expanded tubules. Such foci have been described as "hematoxylin-staining bodies" and correspond to necrotic intratubular germ cell tumor.

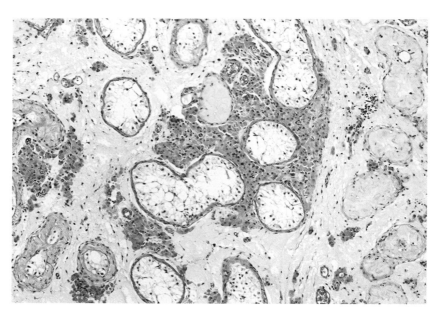

Figure 5-26

TESTIS PERIPHERAL TO A REGRESSED GERM CELL TUMOR

Many tubules are sclerotic or have absent spermatogenesis. Prominent clusters of Leydig cells are seen.

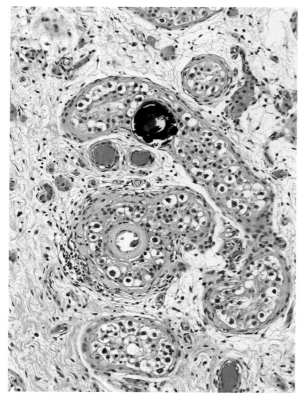

Figure 5-27

TESTIS PERIPHERAL TO A REGRESSED GERM CELL TUMOR

Atrophic tubules with thickened basement membranes show intratubular germ cell neoplasia, unclassified type (IGCNU) and microliths.

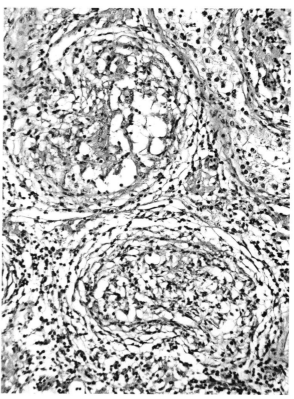

Figure 5-28

TESTIS PERIPHERAL TO A REGRESSED GERM CELL TUMOR

An intratubular granulomatous reaction is present.

MIXED GERM CELL–SEX CORD-STROMAL TUMORS

These are neoplastic germ cells that are admixed with sex cord-stromal elements. There are two types of mixed germ cell–sex cord-stromal tumor: gonadoblastoma and unclassified type.

Gonadoblastoma

General Features. About 20 percent of *gonadoblastomas* occur in phenotypic males, usually under 20 years of age, who also often have cryptorchidism, hypospadias, and gynecomastia, which usually cause the clinical presentation (39). Some cases are seen in children less than 2 years of age (40,41). Surgical exploration of the cryptorchid gonads often reveals female internal genitalia (uterus and fallopian tubes) that result from failure of the müllerian ducts to involute (42). The gonads usually have the features of mixed gonadal dysgenesis (unilateral streak gonad or streak testis and contralateral testis or bilateral streak testis) and karyotypic analysis almost always reveals the presence of a Y chromosome, usually as 45,X/46,XY mosaicism or 46,XY (42). In a series of 101 tumors, 18 occurred in a recognizable testis (39). Overall, about 40 percent of gonadoblastomas are bilateral, but the frequency of bilaterality in phenotypic males may be less (39).

Chromosomal studies have identified a locus on the Y chromosome, the GBY region, that is necessary for the development of gonadoblastoma. A candidate gene within the GBY region, the testis-specific protein on the Y chromosome (*TSPY*) gene, has been implicated as necessary for the development of gonadoblastoma or its progression to an invasive germ cell tumor (43,44). Another gene on the Y chromosome, the sex determining gene Y (*SRY*), has also been thought to be of crucial importance in the development of gonadoblastoma (45). These observations have yet to be worked into a consensus model of pathogenesis.

Many consider gonadoblastoma a form of in situ germ cell tumor since, at the time of diagnosis, about half of the collective cases (including testicular, streak, and gonad of undetermined nature) have progressed to an invasive germinoma (seminoma or dysgerminoma) and 8 percent to another form of germ cell tumor, such as embryonal carcinoma, yolk sac tumor, or teratoma (39).

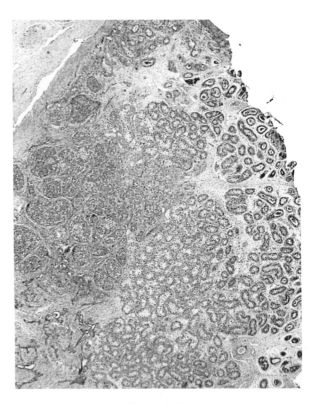

Figure 5-29

GONADOBLASTOMA

Nests of gonadoblastoma cells are present at left above the rete testis, with immature seminiferous tubules on the right.

Gross Findings. About 25 percent of gonadoblastomas are microscopic, but they may measure up to 8 cm in diameter. They are brown to yellow to gray tumors, varying from soft and fleshy to firm and cartilage-like, often flecked with gritty calcifications and, less commonly, showing diffuse calcification (39). Large tumor size, fleshy areas, hemorrhage, or necrosis are suspicious for an invasive germ cell tumor that has arisen from the gonadoblastoma. Thorough sampling is crucial to avoid overlooking an invasive tumor.

Microscopic Findings. The gonadoblastoma is composed of both germ cells and immature sex cord cells that are typically arranged in round nests (figs. 5-29–5-31). Many of the germ cells resemble those of seminoma or IGCNU, but some are similar to spermatogonia or gonocytes (fig. 5-32) (46). The sex cord cells resemble the Sertoli cells of the fetal testis and may contain Charcot-Böttcher filaments on ultrastructural examination (47,48).

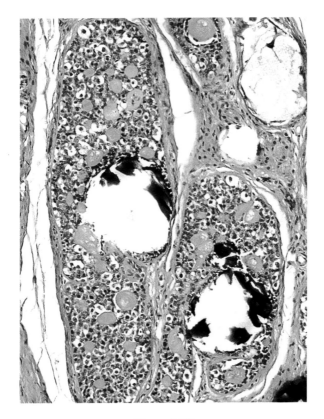

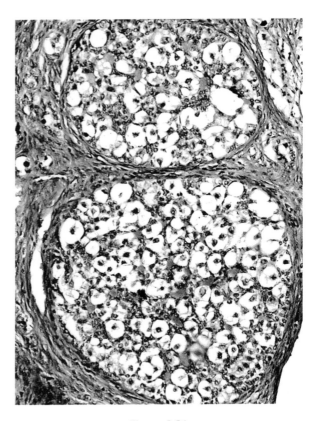

Figure 5-30

GONADOBLASTOMA

Discrete nests are composed of dark sex cord cells that surround germ cells with clear cytoplasm. There are round deposits of basement membrane material and calcifications. (Fig. 6.2 from Young RH, Scully RE. Testicular tumors. Chicago, ASCP Press; 1990:142.)

Figure 5-31

GONADOBLASTOMA

Neoplastic germ cells with clear cytoplasm, resembling seminoma cells, are surrounded by sex cord cells in two rounded nests. There are also interspersed deposits of eosinophilic basement membrane material. (Fig. 6.3 from Young RH, Scully RE. Testicular tumors. Chicago, ASCP Press; 1990:143.)

Figure 5-32

GONADOBLASTOMA

There are both follicular and Call-Exner-like patterns. In the former, sex cord cells surround individual germ cells and in the latter, sex cord cells are arranged in a radial fashion around circular deposits of basement membrane. The germ cells vary in appearance, with some resembling seminoma cells and others spermatogonia or gonocytes.

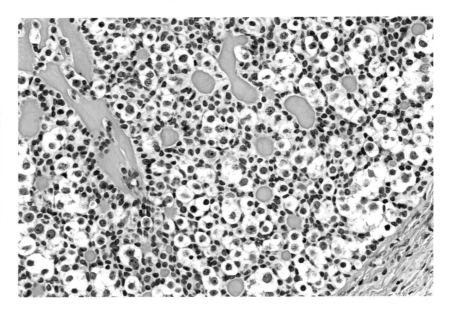

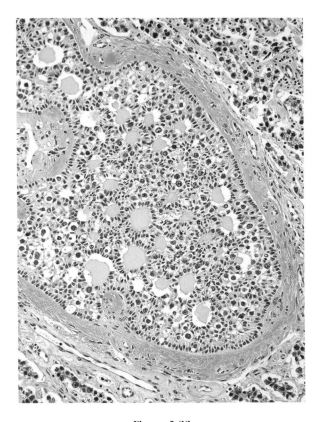

Figure 5-33

GONADOBLASTOMA AND SEMINOMA

There are both coronal and Call-Exner-like patterns in the gonadoblastoma. Invasive seminoma is present at the periphery.

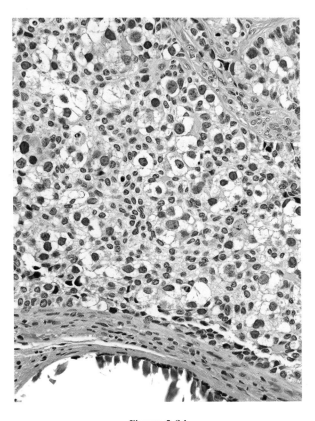

Figure 5-34

GONADOBLASTOMA

A follicular pattern, with sex cord cells surrounding individual germ cells, is seen. Many of the germ cells resemble spermatogonia. Calcification is present (bottom).

Three patterns have been described for gonadoblastoma: coronal, follicular, and Call-Exner-like (39,49). In the coronal pattern, the sex cord cells are mostly arranged at the periphery of the tumor islands (fig. 5-33). In the follicular pattern, they surround one or more germ cells (figs. 5-32, 5-34). In the Call-Exner-like pattern, they are arranged around the globoid basement membrane deposits. Admixture of these patterns is usual (figs. 5-32, 5-33). Calcification occurs in 80 percent of the cases, and starts on the basement membrane deposits; coalescence of calcifications results in irregular, mulberry-shaped calcific islands devoid of tumor cells (39). Peripheral to the tumor nests, Leydig-like cells lacking Reinke crystals are identified in about two thirds of cases, but are more conspicuous in postpubertal cases (39,42). Invasive germ cell tumors developing from gonadoblastoma have the features typical

of those neoplasms. Coarse calcifications in an invasive germ cell tumor are suspicious for origin from a gonadoblastoma (39).

Recently, a putative gonadoblastoma precursor lesion, designated "undifferentiated gonadal tissue," has been described adjacent to gonadoblastomas and in dysgenetic gonads at risk for the development of gonadoblastoma (50). Such areas have a cellular composition similar to gonadoblastoma but with a diffuse rather than nested arrangement (fig. 5-35) (50). Dr. Robert E. Scully recognized this tissue as *dissecting gonadoblastoma* (personal observation) because of its diffuse rather than nested arrangement of germ cells and sex cord cells.

Immunohistochemical Findings. The germ cells show a heterogeneous immunohistochemical pattern. Those resembling seminoma or IGCNU cells are positive for the markers

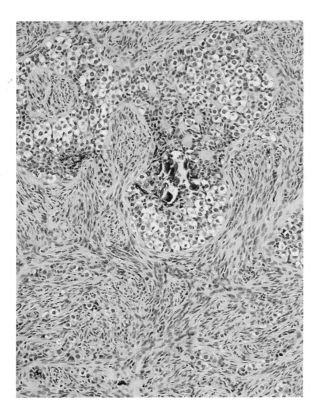 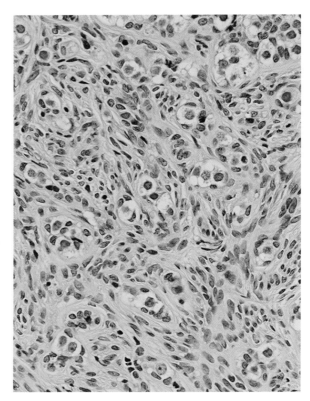

Figure 5-35

GONADOBLASTOMA WITH "UNDIFFERENTIATED GONADAL TISSUE"

Left: A typical round nest of gonadoblastoma is surrounded by a cellular stroma containing germ cells of similar appearance to those in the nest.

Right: The germ cells vary in appearance in the undifferentiated gonadal tissue, and include seminoma-like forms and those resembling spermatogonia.

typically identified in those neoplasms, including OCT3/4, placental-like alkaline phosphatase (PLAP), CD117, and podoplanin (50,51), although CD117 is less consistently reactive than the other markers (50,51). The more mature germ cells, resembling spermatogonia, are typically positive for TSPY and negative for OCT3/4 (44). There is also a population of immature-appearing but non-neoplastic germ cells (resembling gonocytes) that are mostly OCT3/4 positive and TSPY negative (44). These cells have been interpreted as exhibiting delayed maturation, with retention of antigens that are typical of fetal rather than more mature germ cells. The "undifferentiated gonadal tissue" adjacent to some gonadoblastomas shows the same immunoreactivities as the gonadoblastoma (50). The sex cord component of gonadoblastoma stains for S-100 protein beta (52), anti-müllerian hormone (53), inhibin,

vimentin, cytokeratin, and the Wilms tumor gene 1 protein (WT1) (54).

Differential Diagnosis. Sertoli cell nodules, which commonly occur in cryptorchid testes (55,56), may be colonized by IGCNU and mimic gonadoblastoma (fig. 5-36). These lesions, however, occur in phenotypically normal males whose gonads lack dysgenetic features and who do not have internal müllerian genitalia, unlike many patients with gonadoblastoma. The usual microscopic size and the frequently focal distribution of the malignant germ cells of Sertoli cell nodules differ from the features of gonadoblastoma.

The "dissecting" form of gonadoblastoma may be mistaken for seminoma when the sex cord cells that are associated with the germ cells are inconspicuous, the germ cells are predominant, and the associated gonadal stroma minor (fig. 5-37). In that circumstance, large islands of

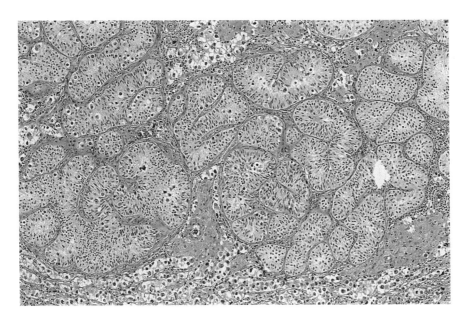

Figure 5-36

SERTOLI CELL NODULE WITH IGCNU AND SEMINOMA POTENTIALLY MIMICKING GONADOBLASTOMA

IGCNU involves a Sertoli cell nodule. The IGCNU cells are focally distributed in the Sertoli cell nodule in contrast to their diffuse distribution in gonadoblastoma. Seminoma is seen at the periphery.

germ cells, many of which may appear atypical, dominate the morphology. Clues to the correct interpretation include the consistent association of the germ cells with the sex cord component, regardless of the subtlety of the latter, and the heterogeneous appearance of the germ cells, which vary from seminoma-like to spermatogonia-like.

Unlike gonadoblastoma, the unclassified form of mixed germ cell–sex cord-stromal tumor is not arranged in the typical small nests with hyaline basement membrane deposits but forms larger, circumscribed to infiltrating nodules of sex cord tumor elements. These elements resemble any of the common types: Sertoli cell, granulosa cell, or unclassified sex cord-stromal elements with admixed germ cells (see below).

Treatment and Prognosis. The usual treatment for gonadoblastoma is bilateral gonadectomy because of the association with gonadal dysgenesis and the high frequency of bilaterality (over 40 percent). Such treatment is curative if prior to the development of an invasive germ cell tumor. If an invasive tumor is present, the treatment and prognosis are determined by its nature and stage.

Unclassified Germ Cell–Sex Cord-Stromal Tumors

General Features. *Unclassified germ cell–sex cord-stromal tumors* are rare. The germ cells

within these neoplasms are considered neoplastic in the literature, but most putative examples that we have seen we have interpreted as sex cord-stromal tumors with entrapped, non-neoplastic germ cells. The reported tumors occurred in patients 30 to 69 years of age. One case was described in a 7-year-old who presented with virilization, but we are uncertain concerning the nature of this case (57). The patients present with testicular masses, in the absence of hormonal symptoms or features of a disorder of sex development (intersex syndrome), including gonadal dysgenesis (58–60).

Gross and Microscopic Findings. Usually, the tumors are fleshy, solid, and gray-white and sometimes show cystic change. On microscopic examination, there is often a sheet-like pattern of sex cord cells with scant cytoplasm and usually angulated, sometimes grooved nuclei (fig. 5-38). Gonadal stromal differentiation may be apparent as a spindle cell component that frequently subtly blends with the sex cord cells (fig. 5-38). Intertubular growth is often present at the periphery. Sertoli cell and granulosa cell differentiation may be apparent in the form of tubules (fig. 5-39), cords, or follicle-like structures, as seen in typical sex cord-stromal tumors (see chapter 6). The germ cell component most frequently occurs in distinct clusters (fig. 5-38), but rarely shows a diffuse arrangement (fig. 5-40). In some of the reported cases, the germ

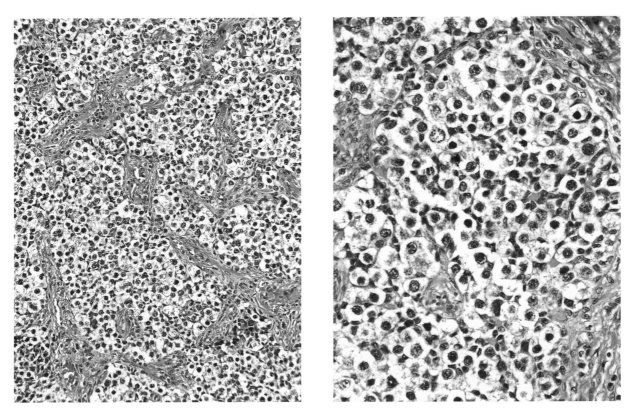

Figure 5-37

GONADOBLASTOMA

Left: The nests are virtually confluent and are germ cell predominant, closely resembling seminoma. This may be termed "dissecting gonadoblastoma" or, alternatively, "undifferentiated gonadal tissue" with a predominance of germ cells.

Right: Close inspection shows a consistent sex cord component and occasional small, non-neoplastic-appearing germ cells.

cells have been described as "seminoma-like," with clear cytoplasm and round nuclei with prominent nucleoli (61), although glycogen and PLAP reactivity may be absent (58,59). More recent studies (62), however, in accord with our observations (63), have noted that the germ cells differed from those of seminoma by having a more mature appearance, with round rather than polygonal nuclei, inconspicuous nucleoli, and fine chromatin (fig. 5-38). Charcot-Böttcher filaments in one case confirmed Sertoli cell differentiation (59).

Differential Diagnosis. A major lesion in the differential diagnosis is the sex cord-stromal tumor with entrapped germ cells (63). Based on our experience, it is more common than the unclassified mixed germ cell–sex cord-stromal tumor, to the extent that we question the legitimacy of the latter. In the sex cord-stromal tumor

with entrapped germ cells, the germ cells have round, uniform, euchromatic nuclei and are interspersed singly or in small nests, usually at the periphery of the tumor but sometimes more centrally (fig. 5-38). The non-neoplastic nature of the germ cells in these cases is supported by their preferential peripheral location, bland nuclear features that are unlike those of the seminoma-like cells of gonadoblastoma, lack of PLAP and cKIT reactivity, and diploid DNA content on static cytophotometry (63).

A rare "collision" tumor consisting of a sex cord-stromal tumor and either seminoma or IGCNU may mimic a mixed germ cell–sex cord-stromal tumor (fig. 5-41). The presence of foci of pure sex cord-stromal tumor or pure seminoma supports the independent nature of the two neoplasms, although this distinction may be problematic in some cases.

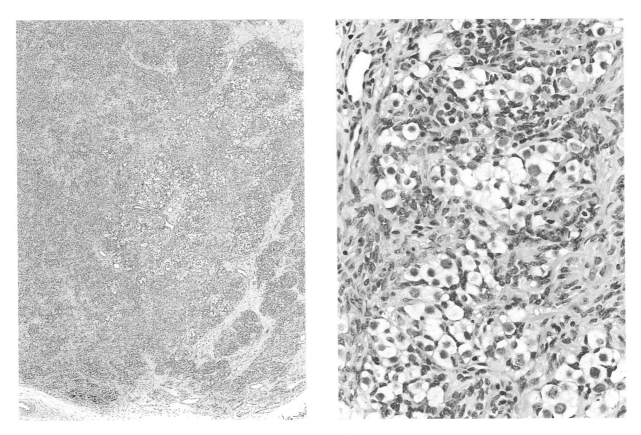

Figure 5-38

UNCLASSIFIED SEX CORD-STROMAL TUMOR WITH ENTRAPPED GERM CELLS

Left: A focus of light-staining germ cells is near the periphery of a tumor composed mainly of sex cord cells.

Right: High magnification shows the admixture of germ cells with sex cord cells. The germ cells have regular, round nuclei with uniform, fine chromatin.

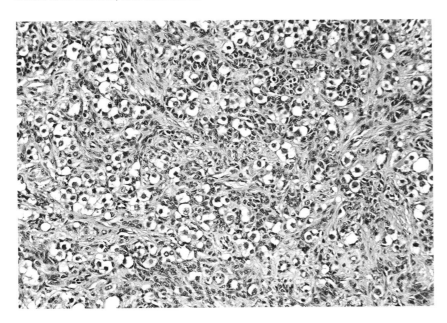

Figure 5-39

UNCLASSIFIED SEX CORD-STROMAL TUMOR WITH ENTRAPPED GERM CELLS

The sex cord cells form nests and solid tubules that enclose non-neoplastic germ cells.

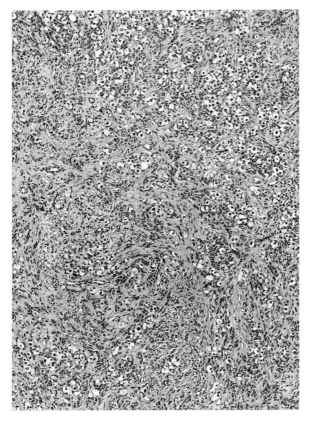

Figure 5-40

UNCLASSIFIED SEX CORD-STROMAL
TUMOR WITH ENTRAPPED GERM CELLS

The germ cells occur diffusely throughout this field.

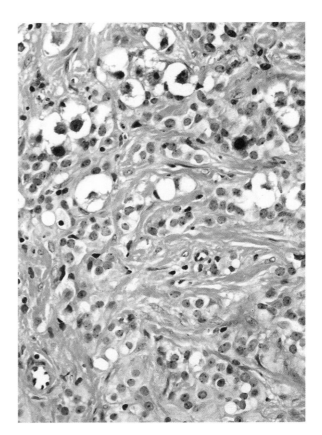

Figure 5-41

"COLLISION TUMOR" OF UNCLASSIFIED
SEX CORD TUMOR AND IGCNU

Neoplastic sex cord cells are admixed with IGCNU. Classification as a mixed germ cell–sex cord-stromal tumor or a collision tumor may be problematic.

The differential diagnosis with gonadoblastoma is discussed with the latter, above. Prominent luteinized cells in a sex cord-stromal tumor may be misinterpreted as neoplastic germ cells, leading to misclassification as mixed germ cell–sex cord-stromal tumor (63). This differential is discussed in chapter 6.

Treatment and Prognosis. Orchiectomy is standard therapy (58). No case is known to have metastasized but experience is limited.

REFERENCES

1. Krag Jacobsen G, Barlebo H, Olsen J, et al. Testicular germ cell tumours in Denmark 1976-1980: pathology of 1058 consecutive cases. Acta Radiol Oncol 1984;23:239-47.

2. Barsky SH. Germ cell tumors of the testis. In: Javadpour N, Barsky SH, eds. Surgical pathology of urologic diseases. Baltimore: Williams & Wilkins; 1987:224-46.

3. Brawn PN. The origin of germ cell tumors of the testis. Cancer 1983;51:1610-4.

4. Rustin GJ, Vogelzang NJ, Sleijfer DT, Nisselbaum JN. Consensus statement on circulating tumour markers and staging patients with germ cell tumours. Prog Clin Biol Res 1990;357:277-84.

5. Beck SD, Foster RS, Bihrle R, Donohue JP. Significance of primary tumor size and preorchiectomy serum tumor marker level in predicting pathologic stage at retroperitoneal lymph node dissection in clinical stage A nonseminomatous germ cell tumors. Urology 2007;69:557-9.

6. Evans RW. Developmental stages of embryolike bodies in teratoma testis. J Clin Pathol 1957;10:31-9.

7. Peyron A. Faits nouveaux relatifs à l'origine et à l'histogenèse des embryomes. Bull Assoc France Cancer 1939;28:658-91.

8. Nakashima N, Murakami S, Fukatsu T, et al. Characteristics of "embryoid body" in human gonadal germ cell tumors. Hum Pathol 1988;19:1144-54.

9. Eble JN, ed. Pathology and genetics of tumours of the urinary system and male genital organs. Lyon: IARC Press; 2004.

10. Cardoso de Almeida PC, Scully RE. Diffuse embryoma of the testis. A distinctive form of mixed germ cell tumor. Am J Surg Pathol 1983;7:633-42.

11. de Peralta-Venturina MN, Ro JY, Ordonez NG, Ayala AG. Diffuse embryoma of the testis: an immunohistochemical study of two cases. Am J Clin Pathol 1994;101:402-5.

12. Jacobsen GK. Histogenetic considerations concerning germ cell tumours. Morphological and immunohistochemical comparative investigation of the human embryo and testicular germ cell tumours. Virchows Arch A Pathol Anat Histopathol 1986;408:509-25.

13. Okamoto T. A human vitelline component in embryonal carcinoma of the testis. Acta Pathol Jap 1986;36:41-8.

14. Brawn PN. The characteristics of embryonal carcinoma cells in teratocarcinomas. Cancer 1987;59:2042-6.

15. Motoyama T, Watanabe H, Yamamoto T, Sekiguchi M. Human testicular germ cell tumors in vitro and in athymic nude mice. Acta Pathol Jap 1987;37:431-48.

16. Pera MF, Blasco Lafita MJ, Mills J. Cultured stem-cells from human testicular teratomas: the nature of human embryonal carcinoma, and its comparison with two types of yolk-sac carcinoma. Int J Cancer 1987;40:334-43.

17. Pera MF, Mills J, Parrington JM. Isolation and characterization of a multipotent clone of human embryonal carcinoma cells. Differentiation 1989;42:10-23.

18. Gels ME, Hoekstra HJ, Sleijfer DT, et al. Detection of recurrence in patients with clinical stage I nonseminomatous testicular germ cell tumors and consequences for further follow-up: a single-center 10-year experience. J Clin Oncol 1995;13:1188-94.

19. Wishnow KI, Johnson DE, Swanson DA, et al. Identifying patients with low-risk clinical stage I nonseminomatous testicular tumors who should be treated by surveillance. Urology 1989;34:339-43.

20. Fung CY, Kalish LA, Brodsky GL, Richie JP, Garnick MB. Stage I nonseminomatous germ cell testicular tumor: prediction of metastatic potential by primary histopathology. J Clin Oncol 1988;6:1467-73.

21. Moul JW, McCarthy WF, Fernandez EB, Sesterhenn IA. Percentage of embryonal carcinoma and of vascular invasion predicts pathological stage in clinical stage I nonseminomatous testicular cancer. Cancer Res 1994;54:362-4.

22. Freedman LS, Parkinson MC, Jones WG, et al. Histopathology in the prediction of relapse of patients with stage I testicular teratoma treated by orchidectomy alone. Lancet 1987;2:294-8.

23. Burt ME, Javadpour N. Germ-cell tumors in patients with apparently normal testes. Cancer 1981;47:1911-5.

24. Meares EM Jr, Briggs EM. Occult seminoma of the testis masquerading as primary extragonadal germinal neoplasm. Cancer 1972;30:300-6.

25. Asif S, Uehling DT. Microscopic tumor foci in testes. J Urol 1968;99:776-9.

26. Bohle A, Studer UE, Sonntag RW, Scheidegger JR. Primary or secondary extragonadal germ cell tumors. J Urol 1986;135:939-43.

27. Abell MR, Fayos JV, Lampe I. Retroperitoneal germinomas (seminomas) without evidence of testicular involvement. Cancer 1965;18:273-90.

28. Daugaard G, von der Maase H, Olsen J, Rorth M, Skakkebaek NE. Carcinoma-in-situ testis in patients with assumed extragonadal germ-cell tumours. Lancet 1987;2:528-30.

29. Rothman J, Greenberg RE, Jaffe WI. Nonseminomatous germ cell tumor of the testis 9 years after a germ cell tumor of the pineal gland: case report and review of the literature. Can J Urol 2008;15:4122-4.

30. Chen KT, Cheng AC. Retroperitoneal seminoma and intratubular germ cell neoplasia. Hum Pathol 1989;20:493-5.

31. Saltzman B, Pitts WR, Vaughan ED Jr. Extragonadal retroperitoneal germ cell tumors without apparent testicular involvement. A search for the source. Urology 1986;27:504-7.

32. Hailemariam S, Engeler DS, Bannwart F, Amin MB. Primary mediastinal germ cell tumor with intratubular germ cell neoplasia of the testis—further support for germ cell origin of these tumors: a case report. Cancer 1997;79:1031-6.

33. Rottinto A, DeBellis H. Extragenital chorioma: its relation to teratoid vestiges in the testicles. Arch Pathol 1944;37:78-80.

34. Bär W, Hedinger C. Comparison of histologic types of primary testicular germ cell tumors with their metastases: consequences for the WHO and the British nomenclatures? Virchows Arch A Pathol Anat Histopathol 1976;370:41-54.

35. Azzopardi JG, Mostofi FK, Theiss EA. Lesions of testes observed in certain patients with widespread choriocarcinoma and related tumors. Am J Pathol 1961;38:207-25.

36. Balzer BL, Ulbright TM. Spontaneous regression of testicular germ cell tumors: an analysis of 42 cases. Am J Surg Pathol 2006;30:858-65.

37. Lopez JI, Angulo JC. Burned-out tumour of the testis presenting as retroperitoneal choriocarcinoma. Int Urol Nephrol 1994;26:549-53.

38. Crook JC. Morphogenesis of testicular tumours. J Clin Pathol 1968;21:71-4.

39. Scully RE. Gonadoblastoma. A review of 74 cases. Cancer 1970;25:1340-56.

40. Pena-Alonso R, Nieto K, Alvarez R, et al. Distribution of Y-chromosome-bearing cells in gonadoblastoma and dysgenetic testis in 45,X/46,XY infants. Mod Pathol 2005;18:439-45.

41. Haddad NG, Walvoord EC, Cain MP, Davis MM. Seminoma and a gonadoblastoma in an infant with mixed gonadal dysgenesis. J Pediatr 2003;143:136.

42. Rutgers JL. Advances in the pathology of intersex syndromes. Hum Pathol 1991;22:884-91.

43. Li Y, Vilain E, Conte F, Rajpert-De ME, Lau YF. Testis-specific protein Y-encoded gene is expressed in early and late stages of gonadoblastoma and testicular carcinoma in situ. Urol Oncol 2007;25:141-6.

44. Kersemaekers AM, Honecker F, Stoop H, et al. Identification of germ cells at risk for neoplastic transformation in gonadoblastoma: an immunohistochemical study for OCT3/4 and TSPY. Hum Pathol 2005;36:512-21.

45. Bianco B, Lipay M, Guedes A, Oliveira K, Verreschi IT. SRY gene increases the risk of developing gonadoblastoma and/or nontumoral gonadal lesions in Turner syndrome. Int J Gynecol Pathol 2009;28:197-202.

46. Jorgensen N, Muller J, Jaubert F, Clausen OP, Skakkebaek NE. Heterogeneity of gonadoblastoma germ cells: similarities with immature germ cells, spermatogonia and testicular carcinoma in situ cells. Histopathology 1997;30:177-86.

47. Roth LM, Eglen DE. Gonadoblastoma: immunohistochemical and ultrastructural observations. Int J Gynecol Pathol 1989;8:72-81.

48. Ishida T, Tagatz GE, Okagaki T. Gonadoblastoma: ultrastructural evidence for testicular origin. Cancer 1976;37:1770-81.

49. Talerman A, Roth LM. Recent advances in the pathology and classification of gonadal neoplasms composed of germ cells and sex cord derivatives. Int J Gynecol Pathol 2007;26:313-21.

50. Cools M, Stoop H, Kersemaekers AM, et al. Gonadoblastoma arising in undifferentiated gonadal tissue within dysgenetic gonads. J Clin Endocrinol Metab 2006;91:2404-13.

51. Sonne SB, Herlihy AS, Hoei-Hansen CE, et al. Identity of M2A (D2-40) antigen and gp36 (Aggrus, T1A-2, podoplanin) in human developing testis, testicular carcinoma in situ and germ-cell tumours. Virchows Arch 2006;449:200-6.

52. Tanaka Y, Carney JA, Ijiri R, et al. Utility of immunostaining for S-100 protein subunits in gonadal sex cord-stromal tumors, with emphasis on the large-cell calcifying Sertoli cell tumor of the testis. Hum Pathol 2002;33:285-9.

53. Rey R, Sabourin JC, Venara M, et al. Anti-mullerian hormone is a specific marker of Sertoli- and granulosa-cell origin in gonadal tumors. Hum Pathol 2000;31:1202-8.

54. Hussong J, Crussi FG, Chou PM. Gonadoblastoma: an immunohistochemical localization of mullerian-inhibiting substance, inhibin, WT-1 and p53. Mod Pathol 1997;10:1101-5.

55. Stalker AL, Hendry WT. Hyperplasia and neoplasia of the Sertoli cell. J Pathol Bacteriol 1952;64:161-8.

56. Hedinger CE, Huber R, Weber E. Frequency of so-called hypoplastic or dysgenetic zones in scrotal and otherwise normal human testes. Virchows Arch Pathol Anat Physical Klin Med 1967;342:165-8.

57. Hettinger CA, Cheville JC, Lteif AN, Bradley NA, Kramer SA. Precocious puberty in a 7-year-old boy: a novel case. J Pediatr Urol 2009;5:412-4.

58. Matoska J, Talerman A. Mixed germ cell-sex cord stroma tumor of the testis. A report with ultrastructural findings. Cancer 1989;64:2146-53.

59. Bolen JW. Mixed germ cell-sex cord stromal tumor. A gonadal tumor distinct from gonadoblastoma. Am J Clin Pathol 1981;75:565-73.

60. Rames RA, Richardson M, Swiger F, Kaczmarek A. Mixed germ cell-sex cord stromal tumor of the testis: the incidental finding of a rare testicular neoplasm. J Urol 1995;154:1479.

61. Jacobsen GK, Talerman A. Atlas of germ cell tumours. Copenhagen: Munksgaard; 1989.

62. Michal M, Vanecek T, Sima R, et al. Mixed germ cell sex cord-stromal tumors of the testis and ovary. Morphological, immunohistochemical, and molecular genetic study of seven cases. Virchows Arch 2006;448:612-22.

63. Ulbright TM, Srigley JR, Reuter VE, Wojno K, Roth LM, Young RH. Sex cord-stromal tumors of the testis with entrapped germ cells: a lesion mimicking unclassified mixed germ cell sex cord-stromal tumors. Am J Surg Pathol 2000;24:535-42.

6 SEX CORD-STROMAL TUMORS

Sex cord-stromal tumors represent about 4 percent of all testicular neoplasms (1) and about 8 percent of those in prepubertal males (2). Their classification is presented in Table 6-1. In well-differentiated tumors, the cells usually resemble, to varying degrees, non-neoplastic Leydig cells (3), Sertoli cells, and nonspecific stromal cells of the testis. In more poorly differentiated tumors, these similarities are generally less conspicuous, but the patterns of differentiation that are usually focally present, such as tubular, are diagnostic clues.

Leydig cell tumors are the most common pure sex cord-stromal tumors, followed by Sertoli cell tumors, granulosa cell tumors, and pure stromal tumors. Occasional tumors in the Sertoli and granulosa cell categories also have a neoplastic stromal component. When the stromal component in such cases is small, the tumors are still classified as Sertoli or granulosa cell tumor. We place tumors with prominent stromal components and with neoplastic sex cord cells in the unclassified sex cord-stromal category in an effort to keep the Sertoli and granulosa cell tumor designations comparatively

pure rather than also including those tumors with a substantial amount of undifferentiated neoplastic gonadal stroma. An exception to this approach is a tumor that resembles the ovarian Sertoli-Leydig cell tumor, in which the stromal component has neoplastic Leydig cells; however, such tumors are rare. The remaining neoplasms contain patterns of two or more of the above types or cannot be specifically placed into any clearly defined category; the former are categorized in the mixed group and the latter in the unclassified group, and, in combination, they account for approximately 5 percent of all sex cord-stromal tumors.

SERTOLI-STROMAL CELL TUMORS

Sertoli Cell Tumor

Sertoli cell tumors usually resemble non-neoplastic Sertoli cells of the testis because they show tubular patterns of differentiation, although some tumors are placed in this group by default when they show no feature enabling placement in another category. There are several subtypes, as discussed in the section below, each of which has distinct morphologic features, and in some instances, particular clinical associations.

Sertoli cell tumors account for less than 1 percent of testicular neoplasms (2,4–7). There are four recognized subtypes: *Sertoli cell tumor, not otherwise specified (NOS), large cell calcifying Sertoli cell tumor, intratubular large cell hyalinizing Sertoli cell neoplasia,* and *sclerosing Sertoli cell tumor.* It is a debatable issue whether the sclerosing form merits a separate classification from the NOS type; we separately recognize it because it appears to have a significantly improved prognosis compared to the tumors in the NOS category. Although a "lipid-rich" variant of Sertoli cell tumor has been described in the literature, there are insufficient valid examples of pure, lipid-rich Sertoli cell tumors to consider them a separate subtype. Teilum's descriptions of this pattern appear to refer to foci within

---

Table 6-1

CLASSIFICATION OF SEX CORD-STROMAL TUMORS OF THE TESTIS

Sertoli-Stromal Cell Tumors
　Sertoli cell tumor
　　Sertoli cell tumor, not otherwise specified
　　Large cell calcifying Sertoli cell tumor
　　Intratubular large cell hyalinizing Sertoli cell
　　　neoplasia
　　Sclerosing Sertoli cell tumor
　　Sertoli-Leydig cell tumor

Leydig Cell Tumor

Granulosa-Stromal Cell Tumors
　Adult-type granulosa cell tumor
　Juvenile-type granulosa cell tumor

Tumors in the Fibroma-Thecoma Group

Mixed and Unclassified Sex Cord-Stromal Tumors

Sertoli-Leydig cell tumors (8–11). Reliable data on the frequency of the various subtypes are unavailable, since all the large series are based on consultation material. In our experience, approximately 70 percent of Sertoli cell tumors are in the NOS group, with most of the remainder evenly split between the large cell calcifying and sclerosing variants. The intratubular large cell hyalinizing type is rare.

Approximately 30 percent of reported "Sertoli cell tumors" have occurred in children, many under 1 year old (12). In our opinion, most of these cases have features of juvenile granulosa cell tumor, with the reports antedating the description of that entity. In support of this view, one subsequent pediatric series contained no Sertoli cell tumors, NOS, but there were four juvenile granulosa cell tumors (13). On the other hand, an element of subjectivity in the distinction of a juvenile granulosa cell tumor from a Sertoli cell tumor, particularly in the pediatric age group, is highlighted by another study that included 18 Sertoli cell tumors and 11 juvenile granulosa cell tumors (14). The predominance of Sertoli cell tumors in that study, in contrast to our experience (7) and that of others (13), suggests that different criteria are being applied for the diagnosis of these tumors. In the largest series of Sertoli cell tumors, only 2 of 60 occurred in patients under 20 years of age (a 15-year-old and an 18-year-old), and the mean age was 46 years (7). According to our approach, only rare cases occur in patients under 10 years of age (15–17).

Noteworthy clinical associations exist in some cases. Occasional tumors develop in patients with the androgen insensitivity syndrome (18). The large cell calcifying variant is sometimes associated with the Carney complex, a constellation of lesions that include myxomas of various sites, including the heart; pigmented lesions of skin and mucosal sites; and several endocrine lesions and tumors (19). Its features may initially bring the patient to medical attention. Boys with the Peutz-Jeghers syndrome may develop a distinctive form of intratubular Sertoli cell tumor, the large cell hyalinizing variant, with most of the patients coming to medical attention because of gynecomastia caused by tumor-produced estrogen (20).

Despite these important features, most patients with Sertoli cell tumors lack any known predisposing conditions or unusual clinical associations and present with a testicular mass. For those uncommon cases that exhibit malignant behavior the presentation may be attributable to the metastatic lesions, including dyspnea. One patient with a malignant tumor presented with bloody ejaculation (21). Only rare patients without the Peutz-Jeghers syndrome have gynecomastia, which is a finding more commonly encountered in those with malignant tumors. Gynecomastia is more common in patients with Leydig cell tumors, Sertoli-Leydig cell tumors, or tumors in the mixed and unclassified sex cord-stromal categories, leading to an overall frequency of about 10 to 20 percent of all patients with sex cord-stromal tumors.

Although some types of Sertoli cell tumor are associated with endocrinologic abnormalities, hormonal production by these tumors is uncommon (22). One review of 72 reported cases of Sertoli cell tumor identified occasional patients with elevated serum testosterone, plasma estradiol, urinary estrogens, and urinary 17-ketosteroids (12). The exact nature, however, of many of these tumors is not clear.

Sertoli Cell Tumor, Not Otherwise Specified (NOS)

Gross Findings. *Sertoli cell tumors, NOS,* are typically well-circumscribed, sometimes lobulated, yellow, tan, or white masses (figs. 6-1–6-4). Cysts are occasionally conspicuous (figs. 6-3, 6-4). Foci of hemorrhage may be present (figs. 6-2, 6-4), but necrosis is rare. The mean diameter is approximately 3.5 cm, and they are almost invariably unilateral; there is only one apparently valid case of bilateral Sertoli cell tumor, NOS (15). Most are confined to the testis at presentation.

Microscopic Findings. Microscopic examination usually shows tubular differentiation but its extent, and hence, the overall low-power appearance of the tumor, is quite variable. Diffuse (fig. 6-5) and nodular (fig. 6-6) patterns often predominate on low-power examination. Some tumors have a major pattern of solid, round to irregular nests (fig. 6-7). Tubular differentiation in varying amounts is usually seen with ease in some areas of the tumor, and often is at least focally conspicuous (figs. 6-6, 6-8, 6-9). The tubules may be hollow (figs. 6-8–6-10), round

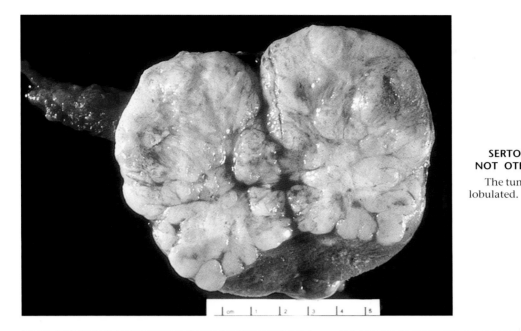

Figure 6-1

SERTOLI CELL TUMOR, NOT OTHERWISE SPECIFIED

The tumor is solid, white, and lobulated.

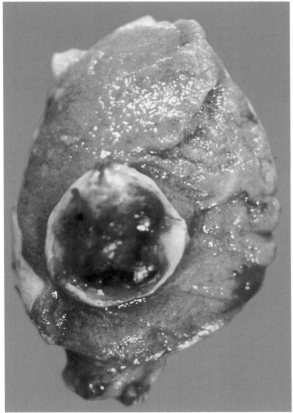

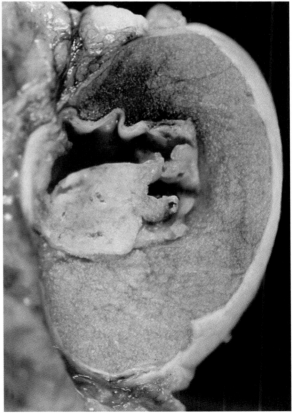

Figure 6-2

SERTOLI CELL TUMOR, NOT OTHERWISE SPECIFIED

The tumor is well circumscribed and hemorrhagic.

Figure 6-3

SERTOLI CELL TUMOR, NOT OTHERWISE SPECIFIED

The sectioned surface shows conspicuous cysts.

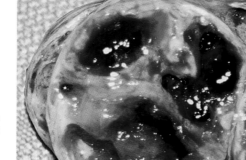

Figure 6-4

SERTOLI CELL TUMOR, NOT OTHERWISE SPECIFIED

The tumor has undergone extensive cystic degeneration with hemorrhage.

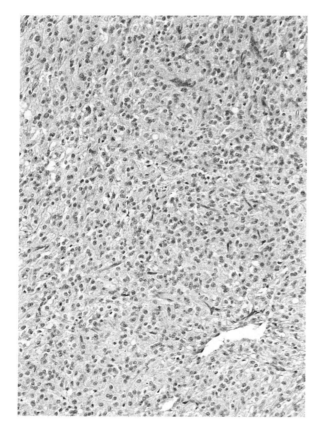

Figure 6-5

SERTOLI CELL TUMOR, NOT OTHERWISE SPECIFIED

The diffuse growth of cells and appreciable eosinophilic cytoplasm resemble a Leydig cell tumor. Tubular differentiation was conspicuous in other areas.

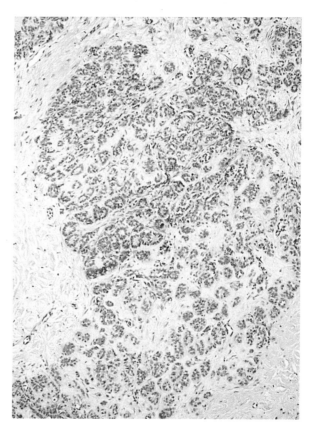

Figure 6-6

SERTOLI CELL TUMOR, NOT OTHERWISE SPECIFIED

Fibrous stroma separates small tubules showing nodular growth.

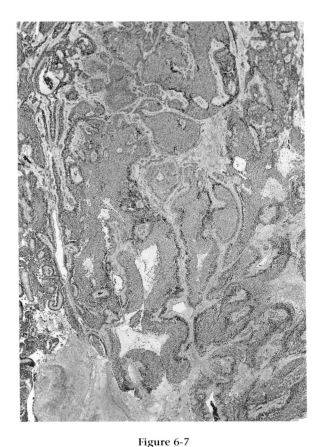

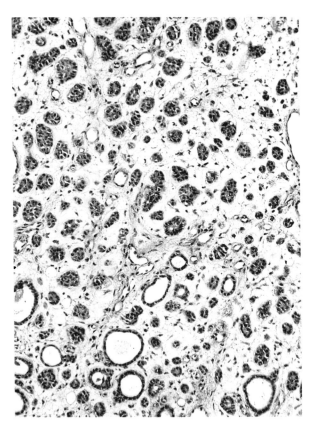

Figure 6-7

SERTOLI CELL TUMOR, NOT OTHERWISE SPECIFIED

Large, interconnecting islands of neoplastic cells are formed.

Figure 6-8

SERTOLI CELL TUMOR, NOT OTHERWISE SPECIFIED

Solid and hollow tubules, some of which are dilated and lined by a single layer of cells, are a common feature.

(figs. 6-6, 6-8, 6-11), irregular (fig. 6-10), solid (figs. 6-6, 6-8, 6-12, 6-13), or elongated (figs. 6-9, 6-12). Rarely, they have a retiform pattern (fig. 6-14). In some tumors, cords and trabeculae are prominent (figs. 6-15–6-17), sometimes yielding a carcinoid-like appearance (fig. 6-16). Some Sertoli cell tumors have large areas of solid growth (figs. 6-5, 6-18), but at least focal tubular differentiation elsewhere facilitates the diagnosis (fig. 6-18). Rare neoplasms that have an entirely solid growth pattern can be diagnosed as Sertoli cell tumor when the appearance is inconsistent with any other plausible diagnosis and is buttressed by appropriate immunohistochemical findings. Thorough sampling to disclose minimal tubular differentiation is crucial in some cases since immunohistochemistry is not always definitive.

The tumor cells usually have moderate to occasionally abundant, lightly eosinophilic cyto-

plasm (figs. 6-5, 6-11, 6-17) that may be pale due to lipid accumulation (figs. 6-12, 6-18). This may take the form of fine droplets (fig. 6-19) or large vacuoles (fig. 6-20) of lipid. The combination of diffuse cytoplasmic pallor and solid growth creates a seminoma-like appearance in rare tumors (fig. 6-21), a resemblance that is further enhanced by the occurrence of a conspicuous lymphocytic infiltrate in some cases (fig. 6-22) (23). Cytoplasmic eosinophilia, to the degree seen in Leydig cell tumors, is occasionally present. The stroma may be scanty or composed of abundant, sometimes hyalinized fibrous tissue (fig. 6-23) that may contain prominent, occasionally dilated blood vessels (figs. 6-15, 6-23). In some cases there are conspicuous zones of hyalinized, perivascular, and peritubular sclerosis (fig. 6-24). Infrequently, tumors with prominent areas of hyaline fibrosis exhibit foci of metaplastic ossification within

243

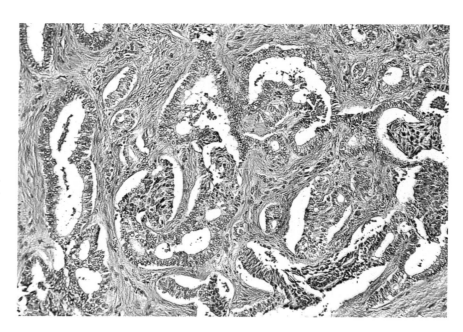

Figure 6-9

SERTOLI CELL TUMOR, NOT OTHERWISE SPECIFIED

Hollow tubules lined by stratified cells resemble an endometrioid neoplasm.

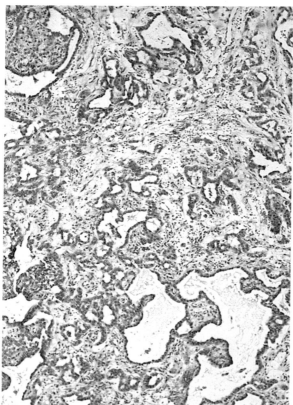

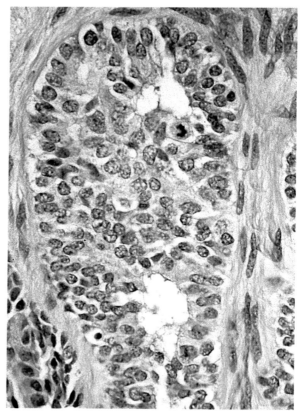

Figure 6-10

SERTOLI CELL TUMOR, NOT OTHERWISE SPECIFIED

Many tubules are dilated and irregular in size and shape.

Figure 6-11

SERTOLI CELL TUMOR, NOT OTHERWISE SPECIFIED

A tubule from the tumor in figure 6-9 is lined by stratified cells. A mitotic figure is seen.

244

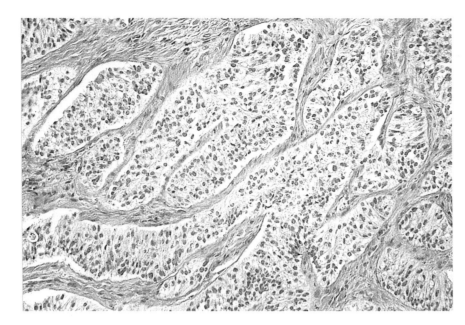

Figure 6-12

SERTOLI CELL TUMOR, NOT OTHERWISE SPECIFIED

The tumor forms solid tubules.

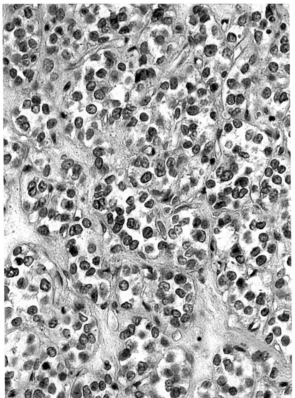

Figure 6-13

SERTOLI CELL TUMOR, NOT OTHERWISE SPECIFIED

Tumor cells exhibit only mild atypicality. Tubular differentiation is seen. This tumor was clinically malignant (see figure 6-35).

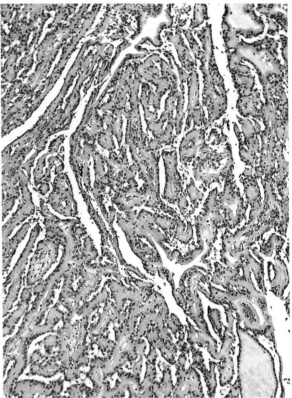

Figure 6-14

SERTOLI CELL TUMOR, NOT OTHERWISE SPECIFIED

This tumor has a prominent retiform pattern.

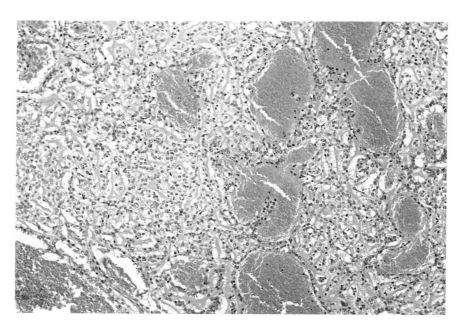

Figure 6-15

SERTOLI CELL TUMOR, NOT OTHERWISE SPECIFIED

Engorged blood vessels are conspicuous. Small tubules and cords are forming.

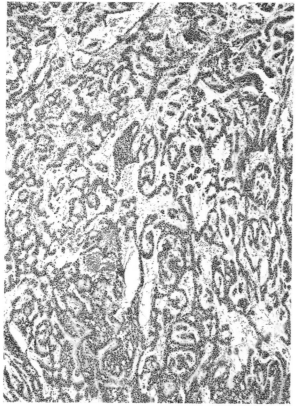

Figure 6-16

SERTOLI CELL TUMOR, NOT OTHERWISE SPECIFIED

This tumor forms long trabeculae, a finding that may suggest carcinoid tumor.

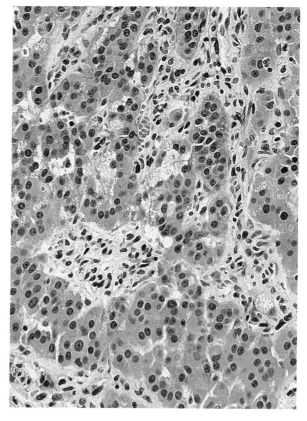

Figure 6-17

SERTOLI CELL TUMOR, NOT OTHERWISE SPECIFIED

Tumor cells with abundant eosinophilic cytoplasm form solid cords and nests.

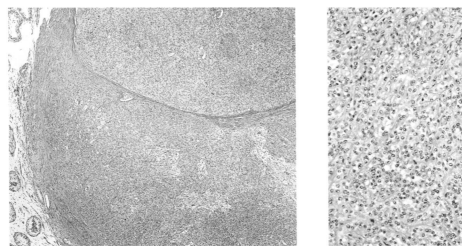
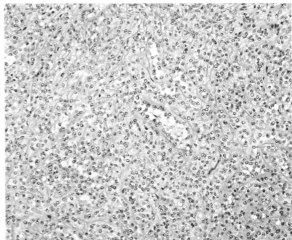

Figure 6-18

SERTOLI CELL TUMOR, NOT OTHERWISE SPECIFIED

Left: There is mostly solid, circumscribed growth of tumor cells.
Right: The pale cells are focally arranged in tubules.

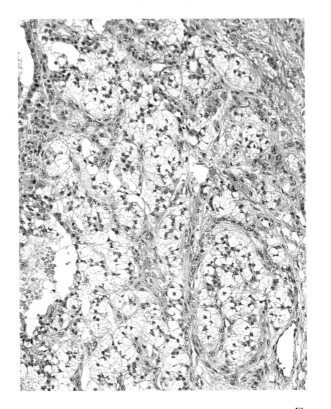
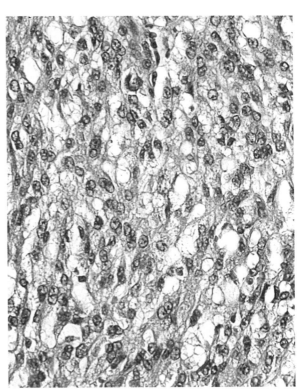

Figure 6-19

SERTOLI CELL TUMOR, NOT OTHERWISE SPECIFIED

Left: The tubules are composed of cells with abundant pale lipid-rich cytoplasm. This lipid-rich pattern of Sertoli cell neoplasia is, in our experience, usually focal.
Right: High magnification of a different case shows tumor cells with finely vacuolated cytoplasm.

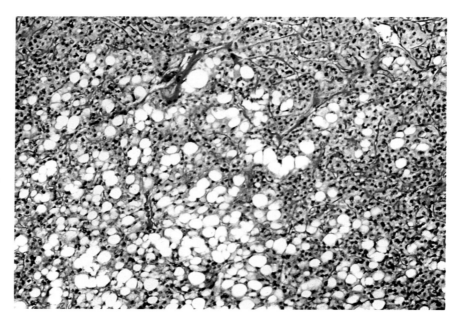

Figure 6-20

SERTOLI CELL TUMOR, NOT OTHERWISE SPECIFIED

Many tumor cells have prominent lipid droplets.

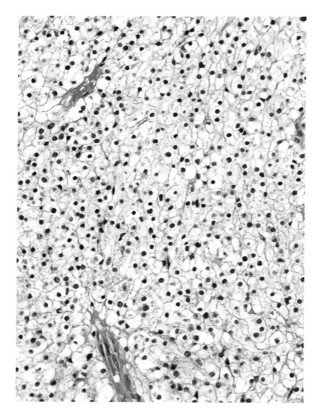

Figure 6-21

SERTOLI CELL TUMOR, NOT OTHERWISE SPECIFIED

The diffuse growth of pale cells with well-defined cytoplasmic membranes and prominent nucleoli may be misinterpreted as seminoma.

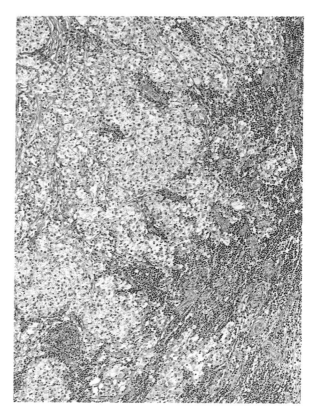

Figure 6-22

SERTOLI CELL TUMOR, NOT OTHERWISE SPECIFIED

There are sheets of cells with lightly eosinophilic cytoplasm in association with a lymphocytic infiltrate, features that led to confusion with seminoma.

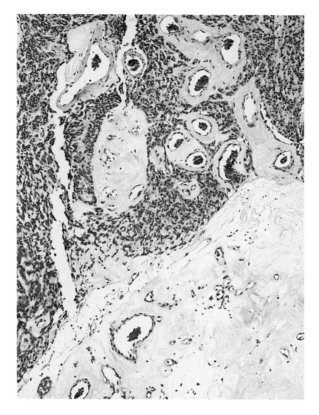

Figure 6-23

SERTOLI CELL TUMOR, NOT OTHERWISE SPECIFIED

This tumor has a prominent hyalinized stroma and many dilated blood vessels.

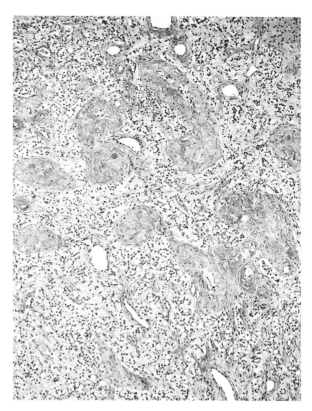

Figure 6-24

SERTOLI CELL TUMOR, NOT OTHERWISE SPECIFIED

Blood vessels are cuffed by sclerotic stroma.

the fibrous zones (fig. 6-25). The potential of the stroma to form bone may be the basis for a single reported case of a Sertoli cell tumor with an osteosarcomatous component (24).

Occasional tumors show foci of patchy calcification and hemosiderin deposits reminiscent of the Gamna-Gandy bodies typically found in the spleen. Rarely, such areas are conspicuous (fig. 6-26). The stroma sometimes has a myxomatous to mucoid appearance (figs. 6-27, 6-28). Most Sertoli cell tumors, NOS, have bland cytologic features and little mitotic activity. The smaller nuclei, less prominent nucleoli, and fewer number of mitotic figures of those tumors having a seminoma-like appearance due to the diffuse growth of pale cells aid in the distinction from seminoma (fig. 6-29). Some tumors with bland cytologic features, however, are clinically malignant. Occasional tumors exhibit overt pleomorphism (fig. 6-30) and conspicuous mitotic figures (fig. 6-31).

Immunohistochemical Findings. Table 6-2 provides a summary of the immunohistochemical staining patterns for tumors in the sex cord-stromal category. Sertoli cell tumors stain for alpha-inhibin in 30 to 90 percent of cases (fig. 6-32) (25–29). Our own experience is that less than 50 percent of Sertoli cell tumors NOS, typically those showing readily appreciated tubular differentiation, react for alpha-inhibin. Some degree of S-100 protein staining is seen in 30 to 100 percent of these tumors (26,29,30), although it is often focal. CD99 is expressed in 15 to 60 percent of Sertoli cell tumors, NOS (25,28). Surprisingly, positivity for chromogranin and synaptophysin (fig. 6-33) has been reported in 0 to 80 percent (25,27) and 45 percent (27) of cases, respectively. Cytokeratins are expressed in many Sertoli cell tumors, NOS (AE1/AE3/CAM 5.2, 80 percent [29]; CAM 5.2, 100 percent [26]), as is vimentin (75 percent [26]). Epithelial membrane antigen

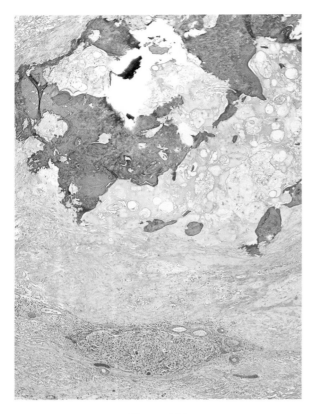

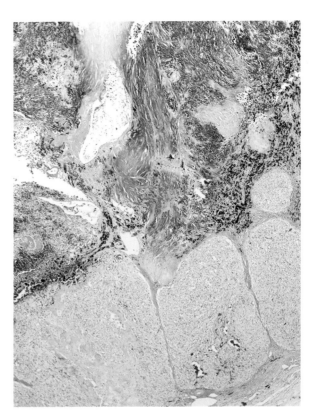

Figure 6-25

SERTOLI CELL TUMOR, NOT OTHERWISE SPECIFIED

Metaplastic bone has formed in a large area of hyaline fibrosis, a finding that may cause confusion with the large cell calcifying variant. Unlike in the latter, however, the calcific foci were confined to densely scarred areas.

Figure 6-26

SERTOLI CELL TUMOR, NOT OTHERWISE SPECIFIED

A dense focus of fibrosis contains calcified elastic fibers and hemosiderin deposits, similar to the Gamna-Gandy bodies often seen in the spleen.

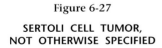

Figure 6-27

SERTOLI CELL TUMOR, NOT OTHERWISE SPECIFIED

Cords of cells are separated by a basophilic, myxoid stroma.

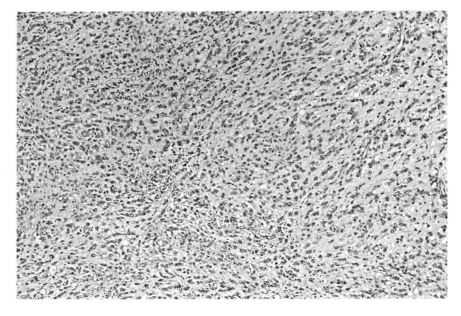

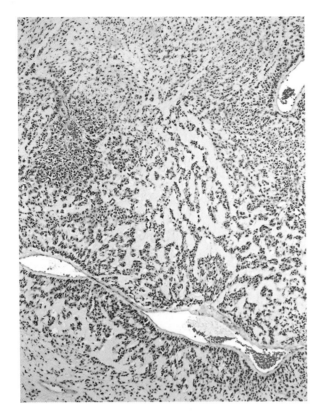

Figure 6-28

SERTOLI CELL TUMOR, NOT OTHERWISE SPECIFIED

This tumor has a lightly staining, mucoid stroma.

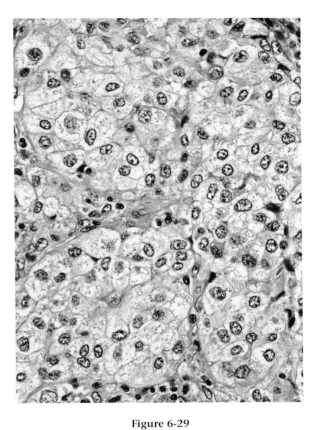

Figure 6-29

SERTOLI CELL TUMOR, NOT OTHERWISE SPECIFIED

The clear cells in this tumor have oval nuclei with inconspicuous nucleoli and infrequent mitotic figures, features that aid in the distinction from seminoma.

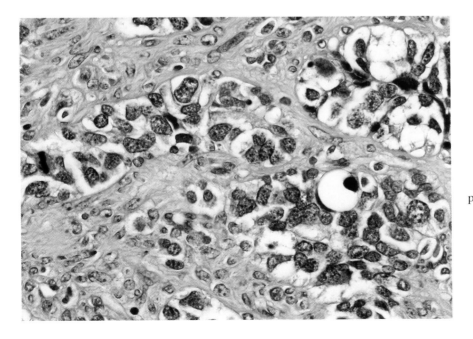

Figure 6-30

SERTOLI CELL TUMOR, NOT OTHERWISE SPECIFIED

Solid tubules of cells have pleomorphic nuclei.

Table 6-2

USUAL IMMUNOHISTOCHEMICAL STAINING REACTIONS IN DIFFERENT TYPES OF TESTICULAR SEX CORD-STROMAL TUMORS[a]

	Inhibin	S-100 Protein	CD99	Chrom[b]	Synapt	EMA	CK	Vim	OCT3/4	Calre-tinin	Melan-A
Sertoli cell tumor, NOS	V[c]	V	V	V	V	–	+	V	–	V	ND
Large cell calcifying Sertoli cell tumor	+	+	–	ND	ND	–	–	+	–	+	ND
Intratubular large cell hyalinizing Sertoli cell tumor	+	ND	ND	ND	ND	ND	+	ND	ND	ND	ND
Sclerosing Sertoli cell tumor	ND	ND	ND	–	ND	ND	–	+	ND	ND	ND
Leydig cell tumor	+	V	V	V	+	–	V	+	–	+	+
Granulosa cell tumor, adult type[d]	+	V	+	ND	ND	–	V	+	–	+	ND
Granulosa cell tumor, juvenile type	+	+	+	–	ND	ND	V	+	–	+	ND
Sex cord-stromal tumor, unclassified type	V	V	V	ND	ND	V	V	+	–	ND	V

[a]Data in the table are supplemented by unpublished, personal observations.
[b]Chrom = chromogranin; Synapt = synaptophysin; EMA = epithelial membrane antigen; CK = cytokeratin; Vim = vimentin; NOS = not otherwise specified.
[c]V = variable expression (20-80% of cases); – = usually negative (<20% of cases); + = usually positive (>80% of cases); ND = no data available.
[d]Based in part on data from ovarian examples.

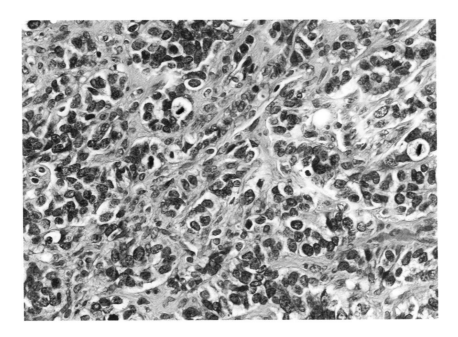

Figure 6-31

**SERTOLI CELL TUMOR,
NOT OTHERWISE SPECIFIED**

Several mitotic figures are evident.

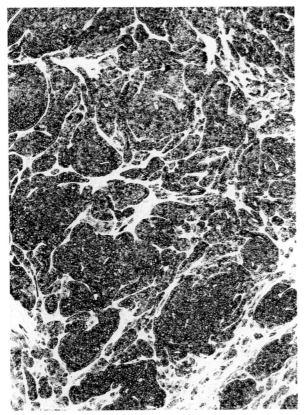

Figure 6-32

SERTOLI CELL TUMOR, NOT OTHERWISE SPECIFIED

Diffuse and intense positivity for alpha-inhibin is seen.

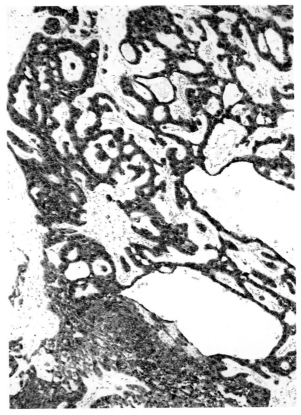

Figure 6-33

SERTOLI CELL TUMOR, NOT OTHERWISE SPECIFIED

There is strong reactivity for synaptophysin.

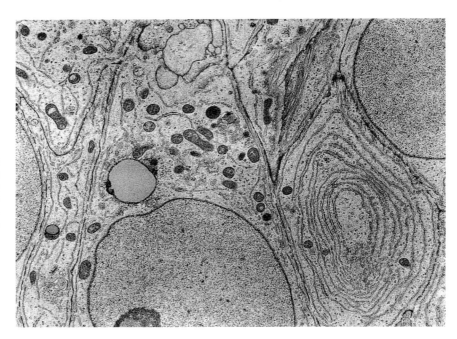

Figure 6-34

SERTOLI CELL TUMOR, NOT OTHERWISE SPECIFIED

A cluster of Sertoli cells shows tight junctions, prominent whorls of smooth and rough endoplasmic reticulum, lipid droplets, and interdigitating cell processes (top). (Courtesy of Dr. R. Erlandson, New York, NY.)

(EMA) is typically negative (26,29), although in our experience, some of the seminoma-like cases demonstrate patchy EMA positivity (23). Anti-müllerian hormone is identified focally in Sertoli cell tumors, although few cases have been studied (31). OCT3/4 and placental-like alkaline phosphatase (PLAP) are negative, and calretinin is often negative (28,32).

Ultrastructural Findings. On ultrastructural examination, Sertoli cell tumors typically have a well-developed Golgi apparatus, variably prominent smooth endoplasmic reticulum, lipid droplets, lateral desmosomes, and a peripheral investment of basement membrane (fig. 6-34) (33). Cisternae of rough endoplasmic reticulum may be prominent in some cases, but convincing Charcot-Böttcher filaments have not been identified in the few cases in the NOS category that have been examined ultrastructurally, unlike the large cell calcifying variant (see next section) (33,34).

Cytologic Findings. There are few reports concerning the cytologic features of Sertoli cell tumor, NOS. These have emphasized the discohesive nature of the tumor cells, the pallor and fragility of the cytoplasm (the latter causing a "naked nucleus"), and the oval to elongated nuclei, sometimes displaying identifiable grooves (35,36).

Special Techniques. Using comparative genomic hybridization, highly variable chromosomal aberrations were found in 9 of 11 cases,

with the most frequent findings being gain of the X chromosome and loss of the entire or part of chromosomes 2 and 19 (37). A clinically malignant Sertoli cell tumor in a 5-year-old boy had loss of the Y chromosome (38).

Differential Diagnosis. Sertoli cell tumors in the NOS category must be distinguished from the focal non-neoplastic clusters of immature tubules referred to as Sertoli cell nodules. The latter are usually of microscopic size but are occasionally visible grossly as white nodules a few millimeters in diameter or, rarely, larger (39). This differential diagnosis is considered in chapter 8.

Pure Sertoli cell tumors are distinguished from unclassified sex cord-stromal tumors by the often prominent cellular stromal component in the latter. This contrasts with the fibrotic to hyalinized, non-neoplastic appearance of the stroma in a pure Sertoli cell tumor.

Sertoli cell tumors generally lack the typical architectural features of adult granulosa cell tumor, a much rarer neoplasm in the testis, although there is some overlap: both, for example, sometimes form cords. The adult granulosa cell tumor has cells with less cytoplasm, and the typical pale, grooved nuclei are never a conspicuous feature of a Sertoli cell tumor. Juvenile granulosa cell tumors exhibit prominent follicle differentiation; the follicles are usually larger than the lumens of the tubules of Sertoli cell tumors and frequently are lined by stratified cells. Many also have a lobular architecture with an intervening fibromatous stroma in contrast to Sertoli cell tumor, NOS. Uncommonly, juvenile granulosa cell tumors have little or no follicular differentiation, and, in such cases, intercellular basophilic fluid may impart a chondroid appearance suggestive of the diagnosis. The juvenile granulosa cell tumor typically has more immature-appearing nuclei and mitotic activity than most Sertoli cell tumors, NOS. Juvenile granulosa cell tumor typically occurs in the first few months of life; in contrast, in the largest series of Sertoli cell tumors, NOS, no patient was under 15 years of age (7).

Areas in some Sertoli cell tumors, NOS, resemble Leydig cell tumors because of a diffuse growth of cells with appreciable eosinophilic cytoplasm. Despite this superficial similarity, many features help distinguish these tumors. Leydig cell tumors are more often yellow or brown on their sectioned surface, whereas Sertoli cell tumors are more often white to tan. On microscopic examination, the most helpful difference is the presence of tubular differentiation in most Sertoli cell tumors, a finding that excludes the diagnosis of Leydig cell tumor, although focal pseudotubules may be seen in rare Leydig cell tumors. Additionally, about one third of testicular Leydig cell tumors contain intracytoplasmic crystals of Reinke, which are absent in Sertoli cell tumors. Immunostaining for cytokeratin is typically stronger and more diffuse in Sertoli cell tumors and usually focal, weak, or absent in Leydig cell tumors. Inhibin immunoreactivity occurs in almost all Leydig cell tumors and is typically more intense and diffuse than in Sertoli cell tumors (26,27,29); a negative stain for alpha-inhibin therefore favors a Sertoli cell tumor.

Sertoli cell tumor, NOS, may be potentially misdiagnosed as seminoma when it has a diffuse pattern. Sertoli cell tumors usually have none or only a scant, nonspecific chronic inflammatory cell infiltrate, lacking the consistent sprinkling of lymphocytes that characterizes most seminomas. Rare cases, however, having diffuse and prominent lymphocytic infiltrates and clear tumor cells, have been misinterpreted as seminoma (23). In such cases, the absence of polygonal nuclei with "flattened" edges and one to four prominent nucleoli, lack of glycogen-rich cytoplasm, and paucity of mitotic

figures help in the distinction from seminoma, as does the absence of associated intratubular germ cell neoplasia, unclassified type (IGCNU) (23). Conversely, the presence of granulomas favors seminoma. Rare seminomas (see chapter 3) have a well-developed, solid tubular pattern that on low-power examination suggests a Sertoli cell tumor. This appears to have been the main confusing feature of five tumors whose distinction from Sertoli cell tumor was problematic, as mentioned by Collins and Symington almost 50 years ago (4). Tubular seminomas, however, have the usual lymphocytes and cytologic features of seminoma, and typical seminoma is usually apparent in other areas. The presence of adjacent IGCNU provides additional evidence that a tubular tumor is a seminoma. Seminoma cells stain strongly for glycogen, PLAP, and OCT3/4 (in contrast to neoplastic Sertoli cells), and Sertoli cells stain for lipid, cytokeratins, and often alpha-inhibin (in contrast to seminoma cells).

Adenomatoid tumors may have solid tubules but there are almost always some foci where the characteristic prominent vacuoles with flattening of the cells and the production of "thread-like bridging strands" (see chapter 7) are seen. The cells of Sertoli cell tumor may also have cytoplasmic vacuoles but these have a lipoblast-like appearance, typically with clear to pale cytoplasm that contrasts with the more eosinophilic cytoplasm of adenomatoid tumor. Rare adenomatoid tumors involve the testis to an appreciable degree but they are primarily paratesticular, in contrast to Sertoli cell tumor. Caution is advisable with the use of immunostains in this differential as both tumors may be reactive for WT1 and calretinin.

Another neoplasm that on microscopic evaluation alone simulates Sertoli cell tumor, NOS, is sertoliform rete cystadenoma, but its usual confinement to the rete should make distinction easy in most instances. A metastatic adenocarcinoma with regular tubular glands, such as one from the stomach, can mimic a Sertoli cell tumor, but such a neoplasm tends to have a more variegated microscopic appearance than a Sertoli cell tumor, a prominent intertubular growth pattern, and lymphatic involvement, and would likely be associated with clinical evidence of tumor elsewhere, or at least tumor in the paratesticular tissues. EMA positivity in most adenocarcinomas

Table 6-3

FINDINGS IN CLINICALLY MALIGNANT AND CLINICALLY BENIGN SERTOLI CELL TUMORS, NOS[a]

	Malignant Cases	Benign Cases
Dimension ≥ 5 cm	25 of 35 (71%)	1 of 9 (11%)
Mitotic rate > 5 MF/10 HPF[b]	8 of 21 (38%)	1 of 9 (11%)
Necrosis	16 of 20 (80%)	0 of 9 (0%)
Vascular invasion	13 of 20 (65%)	0 of 9 (0%)
Nuclear atypia	5 of 8 (63%)	0 of 9 (0%)

[a]Data from this table were abstracted from references 7, 17, 21, 23, and 41.
[b]MF = mitotic figures; HPF = high-power field.

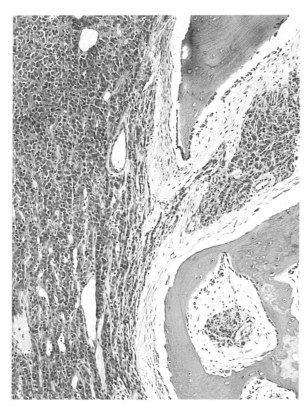

Figure 6-35

SERTOLI CELL TUMOR, NOT OTHERWISE SPECIFIED

This is a bone metastasis from the tumor illustrated in figure 6-13.

provides additional diagnostic aid in difficult cases, but are not entirely specific, and positivity for alpha-inhibin provides support for Sertoli cell tumor (40). These same immunostains are also useful for differentiating the rare endometrioid adenocarcinoma (see chapter 7), whose glands may simulate the hollow tubules of a Sertoli cell tumor. Squamous differentiation may occur in endometrioid adenocarcinoma but is exceptionally rare in Sertoli cell tumor. The distinction of Sertoli cell tumor from carcinoid tumor is discussed in chapter 4.

Spread and Metastasis. Malignant Sertoli cell tumors, NOS, most commonly metastasize to retroperitoneal lymph nodes, with the lung and pleura being the second most frequent sites of involvement (7,17,21,23,41). These are followed by inguinal lymph nodes, bone (fig. 6-35), supraclavicular lymph nodes, liver, mediastinum, pelvic lymph nodes, adrenal gland, heart, and skin.

Treatment and Prognosis. Only two series of Sertoli cell tumors, NOS (7,23) dealt with important prognostic pathologic findings, and one of these studied exclusively malignant tumors. Additional information derives from case reports, but these often have incomplete pathologic details and disproportionately represent malignant tumors. With these caveats, a summary of findings in malignant versus benign tumors is provided in Table 6-3. As is apparent, several features occur with greater frequency in malignant cases than benign ones: a tumor diameter of 5 cm or greater, necrosis, moderate to severe nuclear atypia, vascular invasion, and a mitotic rate over 5 mitotic figures per 10 high-power fields. It is our practice to place those tumors that have only one of these features into an "uncertain malignant potential" category and to regard those with two or more features as malignant Sertoli cell tumors. We do not use the term "benign Sertoli cell tumor" because there are no data to indicate that those tumors lacking all of these features cannot metastasize, but they are certainly at very low risk, which we indicate in our diagnostic report.

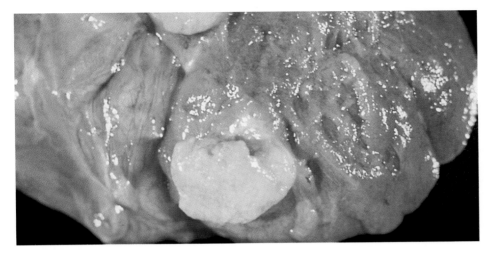

Figure 6-36

LARGE CELL CALCIFYING SERTOLI CELL TUMOR

A well-circumscribed tumor has a glistening, yellow-white sectioned surface.

The proportion of malignant tumors in children appears to be significantly less than in postpubertal patients. We are aware of reports of four cases of metastasizing Sertoli cell tumors in children from 5 to 12 years of age (2,16,17,38), but none were documented by immunohistochemical study and one did not have a pathologic review (2). Additional examples of "malignant" cases have been reported but are based solely on morphologic criteria, without clinical evidence of malignant behavior. We are not aware of a well-documented, clinically malignant Sertoli cell tumor in a child less than 5 years of age, despite some tumors in this age group having high cellularity and frequent mitotic figures (13).

The initial treatment of a Sertoli cell tumor, NOS, is radical orchiectomy. Retroperitoneal lymph node dissection is indicated if the patient has radiographically apparent retroperitoneal involvement. For cases judged to be likely malignant based on pathologic criteria alone, in the absence of known metastatic disease, it remains controversial whether retroperitoneal lymph node dissection should be performed. At the minimum, close follow-up is indicated. Radiation and chemotherapy have not proved consistently effective, although there are sporadic cases that have responded to these modalities (42).

Large Cell Calcifying Sertoli Cell Tumor

General and Clinical Features. About 70 *large cell calcifying Sertoli cell tumors* have been reported in patients from 2 to 73 years of age (average, 21 years) (34,42–49). In approximately one third of the cases, a variety of associated findings resulted in interesting and unusual clinical situations: acromegaly, pituitary gigantism, Cushing syndrome, sexual precocity, spotty mucocutaneous pigmentation, and sudden death. The correlating pathologic findings consisted of pituitary adenomas, bilateral primary adrenocortical hyperplasia, testicular sex cord-stromal tumors, cardiac myxomas, and lentigines (19). These findings are now recognized to be components of the Carney complex, an autosomal dominant, inherited disorder that has, in about half the cases, a germline mutation in the tumor-suppressor gene *PRKAR1A*, which encodes for cAMP-dependent protein kinase type I-alpha regulatory subunit. Most of the patients with the syndrome-associated tumors present at a younger patient age (less than 20 years) than those with sporadically developing tumors, although there are exceptions (42,49). Although many of the tumors described in patients with the Peutz-Jeghers syndrome were classified as large cell calcifying Sertoli cell tumors, our experience is that they are mostly intratubular proliferations having a different morphology (see below) (50).

Gross Findings. The tumors are usually well-circumscribed and 4 cm or less in diameter (mean, 2 cm) (figs. 6-36, 6-37). They may be multifocal, and approximately 20 percent are bilateral; these two features are almost exclusively seen in patients with the Carney complex. Sectioning reveals firm, yellow to tan to white tissue, often with granular, calcific foci (figs. 6-36–6-38). Necrosis is occasionally seen (fig. 6-38), usually in clinically malignant cases, as is hemorrhage (fig. 6-38).

Microscopic Findings. The tumor cells are typically arranged in closely packed nests (figs. 6-39, 6-40), trabeculae (fig. 6-41), cords (fig. 6-42), small clusters (fig. 6-42), or solid tubules (fig. 6-43). Foci of intratubular tumor are found in approximately half of the cases, supporting their Sertoli cell origin (fig. 6-44). The stroma varies from loose and myxoid (fig. 6-41) to densely collagenous (fig. 6-45). Many tumors exhibit a prominent neutrophilic infiltrate (figs. 6-43, 6-46). The characteristic calcification is usually conspicuous (figs. 6-39, 6-42, 6-45) and sometimes massive (fig. 6-39) but may also be minor. It often consists of large, wavy, laminated nodules having a mulberry-like appearance (fig. 6-42). Small psammoma bodies occasionally are seen (figs. 6-40, 6-44), as is ossification (fig. 6-39). The neoplastic cells are large and usually round (figs. 6-40, 6-43, 6-46), but are sometimes cuboidal or columnar, and rarely spindle shaped (fig. 6-47).

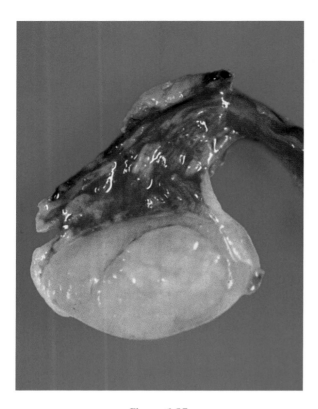

Figure 6-37

LARGE CELL CALCIFYING SERTOLI CELL TUMOR

This tumor is well circumscribed and light tan, with a nodular cut surface. (Courtesy of Dr. J.Y. Ro, Houston, TX.)

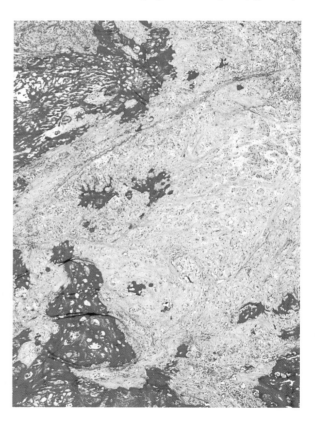

Figure 6-39

LARGE CELL CALCIFYING SERTOLI CELL TUMOR

Large, irregular, plaque-like foci of calcium are conspicuous on low-power examination.

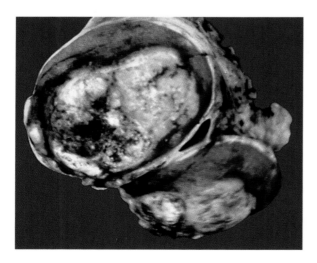

Figure 6-38

LARGE CELL CALCIFYING SERTOLI CELL TUMOR

The large tumor exhibits both hemorrhage and necrosis. It was clinically malignant.

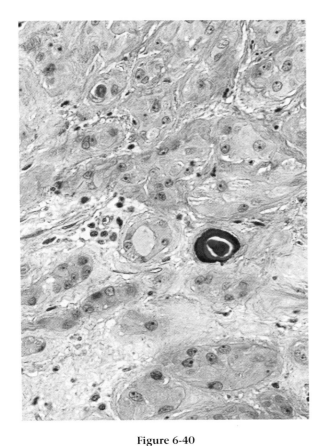

Figure 6-40

LARGE CELL CALCIFYING SERTOLI CELL TUMOR

The tumor cells have abundant eosinophilic cytoplasm.

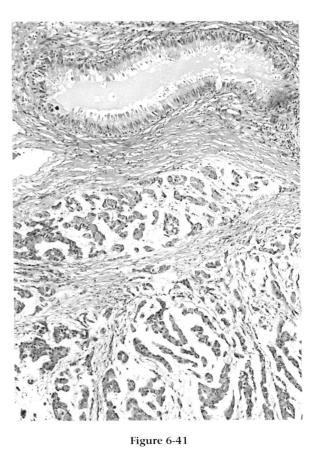

Figure 6-41

LARGE CELL CALCIFYING SERTOLI CELL TUMOR

This clinically malignant tumor has spread to involve the epididymis.

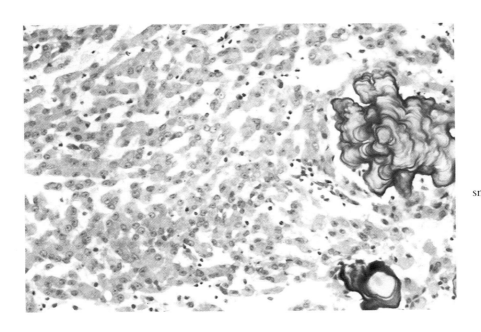

Figure 6-42

LARGE CELL CALCIFYING SERTOLI CELL TUMOR

Tumor cells grow in cords and small clusters.

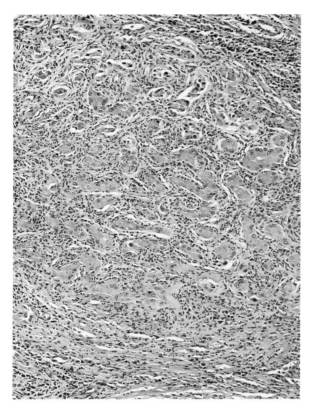

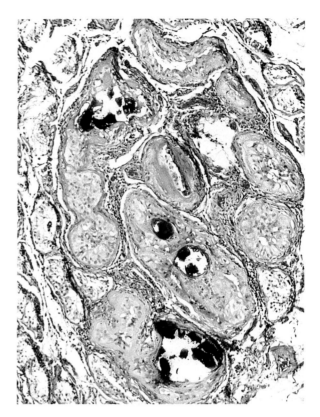

Figure 6-43

LARGE CELL CALCIFYING SERTOLI CELL TUMOR

Solid tubules of tumor cells are separated by a stroma containing a prominent neutrophilic infiltrate. This field lacks the calcifications that were present elsewhere.

Figure 6-44

LARGE CELL CALCIFYING SERTOLI CELL TUMOR

Tumor is present within tubules.

Figure 6-45

LARGE CELL CALCIFYING SERTOLI CELL TUMOR

This tumor has a densely collagenous stroma and laminated calcifications.

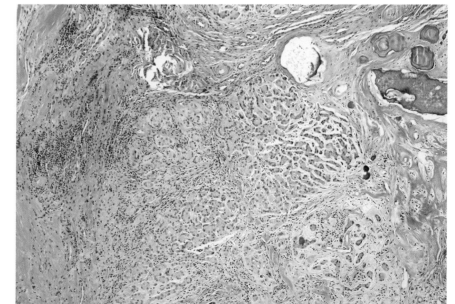

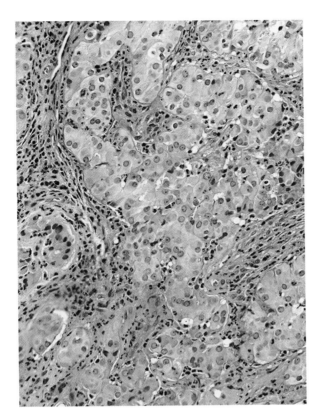

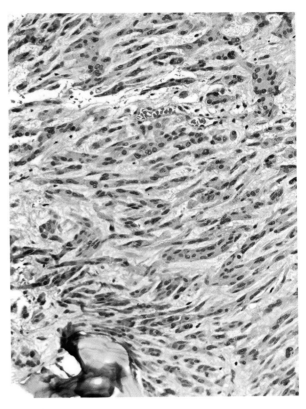

Figure 6-46

LARGE CELL CALCIFYING SERTOLI CELL TUMOR

The tumor cells are round and have pale, eosinophilic cytoplasm. A neutrophilic infiltrate is prominent.

Figure 6-47

LARGE CELL CALCIFYING SERTOLI CELL TUMOR

Many cells are spindle shaped.

In most cases, the cytoplasm is abundant, eosinophilic, and finely granular (figs. 6-40, 6-43), but occasionally it is pale (fig. 6-46), amphophilic, or slightly vacuolated. The nuclei are round or oval, with one or two small to moderate-sized nucleoli (fig. 6-40). Mitotic figures are generally rare.

Immunohistochemical Findings. These tumors differ from Sertoli cell tumors, NOS, by being more consistently reactive for alpha-inhibin (fig. 6-48) (28,51–54), calretinin (28,51), and S-100 protein (fig. 6-49) (30,42,48,51,53,55). Vimentin is also positive (42,51,53-55) whereas CD99 is only rarely reactive (28). Cytokeratins and EMA are either negative (EMA) or focally positive (cytokeratins) in some cases (42,52-54). There are isolated reports of positivity for aromatase (56) and CD10 (51).

Ultrastructural Findings. Clusters of tumor cells are surrounded by basement membrane and sometimes form a central space that is also surrounded by basement membrane (55,57). Adjacent cells are joined by well-developed desmosomes (34,43,57), and the cytoplasm contains stacks of round and smooth endoplasmic reticulum, lipid droplets, and intermediate filaments (34,43,55,57,58). Charcot-Böttcher filament bundles, the specific cytoplasmic inclusions of Sertoli cells, are seen in only a minority of cases (fig. 6-50) (34,47).

Differential Diagnosis. In contrast to most Sertoli cell tumors NOS, large cell calcifying Sertoli cell tumors have calcifications, more abundant eosinophilic cytoplasm, a more frequently myxoid stroma, associated neutrophilic infiltrates, and, at least in some cases, a conspicuous intratubular component. Leydig cell tumor may enter the differential. Calcification, however, is rare in Leydig cell tumor (59,60) and tubular differentiation is absent; its stroma is usually densely fibrous rather than myxoid; it

261

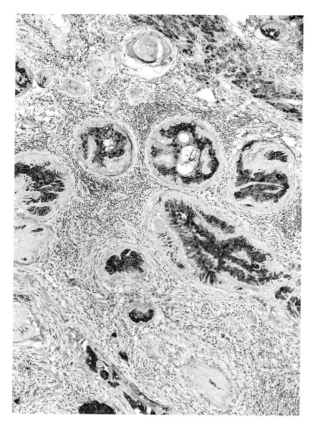

Figure 6-48

LARGE CELL CALCIFYING SERTOLI CELL TUMOR

Both the invasive and intratubular components are positive for alpha-inhibin.

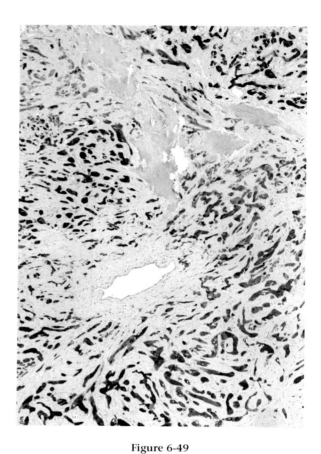

Figure 6-49

LARGE CELL CALCIFYING SERTOLI CELL TUMOR

There is diffuse positivity for S-100 protein. The nonstaining area at upper center represents a focus of calcification.

Figure 6-50

LARGE CELL CALCIFYING SERTOLI CELL TUMOR

There is a perinuclear array of parallel cytoplasmic filaments (Charcot-Böttcher filaments), a feature of Sertoli cells. (Courtesy of Dr. B. Têtu, Québec, Canada.)

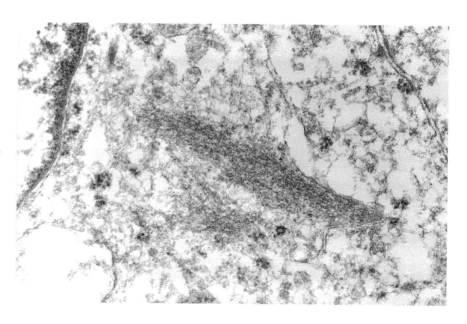

Table 6-4

COMPARISON BETWEEN REPORTED BENIGN AND MALIGNANT CASES OF LARGE CELL CALCIFYING SERTOLI CELL TUMOR[a]

	Benign	Malignant
Mean age	17 years	39 years
Association with syndrome or congenital abnormality (see text)	36%	12.5%
Laterality/Focality	Bilateral and/or multifocal (28%)	All unilateral and unifocal
Mean size	1.4 cm	5.4 cm
Histologic features	No extratesticular spread, size <4 cm, rare mitotic figures, only mild nuclear atypia, no necrosis, no lymphovascular invasion	Contains 2 or more of: extratesticular spread, size >4 cm, mitoses >3/10 HPF[b], significant nuclear atypia, necrosis, lymphovascular invasion

[a]Adapted from reference 42.
[b]HPF = high-power field.

may have identifiable Reinke crystals and cytoplasmic lipofuscin; it almost always lacks a neutrophilic infiltrate; and there is no intratubular component. The distinction from the Sertoli cell neoplasia characteristic of the Peutz-Jeghers syndrome is discussed in the next section.

Treatment and Prognosis. Most large cell calcifying Sertoli cell tumors are benign. In one report, 8 of 47 tumors (17 percent) were clinically malignant (42). This proportion of malignant tumors is almost certainly inflated because of the selection bias associated with the referral of malignant cases to academic centers and the tendency to more frequently report the uncommon malignant variants. Nonetheless, since that study several additional malignant tumors have been described (48,54,55,61). The mean age of patients with malignant tumors is 39 years, compared to 17 years for those with benign tumors. Only one patient with a malignant tumor had any features of the Carney complex. In contrast to the benign tumors, a significant number of which are bilateral and multifocal, all the malignant tumors are unilateral and unifocal. The pathologic features that suggest a malignant course include large size and other features generally similar to those useful in determining prognosis in cases of Sertoli cell tumors, NOS. The features of the reported benign and malignant cases of large cell calcifying Sertoli cell tumors are contrasted in Table 6-4.

The usual treatment of patients with unilateral large cell calcifying Sertoli cell tumor is radical orchiectomy. If there is clinical or radiographic evidence of retroperitoneal spread, a retroperitoneal lymph node dissection is often performed. If the tumor shows malignant features on pathologic examination but lacks clinical and radiographic evidence of metastatic involvement, some urologists proceed with retroperitoneal lymph node dissection because of the possibility of occult metastasis. Only an occasional metastatic large cell calcifying Sertoli cell tumor has responded to radiation or chemotherapy (42).

For young patients with small, bilateral and multifocal tumors, conservative treatment is appropriate. Because some of these patients may have estrogenic symptoms, notably gynecomastia, administration of antiestrogen drugs in conjunction with testicular surveillance has been advocated (62).

Intratubular Large Cell Hyalinizing Sertoli Cell Neoplasia

General and Clinical Features. *Intratubular large cell hyalinizing Sertoli cell neoplasia* is a form of intratubular proliferation so characteristic of the Peutz-Jeghers syndrome that it should prompt investigation for the syndrome whenever the testicular lesion is encountered (50,63,64). Although the neoplastic nature of this process may be questioned, the occasional development of invasive tumors leads us to regard the lesion as neoplastic. In 27 percent of patients with the Peutz-Jeghers syndrome, there is progression to an invasive tumor that may resemble the large cell calcifying Sertoli cell tumor (see prior section) but usually differs from it (see below) (50).

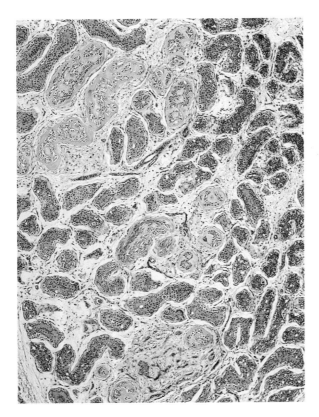

Figure 6-51

**INTRATUBULAR LARGE CELL
HYALINIZING SERTOLI CELL NEOPLASIA**

The lobular clusters of seminiferous tubules show thickened peritubular basement membranes that project into the tubular lumens.

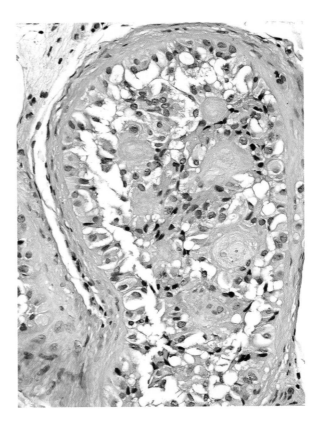

Figure 6-52

**INTRATUBULAR LARGE CELL
HYALINIZING SERTOLI CELL NEOPLASIA**

The tubules are lined by large Sertoli cells with vacuolated, eosinophilic cytoplasm and uniform, round nuclei with small nucleoli. Intraluminal globular deposits of basement membrane are seen.

These tumors are found in young boys (age range, 1.8 to 14.0 years; mean, 7 years) (50). Almost all of the patients present with gynecomastia, which is found on physical examination should it not be the presenting feature. The gynecomastia is attributable to aromatase production by the tumor (65–67). This enzyme is capable of using testosterone and androstenedione as substrates for the synthesis of estradiol and estrone, respectively, which are therefore elevated in the serum. The most common additional manifestation of Peutz-Jeghers syndrome is perioral pigmentation. Advanced bone age is also common.

Gross Findings. A few to numerous small, white to light pink nodules, usually less than 0.4 cm, protrude from the cut surface of the parenchyma (50,68). These small lesions correspond to the intratubular tumor. For the less

common cases with an invasive component, there is a larger, typically circumscribed, yellow to tan, solid mass that may show minor foci of cystic degeneration and have a gritty texture secondary to calcification.

Microscopic Findings. Lobular clusters of expanded seminiferous tubules are typically scattered in the testis (fig. 6-51). The tubules are lined by one or several layers of enlarged Sertoli cells having lightly stained to eosinophilic, frequently vacuolated cytoplasm and ovoid nuclei with fine chromatin and small to moderate-sized nucleoli (fig. 6-52). The tubules are surrounded by an impressively thickened basement membrane, which also invaginates into the lumens of the tubules to produce what appears as intraluminal globoid deposits of pink basement membrane matrix (fig. 6-53).

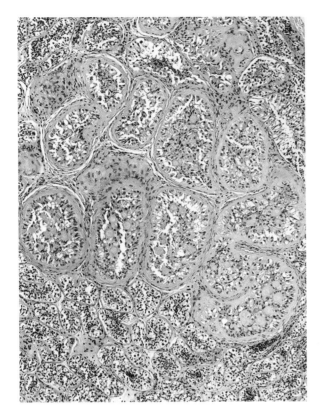

Figure 6-53

**INTRATUBULAR LARGE CELL
HYALINIZING SERTOLI CELL NEOPLASIA**

A cluster of enlarged tubules contains prominent globules of basement membrane.

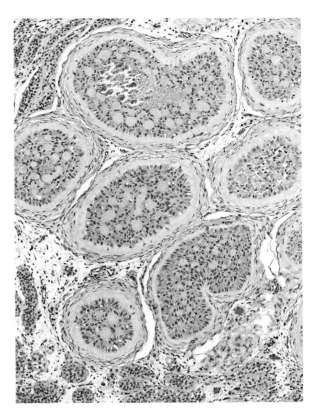

Figure 6-54

**INTRATUBULAR LARGE CELL
HYALINIZING SERTOLI CELL NEOPLASIA**

There is focal comedo necrosis with calcification.

Germ cells are mostly excluded by the Sertoli cell proliferation. Uncommonly, there may be central, comedo-type necrosis and associated dystrophic calcification (fig. 6-54), but calcification is not a conspicuous feature. The surrounding testis maintains a typical prepubertal appearance.

When the tumor is invasive, the features of the large cell calcifying Sertoli cell tumor may be present (fig. 6-55) (69). We have seen one case that had the pattern of the large cell calcifying Sertoli cell but lacked calcification (fig. 6-56). One tumor formed cysts that may have been within intratubular tumor (fig. 6-57).

Immunohistochemical Findings. There is strong and diffuse positivity for alpha-inhibin in the intratubular neoplastic Sertoli cells, which also stain, but more focally, for cytokeratins (fig. 6-58). Aromatase stains are also positive

(67), and the basement membrane deposits are highlighted by stains against laminin and collagen IV (70).

Ultrastructural Findings. The intratubular tumor cells are surrounded by prominent deposits of laminated basement membrane and contain rough endoplasmic reticulum, occasional lamellae of smooth endoplasmic reticulum, lipid droplets, and glycogen particles (55,63,68,70). Charcot-Böttcher filaments have not been identified (68).

Differential Diagnosis. A number of entities enter the differential diagnosis of large cell hyalinizing Sertoli cell neoplasia. A prime consideration is large cell calcifying Sertoli cell tumor. Contrasting features of these two entities are provided in Table 6-5.

Non-neoplastic Sertoli cell nodules (see chapter 8), because of their usually small size,

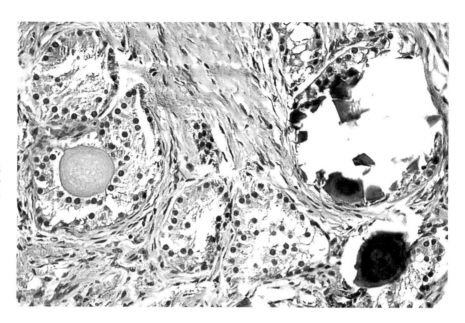

Figure 6-55

SERTOLI CELL TUMOR IN PEUTZ-JEGHERS SYNDROME

This invasive tumor shows some features similar to those of large cell calcifying Sertoli cell tumor.

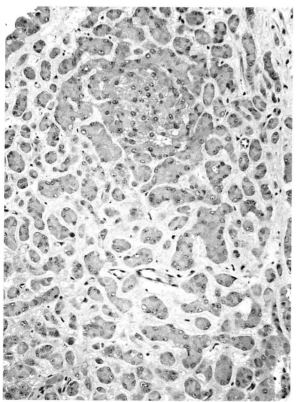

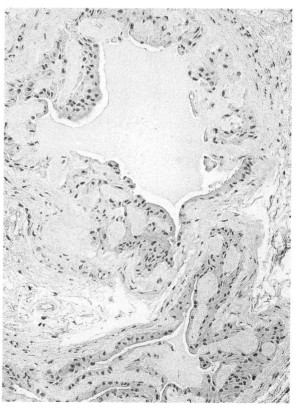

Figure 6-56

SERTOLI CELL TUMOR IN PEUTZ-JEGHERS SYNDROME

The tumor cells grow in solid tubules and have abundant cytoplasm. The appearance is reminiscent of large cell calcifying Sertoli cell tumor but calcification is lacking.

Figure 6-57

SERTOLI CELL TUMOR IN PEUTZ-JEGHERS SYNDROME

Cysts surrounded by basement membrane are lined by Sertoli cells with abundant eosinophilic cytoplasm.

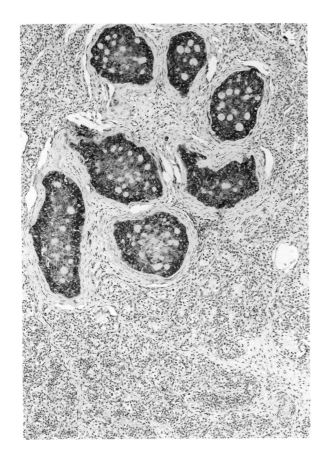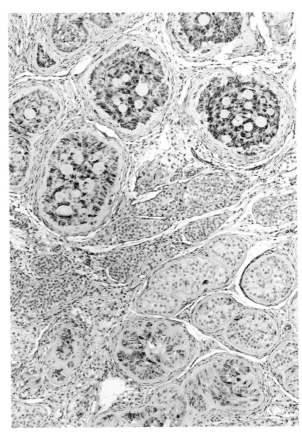

Figure 6-58

INTRATUBULAR LARGE CELL HYALINIZING SERTOLI CELL NEOPLASIA

Left: There is strong and diffuse reactivity for alpha-inhibin.
Right: Patchy reactivity is present for cytokeratins.

Table 6-5

GENERALIZATIONS CONCERNING TESTICULAR LESIONS ASSOCIATED WITH PEUTZ-JEGHERS SYNDROME VERSUS THOSE ASSOCIATED WITH CARNEY SYNDROME[a]

	Peutz-Jeghers	Carney
Presentation	Gynecomastia	Pseudoprecocity
Age at presentation	~ 7 years	~ 9 years
Bilaterality	Yes	Yes
Multifocality	Yes	Yes
Large Sertoli cells	Yes	Yes
Basement membrane deposits	Prominent	Less prominent
Tubular expansion	2-4X	1.5-2X
Calcification	Occasional, focal	Prominent
Intratubular tumor>extratubular tumor	Yes	No
Genetic mutation	*STK11/LKB1* (on 19p)	*PRKAR1A* (on 17q)

[a]Data from reference 187.

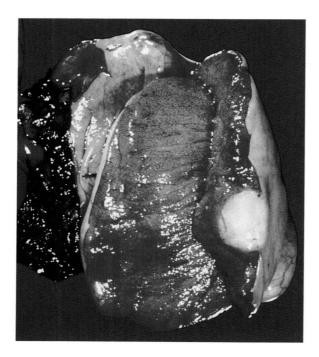

Figure 6-59

SCLEROSING SERTOLI CELL TUMOR

The tumor is well circumscribed and white.

intratubular nature, patchy distribution, and frequently prominent component of globular basement membrane deposits, may be confused with large cell hyalinizing Sertoli cell neoplasia. Unlike the latter, however, the lesional cells are smaller than normal Sertoli cells, displaying a fetal-type phenotype. Also, they often contain a component of non-neoplastic germ cells, whereas these are almost always absent in the Peutz-Jeghers–associated intratubular tumor.

Treatment and Prognosis. No lesion of this type has metastasized. When tumors, based on clinical and radiographic features, are judged to be intratubular (multifocal nodules less than 3 to 4 mm in size), careful follow-up and treatment with aromatase inhibitors is advocated (50,63,71). Orchiectomy remains the standard approach when there is evidence of invasion.

Sclerosing Sertoli Cell Tumor

General and Clinical Features. Some Sertoli cell tumors exhibit extensive sclerosis, placing the neoplasm in the category of a *sclerosing Sertoli cell tumor* (72). This variant is uncommon, with about

40 cases reported in the literature, which includes the 10 patients in the original description of this entity in 1991 (72) and 20 in a recent series (73). Most patients present with a mass, although one sought attention for testicular pain (74). Hormonal symptoms have not been reported. Patient ages range from 18 to 80 years, with a mean of 35 years (72). One patient was positive for the human immunodeficiency virus (HIV) (75).

Gross Findings. Eighty percent of the tumors are 2 cm or less in diameter, but they range up to 4 cm. They are typically circumscribed, firm, white to yellow to tan solitary masses (fig. 6-59). Necrosis is absent. Extratesticular growth has been described in one case (72).

Microscopic Findings. The tumor cells are fairly evenly distributed in a densely collagenous stroma that comprises the majority of the lesion. Most frequently they are arranged in small solid nests, tubules, and cords (figs. 6-60, 6-61). Occasional hollow tubules are seen (fig. 6-62), sometimes arranged in a retiform pattern. The prominence of cellular cords may create an appearance that simulates trabecular carcinoid tumor (fig. 6-63). Entrapped, non-neoplastic seminiferous tubules, often with an appearance similar to that of the immature tubules commonly seen in cryptorchid testes, are frequent. The tumor cells usually have a moderate amount of lightly eosinophilic, sometimes vacuolated, cytoplasm (fig. 6-64). The nuclei vary from small and dark-staining to large and vesicular, with moderate-sized nucleoli (fig. 6-64), although most tumor cells have oval to polygonal nuclei with finely granular, uniform chromatin and small nucleoli. Significant cytologic atypia or more than minimal mitotic activity is lacking, although one tumor was cytologically atypical and had frequent mitotic figures (72). The stroma is hypocellular and varies from finely fibrous (fig. 6-60) to hyalinized (figs. 6-63, 6-64). Thick collagen bundles are frequent. Almost all cases have been well circumscribed.

Immunohistochemical Findings. Vimentin is positive whereas cytokeratins (AE1/AE3 and CAM 5.2) are usually negative but may show weak positivity (72,76). Several other markers (chromogranin, carcinoembryonic antigen, PLAP, alpha-fetoprotein, beta-human chorionic gonadotropin, prostate-specific antigen, and prostate-specific acid phosphatase) have been reported as negative (72).

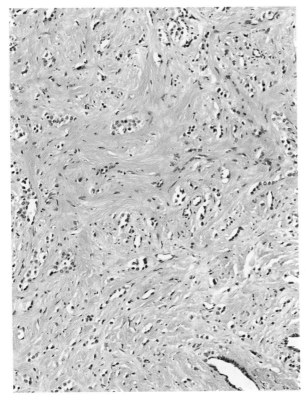

Figure 6-60

SCLEROSING SERTOLI CELL TUMOR

Small tubules are separated by a conspicuous fibrous stroma.

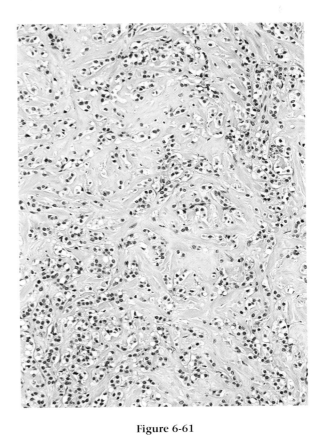

Figure 6-61

SCLEROSING SERTOLI CELL TUMOR

Cords and nests of tumor cells are present in a densely collagenous stroma.

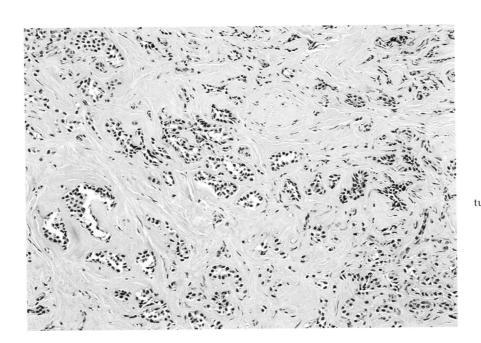

Figure 6-62

SCLEROSING SERTOLI CELL TUMOR

Cords and solid and hollow tubules are formed.

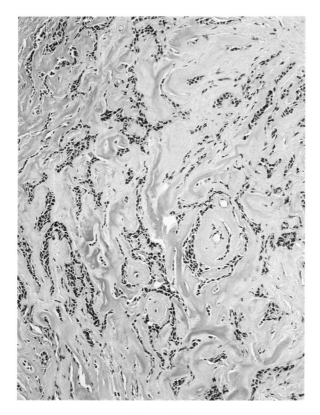

Figure 6-63

SCLEROSING SERTOLI CELL TUMOR

Elongated cords in a densely collagenous stroma are reminiscent of carcinoid tumor.

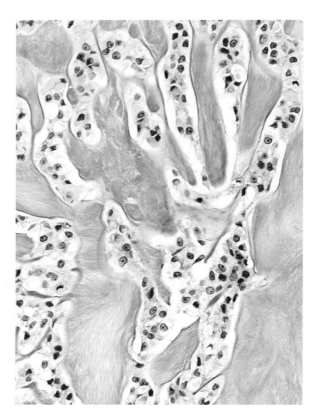

Figure 6-64

SCLEROSING SERTOLI CELL TUMOR

The tumor cells have pale, eosinophilic cytoplasm and uniform, round nuclei with small nucleoli.

Treatment and Prognosis. The standard treatment is orchiectomy. No acceptable cases have metastasized. One tumor that had significant cytologic atypia, an elevated mitotic rate, and extratesticular growth had no evidence of recurrence 5 years after orchiectomy (72). Another tumor that we considered a possible sclerosing Sertoli cell tumor showed 50 percent overall cellularity, clusters of greater cellularity, invasive growth, and size of 3.8 cm. This patient presented with metastases and the features of his tumor (invasive growth, cellularity equivalent to or greater than the amount of stroma, clustered hypercellularity) we now consider exclusionary criteria for sclerosing Sertoli cell tumor and place such cases in the NOS category.

Sertoli-Leydig Cell Tumor

General and Clinical Features. Six reported testicular cases describe a tubular component and patterns similar to those seen in the Sertoli-Leydig cell tumor of the ovary, with an additional Leydig cell component (8,11,77–80). It is difficult to assess these cases; most were published in early literature with images not of contemporary quality and immunohistochemical evidence lacking. We believe that at least some of these cases represent Sertoli-stromal cell tumors or unclassified sex cord-stromal tumors with entrapped, non-neoplastic Leydig cells (fig. 6-65), an idea supported by the Sertoli cell–predominant nature of the tumors and the simultaneous presence of entrapped seminiferous tubules. Of these six reported cases, one was a 3.5-month-old infant; the other patients were 4, 53, 54, 63, and 66 years of age. Two patients had gynecomastia.

Gross Findings. Testicular Sertoli-Leydig cell tumors range from 1.8 to 12.0 cm in diameter. They are usually uniformly or dominantly solid, frequently yellow, and often have a lobulated

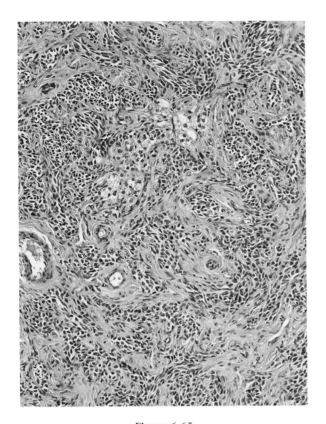

Figure 6-65

UNCLASSIFIED SEX CORD-STROMAL TUMOR

Clusters of entrapped, non-neoplastic Leydig cells (top center) among nests of undifferentiated oval to fusiform sex cord cells may cause confusion with Sertoli-Leydig cell tumor.

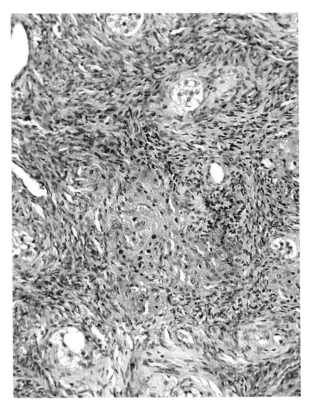

Figure 6-66

SERTOLI-LEYDIG CELL TUMOR

A cellular neoplastic stroma contains aggregates of Leydig cells.

sectioned surface. The single known malignant tumor had areas of hemorrhage and necrosis (79).

Microscopic Findings. Most of the tumors have tubules, cords, and trabeculae in haphazard arrangements with a background stroma that usually contains focal Leydig cells (fig. 6-66). Most tumors are of intermediate differentiation, according to the classification of ovarian cases, but some are poorly differentiated; there is only one report of a well-differentiated tumor (80). Retiform differentiation, with slit-like glands and cysts, is unusual (81). One tumor had areas of osteosarcoma and foci that resembled a malignant giant cell tumor (79). The metastases in that case were composed predominantly of osteosarcoma, but one lung lesion had the features of a malignant Leydig cell tumor with "unmistakable" Reinke crystals.

Typical heterologous elements, as seen in ovarian cases, have not been encountered to date.

Differential Diagnosis. The differential diagnosis for tumors with a prominent tubular pattern is similar to that of pure Sertoli cell tumors. In general, the resemblance to ovarian Sertoli-Leydig cell tumor should facilitate their recognition. The presence of a neoplastic Leydig cell component separates the tumors from pure Sertoli cell tumors and, in contrast to unclassified tumors in the sex cord-stromal category, there is a less conspicuous fibrothecomatous stroma and lack of granulosa cell differentiation.

LEYDIG CELL TUMORS

General and Clinical Features. *Leydig cell tumors* account for about 2 percent of testicular neoplasms (82,83). Approximately 20 percent are detected in the first decade of life, 25 percent between 10 and 30 years, 30 percent between 30

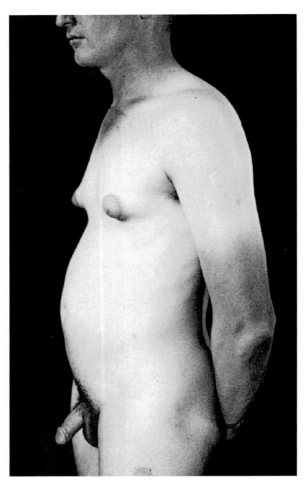

Figure 6-67

LEYDIG CELL TUMOR

The patient has gynecomastia.

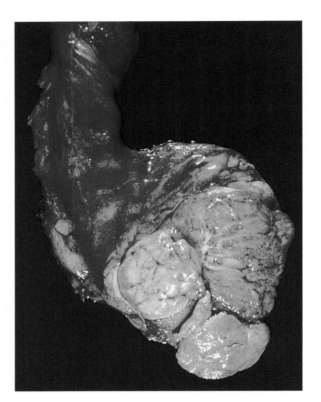

Figure 6-68

LEYDIG CELL TUMOR

The tumor is well demarcated and yellow. (Fig. 5.1 from Young RH, Scully RE. Testicular tumors. Chicago: ASCP Press; 1990:110.)

and 50 years, and 25 percent beyond that age. Bilaterality is seen in only about 3 percent of cases (84–86). Rare tumors are familial (87).

Adults usually complain of testicular swelling, but gynecomastia causes the patient to seek medical attention in 15 percent of the cases (fig. 6-67) and is present in an additional 15 percent of patients on clinical evaluation (86). In some cases an impalpable tumor is detected by ultrasound examination of an adult with gynecomastia (88). A decrease in libido or potency occurs in some patients. Children almost always present with isosexual pseudoprecocity, usually at 5 to 9 years of age (89). They frequently have small tumors requiring special studies, including selective testicular vein sampling, for detec-

tion. Approximately 10 percent of patients are asymptomatic and the tumors are discovered on physical examination. The presence of an undescended testis or a history of it in 5 to 10 percent of the cases in one series (86) suggests that cryptorchidism may predispose to tumor development in some. Germline mutations of the fumarate hydratase gene, which are seen in patients with the hereditary leiomyomatosis and renal cell carcinoma syndrome, are reported in rare patients with Leydig cell tumors (90). One patient with recurrent Leydig cell tumor developed tumor-induced Cushing syndrome (91). Rare examples have occurred in patients with Klinefelter syndrome (92) but these should be distinguished from the Leydig cell hyperplasia that is common in that disorder. One malignant "Leydig cell" tumor was associated with the adrenogenital syndrome, but crystals of Reinke were absent in the tumor cells (93).

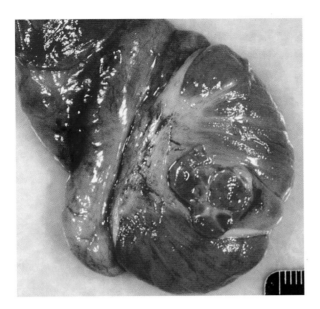

Figure 6-69

LEYDIG CELL TUMOR

Fibrous septa divide a tan-orange tumor into distinct lobules.

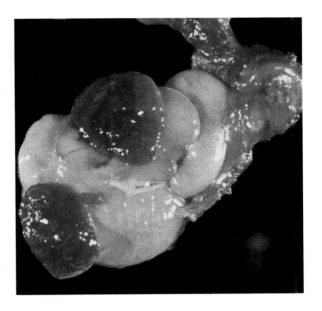

Figure 6-70

LEYDIG CELL TUMOR

This green-brown tumor from a prepubertal boy caused sexual precocity.

Testosterone is the major androgen produced by Leydig cell tumors, but androstenedione and dehydroepiandrosterone are also secreted (89,94). Urinary 17-ketosteroids may be normal or high. Elevated estrogen levels are recorded in patients with and without gynecomastia, and estradiol was present in high concentrations in spermatic vein blood in several cases (95). Testosterone levels and values for gonadotropins, particularly follicle-stimulating hormone (FSH), are low in patients with gynecomastia and elevated estradiol levels (96,97); plasma progesterone or urinary pregnanediol values may be elevated (98,99). The abnormal hormonal levels may return to normal after removal of the tumor (100), but in some cases they persist.

Gross Findings. The tumors are typically sharply circumscribed (figs. 6-68–6-70), usually under 4 cm in diameter, and sometimes lobulated by fibrous septa (fig. 6-69). They are usually uniformly solid and yellow (fig. 6-68) or yellow-tan, but occasionally are red-tan (fig. 6-69), brown (fig. 6-71), green-brown (fig. 6-70), or gray-white. Foci of hemorrhage, necrosis, or both are present in approximately one quarter of the cases (fig. 6-71). Growth beyond the testis is seen in up to 15 percent of the cases (86).

Microscopic Findings. The most common microscopic patterns are diffuse and nodular (figs. 6-72, 6-73). Combinations of diffuse and nodular growth result in cellular lobules of tumor (fig. 6-74). In the diffuse pattern, the stroma is typically inconspicuous and has a nondescript fibrous character (figs. 6-72, 6-75); in nodular tumors, the stroma is prominent and often extensively hyalinized, dividing the nodules by broad fibrous bands (fig. 6-73). Occasionally, the stroma is focally or conspicuously edematous or myxoid, and the tumor cells are dispersed as regular nests, irregular clusters (fig. 6-76), trabeculae, or cords (fig. 6-77). Edema likely also contributes to a striking microcystic arrangement (fig. 6-78), mixed microcystic and macrocystic appearance (fig. 6-79), or pseudotubular pattern (fig. 6-80), which occurs in rare cases. Foci of adipose differentiation are seen in occasional cases (fig. 6-81) (60,101), as are psammomatous calcifications (60,86,102,103) and ossification (60,102,104).

The tumor cells are typically large and polygonal, with abundant, slightly granular, eosinophilic cytoplasm (fig. 6-82). Occasionally, the cytoplasm is extensively vacuolated or spongy due to abundant lipid (fig. 6-83), and

273

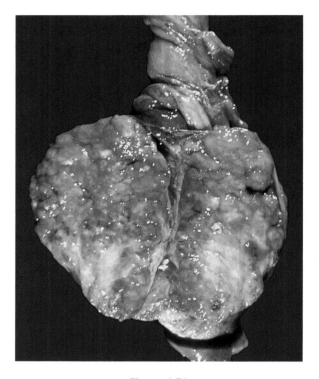

Figure 6-71

LEYDIG CELL TUMOR

The tumor is brown and nodular, and has a few small foci of yellow necrosis. The testis is completely replaced by this tumor, which was clinically malignant. (Fig. 5.3 from Young RH, Scully RE. Testicular tumors. Chicago: ASCP Press; 1990:112.)

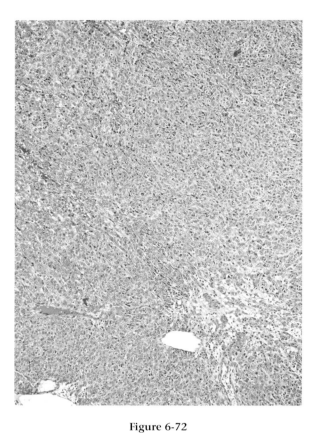

Figure 6-72

LEYDIG CELL TUMOR

There is a diffuse growth of eosinophilic cells with scant stroma.

Figure 6-73

LEYDIG CELL TUMOR

A prominent, hyalinized stroma separates the tumor into distinct nodules.

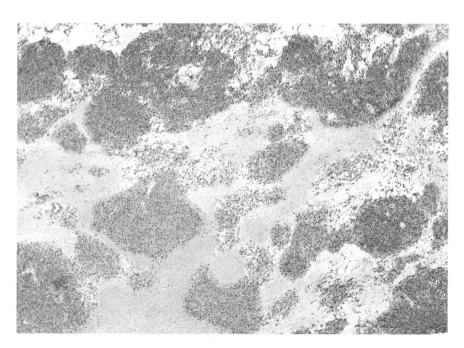

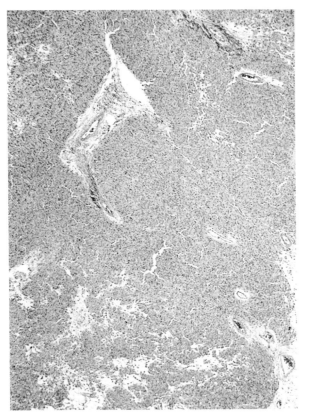

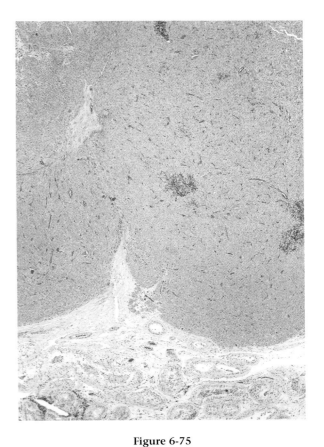

Figure 6-74

LEYDIG CELL TUMOR

Cells with abundant eosinophilic cytoplasm grow in lobular aggregates.

Figure 6-75

LEYDIG CELL TUMOR

A large, solid tumor has a circumscribed interface with the surrounding testis.

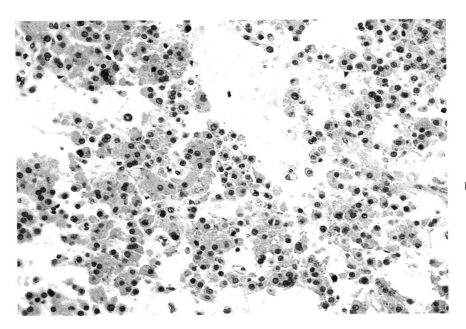

Figure 6-76

LEYDIG CELL TUMOR

Clusters of cells are separated by an edematous stroma.

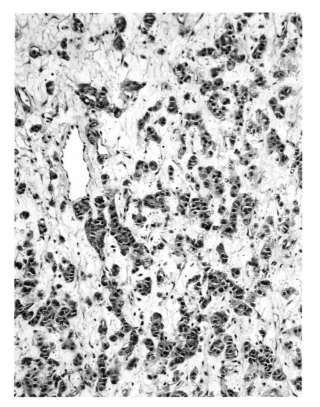

Figure 6-77

LEYDIG CELL TUMOR

This tumor grows in cellular cords.

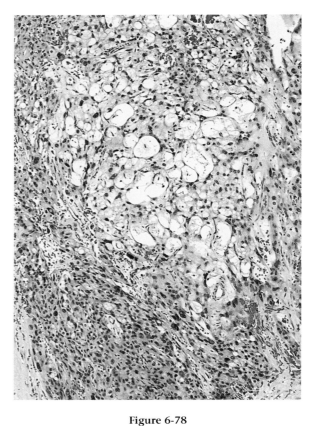

Figure 6-78

LEYDIG CELL TUMOR

Prominent cytoplasmic vacuoles create a microcystic pattern, mimicking yolk sac tumor. The focus at the bottom left has the usual appearance.

Figure 6-79

LEYDIG CELL TUMOR

Large and small cysts are formed.

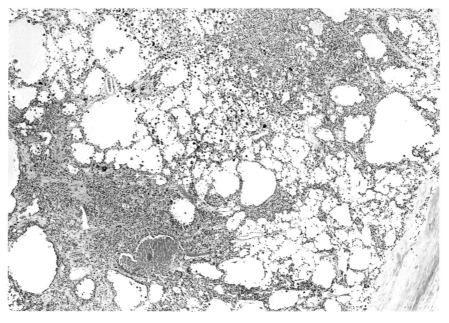

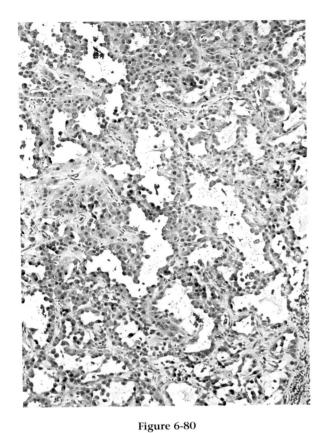

Figure 6-80

LEYDIG CELL TUMOR

Faintly staining edema fluid is present within pseudo-tubular structures.

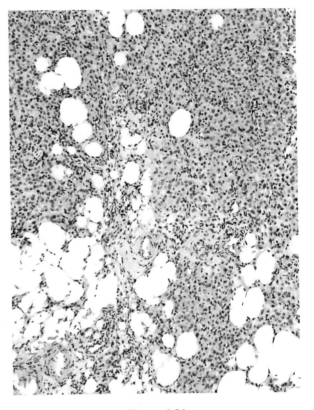

Figure 6-81

LEYDIG CELL TUMOR

There is prominent fatty metaplasia, a rare feature.

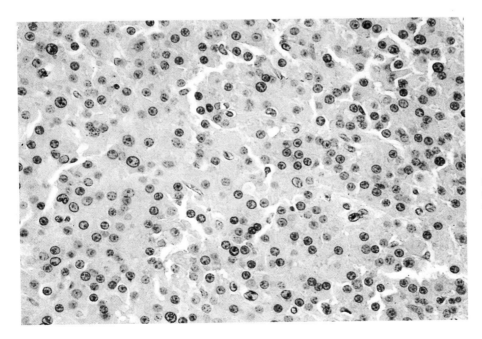

Figure 6-82

LEYDIG CELL TUMOR

The tumor cells have abundant eosinophilic cytoplasm and regular round nuclei, some with visible nucleoli.

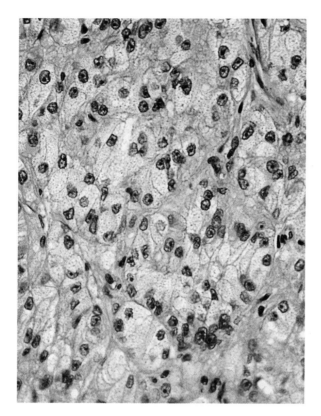

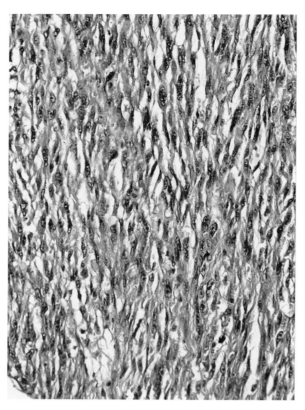

Figure 6-83

LEYDIG CELL TUMOR

The abundant pale cytoplasm in the tumor cells is due to lipid accumulation.

Figure 6-84

LEYDIG CELL TUMOR

The tumor cells are spindle shaped.

appears pale to clear. Rarely, the cells are small with scanty cytoplasm and nuclei containing grooves, and exceptionally, the tumor cells are spindle shaped (fig. 6-84) (105). The combination of spindle cells and a fascicular growth pattern may cause concern for a neoplasm of soft tissue type (fig. 6-85); however, both the spindle cell and small cell variants are usually associated with the characteristic polygonal cell type. Crystals of Reinke are identified in the cytoplasm in approximately one third of the cases (figs. 6-86–6-88) (106). In occasional tumors, some of the Reinke crystals are intranuclear (fig. 6-89). Some Leydig cell tumors show globular cytoplasmic inclusions rather than polygonal ones (fig. 6-90); these are likely precrystalline material. Cytoplasmic lipochrome pigment is present in 10 to 15 percent of the tumors (fig. 6-91), but not usually in the pediatric cases. The nuclei are typically round and contain a single

prominent nucleolus (figs. 6-82, 6-85). A distinctive "ground glass" nuclear change occurs in some (fig. 6-92). Nuclear atypicality is usually absent or slight, but is marked in approximately 30 percent of the cases (fig. 6-93).

The mitotic rate varies greatly: it is usually low, in accord with the bland cytology of most tumors, but is typically appreciable in cases with striking nuclear atypia (fig. 6-94). We have seen one highly atypical and mitotically active tumor with a spindle cell morphology that was indistinguishable from a pleomorphic sarcoma (fig. 6-95) except for an adjacent component with a conventional appearance; rare similar cases have been reported (60,105,107).

Immunohistochemical Findings. The single most useful marker for Leydig cell tumor is alpha-inhibin, which is positive in about 95 percent of cases (fig. 6-96) (25–27,60). Calretinin and vimentin are reactive in 90 percent of the tumors

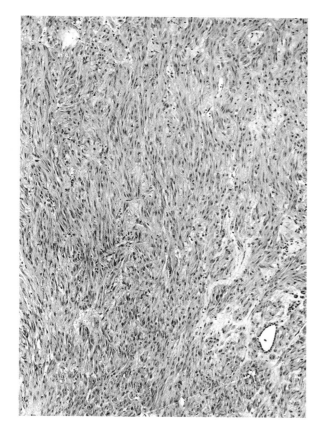

Figure 6-85

LEYDIG CELL TUMOR

T he predominant spindle cell morphology in this tumor causes it to resemble a neoplasm of soft tissue type.

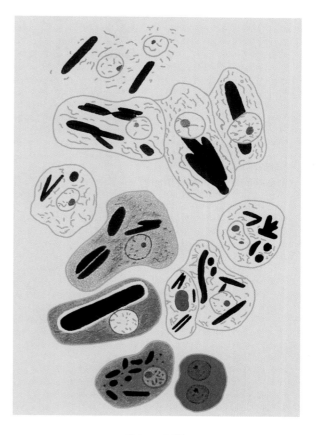

Figure 6-86

REINKE CRYSTALS

Reinke's drawing of the intracytoplasmic crystalloids in Leydig cells (1896) at high magnification. Absolute alcohol fixation and Weigert fibrin stain were used. The crystalloids stain bright royal blue and the cytoplasm light claret lake. (Legend and photograph courtesy of the late Dr. W. Ober.)

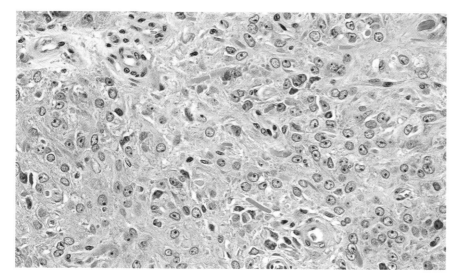

Figure 6-87

LEYDIG CELL TUMOR

Numerous Reinke crystals appear as rod-shaped, eosinophilic cytoplasmic inclusions.

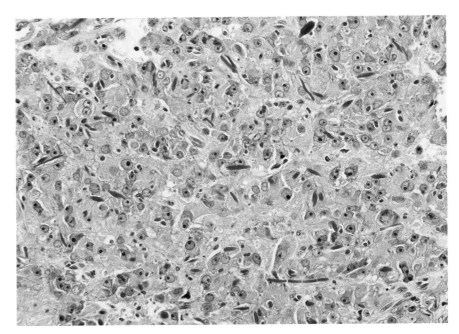

Figure 6-88

LEYDIG CELL TUMOR

The Reinke crystals are bright red with the trichrome stain.

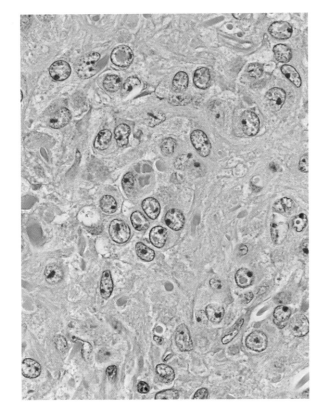

Figure 6-89

LEYDIG CELL TUMOR

Some cells have intranuclear Reinke crystals.

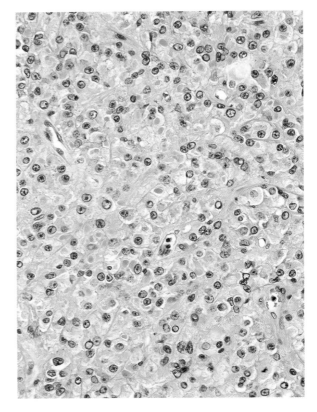

Figure 6-90

LEYDIG CELL TUMOR

Globular, eosinophilic cytoplasmic inclusions are apparent.

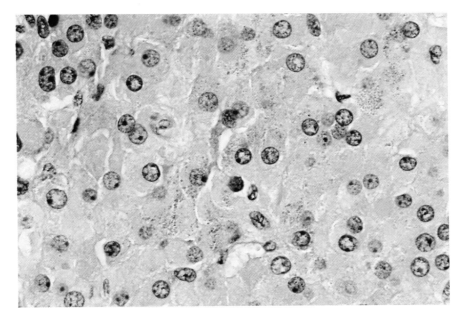

Figure 6-91

LEYDIG CELL TUMOR

Granules of lipochrome pigment are present in the cytoplasm of the tumor cells.

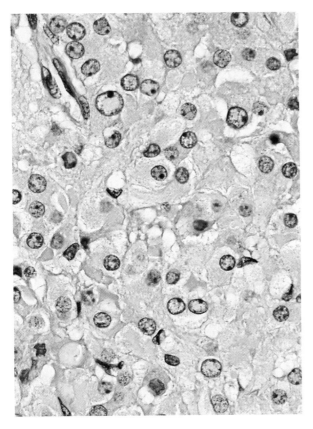

Figure 6-92

LEYDIG CELL TUMOR

"Ground glass" change is seen in several nuclei.

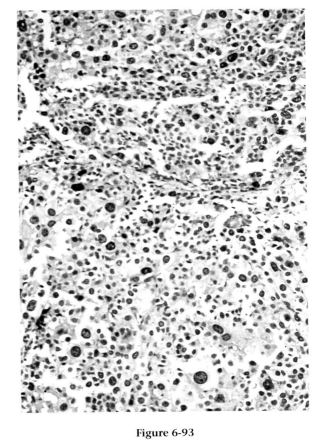

Figure 6-93

LEYDIG CELL TUMOR

There is marked nuclear pleomorphism in a tumor that was clinically malignant.

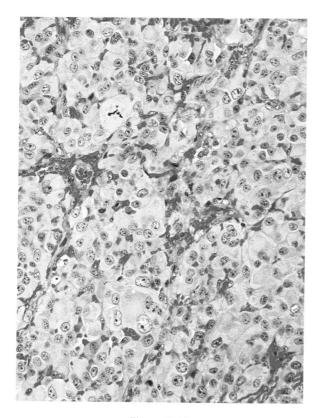

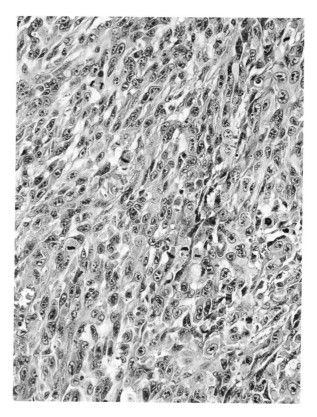

Figure 6-94

LEYDIG CELL TUMOR

Moderate nuclear pleomorphism is accompanied by an atypical mitotic figure.

Figure 6-95

LEYDIG CELL TUMOR

Highly atypical fusiform tumor cells and numerous mitotic figures make this area indistinguishable from a pleomorphic sarcoma.

Figure 6-96

LEYDIG CELL TUMOR

There is strong positivity for alpha-inhibin in a Leydig cell tumor. Non-neoplastic Sertoli cells and Leydig cells (right) also are reactive (anti-inhibin immunoperoxidase stain).

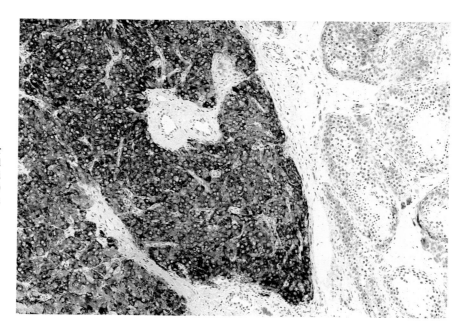

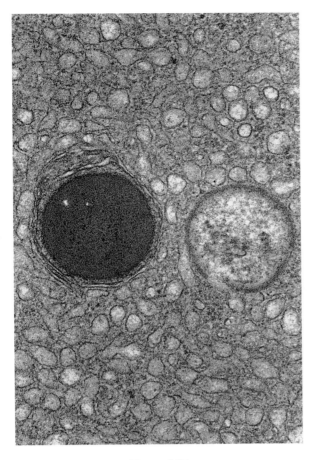

Figure 6-97

LEYDIG CELL TUMOR

There are numerous vesicles of smooth endoplasmic reticulum, occasionally surrounding lipid droplets. (Courtesy of Dr. R. Erlandson, New York, NY.)

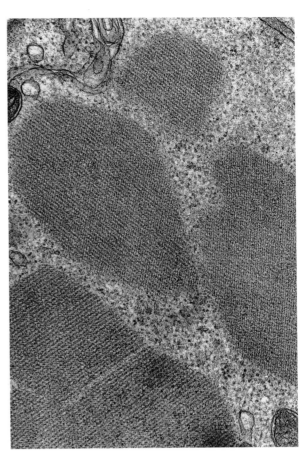

Figure 6-98

LEYDIG CELL TUMOR

Geometrically shaped Reinke crystals have a striking periodicity. (Courtesy of Dr. R. Erlandson, New York, NY.)

(26,108–110) and melan-A (MART-1) in 85 percent (60,111,112). CD99 stains about two thirds of cases (25) and S-100 protein approximately 10 percent (27). OCT3/4 is negative (113,114).

Ultrastructural Findings. Ultrastructurally, there are features of steroid-secreting cells, including prominent vesicles of smooth endoplasmic reticulum that are sometimes arranged in concentric whorls around lipid droplets (fig. 6-97) (115), mitochondria with either tubular or lamellar cristae, and lipid droplets (33). In some cases, Reinke crystals, showing the distinctive periodicity, are identified (fig. 6-98).

Cytologic Findings. Fine needle aspiration of Leydig cell tumors produces both two-dimensional cohesive clusters of cells as well as isolated cells (116,117). The cytoplasm is abundant and gray-blue in Papanicolaou-stained preparations. The nuclei are round and sometimes grooved, and have distinct nucleoli (117,118). Reinke crystals are best appreciated in air-dried specimens stained with a Romanovsky-type stain where they may appear as either intracytoplasmic or intranuclear inclusions (119), although only seen in a minority of cases.

Special Techniques. Molecular biological analysis of Leydig cell tumors has shown some with acquired (rather than germline) mutations in the gene for the luteinizing hormone receptor, thereby permitting gonadotropin-independent hypersecretion of testosterone from the neoplastic cells (120–123). These occur as missense mutations in codon 578, which results in the substitution of histidine for aspartic acid in the translated protein. These acquired mutations occur in tumors of children rather than adults, and likely occur only in a fraction of such cases (124), although there is one report in an adult tumor (90).

As mentioned, germline mutations in the fumarate hydratase gene are characteristic of hereditary leiomyomatosis and renal cell carcinoma syndrome, and rarely associated with Leydig cell tumor (90). In a study of 29 sporadic Leydig cell tumors in adult patients, one was found to have a different fumarate hydratase gene mutation than that seen as the germline abnormality (90).

Comparative genomic hybridization of Leydig cell tumors has demonstrated chromosomal imbalance in 84 percent of cases. The most common findings were gain of chromosomes X, 19, or 19p and losses involving chromosomes 8 and 16 (125).

Differential Diagnosis. A Leydig cell tumor may be confused with three non-neoplastic lesions. The first is Leydig cell hyperplasia, which may be florid, particularly in cryptorchid testes. However, the usual lack of a discrete mass on gross inspection and the presence of atrophic tubules in the midst of the Leydig cells suggest the correct diagnosis. When grossly apparent, Leydig cell hyperplasia is usually multifocal, and the nodules are small.

Malakoplakia is more likely to be a problem because it may result in the formation of a single, homogeneous, yellow or brown mass that is grossly indistinguishable from a Leydig cell tumor, although in many cases the presence of an abscess is a clue to the diagnosis of malakoplakia. On low-power microscopic examination, the eosinophilic histiocytes (von Hansemann cells) of malakoplakia may be misconstrued as Leydig cells, but they typically involve tubules as well as the interstitium and are admixed with other inflammatory cells. The presence of Michaelis-Gutmann bodies is diagnostic of malakoplakia.

The testicular "tumors" that develop in patients with the adrenogenital syndrome closely resemble Leydig cell tumors but differ from them in their usual bilaterality, multifocality, and dark brown color, although occasional Leydig cell tumors are brown. More reliable is the finding of seminiferous tubules within the non-neoplastic lesion; they are found only rarely within a Leydig cell tumor. Another characteristic finding in adrenogenital lesions is a prominent fibrous tissue component represented by thick collagen bands that dissect throughout the nodule. While these are not specific, this pattern should raise concern for an adrenogenital-associated lesion. The cells of the adrenogenital tumor tend to be larger, with more abundant cytoplasm, than seen in Leydig cell tumors and contain lipochrome pigment (responsible for the dark color) more frequently and in greater amounts. Reinke crystals have not been identified within the cells of the tumors of the adrenogenital syndrome. Significant variation in nuclear size occurs in one third of the adrenogenital-associated lesions, with scattered large nuclei in half of these; mitotic figures are rare (126). In contrast, the nuclei in Leydig cell tumors are usually more uniform and mitotic activity is apparent in the majority. Reactivity for synaptophysin and CD56 and negativity for the androgen receptor favor the adrenogenital tumor over Leydig cell tumor (127,128). Similar criteria are helpful for differentiating Leydig cell tumor from the hyperplastic nodules of steroid cells that may be seen in patients with Nelson syndrome.

Leydig cell tumors are generally easily distinguished from Sertoli cell tumors and other tumors in the sex cord-stromal category because the resemblance of the neoplastic cells to Leydig cells is usually sufficiently striking to suggest the correct diagnosis. The differential diagnosis with Sertoli cell tumors, including the large cell calcifying subtype, is discussed with Sertoli cell tumors. The rare Leydig cell tumor that contains cells with nuclear grooves and focally resembles a granulosa cell tumor has other areas characteristic of Leydig cell tumor that are easily found.

Leydig cell tumors rarely may be confused with malignant lymphomas when their cells have scant cytoplasm and atypical nuclei. Lymphomas have a much higher frequency of bilaterality, common involvement of the epididymis and spermatic cord, characteristic intertubular infiltration of the tumor cells, invasion of the tubules in one third of the cases, and the distinctive cytologic features of the neoplastic cells. Appropriate immunostains resolve this differential, but they are rarely necessary.

The differential diagnosis with plasmacytoma is considered with that tumor.

Occasional Leydig cell tumors have foci with small cytoplasmic vacuoles and rare cases have prominent large vacuoles, which may be confused with the microcystic pattern of yolk sac tumor (see fig. 6-78) (129). The presence of areas of typical Leydig cell tumor, the generally low mitotic rate, the occurrence of cells with foamy cytoplasm, and the absence of other patterns reminiscent of yolk sac tumor and of associated IGCNU are helpful distinguishing features in these cases. Additional support can be obtained with immunostains: inhibin is positive in Leydig cell tumor (fig. 6-96), alpha-fetoprotein, SALL4, and glypican 3 are negative, and cytokeratins (AE1/AE3) are weak or negative (27,130,130a); opposite patterns of reactivity are expected in yolk sac tumor.

The uncommon Leydig cell tumors with a prominent spindle cell component, including the "sarcomatoid" variants (60,105), have conventional foci that are crucial in establishing their nature. If a tumor is not well sampled, a mistaken diagnosis of sarcoma may result. Such cases may also be misinterpreted as mixed sex cord-stromal tumor if the spindled cells are not recognized as Leydig cell variants, although this is not an important clinical distinction. Although positivity for alpha-inhibin supports the Leydig cell nature of such neoplasms, this reactivity may be lost in the spindle cell areas (60).

Metastatic carcinoma, particularly from the prostate, may be mistaken for a Leydig cell tumor when the former has a diffuse pattern and cells with appreciable eosinophilic cytoplasm. In such cases, the clinical history is usually helpful, and, in the rare cases with an occult primary, other areas characteristic of prostatic adenocarcinoma are usually present. Immunostains for prostate-specific acid phosphatase and prostate-specific antigen are diagnostic. Alpha-inhibin positivity in Leydig cell tumor (26,27,29,131,132) and its usual negativity in metastatic adenocarcinoma should clarify the diagnosis. The history, presence of melanin pigment, and immunopositivity with HMB45 aid in the rare differential with metastatic malignant melanoma. S-100 protein and melan-A are sometimes demonstrated in Leydig cell tumors and therefore immunopositivity for these markers is not helpful in this situation (27,130,133), and similar comments pertain to alpha-inhibin, which occasionally is reactive in melanoma (134).

Treatment and Prognosis. In the largest series of Leydig cell tumors, 5 of 30 patients with follow-up (17 percent) developed metastases (86). There is one report of bilateral malignant Leydig cell tumor (135). A number of features viewed in aggregate are helpful in assessing the likelihood of a malignant course. The average age of patients with malignant tumors is 62 to 63 years, in contrast to the late thirties for those with benign Leydig cell tumors (86,130,136). Only an occasional patient with a malignant tumor has presented with endocrine manifestations (102,137), despite frequently elevated levels of various hormones or their metabolites. A malignant course in a prepubertal patient with a Leydig cell tumor is exceptional (22). Tumors that metastasize are typically larger than those with a benign course. In three series, benign tumors averaged 1.8 to 2.7 cm compared to 4.7 to 6.9 cm for malignant ones (86,130,136). The latter characteristically have infiltrative margins, invade lymphatics or blood vessels, and contain foci of necrosis. They also usually have a high mitotic rate (over 3 mitotic figures per 10 high-power fields) and exhibit significant nuclear atypicality much more often than benign tumors (86,136). All five clinically malignant tumors in a series of 40 had four or more of the above features, while 12 of the 14 tumors that were benign on the basis of follow-up of 2 or more years had none of them (86).

It has been suggested that ancillary methods may assist with the prediction of clinical behavior of Leydig cell tumor. Aneuploidy was consistently observed in metastasizing Leydig cell tumors (and occasionally in benign tumors) in two studies (136,138), but not in a third (130). Significantly higher MIB-1 staining indices were seen in the malignant cases, but with some overlap of values with benign cases (130,136). Staining for p53 protein highlighted 50 percent of the nuclei of two malignant cases and 2 percent or less of benign cases, but p53 was positive in only 1 percent of cells of two additional malignant tumors (130).

Malignant Leydig cell tumors spread most commonly to regional lymph nodes (72 percent), lung (43 percent), liver (38 percent), and bone (28 percent) (54). About 20 percent of the patients with clinically malignant tumors have metastases at the time of diagnosis (139). The treatment of a Leydig cell tumor is inguinal orchiectomy. If the gross or histologic features indicate a likelihood of malignancy, a retroperitoneal lymphadenectomy should be considered. The treatment of metastatic Leydig cell tumor has been generally unsatisfactory (139–141). Most patients with a clinically malignant Leydig cell tumor die within 5 years, but occasionally there is a prolonged course.

GRANULOSA-STROMAL CELL TUMORS

Granulosa cell tumors, like their ovarian counterparts, are now subdivided into two categories, adult and juvenile. The adult type is rare if strict criteria for its recognition are applied (see below). The juvenile type, in our experience, is more common, although as alluded to earlier, it is also apparent that some pathologists regard cases we would consider as juvenile granulosa cell tumors as either Sertoli cell tumors or unclassified sex cord-stromal tumors.

Adult-Type Granulosa Cell Tumor

General and Clinical Features. There are about 25 cases of *adult granulosa cell tumor* reported (5,142–148). Several of the reported examples, in our opinion, are better classified as either Sertoli cell tumor or a neoplasm in the mixed or unclassified category of sex cord-stromal tumor. The tumors typically occur in adults ranging from 16 to 83 years of age (mean, 42 years) (143,147). Twenty percent of the reported cases are associated with gynecomastia (fig. 6-99). Some patients have a history of testicular enlargement of several years' duration.

Gross Findings. The tumors are usually 3 to 5 cm but tumors up to 18 cm in diameter have been recorded. They typically are homogeneous, yellow to yellow-gray or white, firm, and lobulated (fig. 6-100). Cysts are sometimes present.

Microscopic Findings. The patterns are usually either microfollicular, with Call-Exner bodies (figs. 6-101, 6-102), or diffuse (fig. 6-103), but other patterns, as seen in the ovary, may be observed. The cytoplasm is typically scanty, and the nuclei are pale with variably prominent grooves (fig. 6-104). If the architectural features are typical of adult granulosa cell tumor, a paucity of nuclear

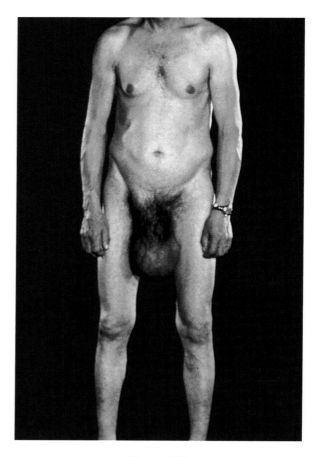

Figure 6-99

GRANULOSA CELL TUMOR, ADULT TYPE

Prominent scrotal enlargement and gynecomastia are seen. The tumor is shown in figure 6-100.

grooves is still consistent with the diagnosis. The mitotic rate is generally low, but a high rate is seen in occasional tumors (69). The tumors may have the prominent fibrous stroma that characterizes the better-known ovarian counterpart. It is only rarely thecomatous. Exceptionally, the stromal cells have abundant pale to eosinophilic cytoplasm but lack crystals of Reinke (fig. 6-105). The occasional cases in which immunohistochemistry was done report positive reactions for vimentin, alpha-inhibin, actin, estrogen and progesterone receptors, and, variably, cytokeratins but negativity for EMA (143,147,149).

Differential Diagnosis. Unclassified tumors in the sex cord-stromal category often have a focal appearance compatible with a granulosa cell tumor, but a specific diagnosis of granulosa cell

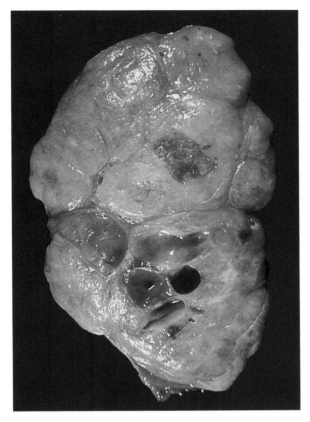

Figure 6-100

GRANULOSA CELL TUMOR, ADULT TYPE

The tumor is lobulated, brownish yellow, and mostly solid with focal hemorrhage. (Fig. 5.33 from Young RH, Scully RE. Testicular tumors. Chicago: ASCP Press; 1990:127.)

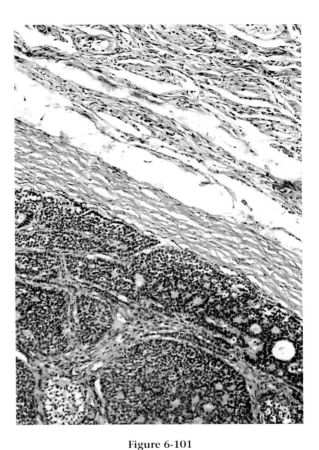

Figure 6-101

GRANULOSA CELL TUMOR, ADULT TYPE

The tumor is well circumscribed and contains numerous Call-Exner bodies. (Courtesy of Dr. A. Talerman, Philadelphia, PA.)

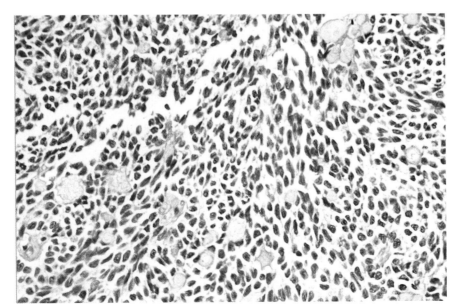

Figure 6-102

GRANULOSA CELL TUMOR, ADULT TYPE

Many of the nuclei have nuclear grooves. Call-Exner bodies are seen.

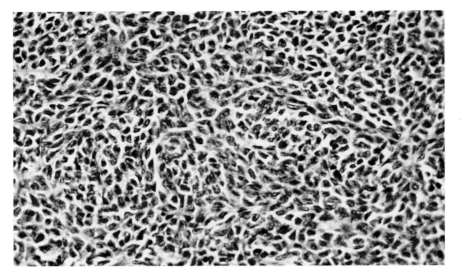

Figure 6-103

GRANULOSA CELL TUMOR, ADULT TYPE

The tumor has a diffuse pattern.

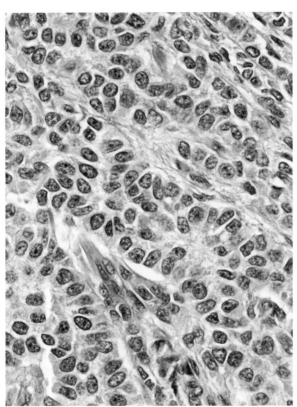

Figure 6-104

GRANULOSA CELL TUMOR, ADULT TYPE

The nuclei are oval to angulated and pale, and occasionally show grooves.

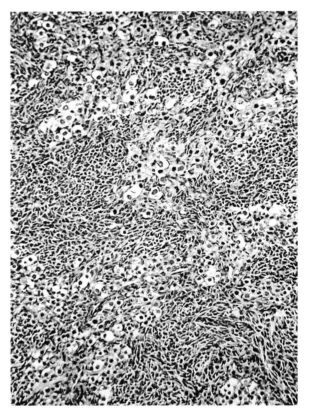

Figure 6-105

GRANULOSA CELL TUMOR, ADULT TYPE

Many tumor cells have abundant cytoplasm that ranges from eosinophilic to pale. The juxtaposition of these lutein-type cells with typical granulosa cells with scant cytoplasm may cause the erroneous diagnosis of a mixed germ cell-sex cord-stromal tumor, with the lutein-type cells misinterpreted as germ cells because of their abundant pale cytoplasm.

tumor should only be made when all, or almost all, the neoplasm has granulosa cell features. Tubular differentiation indicates Sertoli cell features and is, therefore, a Sertoli cell tumor or mixed or unclassified sex cord-stromal tumor. Rare Leydig cell tumors have cells with nuclear grooves, but other features of Leydig cell tumor are present. Abundant pale cytoplasm in the cells of the stromal component of an adult granulosa cell tumor may simulate the germ cell component of the rare mixed germ cell-sex cord-stromal tumor; however, the nuclei in the latter are typically smaller and may be irregular, unlike the larger, round nuclei of germ cells. Since we have seen such cells lead to the erroneous diagnosis of a mixed germ cell-sex cord-stromal tumor, it is ideal that the putative neoplastic germ cell nature of such cells be confirmed by appropriate immunoreactivity for markers such as PLAP and OCT3/4. As detailed in chapter 5, we believe many of these supposed "mixed" tumors actually represent a sex cord-stromal tumor with entrapped, non-neoplastic germ cells.

Treatment and Prognosis. Four patients with granulosa cell tumor had metastases. In two, retroperitoneal lymph node spread was present at presentation (143,144). One patient was alive after 14 months and the other after 14 years. One received radiation therapy and the other chemotherapy. The other two patients with malignant tumors died of disease, at 5 months (5) and just over 11 years (143). Size greater than 7 cm, vascular or lymphatic invasion, and hemorrhage or necrosis are features of malignant tumors (143). Treatment is similar to that for Sertoli cell tumors, NOS.

Juvenile-Type Granulosa Cell Tumor

General and Clinical Features. *Juvenile-type granulosa cell tumor* is the most common neoplasm of the testis in the first 6 months of life and is uncommon in children beyond that age (14,150–159). Two possible examples in a 4-year-old boy and a 27-year-old man, in our opinion, are better regarded as unclassified sex cord-stromal tumors (160,161). Occasional juvenile granulosa cell tumors occur in the undescended testes of infants with disorders of sex development (intersex disorders) (156,159,162), and one developed in a patient with the Drash syndrome (163). Such cases may be associated with karyotypic

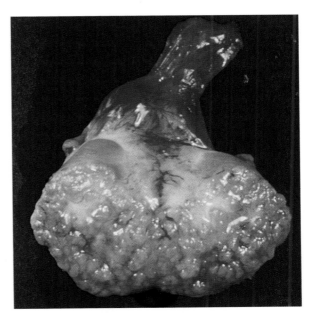

Figure 6-106

GRANULOSA CELL TUMOR, JUVENILE TYPE

The tumor is solid, lobulated, and orange-tan. (Courtesy of Dr. J. Henley, Columbus, IN.)

anomalies, including 45X/46XY mosaicism or, in a fetal case, XXY triploidy (162,164).

A testicular mass is almost always the presenting feature, although torsion is the presenting feature on rare occasion (153,154). There are no associated hormonal features, and all of the reported cases have had a benign outcome.

Gross Findings. The tumors measure up to 6 cm in diameter. They may be solid (fig. 6-106), cystic (fig. 6-107), or both (fig. 6-108). The solid tissue may be nodular and yellow-orange (fig. 6-106) or tan-white (fig. 6-108). The cysts are usually thin-walled and contain viscid or gelatinous fluid (fig. 6-107) or clotted blood.

Microscopic Findings. Microscopic examination reveals variably prominent follicular (fig. 6-109), solid (fig. 6-110), or mixed follicular and solid (fig. 6-111) patterns, typically with a lobular arrangement, with the tumor lobules sometimes separated by a spindle cell stroma (figs. 6-109–6-112). The follicles vary from large and round (fig. 6-109), to oval, to small (fig. 6-113) and irregular (fig. 6-112). They typically are lined by several layers of polygonal cells and contain basophilic (figs. 6-109, 6-112, 6-113) or

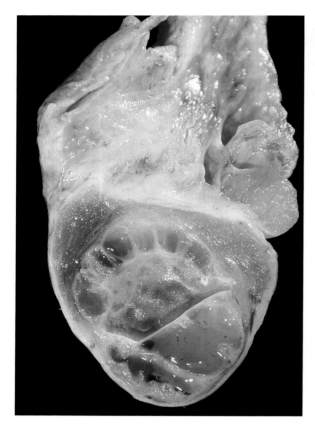

Figure 6-107

GRANULOSA CELL TUMOR, JUVENILE TYPE

The sectioned surface of this predominantly cystic tumor shows several smaller cysts and one larger one that contains gelatinous fluid.

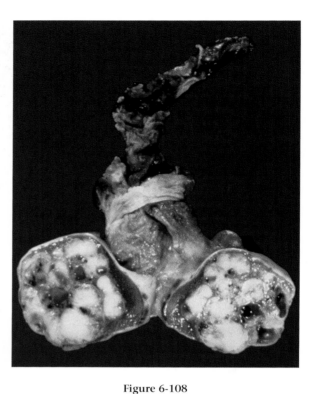

Figure 6-108

GRANULOSA CELL TUMOR, JUVENILE TYPE

The sectioned surface of the tumor is composed of multiple nodules of solid white tissue with several interspersed cysts. (Fig. 5.36 from Young RH, Scully RE. Testicular tumors. Chicago: ASCP Press; 1990:128.)

Figure 6-109

GRANULOSA CELL TUMOR, JUVENILE TYPE

Large follicles contain basophilic intraluminal material.

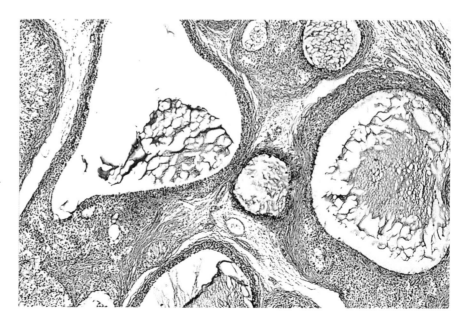

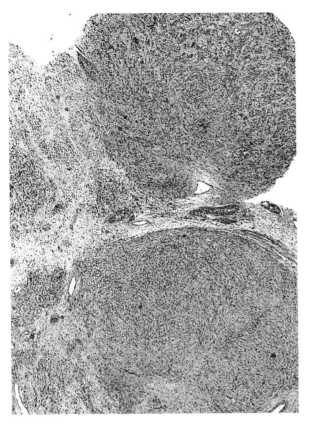

Figure 6-110

GRANULOSA CELL TUMOR, JUVENILE TYPE

Tumor cells grow in large nodular aggregates.

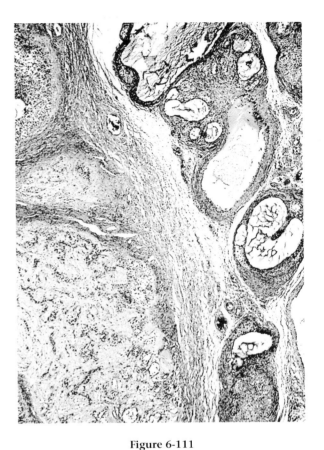

Figure 6-111

GRANULOSA CELL TUMOR, JUVENILE TYPE

Mixed follicular and solid patterns are seen. A predominantly solid area (bottom left) is basophilic and has a vaguely chondroid appearance.

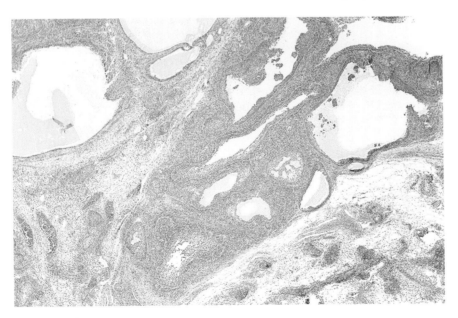

Figure 6-112

GRANULOSA CELL TUMOR, JUVENILE TYPE

Tumor lobules containing round to irregular follicles with lightly basophilic fluid are separated by a spindle cell stroma.

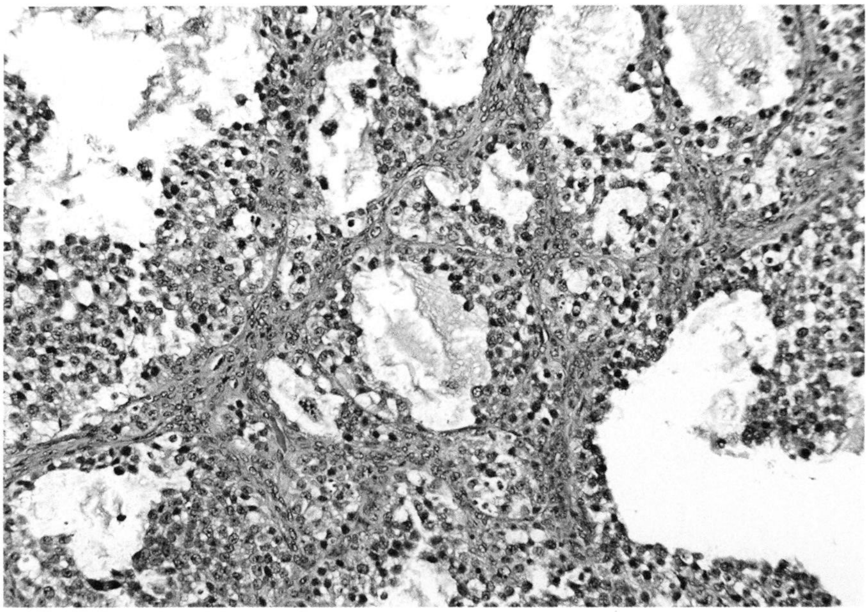

Figure 6-113

GRANULOSA CELL TUMOR, JUVENILE TYPE

Small follicles contain basophilic fluid.

eosinophilic fluid that is stained by mucicarmine (fig. 6-114). In nonfollicular areas the cells grow in sheets, nodules (fig. 6-110), trabeculae (fig. 6-115), and irregular clusters. A retained lobular pattern is often appreciable in these areas, even in the absence of distinct follicles, and more typical features are seen elsewhere. Hyalinization is sometimes extensive, and in some cases intercellular basophilic mucinous fluid is conspicuous and may result in a vaguely "chondroid" appearance (fig. 6-111). Where the tumor cells are dispersed loosely in a myxoid stroma, some foci simulate the reticular pattern of yolk sac tumor (fig. 6-116). Uncommonly, there is appreciable intratubular growth at the periphery (fig. 6-117). Marked cystic degeneration, as described in a congenital intra-abdominal tumor (151), may be seen (fig. 6-118). The tumor cells have moderate to large amounts of pale to occasionally eosinophilic cytoplasm and hyperchromatic, round to oval nuclei, some of which contain nucleoli (fig. 6-119). Mitotic activity and cellular apoptosis are usually evident and often prominent (fig. 6-119).

Immunohistochemical Findings. Immunostains for alpha-inhibin are positive in the polyhedral cells in most cases (25,165). The spindle cells that separate tumor lobules are positive for muscle-specific actin, vimentin, and, focally, desmin (166,167). Low molecular weight cytokeratins may also be focally positive (167). Alpha-fetoprotein is negative.

Ultrastructural Findings. Three cell types have been identified on ultrastructural examination: polyhedral granulosa cells, spindled cells with smooth muscle differentiation, and theca-like cells (155,167). Continuous basal lamina invests clusters of the granulosa cells, which contain cytoplasmic bundles of filaments with dense bodies, cisternae of rough endoplasmic reticulum, a Golgi complex, and fat droplets (167). The mitochondria contain lamellar cristae; Charcot-Böttcher filaments have not been identified (155,167).

Cytologic Findings. There is a single case report of the cytologic findings of a fine needle aspiration (165). Single and cohesive groups of spindle cells with uniform fine chromatin, regular nuclei, and inconspicuous nucleoli were identified. This case was positive for alpha-inhibin, S-100 protein, and vimentin.

Differential Diagnosis. Juvenile granulosa cell tumor may be misinterpreted as a yolk sac tumor, one of the other frequent tumors of infants, particularly when it exhibits a "reticular" pattern and brisk mitotic activity. The patient age is often helpful in this situation since juvenile granulosa cell tumors rarely present after 6 months of age and yolk sac tumors are mostly seen in children beyond this age. Juvenile

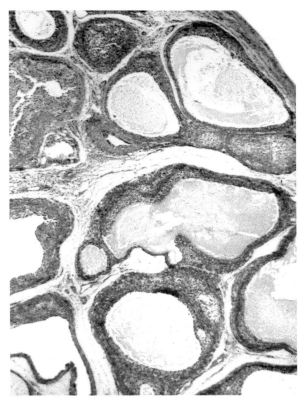

Figure 6-114

GRANULOSA CELL TUMOR, JUVENILE TYPE

The material within follicles of the type seen in figure 6-109 is positive with the mucicarmine stain.

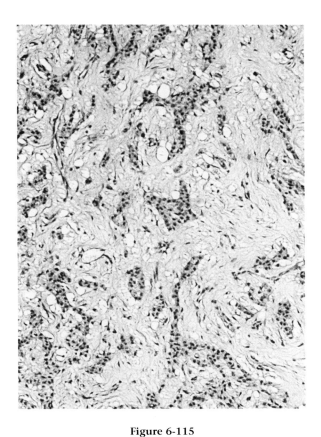

Figure 6-115

GRANULOSA CELL TUMOR, JUVENILE TYPE

Trabeculae, nests, and single tumor cells are irregularly distributed in a stroma that varied from hyaline to slightly basophilic.

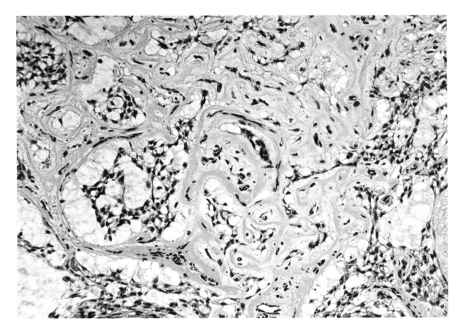

Figure 6-116

GRANULOSA CELL TUMOR, JUVENILE TYPE

A lace-like arrangement of tumor cells in a mucoid stroma resembles the reticular pattern of yolk sac tumor to a limited degree.

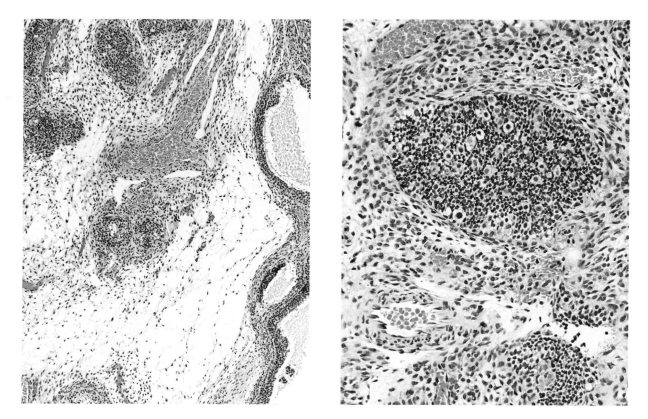

Figure 6-117

GRANULOSA CELL TUMOR, JUVENILE TYPE

Left: Nests of intratubular neoplasm are seen at the periphery of a tumor with the usual appearance (right).
Right: The intratubular cells are admixed with non-neoplastic germ cells and have less cytoplasm than is typical.

Figure 6-118

GRANULOSA CELL TUMOR, JUVENILE TYPE

There is marked cystic change.

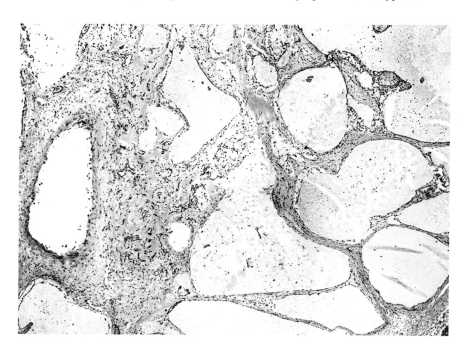

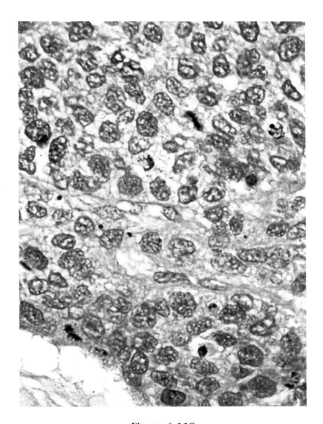

Figure 6-119

GRANULOSA CELL TUMOR, JUVENILE TYPE

The nuclei are immature and exhibit brisk mitotic activity.

granulosa cell tumors are commonly congenital and, to the best of our knowledge, no testicular yolk sac tumor has been congenital. The presence of follicles in most juvenile granulosa cell tumors, the absence of the various characteristic patterns of yolk sac tumor, positivity for alpha-inhibin, and absence of immunoreactivity for alpha-fetoprotein, glypican 3, and diffuse cytokeratin, should help in diagnosis.

Juvenile granulosa cell tumors are distinguished from the adult form by the greater degree of irregularity in size and shape of the follicles, which usually show intraluminal basophilic fluid that is typically absent in the adult tumors. Also, the juvenile cases have more abundant cytoplasm, a more immature nuclear appearance, and a greater degree of mitotic activity. The age of the patient is again helpful because of the great tendency for the juvenile variant to be found in infants.

The differential with Sertoli cell tumors is discussed with that tumor. There is some morphologic overlap of juvenile granulosa cell tumors and unclassified sex cord-stromal tumors. Our guidelines for the distinction of these two entities include follicle formation or a lobular growth pattern in the former and absence of both of these features in the latter.

The primitive nuclei, mitotic activity, and eosinophilic cytoplasm of the juvenile granulosa cell tumor may suggest embryonal rhabdomyosarcoma with scattered rhabdomyoblastic cells. Embryonal rhabdomyosarcoma, however, is almost always a paratesticular tumor and usually found in older children (mean age, 7 years). Rare testicular cases do occur, probably representing sarcomatous overgrowth in teratomas, but have not, to our knowledge, been reported in infants. Although cystic degeneration may occur, the characteristic fluid-filled follicles of juvenile granulosa cell tumor are not a feature. Immunostains for markers of skeletal muscle resolve this differential.

Treatment and Prognosis. Most patients receive standard orchiectomy, although local tumor excision with sparing of the testis has also been advocated (168). All tumors to date have exhibited benign behavior.

TUMORS IN THE FIBROMA-THECOMA GROUP

General and Clinical Features. Tumors in the *fibroma-thecoma* category are uncommon, and, in most cases, resemble either a typical ovarian fibroma or the cellular variant (169). We have not personally seen a convincing example of testicular thecoma, and the one tumor reported in the literature as "thecoma" (170) is best placed in the fibroma category according to our criteria. Collins and Symington (4), who reported four tumors of the testicular parenchyma in this group and noted a resemblance to ovarian fibroma, suggested, however, that "the analogy not be too far pressed." There are occasional tumors that are reported as "testicular fibromas with minor sex cord elements" (171) but we feel these are better placed in the unclassified sex cord-stromal group. It is possible that some fibromas are not of gonadal stromal origin but arise from nonspecific soft tissue fibroblasts, but it is convenient to consider them together here.

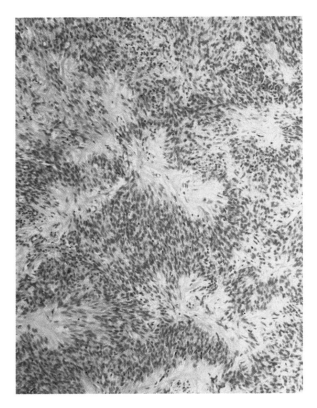

Figure 6-120

CELLULAR FIBROMA

The testicular tumor is similar to the ovarian tumor of the same name.

The 20 patients whose tumors appear to definitely or probably fit in this category ranged from 5 to 67 (mean, 34) years of age (4,133,170,172–179). They typically presented with a testicular mass (4,170,172–177). Although follow-up is limited, it has been unremarkable.

Gross Findings. The tumors range from 0.9 to 7.0 cm (mean, 3.0 cm) in maximum dimension and are typically well circumscribed, firm, and tan-white to, more commonly, yellow. Hemorrhage and necrosis are absent.

Microscopic Findings. These tumors are, by definition, indistinguishable from a typical or cellular fibroma of the ovary. They are characterized by spindle-shaped fibroblasts associated with variable amounts of collagen that often grow in a storiform pattern, sometimes associated with mild edema and modest vascularity (fig. 6-120). The cellular tumors are often strikingly so, and occasional cellular tumors have up to 2 mitotic figures per 10 high-power fields. Conspicuous zones of hyalinized collagen may show calcification.

Immunohistochemical studies yield variable results. The most consistently positive immunostains are vimentin and actin; reactivity for focal desmin, keratin, and S-100 protein is also reported. Ultrastructural studies show fibroblastic or myofibroblastic differentiation, with the tumor cells containing filaments, subplasmalemmal electron-dense bodies, pinocytotic vesicles, discontinuous basal lamina, and intercellular desmosomes. Although ultrastructural and immunohistochemical studies are of academic interest, in our opinion they are not indicated for routine evaluation.

Differential Diagnosis. Noncellular fibromas are similar to fibromatous tumors of the testicular tunics and are distinguished from them on the basis of the gross characteristics (see chapter 7, Table 7-1). Cellular fibromas may simulate the exceptionally rare fibrosarcoma of the testis (see chapter 7). There are no established criteria for the distinction of these two tumors in the testis, but it appears reasonable to apply similar criteria to those used in the ovary (180). Leiomyomas of both typical and cellular type (each exceptionally rare in the testis) are differentiated using criteria applicable in the ovary and soft tissues, including the more abundant eosinophilic cytoplasm and blunt-ended nuclei of the smooth muscle tumors. We have not found actin staining reliable in this differential.

Unclassified sex cord-stromal tumors may have prominent fibromatous areas but, by definition, have at least some focal epithelial differentiation that permits distinction from pure fibromas. Such elements are often enhanced by reticulum stains that surround distinct cellular groupings rather than the individual cells as seen in fibromas. This distinction is important because of the benign course of all reported fibromas, whereas occasional tumors in the unclassified sex cord-stromal tumor category are malignant.

SEX CORD-STROMAL TUMORS, MIXED AND UNCLASSIFIED

General and Clinical Features. Some testicular sex cord-stromal tumors have patterns of two or more of the above discussed specific subtypes, but distinguishing them in the literature from

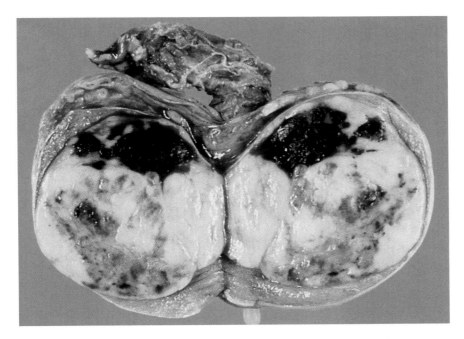

Figure 6-121

SEX CORD–STROMAL TUMOR, UNCLASSIFIED

The well-circumscribed tumor is white and shows focal hemorrhage.

cases in the unclassified category is often impossible. It is, therefore, unrealistic to cover separately the mixed and unclassified tumors on the basis of the available information. All patterns in a mixed tumor should be recorded, and the behavior of the tumor is most likely to be that of the predominant pattern or that which is most histologically atypical. Tumors in the unclassified category frequently lack specific differentiation or contain patterns and cells resembling, to varying degrees, both testicular and ovarian elements (5,181). Many of these cases, in our experience, consist of a mixture of epithelial sex cord elements that may focally form tubules and a neoplastic spindle cell component.

Unclassified sex cord-stromal tumors occur at all ages. In a registry of tumors in children, 62 percent of sex cord tumors were considered unclassified (83). From another viewpoint, approximately one third of the reported tumors have been in children. The most common clinical symptom is painless testicular enlargement, but gynecomastia is present in about 10 percent of patients.

Gross Findings. The tumors vary greatly in size, with many replacing most or the entire testis. They are usually well circumscribed (fig. 6-121) and composed of white to yellow, often lobulated tissue, sometimes traversed by gray-white fibrous septa. The low-grade spindle cell–

predominant cases have a tendency to be smaller and preferentially localized in proximity to the rete testis (133). Cysts are occasionally present; hemorrhage and necrosis are uncommon.

Microscopic Findings. The appearance of the individual patterns in mixed tumors is similar to that observed when such patterns are seen in pure form, as discussed above.

A spectrum of patterns is seen in the unclassified tumors, ranging from predominantly epithelial to predominantly stromal. The better-differentiated tumors typically contain solid to hollow tubules, or cords composed of or lined by cells resembling Sertoli cells (fig. 6-122). The cytoplasm of cells lining sertoliform tubules varies from scanty to abundant, and may be eosinophilic, amphophilic, or vacuolated and lipid-laden; the nuclei are round to oval and often vesicular, and sometimes contain single small nucleoli. Mitotic figures are variably prominent.

Some tumors exhibit a microcystic pattern (fig. 6-123). Islands and masses of cells resembling granulosa cells (fig. 6-124) and containing Call-Exner–like bodies may also be present, but usually the nuclei lack grooves and, although often suggestive of granulosa cell tumor, the overall architectural and cytologic features are usually not typical of that tumor. An admixture of such foci with a spindle cell stromal component is common (fig. 6-124).

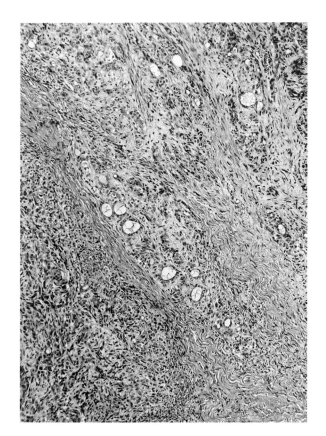

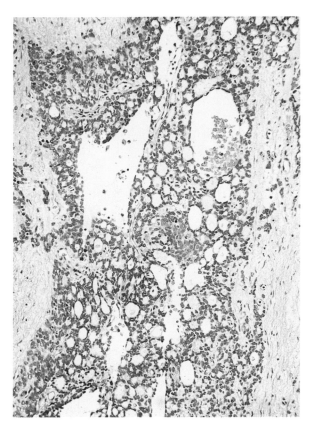

Figure 6-122

SEX CORD–STROMAL TUMOR, UNCLASSIFIED

This tumor has a mostly solid appearance with a small focus of tubular differentiation.

Figure 6-123

SEX CORD–STROMAL TUMOR, UNCLASSIFIED

The epithelial component of this tumor exhibits a prominent microcystic pattern.

Some tumors exhibit foci of pure sex cord type and other areas are composed exclusively of a neoplastic stroma that may be densely cellular or fibromatous (fig. 6-125). More commonly, however, sex cord cells and spindled stromal cells are intimately admixed (figs. 6-126, 6-127) and sometimes difficult to distinguish (fig. 6-127). In such tumors, the sex cord foci may be better delineated with a reticulum stain, which accentuates the nested nature of the sex cord component (133). Many of the spindle cell–predominant tumors have uniform cells with low mitotic rates, and are circumscribed, small (under 2 cm), and close to the rete testis (fig. 6-128). Some stromal cells have abundant vacuolated or eosinophilic cytoplasm. The less-differentiated tumors exhibit varying degrees of nuclear pleomorphism and mitotic activity. Diffuse and sarcomatoid patterns may be seen. Rare features

include heterologous mesenchymal elements, as in one case we have seen that formed atypical bone and cartilage (fig. 6-129), or squamous metaplasia of the sex cord elements (fig. 6-130). Spindle cell–predominant cases are often reactive for S-100 protein and smooth muscle actin, similar to granulosa cell tumors (133).

Differential Diagnosis. It should be readily evident in most cases that these tumors are in the sex cord-stromal category as opposed to, for example, any other more common form of testicular neoplasm such as a germ cell tumor. The greatest problem is the distinction of tumors in the unclassified and mixed category from pure tumors of the various subtypes discussed earlier. Strict adherence to the morphologic features and criteria discussed in those sections should, in the majority of cases, enable the pure tumors to be separated from those in the mixed and

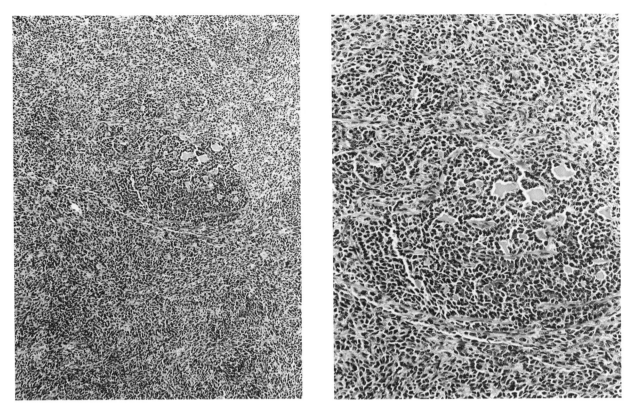

Figure 6-124

SEX CORD–STROMAL TUMOR, UNCLASSIFIED

Left: A focus of sex cord cells with granulosa-like features is surrounded by a nonspecific solid pattern of growth including spindle cells. The distinction from granulosa cell tumor was based on the confinement of granulosa cell features to a few small foci.

Right: Higher magnification shows that the focus contains Call-Exner body-like structures surrounded by a spindle cell proliferation.

unclassified categories. Of particular note are the prominent cellular stromal component of many unclassified tumors and the typical presence of both granulosa-like and Sertoli-like areas. When the epithelial component is small, areas of the tumor may resemble one or other form of pure sarcoma of the testis, and such a diagnosis should only be made after thorough sampling, supplemented by reticulum stains, has ruled out epithelial elements that are consistent with a sex cord nature.

Treatment and Prognosis. An important aspect of these tumors is the rarity of malignant behavior in children compared to an approximately 25 percent frequency in adults. Features that generally correlate with aggressive behavior are similar to those that suggest malignant behavior in pure sex cord-stromal tumors, namely,

large size, extratesticular spread, necrosis, vascular invasion, marked nuclear pleomorphism, and brisk mitotic activity. The patterns of spread are predominantly to retroperitoneal lymph nodes, but visceral metastases are not rare. In cases with overt malignant features on microscopic examination, a staging lymph node dissection is indicated.

IMMUNOHISTOCHEMISTRY OF SEX CORD-STROMAL TUMORS

A summary of the immunohistochemical data concerning testicular sex cord-stromal tumors is provided here (26,27,29,40,42,133,167,182–185), with some comments regarding their application. These results are also summarized in Table 6-2. Although the expression of various markers by these tumors may be helpful, there are frequent

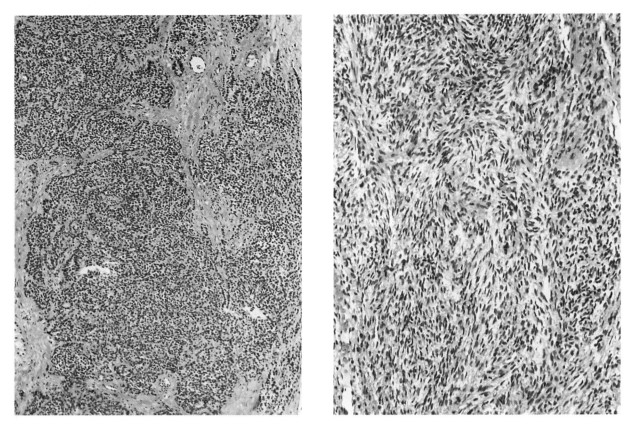

Figure 6-125

SEX CORD–STROMAL TUMOR, UNCLASSIFIED

Left: There is an epithelial pattern in this portion of the tumor.
Right: Other areas of the same tumor show prominent cellular mesenchymal growth.

Figure 6-126

SEX CORD–STROMAL TUMOR, UNCLASSIFIED

Small foci of sex cord cells are admixed with a more prominent stromal proliferation.

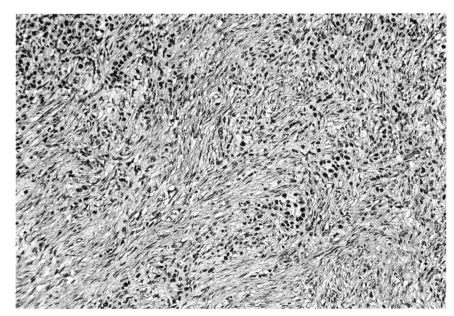

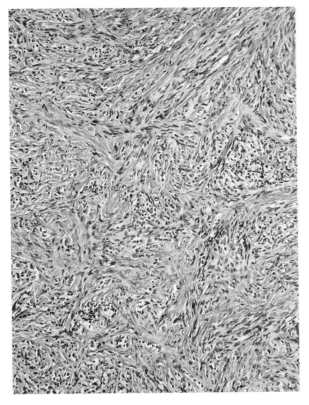

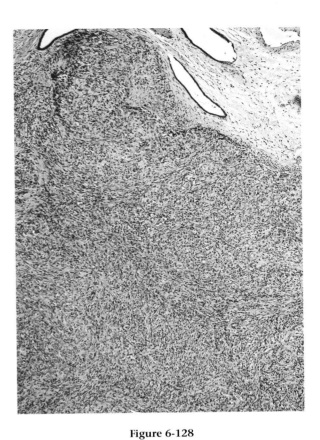

Figure 6-127

SEX CORD–STROMAL TUMOR, UNCLASSIFIED

Sex cord cells and stromal cells subtly blend together.

Figure 6-128

SEX CORD–STROMAL TUMOR, UNCLASSIFIED

This tumor has a predominantly spindle cell pattern and is located close to the rete testis.

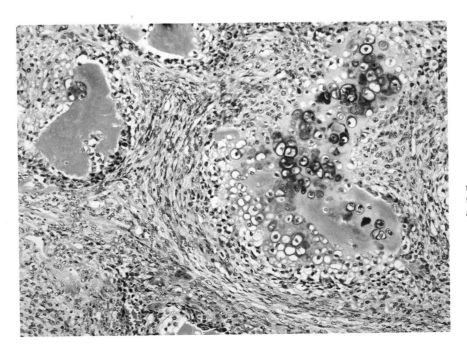

Figure 6-129

SEX CORD–STROMAL TUMOR, UNCLASSIFIED

This tumor formed differentiated mesenchymal elements that included atypical cartilage and bone.

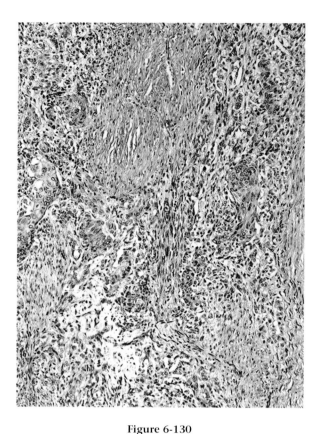

Figure 6-130

SEX CORD–STROMAL TUMOR, UNCLASSIFIED

There are foci of squamous metaplasia within the sex cord component of this unusual tumor.

exceptions to many of the generalizations and, for that reason, immunohistochemical data must always be interpreted in the context of standard light microscopic morphology.

Important findings that aid in diagnosing Leydig cell tumors include their positivity for inhibin, negativity for EMA and HMB45, and usually negative or weak and focal staining for cytokeratin. The tumors are vimentin positive, which, in conjunction with inhibin positivity, negative staining for EMA, and variable cytokeratin immunoreactivity, is helpful in differentiating them from metastatic carcinoma. Some Leydig cell tumors are S-100 protein positive, and there is more frequent positivity with

melan-A, so these stains have limited value when considering melanoma (26,27,167,182,186). A potential immunohistochemical pitfall is the reported positivity of some Leydig cell tumors for chromogranin and synaptophysin.

Sertoli cell tumors, NOS, are often positive for cytokeratin and vimentin, and negative for EMA (26,27,29). Inhibin is variably positive, although often focal, and such positivity favors Sertoli cell tumor over germ cell tumor or metastatic carcinoma. The negativity for OCT3/4 or SALL4 helps prevent the unfortunate circumstance of a Sertoli cell tumor being misinterpreted as a germ cell tumor, usually seminoma. Inhibin may also help to identify the sex cord component of biphasic neoplasms in the unclassified category in which the epithelial component is indistinct (24). The large cell calcifying variant of Sertoli cell tumor often stains more robustly for S-100 protein (42) and inhibin than does Sertoli cell tumor, NOS (26,27,29).

Within the granulosa cell group, staining for cytokeratin is usually absent or only focally positive, and vimentin is usually strongly positive. S-100 protein and smooth muscle actin may be demonstrated in both the juvenile and adult types (133,167), and desmin has also been demonstrated in the juvenile variant (167). Juvenile granulosa cell tumors reportedly stain for inhibin (25), but we are not aware of inhibin studies on testicular tumors we consider legitimate pure granulosa cell tumor of adult type. The spindle cell areas of granulosa cell tumors may stain for desmin, while these areas in unclassified tumors may be S-100 protein and smooth muscle actin immunoreactive, and focally positive for cytokeratin, in keeping with the myoepithelial or myofibroblastic differentiation of some of the cells.

Immunohistochemical staining of fibromatous tumors is rarely indicated, but a potentially useful finding is its typical negativity for desmin, which provides evidence against a smooth muscle tumor. Weak desmin staining and actin staining have to be interpreted in light of the overall microscopic findings. Actin staining is not reliable in the distinction of fibromatous from myogenic tumors.

REFERENCES

1. Scully RE. Testicular tumors with endocrine manifestations. In: DeGroot LJ, ed. Endocrinology. 3rd ed. Philadelphia: WB Saunders Co; 1995:2442-8.
2. Kaplan GW, Cromie WJ, Kelalis PP, Silber I, Tank ES Jr. Gonadal stromal tumors: a report of the Prepubertal Testicular Tumor Registry. J Urol 1986;136:300-2.
3. Ober WB, Sciagura C. Leydig, Sertoli, and Reinke: three anatomists who were on the ball. Pathol Annu 1981;16 (Pt.1):1-13.
4. Collins DH, Symington T. Sertoli-cell tumor. Br J Urol 1964;36 (suppl):52-61.
5. Mostofi FK, Theiss EA, Ashley DJ. Tumors of specialized gonadal stroma in human male patients. Cancer 1959;12:944-57.
6. Talerman A. Malignant Sertoli cell tumor of the testis. Cancer 1971;28:446-54.
7. Young RH, Koelliker DD, Scully RE. Sertoli cell tumors of the testis, not otherwise specified: a clinicopathologic analysis of 60 cases. Am J Surg Pathol 1998;22:709-21.
8. Teilum G. Arrhenoblastoma—androblastoma. Homologous ovarian and testicular tumors. II. Including the so-called luteomas and adrenal tumors of the ovary and the interstitial cell tumors of the testis. Acta Pathol Microbiol Scand 1943;23:252-64.
9. Teilum G. Classification of testicular and ovarian androblastoma and Sertoli cell tumors. A survey of comparative studies with consideration of histogenesis, endocrinology, and embryological theories. Cancer 1958;11:769-82.
10. Teilum G. Estrogen producing Sertoli-cell tumors (androblastoma tubulare lipoides) of the human testis and ovary: homologous ovarian and testicular tumors. J Clin Endocrinol Metab 1949;9:301-18.
11. Teilum G. Homologous tumors in the ovary and testis. Contributions to classification of the gonadal tumors. Acta Obstet Gynecol 1944;24:480-503.
12. Gabrilove JL, Freiberg EK, Leiter E, Nicolis GL. Feminizing and non-feminizing Sertoli cell tumors. J Urol 2010;124:767.
13. Goswitz JJ, Pettinato G, Manivel JC. Testicular sex cord-stromal tumors in children: clinicopathologic study of sixteen children with review of the literature. Pediatr Pathol Lab Med 1996;16:451-70.
14. Harms D, Kock LR. Testicular juvenile granulosa cell and Sertoli cell tumours: a clinicopathological study of 29 cases from the Kiel Paediatric Tumour Registry. Virchows Arch 1997;430:301-9.
15. Adlington SR, Salm R. A case of bilteral tubular adenoma of the testis. Br J Surg 1960;48:152-5.
16. Rosvoll R, Woodard JR. Malignant Sertoli cell tumor of the testis. Cancer 1968;22:8-13.
17. Sharma S, Seam RK, Kapoor HL. Malignant Sertoli cell tumour of the testis in a child. J Surg Oncol 1990;44:129-31.
18. Rutgers JL, Scully RE. The androgen insensitivity syndrome (testicular feminization): a clinicopathologic study of 43 cases. Int J Gynecol Pathol 1991;10:126-44.
19. Carney JA, Gordon H, Carpenter PC, Shenoy BV, Go VL. The complex of myxomas, spotty pigmentation, and endocrine overactivity. Medicine 1985;64:270-83.
20. Ferlin A, Pengo M, Selice R, et al. Analysis of single nucleotide polymorphisms of FSH receptor gene suggests association with testicular cancer susceptibility. Endocr Relat Cancer 2008;15:429-37.
21. Jacobsen GK. Malignant Sertoli cell tumors of the testis. J Urol Pathol 1993;1:233-55.
22. Freeman DA. Steroid hormone-producing tumors in man. Endocr Rev 1986;7:204-20.
23. Henley JD, Young RH, Ulbright TM. Malignant Sertoli cell tumors of the testis: a study of 13 examples of a neoplasm frequently misinterpreted as seminoma. Am J Surg Pathol 2002;26:541-50.
24. Gilcrease MZ, Delgado R, Albores-Saavedra J. Testicular Sertoli cell tumor with a heterologous sarcomatous component: immunohistochemical assessment of Sertoli cell differentiation. Arch Pathol Lab Med 1998;122:907-11.
25. Kommoss F, Oliva E, Bittinger F, et al. Inhibin-alpha CD99, HEA125, PLAP, and chromogranin immunoreactivity in testicular neoplasms and the androgen insensitivity syndrome. Hum Pathol 2000;31:1055-61.
26. McCluggage WG, Shanks JH, Whiteside C, Maxwell P, Banerjee SS, Biggart JD. Immunohistochemical study of testicular sex cord-stromal tumors, including staining with anti-inhibin antibody. Am J Surg Pathol 1998;22:615-9.
27. Iczkowski KA, Bostwick DG, Roche PC, Cheville JC. Inhibin A is a sensitive and specific marker for testicular sex cord-stromal tumors. Mod Pathol 1998;11:774-9.
28. Bennett AK, Ulbright TM, Ramnani DM, Young RH, Mills SE. Immunohistochemical expression of calretinin, CD99, and alpha-inhibin in Sertoli and Leydig cells and their lesions, emphasizing large cell calcifying Sertoli cell tumor. Mod Pathol 2005;18:128A.

29. Amin MB, Young RH, Scully RE. Immunohisto-chemical profile of Sertoli and Leydig cell tumors of the testis. Mod Pathol 1998;11:76A.

30. Tanaka Y, Carney JA, Ijiri R, et al. Utility of immunostaining for S-100 protein subunits in gonadal sex cord-stromal tumors, with emphasis on the large-cell calcifying Sertoli cell tumor of the testis. Hum Pathol 2002;33:285-9.

31. Rey R, Sabourin JC, Venara M, et al. Anti-Mulle-rian hormone is a specific marker of sertoli- and granulosa-cell origin in gonadal tumors. Hum Pathol 2000;31:1202-8.

32. Augusto D, Leteurtre E, De La Taille A, Gosselin B, Leroy X. Calretinin: a valuable marker of normal and neoplastic Leydig cells of the testis. Appl Immunohistochem Mol Morphol 2002;10:159-62.

33. Erlandson RA. Diagnostic transmission electron microscopy of tumors with clinicopathological, immunohistochemical, and cytogenetic correla-tions. New York: Raven Press; 1994.

34. Tetu B, Ro JY, Ayala AG. Large cell calcifying Ser-toli cell tumor of the testis: a clinicopathologic, immunohistochemical, and ultrastructural study of two cases. Am J Clin Pathol 1991;96:717-22.

35. Kronz JD, Nicol TL, Rosenthal DL, Ali SZ. Meta-static testicular Sertoli-cell tumor: cytopatho-logic findings on fine-needle aspiration. Diagn Cytopathol 1998;19:127-30.

36. Terayama K, Hirokawa M, Shimizu M, Kanahara T, Manabe T. Sertoli cell tumor of the testis. Re-port of a case with imprint cytology findings. Acta Cytol 1998;42:1458-60.

37. Verdorfer I, Hollrigl A, Strasser U, et al. Molecular-cytogenetic characterisation of sex cord-stromal tumours: CGH analysis in sertoli cell tumours of the testis. Virchows Arch 2007;450:425-31.

38. Aly MS, Dal Cin P, Moerman P, et al. Loss of the Y-chromosome in a malignant Sertoli tumor. Cancer Genet Cytogenet 1993;65:104-6.

39. Vallangeon BD, Eble JN, Ulbright TM. Macro-scopic Sertoli cell nodule: a study of 6 cases that presented as testicular masses. Am J Surg Pathol 2010;34:1874-80.

40. Rishi M, Howard LN, Bratthauer GL, Tavassoli FA. Use of monoclonal antibody against inhibin as a marker for sex cord-stromal tumors of the ovary. Am J Surg Pathol 1997;21:583-9.

41. Lindegaard ME, Madsen E, Morck Hultberg B. Metastasizing Sertoli cell tumours of the human testis--a report of two cases and a review of the literature. Acta Oncol 1990;29:946-9.

42. Kratzer SS, Ulbright TM, Talerman A, et al. Large cell calcifying Sertoli cell tumor of the testis: contrasting features of six malignant and six benign tumors and a review of the literature. Am J Surg Pathol 1997;21:1271-80.

43. Horn T, Jao W, Keh PC. Large-cell calcifying Sertoli cell tumor of the testis: a case report with ultrastructural study. Ultrastruc Pathol 1983;4:359-64.

44. Plata C, Algaba F, Andujar M, et al. Large cell calcifying Sertoli cell tumour of the testis. His-topathology 1995;26:255-9.

45. Proppe KH, Scully RE. Large-cell calcifying Ser-toli cell tumor of the testis. Am J Clin Pathol 1980;74:607-19.

46. Rosenzweig JL, Lawrence DA, Vogel DL, Costa J, Gorden P. Adrenocorticotropin-independent hypercortisolemia and testicular tumors in a patient with a pituitary tumor and gigantism. J Clin Endocrinol Metab 1982;55:421-7.

47. Waxman M, Damjanov I, Khapra A, Landau SJ. Large cell calcifying Sertoli tumor of the testis. Light microscopic and ultrastructural study. Cancer 1984;54:1574-81.

48. Bufo P, Pennella A, Serio G, et al. Malignant large cell calcifying Sertoli cell tumor of the testis (LCCSCTT). Report of a case in an elderly man and review of the literature. Pathologica 1999;91:107-14.

49. Washecka R, Dresner MI, Honda SA. Tes-ticular tumors in Carney's complex. J Urol 2002;167:1299-302.

50. Ulbright TM, Amin MB, Young RH. Intratubular large cell hyalinizing sertoli cell neoplasia of the testis: a report of 8 cases of a distinctive lesion of the Peutz-Jeghers syndrome. Am J Surg Pathol 2007;31:827-35.

51. Sato K, Ueda Y, Sakurai A, et al. Large cell calcify-ing Sertoli cell tumor of the testis: comparative immunohistochemical study with Leydig cell tumor. Pathol Int 2005;55:366-71.

52. Evans TN, Carter JE. Pathologic quiz case: testicu-lar pain and scrotal swelling in a 25-year-old man. Large cell calcifying Sertoli cell tumor of the testis. Arch Pathol Lab Med 2004;128:e137-e138.

53. Aydin H, Omeroglu G, Omeroglu A. Pathologic quiz case: incidental bilateral testicular nodules in an African American man. Large cell calci-fying Sertoli cell tumor. Arch Pathol Lab Med 2004;128:587-8.

54. De Raeve H, Schoonooghe P, Wibowo R, Van Marck E, Goossens A. Malignant large cell calci-fying Sertoli cell tumor of the testis. Pathol Res Pract 2003;199:113-7.

55. Cano-Valdez AM, Chanona-Vilchis J, Domin-guez-Malagon H. Large cell calcifying Sertoli cell tumor of the testis: a clinicopathological, im-munohistochemical, and ultrastructural study of two cases. Ultrastruct Pathol 1999;23:259-65.

56. Saraco N, Berensztein E, Sciara M, et al. High TGFbeta1, estrogen receptor, and aromatase gene expression in a large cell calcifying sertoli cell tumor (LCCSCT): implications for the mechanism of oncogenesis. Pediatr Dev Pathol 2006;9:181-9.

57. Proppe KH, Dickersin GR. Large-cell calcifying Sertoli cell tumor of the testis: light microscopic and ultrastructural study. Hum Pathol 1982;13:1109-14.

58. Perez-Atayde AR, Nunez AE, Carroll WL, et al. Large-cell calcifying Sertoli cell tumor of the testis. An ultrastructural, immunocytochemical, and biochemical study. Cancer 1983;51:2287-92.

59. Malik R, Malik TK, Shinghal RN, Yadav R, Chandra K. Leydig-cell tumour of the testis. Int Urol Nephrol 1980;12:55-8.

60. Ulbright TM, Srigley JR, Hatzianastassiou DK, Young RH. Leydig cell tumors of the testis with unusual features. Adipose differentiation, calcification with ossification, and spindle-shaped tumor cells. Am J Surg Pathol 2002;26:1424-33.

61. Tanaka Y, Yamaguchi M, Ijiri R, Kondo I. Malignant large cell calcifying sertoli cell tumor with endocrine overactivity. J Urol 1999;161:1575.

62. Brown B, Ram A, Clayton P, Humphrey G. Conservative management of bilateral Sertoli cell tumors of the testicle in association with the Carney complex: a case report. J Pediatr Surg 2007;42:E13-E15.

63. Venara M, Rey R, Bergada I, Mendilaharzu H, Campo S, Chemes H. Sertoli cell proliferations of the infantile testis: an intratubular form of Sertoli cell tumor? Am J Surg Pathol 2001;25:1237-44.

64. Small EJ, Torti FM. Testes. In: Abeloff MD, Armitage JO, Lichter AS, Niederhuber JE, eds. Clinical oncology. New York: Churchill-Livingstone; 1995:1493-526.

65. Brodie A, Inkster S, Yue W. Aromatase expression in the human male. Mol Cell Endocrinol 2001;178:23-8.

66. Bulun SE, Rosenthal IM, Brodie AM, et al. Use of tissue-specific promoters in the regulation of aromatase cytochrome P450 gene expression in human testicular and ovarian sex cord tumors, as well as in normal fetal and adult gonads. J Clin Endocrinol Metab 1993;77:1616-21.

67. Coen P, Kulin H, Ballantine T, et al. An aromatase-producing sex-cord tumor resulting in prepubertal gynecomastia. N Engl J Med 1991;324:317-22.

68. Young S, Gooneratne S, Straus FH, Zeller WP, Bulun SE, Rosenthal IM. Feminizing Sertoli cell tumors in boys with Peutz-Jeghers syndrome. Am J Surg Pathol 1995;19:50-8.

69. Dreyer L, Jacyk WK, du Plessis DJ. Bilateral large-cell calcifying Sertoli cell tumor of the testes with Peutz-Jeghers syndrome: a case report. Pediatr Dermatol 1994;11:335-7.

70. Ros P, Nistal M, Alonso M, Calvo de Mora J, Yturriaga R, Barrio R. Sertoli cell tumour in a boy with Peutz-Jeghers syndrome. Histopathology 1999;34:84-6.

71. Kara C, Kutlu AO, Tosun MS, Apaydin S, Senel F. Sertoli cell tumor causing prepubertal gynecomastia in a boy with Peutz-Jeghers syndrome: the outcome of 1-year treatment with the aromatase inhibitor testolactone. Horm Res 2005;63:252-6.

72. Zukerberg LR, Young RH, Scully RE. Sclerosing Sertoli cell tumor of the testis: a report of 10 cases. Am J Surg Pathol 1991;15:829-34.

73. Kum JB, Idrees MT, Ulbright TM. Sclerosing Sertoli cell tumor of the testis: a study of 20 cases. Mod Pathol 2012;24(Suppl 1):401A.

74. Shimomura T, Kiyota H, Kato N, et al. [Sclerosing Sertoli cell tumor of the testis: a case report.] Hinyokika Kiyo 2001;47:293-5. [Japanese]

75. De Diego Rodriguez E, Pascual Soria C, Portillo Martin JA, Martin Garcia B, Villanueva Pena A. [Sclerosing Sertoli cell tumor of the testis in an HIV patient.] Arch Esp Urol 2001;54:1129-32. [Spanish]

76. Gravas S, Papadimitriou K, Kyriakidis A. Sclerosing sertoli cell tumor of the testis—a case report and review of the literature. Scand J Urol Nephrol 1999;33:197-9.

77. Fam A, Ishak KG. Androblastoma of the testicle: report of a case in an infant 3 1/2 months old. J Urol 1958;79:859-62.

78. Fuglsang F, Ohlse NS. Androblastoma predominantly feminizing. With report of a case. Acta Chir Scand 1957;112:405-10.

79. Oosterhuis JW, Castedo SM, de Jong B, et al. A malignant mixed gonadal stromal tumor of the testis with heterologous components and i(12p) in one of its metastases. Cancer Genet Cytogenet 1989;41:105-14.

80. Perito PE, Ciancio G, Civantos F, Politano VA. Sertoli-Leydig cell testicular tumor: case report and review of sex cord/gonadal stromal tumor histogenesis. J Urol 1992;148:883-5.

81. Young RH, Scully RE. Ovarian Sertoli-Leydig cell tumors with a retiform pattern: a problem in histopathologic diagnosis. A report of 25 cases. Am J Surg Pathol 1983;7:755-71.

82. Dilworth JP, Farrow GM, Oesterling JE. Non-germ cell tumors of testis. Urology 1991;37:399-417.

83. Kay R. Prepubertal testicular tumor registry. J Urol 1993;150(Pt 2):671-4.

84. Battaglia M, Ditonno P, Palazzo S, et al. Bilateral tumors of the testis in 21-alpha hydroxylase deficiency without adrenal hyperplasia. Urol Oncol 2005;23:178-80.

85. Leotta A, Lio SG. Bilateral interstitial cell tumor of the testis: a report of a case in an adult. Pathologica 1994;86:557-9.

86. Kim I, Young RH, Scully RE. Leydig cell tumors of the testis. A clinicopathological analysis of 40 cases and review of the literature. Am J Surg Pathol 1985;9:177-92.

87. Bokemeyer C, Kuczyk M, Schoffski P, Schmoll HJ. Familial occurrence of Leydig cell tumors: a report of a case in a father and his adult son. J Urol 1993;150(Pt 1):1509-10.

88. Haas GP, Pittaluga S, Gomella L, et al. Clinically occult Leydig cell tumor presenting with gynecomastia. J Urol 1989;142:1325-7.

89. Wilson BE, Netzloff ML. Primary testicular abnormalities causing precocious puberty Leydig cell tumor, Leydig cell hyperplasia, and adrenal rest tumor. Ann Clin Lab Sci 1983;13:315-20.

90. Carvajal-Carmona LG, Alam NA, Pollard PJ, et al. Adult Leydig cell tumors of the testis caused by germline fumarate hydratase mutations. J Clin Endocrinol Metab 2006;91:3071-5.

91. Papadimitris C, Alevizaki M, Pantazopoulos D, Nakopoulou L, Athanassiades P, Dimopoulos MA. Cushing syndrome as the presenting feature of metastatic Leydig cell tumor of the testis. Urology 2000;56:153.

92. Poster RB, Katz DS. Leydig cell tumor of the testis in Klinefelter syndrome: MR detection. J Comp Assist Tomogr 1993;17:480-1.

93. Davis JM, Woodroof J, Sadasivan R, Stephens R. Case report: congenital adrenal hyperplasia and malignant Leydig cell tumor. Am J Med Sci 1995;309:63-5.

94. Boulanger P, Somma M, Chevalier S, Bleau G, Roberts KD, Chapdelaine A. Elevated secretion of androstenedione in a patient with a Leydig cell tumour. Acta Endocrinol 1984;107:104-9.

95. Gabrilove JL, Nicolis GL, Mitty HA, Sohval AR. Feminizing interstitial cell tumor of the testis: personal observations and a review of the literature. Cancer 1975;35:1184-202.

96. Bercovici JP, Nahoul K, Tater D, Charles JF, Scholler R. Hormonal profile of Leydig cell tumors with gynecomastia. J Clin Endocrinol Metab 1984;59:625-30.

97. Mineur P, De Cooman S, Hustin J, Verhoeven G, De Hertogh R. Feminizing testicular Leydig cell tumor: hormonal profile before and after unilateral orchidectomy. J Clin Endocrinol Metab 1987;64:686-91.

98. Czernobilsky H, Czernobilsky B, Schneider HG, Franke WW, Ziegler R. Characterization of a feminizing testicular Leydig cell tumor by hormonal profile, immunocytochemistry, and tissue culture. Cancer 1985;56:1667-76.

99. Perez C, Novoa J, Alcaniz J, Salto L, Barcelo B. Leydig cell tumour of the testis with gynaecomastia and elevated oestrogen, progesterone and prolactin levels: case report. Clin Endocrinol 1980;13:409-12.

100. Bercovici JP, Nahoul K, Ducasse M, Tater D, Kerlan V, Scholler R. Leydig cell tumor with gynecomastia: further studies—the recovery after unilateral orchidectomy. J Clin Endocrinol Metab 1985;61:957-62.

101. Santonja C, Varona C, Burgos FJ, Nistal M. Leydig cell tumor of testis with adipose metaplasia. Appl Pathol 1989;7:201-4.

102. Balsitis M, Sokal M. Ossifying malignant Leydig (interstitial) cell tumour of the testis. Histopathology 1990;16:599-601.

103. Symington T, Cameron KM. Endocrine and genetic lesions. In: Pugh RC, ed. Pathology of the testis. Oxford: Blackwell Scientific; 1976.

104. Minkowitz S, Soloway H, Soscia J. Ossifying interstitial cell tumor of the testes. J Urol 1965;94:592-5.

105. Richmond I, Banerjee SS, Eyden BP, Sissons MC. Sarcomatoid Leydig cell tumour of testis. Histopathology 1995;27:578-80.

106. Reinke F. Beiträge zur Histologie des Menschen. Arch Mikr Anat 1896;47:34-44.

107. Gulbahce HE, Lindeland AT, Engel W, Lillemoe TJ. Metastatic Leydig cell tumor with sarcomatoid differentiation. Arch Pathol Lab Med 1999;123:1104-7.

108. Lugli A, Forster Y, Haas P, et al. Calretinin expression in human normal and neoplastic tissues: a tissue microarray analysis on 5233 tissue samples. Hum Pathol 2003;34:994-1000.

109. Doglioni C, Dei Tos AP, Laurino L, et al. Calretinin: a novel immunocytochemical marker for mesothelioma. Am J Surg Pathol 1996; 20:1037-46.

110. Gordon MD, Corless C, Renshaw AA, Beckstead J. CD99, keratin, and vimentin staining of sex cord-stromal tumors, normal ovary, and testis. Mod Pathol 1998;11:769-73.

111. McCluggage WG, Maxwell P. Immunohistochemical staining for calretinin is useful in the diagnosis of ovarian sex cord-stromal tumours. Histopathology 2001;38:403-8.

112. Kaufmann O, Koch S, Burghardt J, Audring H, Dietel M. Tyrosinase, melan-A, and KBA62 as markers for the immunohistochemical identification of metastatic amelanotic melanomas on paraffin sections. Mod Pathol 1998;11:740-6.

113. Looijenga LH, Stoop H, de Leeuw HP, et al. POU5F1 (OCT3/4) identifies cells with pluripotent potential in human germ cell tumors. Cancer Res 2003;63:2244-50.

114. Jones TD, Ulbright TM, Eble JN, Baldridge LA, Cheng L. OCT4 staining in testicular tumors: a sensitive and specific marker for seminoma and embryonal carcinoma. Am J Surg Pathol 2004;28:935-40.

115. Dickersin GR. Diagnostic electron microscopy: a text/atlas. New York: Igaku-Shoin; 1988.

116. Burton GV, Bullard DE, Walther PJ, Burger PC. Paraneoplastic encephalopathy with testicular carcinoma: a reversible neurologic syndrome. Cancer 1988;62:2248-51.

117. Assi A, Sironi M, Bacchioni AM, Declich P, Cozzi L, Pasquinelli G. Leydig cell tumor of the testis: a cytohistological, immunohistochemical, and ultrastructural case study. Diagn Cytopathol 1997;16:262-6.

118. Ortiz DJ, Silva J, Abad M, Garcia-Macias MC, Bulon YA. Leydig cell tumour of the testis: cytological findings on fine needle aspiration. Cytopathology 1999;10:217-8.

119. Gupta SK, Francis IM, Sheikh ZA, al-Rubah NA, Das DK. Intranuclear Reinke's crystals in a testicular Leydig cell tumor diagnosed by aspiration cytology. A case report. Acta Cytol 1994;38:252-6.

120. Canto P, Soderlund D, Ramon G, Nishimura E, Mendez JP. Mutational analysis of the luteinizing hormone receptor gene in two individuals with Leydig cell tumors. Am J Med Genet 2002;108:148-52.

121. d'Alva CB, Brito VN, Palhares HM, et al. A single somatic activating Asp578His mutation of the luteinizing hormone receptor causes Leydig cell tumour in boys with gonadotropin-independent precocious puberty. Clin Endocrinol (Oxf)2006;65:408-10.

122. Liu G, Duranteau L, Carel JC, Monroe J, Doyle DA, Shenker A. Leydig-cell tumors caused by an activating mutation of the gene encoding the luteinizing hormone receptor. N Engl J Med 1999;341:1731-6.

123. Richter-Unruh A, Wessels HT, Menken U, et al. Male LH-independent sexual precocity in a 3.5-year-old boy caused by a somatic activating mutation of the LH receptor in a Leydig cell tumor. J Clin Endocrinol Metab 2002;87:1052-6.

124. Petkovic V, Salemi S, Vassella E, et al. Leydig-cell tumour in children: variable clinical presentation, diagnostic features, follow-up and genetic analysis of four cases. Horm Res 2007;67:89-95.

125. Verdorfer I, Horst D, Hollrigl A, et al. Leydig cell tumors of the testis: a molecular-cytogenetic study based on a large series of patients. Oncol Rep 2007;17:585-9.

126. Rutgers JL, Young RH, Scully RE. The testicular "tumor" of the adrenogenital syndrome. A report of six cases and review of the literature on testicular masses in patients with adrenocortical disorders. Am J Surg Pathol 1988;12:503-13.

127. Wang Z, Yang S, Shi H, et al. Histopathological and immunophenotypic features of testicular tumour of the adrenogenital syndrome. Histopathology 2011;58:1013-8.

128. Ashley RA, McGee SM, Isotaolo PA, Kramer SA, Cheville JC. Clinical and pathological features associated with the testicular tumor of the adrenogenital syndrome. J Urol 2007;177:546-9.

129. Billings SD, Roth LM, Ulbright TM. Microcystic Leydig cell tumors mimicking yolk sac tumor: a report of four cases. Am J Surg Pathol 1999;23:546-51.

130. McCluggage WG, Shanks JH, Arthur K, Banerjee SS. Cellular proliferation and nuclear ploidy assessments augment established prognostic factors in predicting malignancy in testicular Leydig cell tumours. Histopathology 1998;33:361-8.

130a. Cao D, Li J, Guo CC, Allen RW, Humphrey PA. SALL4 is a novel diagnostic marker for testicular germ cell tumors. Am J Surg Pathol 2009;33:1065-77.

131. Bergh A, Cajander S. Immunohistochemical localization of inhibin-alpha in the testes of normal men and in men with testicular disorders. Int J Androl 1990;13:463-9.

132. Mehta MK, Garde SV, Sheth AR. Occurrence of FSH, inhibin and other hypothalamic-pituitary-intestinal hormones in normal fertility, subfertility, and tumors of human testes. Int J Fertil Menopausal Stud 1995;40:39-46.

133. Renshaw AA, Gordon M, Corless CL. Immunohistochemistry of unclassified sex cord-stromal tumors of the testis with a predominance of spindle cells. Mod Pathol 1997;10:693-700.

134. Gupta D, Deavers MT, Silva EG, Malpica A. Malignant melanoma involving the ovary: a clinicopathologic and immunohistochemical study of 23 cases. Am J Surg Pathol 2004;28:771-80.

135. Sugimura J, Suzuki Y, Tamura G, Funaki H, Fujioka T, Satodate R. Metachronous development of malignant Leydig cell tumor. Hum Pathol 1997;28:1318-20.

136. Cheville JC, Sebo TJ, Lager DJ, Bostwick DG, Farrow GM. Leydig cell tumor of the testis: a clinicopathologic, DNA content, and MIB-1 comparison of nonmetastasizing and metastasizing tumors. Am J Surg Pathol 1998;22:1361-7.

137. Shapiro CM, Sankovitch A, Yoon WJ. Malignant feminizing Leydig cell tumor. J Surg Oncol 1984;27:73-5.

138. Palazzo JP, Petersen RO, Young RH, Scully RE. Deoxyribonucleic acid flow cytometry of testicular Leydig cell tumors. J Urol 1994;152:415-7.

139. Grem JL, Robins HI, Wilson KS, Gilchrist K, Trump DL. Metastatic Leydig cell tumor of the testis. Report of three cases and review of the literature. Cancer 1986;58:2116-9.

140. Bertram KA, Bratloff B, Hodges GF, Davidson H. Treatment of malignant Leydig cell tumor. Cancer 1991;68:2324-9.

141. Bokemeyer C, Harstrick A, Gonnermann O, et al. Metastatic Leydig cell tumours of the testis: report of four cases and review of the literature. Int J Oncol 1993;2:241-4.

142. Gaylis FD, August C, Yeldandi A, Nemcek A, Garnett J. Granulosa cell tumor of the adult testis: ultrastructural and ultrasonographic characteristics. J Urol 1989;141:126-7.

143. Jimenez-Quintero LP, Ro JY, Zavala-Pompa A, et al. Granulosa cell tumor of the adult testis: a clinicopathologic study of seven cases and a review of the literature. Hum Pathol 1993;24:1120-6.

144. Matoska J, Ondrus D, Talerman A. Malignant granulosa cell tumor of the testis associated with gynecomastia and long survival. Cancer 1992;69:1769-72.

145. Nistal M, Läzaro R, Garcïa J, Paniagua R. Testicular granulosa cell tumor of the adult type. Arch Pathol Lab Med 1992;116:284-7.

146. Talerman A. Pure granulosa cell tumour of the testis. Report of a case and review of the literature. Appl Pathol 1985;3:117-22.

147. Due W, Dieckmann KP, Niedobitek G, Bornhoft G, Loy V, Stein H. Testicular sex cord stromal tumour with granulosa cell differentiation: detection of steroid hormone receptors as a possible basis for tumour development and therapeutic management. J Clin Pathol 1990;43:732-7.

148. Hammerich KH, Hille S, Ayala GE, et al. Malignant advanced granulosa cell tumor of the adult testis: case report and review of the literature. Hum Pathol 2008;39:701-9.

149. Hisano M, Souza FM, Malheiros DM, Pompeo AC, Lucon AM. Granulosa cell tumor of the adult testis: report of a case and review of the literature. Clinics (Sao Paulo) 2006;61:77-8.

150. Lawrence WD, Young RH, Scully RE. Sex cord-stromal tumors. In: Talerman A, Roth LM, eds. Pathology of the testis and its adnexa. New York: Churchill Livingstone; 1986:67-92.

151. Chan JK, Chan VS, Mak KL. Congenital juvenile granulosa cell tumour of the testis: report of a case showing extensive degenerative changes. Histopathology 1990;17:75-80.

152. Crump WD, C. Juvenile granulosa cell (sex cord-stromal) tumor of fetal testis. J Urol 1983;129:1057-8.

153. Lawrence WD, Young RH, Scully RE. Juvenile granulosa cell tumor of the infantile testis. A report of 14 cases. Am J Surg Pathol 1985;9:87-94.

154. Nistal M, Redondo E, Paniagua R. Juvenile granulosa cell tumor of the testis. Arch Pathol Lab Med 1988;112:1129-32.

155. Pinto MM. Juvenile granulosa cell tumor of the infant testis: case report with ultrastructural observations. Pediatr Pathol 1985;4:277-89.

156. Raju U, Fine G, Warrier R, Kini R, Weiss L. Congenital testicular juvenile granulosa cell tumor in a neonate with X/XY mosaicism. Am J Surg Pathol 1986;10:577-83.

157. Uehling DT, Smith JE, Logan R, et al. Newborn granulosa cell tumor of the testis. J Urol 1987;138:385-6.

158. White JM, McCarthy MP. Testicular gonadal stromal tumors in newborns. Urology 1982;20:121-4.

159. Young RH, Lawrence WD, Scully RE. Juvenile granulosa cell tumor—another neoplasm associated with abnormal chromosomes and ambiguous genitalia. A report of three cases. Am J Surg Pathol 1985;9:737-43.

160. Lin KH, Lin SE, Lee LM. Juvenile granulosa cell tumor of adult testis: a case report. Urology 2008;72:230-3.

161. Fidda N, Weeks DA. Juvenile granulosa cell tumor of the testis: a case presenting as a small round cell tumor of childhood. Ultrastruct Pathol 2003;27:451-5.

162. Tanaka Y, Sasaki Y, Tachibana K, Suwa S, Terashima K, Nakatani Y. Testicular juvenile granulosa cell tumor in an infant with X/XY mosaicism clinically diagnosed as true hermaphroditism. Am J Surg Pathol 1994;18:316-22.

163. Manivel JC, Sibley RK, Dehner LP, Manivel JC, Sibley RK, Dehner LP. Complete and incomplete Drash syndrome: a clinicopathologic study of five cases of a dysontogenetic-neoplastic complex. Hum Pathol 1987;18:80-9.

164. Kos M, Nogales FF, Kos M, Stipoljev F, Kunjko K. Congenital juvenile granulosa cell tumor of the testis in a fetus showing full 69,XXY triploidy. Int J Surg Pathol 2005;13:219-21.

165. Barroca H, Gil-da-Costa MJ, Mariz C. Testicular juvenile granulosa cell tumor: a case report. Acta Cytol 2007;51:634-6.

166. Groisman GM, Dische MR, Fine EM, Unger PD. Juvenile granulosa cell tumor of the testis: a comparative immunohistochemical study with normal infantile gonads. Pediatr Pathol 1993;13:389-400.

167. Perez-Atayde AR, Joste N, Mulhern H. Juvenile granulosa cell tumor of the infantile testis. Evidence of a dual epithelial-smooth muscle differentiation. Am J Surg Pathol 1996;20:72-9.

168. Shukla AR, Huff DS, Canning DA, et al. Juvenile granulosa cell tumor of the testis: contemporary clinical management and pathological diagnosis. J Urol 2004;171:1900-2.

169. Prat J, Scully RE. Cellular fibromas and fibrosarcomas of the ovary: a comparative clinicopathologic analysis of seventeen cases. Cancer 1981;47:2663-70.

170. Schenkman NS, Moul JW, Nicely ER, Maggio MI, Ho CK. Synchronous bilateral testis tumor: mixed germ cell and theca cell tumors. Urology 1993;42:593-5.

171. de Pinieux G, Glaser C, Chatelain D, Perie G, Flam T, Vieillefond A. Testicular fibroma of gonadal stromal origin with minor sex cord elements: clinicopathologic and immunohistochemical study of 2 cases. Arch Pathol Lab Med 1999;123:391-4.

172. Allen PR, King AR, Sage MD, Sorrell VF. A benign gonadal stromal tumor of the testis of spindle fibroblastic type. Pathology 1990;22:227-9.

173. Greco MA, Feiner HD, Theil KS, Mufarrij AA. Testicular stromal tumor with myofilaments: ultrastructural comparison with normal gonadal stroma. Hum Pathol 1984;15:238-43.

174. Jones MA, Young RH, Scully RE. Benign fibromatous tumors of the testis and paratesticular region: a report of 9 cases with a proposed classification of fibromatous tumors and tumor-like lesions. Am J Surg Pathol 1997;21:296-305.

175. Miettinen M, Salo J, Virtanen I. Testicular stromal tumor: ultrastructural, immunohistochemical, and gel electrophoretic evidence of epithelial differentiation. Ultrastruc Pathol 1986;10:515-28.

176. Nistal M, Puras A, Perna C, Guarch R, Paniagua R. Fusocellular gonadal stromal tumour of the testis with epithelial and myoid differentiation. Histopathology 1996;29:259-64.

177. Weidner N. Myoid gonadal stromal tumor with epithelial differentiation (? testicular myoepithelioma). Ultrastruct Pathol 1991;15:409-16.

178. Deveci MS, Deveci G, Onguru O, Kilciler M, Celasun B. Testicular (gonadal stromal) fibroma: case report and review of the literature. Pathol Int 2002;52:326-30.

179. Nistal M, Martinez-Garcia C, Paniagua R. Testicular fibroma. J Urol 1992;147:1617-9.

180. Irving JA, Alkushi A, Young RH, Clement PB. Cellular fibromas of the ovary: a study of 75 cases including 40 mitotically active tumors emphasizing their distinction from fibrosarcoma. Am J Surg Pathol 2006;30:929-38.

181. Eble JN, Hull MT, Warfel KA, Donohue JP. Malignant sex cord-stromal tumor of testis. J Urol 1984;131:546-50.

182. McLaren K, Thomson D. Localization of S-100 protein in a Leydig and Sertoli cell tumour of testis. Histopathology 1989;15:649-52.

183. Nielsen K, Jacobsen GK. Malignant Sertoli cell tumour of the testis: an immunohistochemical study and a review of the literature. APMIS 1988;96:755-60.

184. Sasano H, Nakashima N, Matsuzaki O, et al. Testicular sex cord-stromal lesions: immunohistochemical analysis of cytokeratin, vimentin and steroidogenic enzymes. Virchows Arch A Pathol Anat Histol 1992;421:163-9.

185. Ventura T, Discepoli S, Coletti G, et al. Light microscopic, immunocytochemical and ultrastructural study of a case of Sertoli cell tumor of the testis. Tumori 1987;73:649-53.

186. Busam KJ, Iversen K, Coplan KA, et al. Immunoreactivity for A103, an antibody to melan-A (Mart-1), in adrenocortical and other steroid tumors. Am J Surg Pathol 1998;22:57-63.

MISCELLANEOUS PRIMARY TUMORS OF THE TESTIS, ADNEXA, AND SPERMATIC CORD; HEMATOPOIETIC TUMORS; AND SECONDARY TUMORS

OVARIAN-TYPE EPITHELIAL TUMORS

Definition. *Ovarian-type epithelial tumors* are tumors that are identical to the surface epithelial-stromal tumors of the ovary.

General and Clinical Features. Most of these tumors are either *serous tumors of borderline malignancy* (figs. 7-1, 7-2) (1–7), with fewer *serous carcinomas* (figs. 7-3–7-5) (3,8–10), or *mucinous*

cystic tumors ranging from benign (cystadenoma) (fig. 7-6) (11-14) to borderline (figs. 7-7, 7-8) (12,15) to carcinoma (figs. 7-9, 7-10) (11,16–18). About 15 mucinous tumors have been reported (12) and slightly more serous tumors. Serous tumors may be more common than the literature suggests, as a critical review of the reported cases of "carcinoma of the rete testis" (19) uncovered

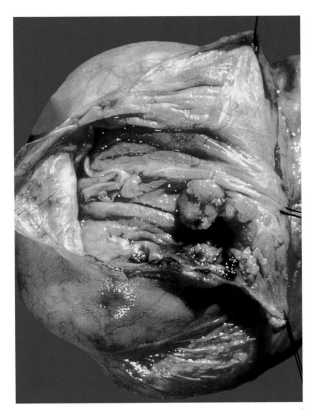

Figure 7-1

SEROUS PAPILLARY CYSTIC TUMOR OF BORDERLINE MALIGNANCY

A unilocular cyst with several small foci of velvety nodular tumor tissue overlies a smooth tunica vaginalis.

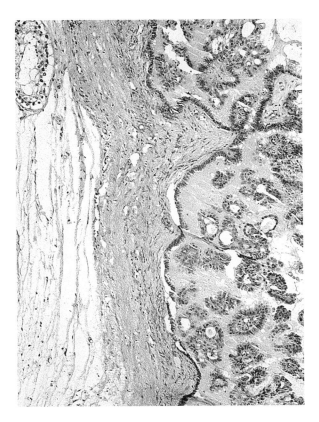

Figure 7-2

SEROUS PAPILLARY CYSTIC TUMOR OF BORDERLINE MALIGNANCY

An intratesticular cyst is lined by tubal-type epithelium from which arise many papillae that exhibit the characteristic pattern of this tumor.

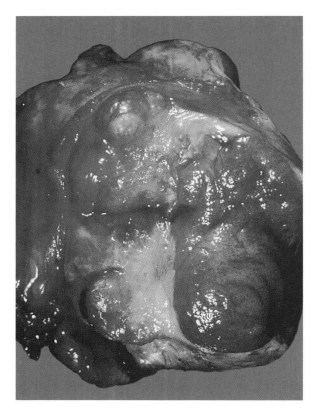

Figure 7-3

SEROUS CARCINOMA OF PARATESTICULAR REGION

Yellow-white sclerotic tumor tissue lies between the testis and epididymis in the testiculoepididymal groove.

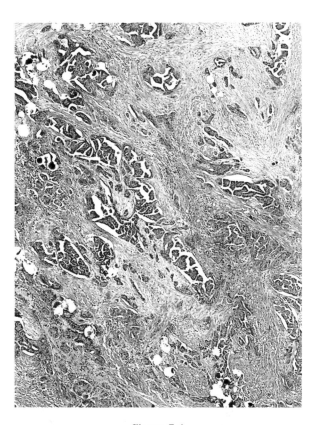

Figure 7-4

SEROUS CARCINOMA OF TESTIS

Small clusters of neoplastic serous cells infiltrate irregularly in a desmoplastic stroma. Psammomatous calcification is seen.

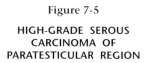

Figure 7-5

HIGH-GRADE SEROUS CARCINOMA OF PARATESTICULAR REGION

Numerous psammoma bodies, a solid growth pattern, and desmoplastic stroma are seen.

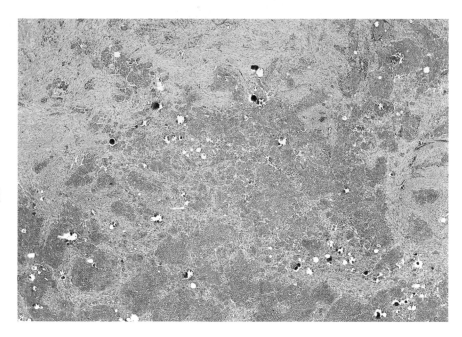

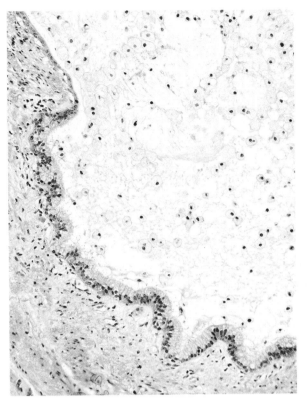

Figure 7-6

**MUCINOUS CYSTADENOMA
OF PARATESTICULR REGION**

Cytologically bland mucinous epithelial cells are arranged in a "picket fence" pattern.

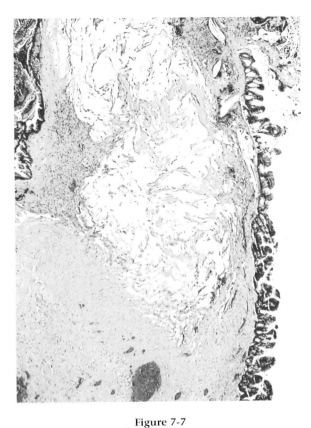

Figure 7-7

**MUCINOUS PAPILLARY CYSTIC TUMOR
OF TESTIS OF BORDERLINE MALIGNANCY**

There is a filigree arrangement of mucinous epithelium lining the wall of a cyst, with extravasated mucin in the stroma secondary to cyst rupture.

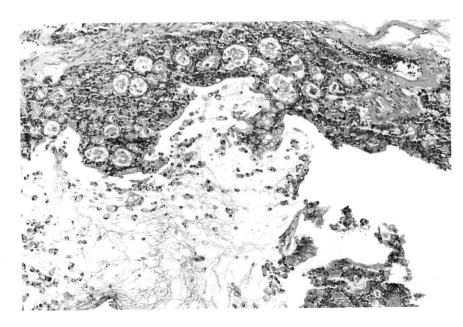

Figure 7-8

**MUCINOUS CYSTIC
NEOPLASM OF TESTIS OF
BORDERLINE MALIGNANCY
WITH INTRAEPITHELIAL
CARCINOMA**

There is a cribriform, intracystic proliferation of highly atypical mucinous epithelium, but stromal invasion was absent.

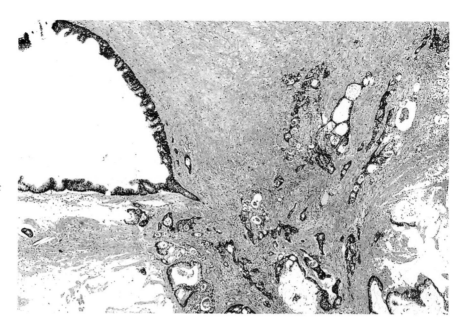

Figure 7-9

INVASIVE MUCINOUS ADENOCARCINOMA OF THE TESTIS

Foci of mucinous cystic borderline tumor are present.

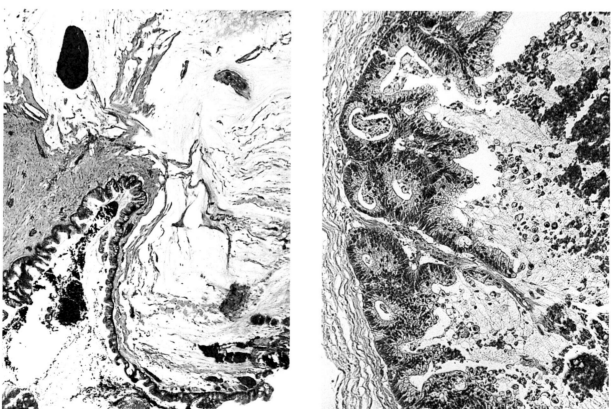

Figure 7-10

LOW-GRADE MUCINOUS CYSTADENOCARCINOMA OF TESTIS

Left: There is prominent extravasated mucin. Abundant mucoid tissue filled the scrotal sac.
Right: A high-power view of a different case shows basally oriented nuclei and apical cytoplasmic mucin.

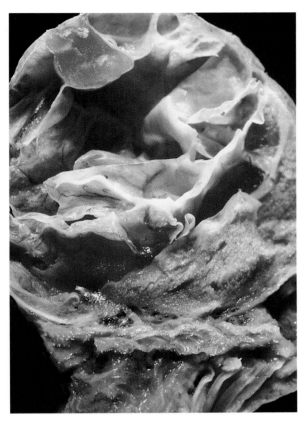

Figure 7-11

BRENNER TUMOR OF TESTIS

The sectioned surface shows a multiloculated cystic neoplasm that replaced the testis. (Courtesy of Dr. J.R. Srigley, Toronto, Canada.)

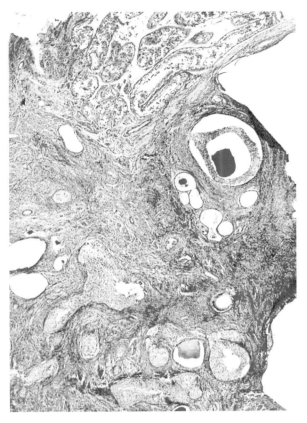

Figure 7-12

BRENNER TUMOR OF TESTIS

Nests of transitional cell epithelium, some with central lumen formation, lie in a fibrous stroma. Unremarkable seminiferous tubules are at the top.

nine cystic tumors that closely resembled ovarian serous borderline tumors on both gross and microscopic examination. Other ovarian-type tumors have been reported as *Brenner tumor* (figs. 7-11, 7-12) (20–25), *endometrioid adenocarcinoma* (figs. 7-13, 7-14) (5), or *clear cell adenocarcinoma* (5,26). A *mesodermal adenosarcoma* has been reported (27), and we have seen a tumor resembling a malignant mixed mesodermal tumor (fig. 7-15).

The average age in one series of six patients with serous carcinoma was 31 years (8); in a series of seven patients with serous borderline tumors, 56 years (6); and in a series and review of mucinous tumors, 56 years (12). The symptoms are the usual ones of a testicular or paratesticular mass; there may be an associated hydrocele. One serous carcinoma was associated with an elevated serum CA125 level (8). In one case of mucinous cystadenocarcinoma of the testis a similar tumor involved the contralateral epididymis (16).

Some of these tumors appear to arise by müllerian metaplasia of the peritoneal lining of the tunica vaginalis, and others probably originate from the appendix testis (2) or müllerian remnants in the connective tissue between the testis and epididymis or in the spermatic cord (28). An origin from the appendix testis is supported by a study of six serous carcinomas (8), which included four tumors centered on the epididymotesticular groove, the location of the appendix testis in the majority of the cases (29). Stronger evidence is provided by a case of endometrioid carcinoma that arose at the site of the appendix testis in a man treated for many years

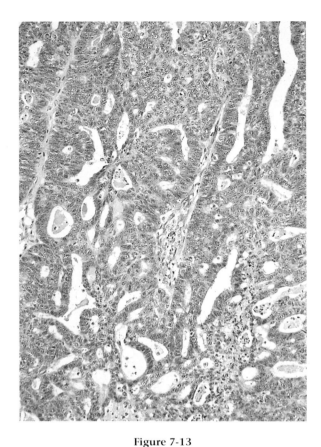

Figure 7-13

**ENDOMETRIOID ADENOCARCINOMA
OF PARATESTICULAR REGION**

The tumor has the typical glandular pattern. (Courtesy of Dr. N.M. Kernohan, Aberdeen, UK.) (Same tumor as figure 7-14.)

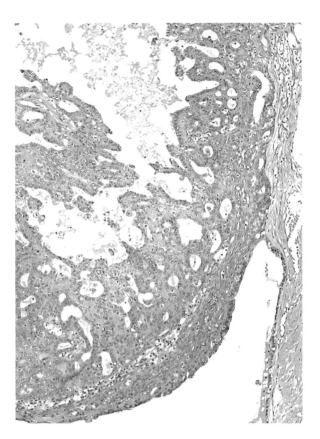

Figure 7-14

**ENDOMETRIOID ADENOCARCINOMA
OF PARATESTICULAR REGION**

This tumor projected into a cyst, the lining of which is seen at the bottom. The tumor in this region is composed of cells with appreciable eosinophilic cytoplasm; some of the tumor cells were spindle shaped. (Courtesy of Dr. N.M. Kernohan, Aberdeen, UK.)

with estrogen (figs. 7-11, 7-12) (2). Origin from persistent müllerian structures is documented in occasional other cases (14,26). Intratesticular mucinous tumors may represent monodermal teratomas, analogous to the presumed origin of a subset of ovarian mucinous cystic tumors, but the generally older patient age argues against this. Some Brenner tumors probably arise from the common Walthard nests of the tunica vaginalis (29). A final possible origin is the ovarian component of an ovotestis or the ovarian streak component of a dysgenetic gonad, such as one case of mucinous cystadenoma that was associated with adjacent tubal tissue (30). In accord with their variable histogeneses, some of these tumors are entirely intratesticular, whereas others are entirely paratesticular.

Gross Findings. The serous tumors of borderline malignancy are typically cystic; fleshy papillae line the cysts (fig. 7-1). The serous carcinomas are usually firm, gritty masses with indistinct margins (fig. 7-3). The mucinous tumors are prominently cystic and may be associated with conspicuous luminal mucin. The rare clear cell and endometrioid tumors have no specific features; one Brenner tumor had a solid and cystic sectioned surface (fig. 7-11) (20).

Microscopic Findings. The microscopic features are identical to those of the well-known ovarian counterparts and will not be reiterated in detail here (figs. 7-2, 7-4–7-10, 7-12–7-15) (31). Occasional serous tumors are predominantly borderline, with only small foci of invasion (3,8),

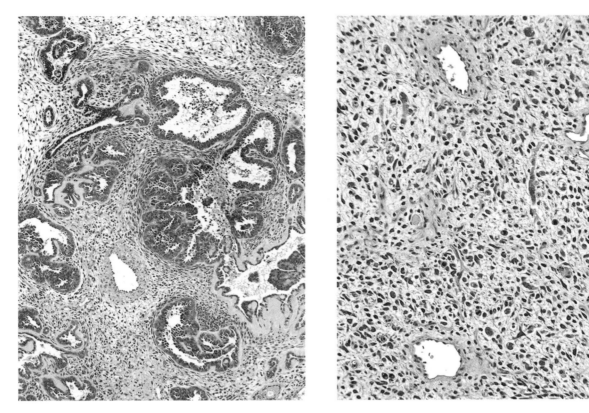

Figure 7-15

MALIGNANT MIXED MESODERMAL TUMOR OF PARATESTICULAR REGION

Left: Glands lined by malignant epithelium are set in a cellular, neoplastic stroma.
Right: At higher magnification, the stroma shows rhabdomyosarcomatous differentiation.

but at least one of these had a malignant course (8), in contrast to most ovarian tumors with "microinvasion." Psammoma body formation may be prominent in some cases of borderline or carcinomatous type (figs. 7-4, 7-5) (6).

The mucinous tumors may generate a prominent fibrotic reaction to extravasated mucin from ruptured cysts, with associated dystrophic calcification or even ossification (15). Some of the borderline mucinous tumors have an intracystic cribriform proliferation of highly atypical cells, justifying subclassification as "borderline mucinous tumor with intraepithelial carcinoma" (fig. 7-8) (12). One endometrioid carcinoma, which we examined, had typical areas as well as other foci with spindle cells felt to represent abortive squamous differentiation (fig. 7-14) (2).

The sex cord–like foci so common in endometrioid carcinoma of the ovary may be encountered in a tumor of the testis or para-

testis. One Brenner tumor was associated with an adenomatoid tumor (23), and another had areas of malignant degeneration (squamous cell and transitional cell carcinoma) and para-aortic lymph node metastases (21).

Immunohistochemical Findings. The serous borderline tumors stain for carcinoembryonic antigen (CEA), CD15, TAG-72 (B72.3 antibody), CA125, cytokeratin (CK)7, S-100 protein, estrogen receptor, and progesterone receptor (1,6,32). We have seen nuclear staining for WT1 in one case (fig. 7-16). The serous carcinomas share many of these immunoreactivities, with frequent positivity for S-100 protein, epithelial membrane antigen (EMA), Ber-EP4, CD15, and TAG-72 and, less commonly, CEA (8).

Little information is available concerning the mucinous tumors. One mucinous cystadenocarcinoma showed diffuse positivity for CK20 and MUC2 and focal reactivity for CK7 and

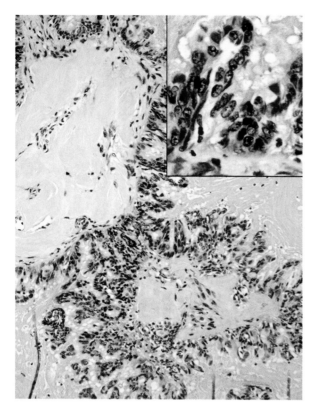

Figure 7-16

**SEROUS PAPILLARY CYSTIC TUMOR
OF BORDERLINE MALIGNANCY**

There is nuclear staining for WT1.

MUC5AC (17). One clear cell carcinoma was positive for CK7, EMA, bcl-2, HER2/neu, and CA125 but negative for CK20, CD15, estrogen receptor, and progesterone receptor (26).

Special Techniques. Image analysis of Feulgen-stained sections of serous borderline tumors demonstrated diploid values in 8 of 10 cases (6,33,34), a tetraploid result in 1 (6), and aneuploidy in 1 (1).

Differential Diagnosis. Serous tumors are easily confused with carcinomas of the rete testis (19), and they are also misinterpreted as mesotheliomas. The typical location of rete carcinomas in the hilus and the presence on microscopic examination of tumor nests in dilated rete channels are helpful in the differential diagnosis, as is the characteristic papillary budding of serous borderline tumors. The serous tumors are more commonly cystic and, in the case of borderline serous tumors, may have obviously ciliated cells and less cellular atypia than rete carcinomas. Conspicuous intrarete growth is usually absent and many cases predominantly involve the testicular surface or the parietal layer of the tunica vaginalis. Psammoma body formation also tends to be more prominent than in rete carcinoma.

Although serous borderline tumors of the tunica vaginalis may be grossly indistinguishable from mesotheliomas, the papillae in well-differentiated mesotheliomas are not as "bud-like" as those of serous borderline tumors, do not exhibit the same degree of cellular stratification, and are lined by more uniform cuboidal cells; psammoma bodies are typically rare, and cilia are absent. Similar features distinguish mesothelioma from serous carcinoma. Immunohistochemistry is helpful since serous papillary tumors are frequently positive for CD15, TAG-72 (B72.3), and CEA, and negative for calretinin whereas mesotheliomas have an opposite pattern.

Mucinous and endometrioid carcinomas must be distinguished on the basis of both clinical and pathologic findings from metastatic adenocarcinoma. Multinodular growth, bilateral testicular involvement, and prominent lymphovascular invasion favor metastasis. Clear cell carcinoma should be differentiated from the rare clear cell adenocarcinoma of the epididymis; the distinction depends on careful gross evaluation and is not always resolvable with certainty. The presence of benign-appearing endometrial tissue in association with the tumor supports primary ovarian-type clear cell (26) or endometrioid (5) carcinoma.

Intratesticular mucinous tumors should be distinguished from teratoma with a prominent mucinous component, as teratoma may be associated with other germ cell tumor types in contrast to the mucinous tumors, which have no such association. Thorough sampling will aid. Even the gross features are helpful because teratomas are generally solid and cystic and not uniformly or dominantly cystic like mucinous tumors. Teratoma is often associated with intratubular germ cell neoplasia, unclassified (IGCNU). It also tends to occur in younger patients (median, 23 to 29 years) than the mucinous tumors (median, 64 years) (12).

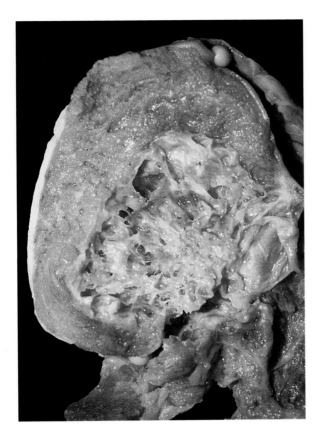 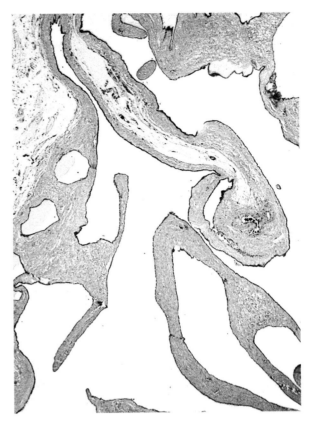

Figure 7-17

CYSTADENOMA OF RETE TESTIS

Left: A multilocular cystic mass involves the rete testis.
Right: The locules are lined by a single layer of epithelial cells.

Treatment and Prognosis. Experience with these tumors is limited because of their rarity, but nonetheless patients with borderline serous and mucinous tumors have favorable outcomes, with no known instance of metastasis or death in those with pure borderline tumors of either type, even when intraepithelial carcinoma is identified (6,12). They are, therefore, appropriately treated by radical orchiectomy alone. On the other hand, the invasive carcinomas may be aggressive, with metastases reported in serous, mucinous, and clear cell types (5,8,10,12,26). There may be a role for chemotherapy similar to that used in ovarian carcinomas for such patients (35). One serous borderline tumor with only focal invasion was associated with abdominal metastases after 7 years (8), indicating that even minimal invasion may be clinically consequential.

BENIGN TUMORS OF THE RETE TESTIS

General Features. Fewer than 20 *benign neoplasms of the rete testis* have been reported in patients from 6 to 79 years old, who almost always presented with a mass (36–43). These have included lesions designated as *adenoma, cystadenoma of usual type, sertoliform cystadenoma,* and *adenofibroma*. One lesion reported as "complex multilocular cystic lesion of the rete testis accompanied by smooth muscle hyperplasia" (42) probably represents *adenomyoma* with prominent cysts.

Gross and Microscopic Findings. On gross examination, the tumors vary from solid to cystic and are centered in the testicular hilum (fig. 7-17). On microscopic examination, cystadenomas of usual type consist of multilocular cysts lined by a single layer of cytologically bland,

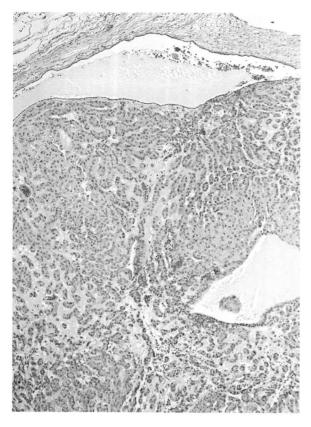

Figure 7-18

SERTOLIFORM CYSTADENOMA OF RETE TESTIS

A nodular proliferation of solid tubules grows within a dilated rete testis (top).

cuboidal to flattened epithelium and separated by septa of fibrous tissue. Tumors that have a greater degree of cellularity of the intervening stroma are appropriately designated as "cystadenofibroma"; if the epithelial component is present as noncystic tubular structures in a cellular stroma, the term "adenofibroma" is apt.

The sertoliform cystadenoma is distinct, consisting of a proliferation of sertoliform tubules with a scant accompanying fibrous stroma within dilated channels of the rete testis (figs. 7-18, 7-19). The tubules are mostly solid but may have central luminal spaces; they are lined by cuboidal to columnar cells with pale, eosinophilic cytoplasm and round, basally oriented nuclei that stain for inhibin and calretinin (39). The probable cystic adenomyoma described under General Features was a 4.5-cm multiloculated cyst lined

by flattened rete epithelium with intervening septa containing a prominent component of epithelioid smooth muscle cells (42).

Differential Diagnosis. Adenomatous hyperplasia of the rete testis (see chapter 8) is a non-neoplastic condition that usually does not present as a mass, unlike the benign neoplasms (44–46). It characteristically retains the arborizing configuration of the normal rete testis, although in an expanded profile, with normal-appearing rete cells lining the retiform tubules (47).

Rete testis hyperplasia with hyaline globule formation (see chapter 8) is a reactive lesion secondary to tumor invasion of the rete testis (48). It, therefore, is seen in testes harboring neoplasms, usually germ cell tumors, unlike the benign neoplasms. Although it causes the rete to appear more prominent, the arborizing architecture of the rete is retained, in contrast to the benign rete neoplasms, which also lack the hyaline globules.

Sertoli cell tumors are distinguished from sertoliform cystadenoma of the rete based on restriction of the latter to dilated rete testis channels. However, the cytologic and immunohistochemical features of these two lesions overlap.

CARCINOMA OF THE RETE TESTIS

General and Clinical Features. *Carcinomas of the rete testis* are rare: approximately 60 legitimate examples have been reported in patients ranging from 8 to 91 years of age (40,49), with a mean age in the sixth decade. More than 80 percent of patients present with a scrotal mass, sometimes associated with pain, although some present with metastases involving lung, bone, or skin (50,51). Direct tumor spread to involve scrotal skin is common. Up to 30 percent of patients have a concomitant or, less frequently, preceding hydrocele that may mask the underlying neoplasm.

Because other histologically similar tumors may involve the paratestis, a number of criteria have been proposed to ensure accurate diagnosis of rete testis carcinoma (47,52). These include: 1) absence of a neoplasm elsewhere that microscopically resembles rete carcinoma; 2) tumor grossly centered at the testicular hilum; 3) morphologic and/or immunohistochemical features incompatible with other forms of primary testicular and paratesticular neoplasms; and 4)

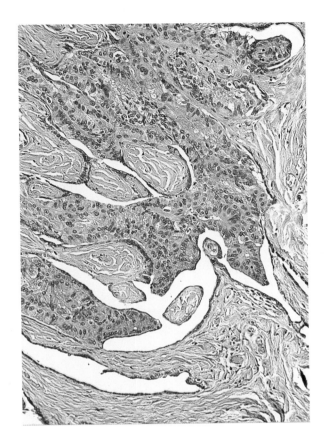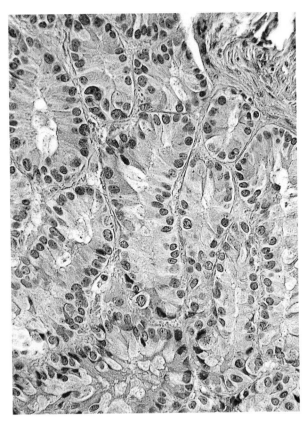

Figure 7-19

SERTOLIFORM CYSTADENOMA OF RETE TESTIS

Left: An epithelial proliferation exhibiting tubular differentiation protrudes into dilated rete channels.
Right: High-power view demonstrates the resemblance of the tubules to those of a Sertoli cell tumor.

at least partial tumor growth within channels of the rete testis. It has also been proposed that the identification of a "transition" from benign to malignant epithelium within the rete testis should be a required criterion (fig. 7-20), but we feel this is too restrictive and does not permit the establishment of a firm diagnosis in cases that are unequivocally primary tumors that have obliterated the non-neoplastic rete epithelium. Furthermore, metastatic carcinomas may grow within the rete and replace its epithelium, thereby mimicking a transition from benign to malignant (see fig. 7-127) (53).

Gross Findings. The tumors range from 1 to 12 cm and are typically solid, firm, and rubbery. They may have a minor cystic component and, rarely, are predominantly cystic (fig. 7-21). The tissue is usually white but may be yellow or gray. In addition to the dominant mass, smaller

tumor nodules may be present on the tunica albuginea, and, in 30 percent of the cases, there is gross involvement of the spermatic cord.

Microscopic Findings. Microscopic examination reveals tubular, papillary, and solid patterns. Low-power magnification often shows large cellular nodules and smaller irregular clumps. The tubules are typically elongated, compressed, and slit-like (fig. 7-22). The papillae, which are present in three quarters of the cases, may project into cysts, and may be small or large with fibrous or hyalinized cores (fig. 7-23). In some cases they resemble the chordae retis of the non-neoplastic rete testis (fig. 7-23). Growth within dilated channels of the rete testis is apparent (fig. 7-24), as are foci of stromal invasion. Occasional tumors have psammoma bodies (51). Varying amounts of necrosis may be present. There may be solid areas

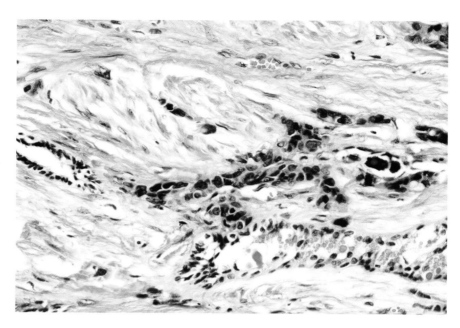

Figure 7-20

HIGH-GRADE EPITHELIAL DYSPLASIA OF RETE TESTIS

This focus was seen adjacent to an invasive rete adenocarcinoma. Both benign and malignant-appearing epithelial cells coexist within the tubules of the rete.

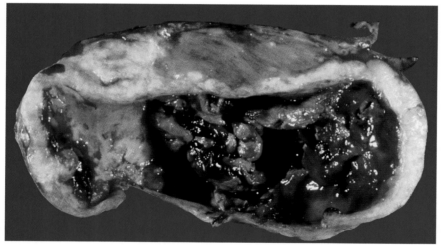

Figure 7-21

CARCINOMA OF RETE TESTIS

Abundant hemorrhagic tumor fills most of this cystic neoplasm. (Courtesy of J.Y. Ro, Houston, TX.)

with a nonspecific appearance and focal tubular differentiation. Rarely, a sertoliform appearance is conspicuous (54). Occasional tumors have a cellular spindle cell component that results in a biphasic pattern (55,56). The stroma is often prominent and may be extensively hyalinized. The neoplastic cells are typically small and cuboidal with scanty cytoplasm (figs. 7-23, 7-24); nuclear stratification and at least moderate nuclear pleomorphism and mitotic activity are usually present. Spread into the testicular parenchyma may be conspicuous (57).

Immunohistochemical Findings. The tumors are positive for cytokeratins (AE1/AE3,

CAM5.2, CK7), EMA, and Ber-EP4 (49,50,58-62). Calretinin, PAX2, and PAX8 were positive in one case each and CK5/6 negative (51,63). Variable results have been obtained for CEA (fig. 7-25), CD15, and CK20 (49,51,60,62,64).

Ultrastructural Findings. On electron microscopic study (51,56,65-67), the tumor forms glands or papillary structures lined by cells that usually have short apical microvilli with an intervening glycocalyx. A prominent Golgi apparatus is characteristic, as are scattered lipid droplets. The nuclei vary from round to deeply clefted. Adjacent cells are joined by variably developed junctions that may include pentalaminate desmosomes.

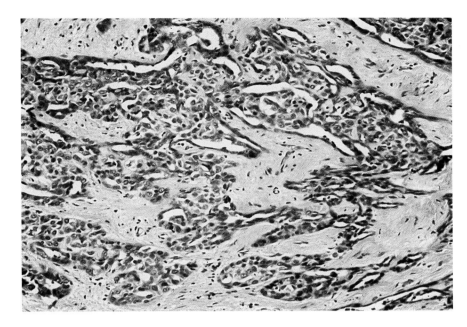

Figure 7-22

ADENOCARCINOMA OF RETE TESTIS

The typical slit-like glandular pattern is seen.

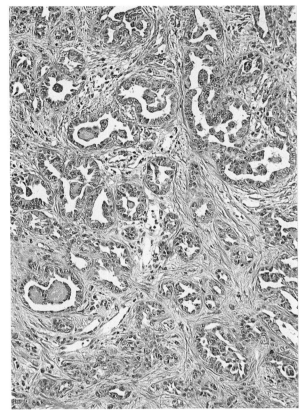

Figure 7-23

ADENOCARCINOMA OF RETE TESTIS

This metastatic focus of tumor shows distinctive papillae with hyalinized cores.

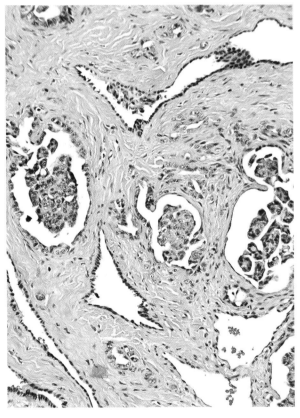

Figure 7-24

ADENOCARCINOMA OF RETE TESTIS

The tumor grows as nests within dilated channels of the rete testis.

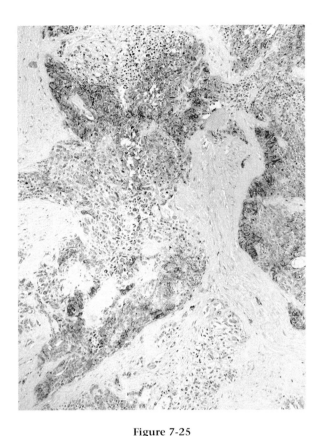

Figure 7-25

ADENOCARCINOMA OF RETE TESTIS

There is patchy reactivity for carcinoembryonic antigen.

Differential Diagnosis. Metastatic adenocarcinomas from various sites may simulate adenocarcinoma of the rete testis and, as noted under the diagnostic criteria, an extratesticular primary must be excluded before the latter is diagnosed. Carcinomas of the prostate gland, kidney, and lung are among the most problematic. The tendency of some metastatic carcinomas, especially prostatic (53), to grow predominantly or exclusively within the channels of the rete testis can be especially misleading. The morphology of these tumors is usually at least somewhat different from those of rete carcinoma. The prostatic carcinomas we have seen that extensively involved the rete had the morphologic features of prostatic ductal carcinoma, consisting of radial arrangements of columnar cells on villus-like fibrovascular cores. This contrasts with the glands and papillae lined by cuboidal cells or the solid arrangements with slit-like glands that

characterize many rete testis carcinomas. Utilization of specific markers of various metastatic carcinomas, including prostate-specific antigen, prostatic acid phosphatase, renal cell carcinoma marker (RCC), TFE3, and TTF-1 is helpful.

Distinction of rete adenocarcinomas from serous tumors of the testis is discussed with the latter.

Mesotheliomas may simulate rete testis carcinomas because of their elongated, slit-like tubules. The distribution of mesothelioma on the surfaces of the tunica vaginalis and the presence of other distinctive patterns (see Malignant Mesothelioma), however, should help in the differential diagnosis. Histochemical and immunostains assist with this differential diagnosis, since mesotheliomas are typically negative for neutral mucins, CEA, CD15, Ber-EP4, TAG-72 (B72.3), PAX2, and PAX8, and many rete adenocarcinomas stain for one or more of these (19,52,63). Furthermore, most mesotheliomas are positive for calretinin and CK5/6 and there is at least one report of negative results for these markers in a rete carcinoma (51). The presence of long microvilli on ultrastructural examination is considered diagnostic of mesothelioma in this context (19,52), whereas rete carcinomas have stubby or absent surface microvilli (51,56,65,67).

In some atrophic testes, a prominent and seemingly hyperplastic rete may result in an erroneous suspicion of adenoma or carcinoma. Rarely, true hyperplasia of the rete testis occurs, but this is usually a consequence of invasion of the rete by some other tumor; the cytologic features of malignancy are lacking in the rete epithelium in such cases and there are often hyaline globules within the rete channels (see chapter 8).

Spread and Metastasis. Carcinomas of the rete testis initially spread locally and then via lymphatics to para-aortic and iliac lymph nodes. Hematogenous spread to many sites, including lung, liver, and bone, may be seen. Involvement of scrotal skin is common.

Treatment and Prognosis. Radical orchiectomy is the initial treatment of choice. There may also be a role for retroperitoneal lymph node dissection (49,66). There is no proven benefit for chemotherapy and radiation (49). The overall prognosis is poor. In one review, the 3-year survival rate was 49 percent and the 5-year rate was 13 percent (49). No patient whose initial tumor was larger than 5 cm survived 1 year, whereas the 3-year survival rate for those whose tumors were less than 5 cm was 75 percent (49).

ADENOMATOID TUMOR

General and Clinical Features. *Adenomatoid tumor* is of mesothelial origin and is the most common benign neoplasm of the testicular adnexa, accounting for about 60 percent of the cases. It occurs at any age but is rare in children (68). More than 90 percent of the patients present with a mass (69). Although it usually is located in the epididymis, often at the lower pole, it also arises in the tunica albuginea and extends into the testicular parenchyma (70,71) or, rarely, arises in the spermatic cord (72). Despite the infiltrative borders of some tumors, the clinical course is invariably benign (68,70-83).

Gross Findings. The adenomatoid tumor is almost always unilateral and solitary, and rarely exceeds 5 cm in diameter (fig. 7-26). Although typically round or oval and well demarcated (fig. 7-26A), it may be plaque-like (fig. 7-26B) and have ill-defined margins. It is composed of solid, white, tan to gray-white, glistening tissue; when it involves the testis prominently, it may resemble a seminoma (fig. 7-26C).

Microscopic Findings. The cardinal features are tubules, cords, and clusters of vacuolated cells (figs. 7-27, 7-28). Although in most cases the tubules have round to oval lumens, they may also be cystic or slit-like. The neoplastic cells lining the tubules vary from flat to columnar and contain moderate to large amounts of dense, eosinophilic cytoplasm. Infrequently, the cells lack vacuoles, resulting in solid tubules and cords that, when densely packed, cause a diffuse pattern that may lead to diagnostic confusion (fig. 7-29). The nuclei are oval to elongated, with uniform chromatin, and often have a single conspicuous nucleolus. Mitotic figures are rare.

One emphasized feature is the occurrence of "thread-like bridging strands" of cytoplasm that cross the luminal spaces (fig. 7-30), a finding identified in all 41 cases in one study (84). This feature may be inconspicuous in those tumors in which vacuoles are scant, and should not be considered specific, as similar structures may be seen in epithelioid hemangiomas (85).

The stroma, which is often prominent (figs. 7-31, 7-32), is usually fibrous and sometimes hyalinized (fig. 7-31); it may contain smooth muscle (fig. 7-32) (86), which rarely predominates, and lymphoid aggregates, which may be prominent (fig. 7-32) (87). Focal papillae are rare (fig. 7-33). One unusual tumor had a cellular mesenchymal component with atypical cytologic features (68). The interface with adjacent testicular tissue may be sharp (fig. 7-34) or irregular (fig. 7-35), with prominent infiltration between preserved, compressed seminiferous tubules (71,88).

Infarction of the tumor can result in a confusing morphology. Central foci of necrosis containing mummified tumor are surrounded by a reactive myofibroblastic or granulation tissue response, with sometimes inconspicuous foci of residual typical adenomatoid tumor (fig. 7-36). Irregular peripheral extension of reactive myofibroblasts and the occurrence of this phenomenon in tumors with a solid, cellular appearance may cause concern for malignancy (89).

Immunohistochemical Findings. Adenomatoid tumors stain in a manner that reflects their mesothelial nature. They are positive for cytokeratins (AE1/AE3, CAM5.2), calretinin, podoplanin (D2-40), thrombomodulin, human mesothelial cell membrane (HBME)-1, EMA, WT1 (nuclear), and GLUT-1, whereas CK5/6 is usually negative or only focally reactive (69,87,90). They are negative for factor VIII-related antigen, CD34, Ber-EP4, CEA, alpha-inhibin, TAG-72, CD15, PAX2, PAX8, androgen receptor, and p53 (63,69,73,90–95).

Ultrastructural Findings. Cuboidal to flattened cells line variably prominent luminal spaces and are conjoined by tight junctional complexes. Abluminal basal laminar material separates the cells from the collagenous stroma. Long, slender microvilli project from the cell surface into the lumen (80,82,96).

Cytologic Findings. Cytologic preparations show fairly uniform cells with sheet-like, corded, and glandular arrangements (97–99). The nuclei are eccentric, with finely granular chromatin and small nucleoli. The cytoplasm is lightly staining and often prominently vacuolated. In one report, a fine needle aspiration preparation showed the "tigroid" background that is a common feature of seminoma (98), a finding that may cause diagnostic confusion.

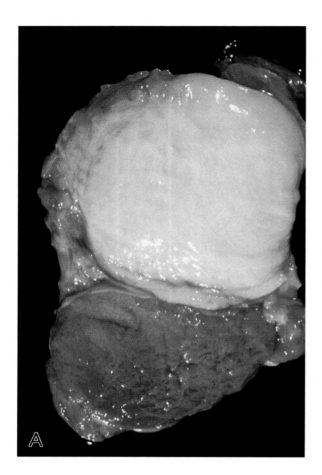

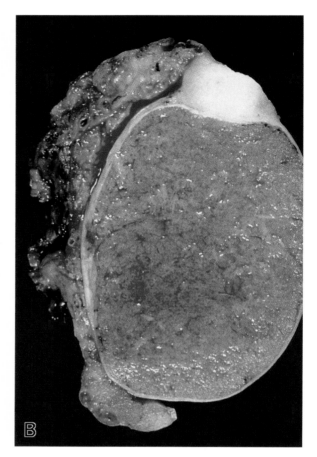

Figure 7-26

ADENOMATOID TUMOR

A: The epididymis is replaced by a large, cream-colored, bulging mass. (Fig. 8.1 from Young RH, Scully RE. Testicular tumors. Chicago: ASCP Press; 1990:169.)

B: A cap-like grayish white tumor involves and expands the tunica albuginea. (Courtesy of Dr. F.B. Askin, Baltimore, MD.)

C: This tumor lies mostly in the testis and resembles seminoma. (Courtesy of Dr. B. Delahunt, Wellington, New Zealand.)

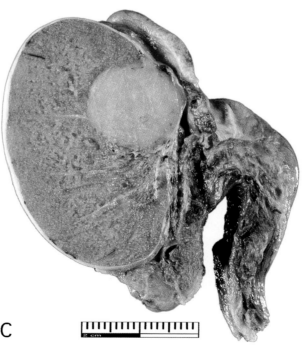

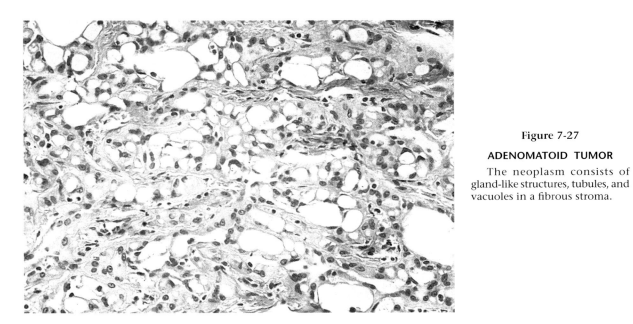

Figure 7-27

ADENOMATOID TUMOR

The neoplasm consists of gland-like structures, tubules, and vacuoles in a fibrous stroma.

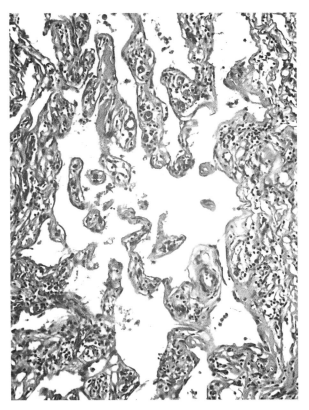

Figure 7-28

ADENOMATOID TUMOR

The tubules in this neoplasm are focally cystic.

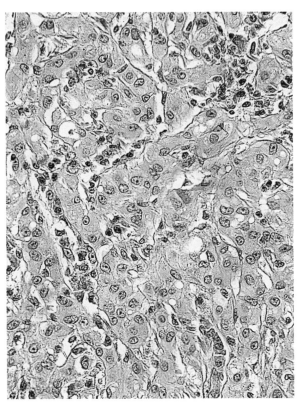

Figure 7-29

ADENOMATOID TUMOR

There is a solid proliferation of cells with appreciable eosinophilic cytoplasm and lack of the characteristic conspicuous vacuoles.

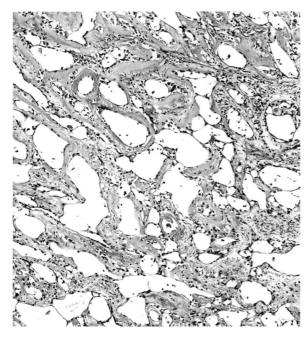

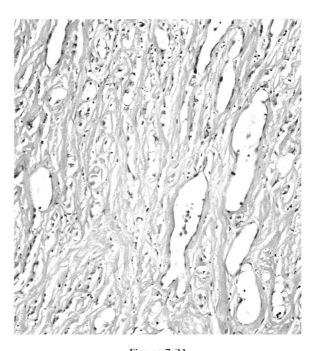

Figure 7-30

ADENOMATOID TUMOR

In this case, many of the tubules have thread-like bridging strands of cytoplasm across the lumens.

Figure 7-31

ADENOMATOID TUMOR

There is prominent stromal hyalinization.

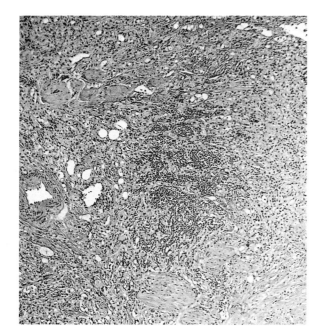

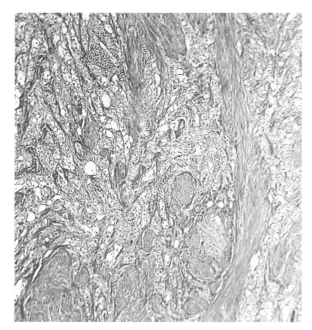

Figure 7-32

ADENOMATOID TUMOR

Left: This low-power view shows a focally prominent lymphoid infiltrate and scattered bundles of smooth muscle.
Right: A Masson trichrome stain shows that the stroma contains both smooth muscle and collagen.

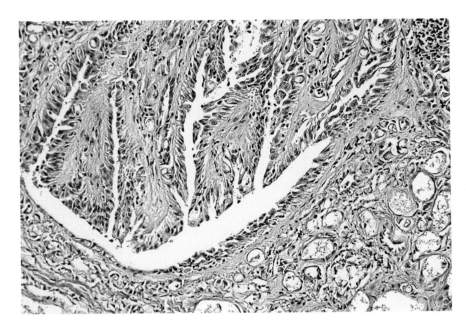

Figure 7-33

ADENOMATOID TUMOR

This unusual example has focal papillae with areas of typical appearance (bottom) elsewhere.

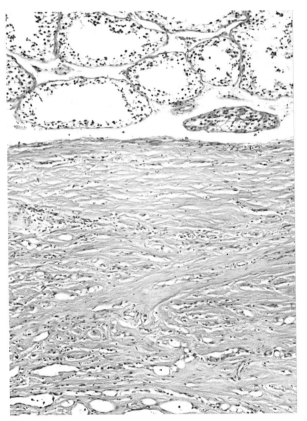

Figure 7-34

ADENOMATOID TUMOR

There is a sharp interface with the adjacent seminiferous tubules.

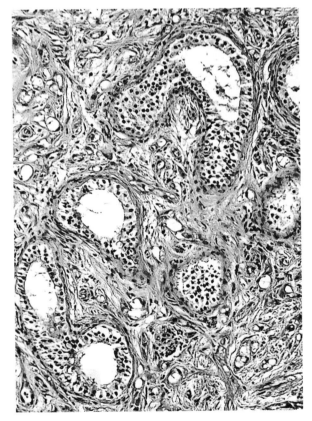

Figure 7-35

ADENOMATOID TUMOR

This tumor infiltrated irregularly between the seminiferous tubules.

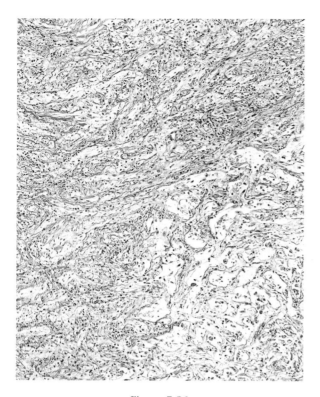

Figure 7-36

ADENOMATOID TUMOR

An area of tumor infarction (lower right) is surrounded by a proliferation of adenomatoid tubules and myofibroblastic cells.

Differential Diagnosis. The plethora of histologic patterns of adenomatoid tumors raise diverse considerations in the differential diagnosis, ranging from sex cord tumors, to vascular tumors, to signet ring cell tumors, to benign mesenchymal neoplasms (for stroma-predominant cases or those with infarction), to malignant mesothelioma, and other rare considerations. Entirely removed adenomatoid tumors are only occasionally the source of diagnostic problems because of their typically innocuous gross appearance and the awareness of their common occurrence in this region. If an adenomatoid tumor is only biopsied, usually in the frozen section setting, initial confusion with malignant mesothelioma may occur and the gross features of the tumor should be ascertained. It is helpful that malignant mesotheliomas are often large and typically diffuse in contrast to adenomatoid tumors. The biphasic pattern of some mesotheliomas is incompatible

with an adenomatoid tumor, and the atypia and diffuse papillae of many mesotheliomas exceeds that of an adenomatoid tumor.

The vacuolated cells of an adenomatoid tumor may suggest the reticular pattern of yolk sac tumor, but the cells do not have the primitive nuclear features, mitotic activity, or other patterns of the latter; in rare cases where doubt persists immunohistochemical positivity of the yolk sac tumor for alpha-fetoprotein, glypican 3, and SALL4 is helpful. Also, yolk sac tumor is rarely primary in the paratestis, although we have seen one such case.

The vacuoles and gland-like differentiation may also simulate a metastatic adenocarcinoma, particularly signet ring cell adenocarcinoma. Appreciation of the overall pattern of the tumor is almost invariably helpful in this regard, and the quiescent appearance of the stroma in an adenomatoid tumor contrasts with the desmoplasia often seen in the stroma of a metastatic signet ring cell carcinoma. Also, adenomatoid tumors are only weakly reactive in luminal spaces for neutral mucins and in only a minority of cases (82), whereas signet ring carcinomas are frequently strongly positive for them. Immunopositivity for calretinin, podoplanin, and WT1 in the adenomatoid tumor is also helpful.

Adenomatoid tumor should be distinguished from rare examples of epithelioid (histiocytoid) hemangioma that involve the testis. It is probable that some of the reported cases of "adenomatoid tumor" that exhibited immunohistochemical staining for vascular markers are examples of this neoplasm. Distinction between the two may be difficult on routine microscopic examination, but the cells lining the spaces in an epithelioid hemangioma typically are plumper than in adenomatoid tumor, and their nuclei frequently have a very irregular, cleaved contour. Both entities may have thin strands of cytoplasm that bridge luminal spaces. Some epithelioid hemangiomas are associated with a prominent infiltrate of eosinophils. Finally, in some of the vascular tumors, the lesional spaces are clearly vessel lumens filled with blood, unlike the spaces in adenomatoid tumor. In a problematic case, immunohistochemical staining for vascular markers resolves the dilemma.

Appreciation of the primarily paratesticular location of an adenomatoid tumor is particularly important in cases that simulate primary tumors of the testicular parenchyma because of the prominently solid, cellular growth with inconspicuous vacuoles of the later. If such a tumor is thought "testicular" rather than paratesticular, problems may ensue. Furthermore, some adenomatoid tumors involve the testicular parenchyma to an appreciable degree and whether the tumor actually arose in the testis or paratestis may not be obvious.

Two primary testicular tumors that are occasionally simulated because of a tubular pattern or diffuse growth of cells with eosinophilic cytoplasm are the Sertoli cell tumor and Leydig cell tumor. When Sertoli cell tumors have conspicuous vacuoles they tend to be more patchily distributed than in adenomatoid tumors, and most have more lightly staining cytoplasm. Focal sertoliform tubules and, rarely, intratubular growth favor a Sertoli cell tumor. Inhibin may be positive in Sertoli cell tumors but is negative in adenomatoid tumors (92). Although calretinin and WT1 may be positive in Sertoli cell tumors, negativity for these markers favors Sertoli cell tumor over adenomatoid tumor. Features favoring Leydig cell tumor include prominent cytoplasmic lipofuscin, foamy cytoplasm, and absence of cytoplasmic vacuoles. Reinke crystals are pathognomonic of Leydig cell tumor. The strong and diffuse cytokeratin reactivity in adenomatoid tumors contrasts with its usual absence in Leydig cell tumors, as does the inhibin negativity of the former (92).

MALIGNANT MESOTHELIOMA

General and Clinical Features. *Malignant mesothelioma* of the tunica vaginalis is uncommon, with approximately 220 cases reported in the literature (100). They comprise less than 1 percent of all malignant mesotheliomas (101). Although two thirds occur in patients older than 45 years (median, 60 years), occurrence in children as young as age 6 years is documented (102-104). Many are associated with a hydrocele, which may recur repeatedly after tapping; in several patients with recurrent hydrocele, the mesothelioma was overlooked for months, or rarely, even years (105,106). The tumor occasionally presents as an incidental finding in a hernia sac. A mass or ill-defined firmness may be palpated, but the diagnosis of a neoplasm is usually not established until the time of explo-

ration (101). A history of asbestos exposure is present in 40 percent of the patients in whom information on exposure, or lack thereof, is available (107). Some very papillary tumors have been equated to the "well-differentiated papillary mesothelioma" of the peritoneum (108), but we caution against use of that term as a diagnostic label because it has led to the conclusion that the neoplasm is benign, which it is not. If completely resected the prognosis may be good, but in our opinion even low-grade papillary mesotheliomas are malignant neoplasms.

Gross Findings. The tumor either coats the tunica vaginalis (fig. 7-37) or multiple nodules of tumor stud it (fig. 7-38). An associated hydrocele and reactive changes may result in gross features that are inconclusive for a neoplasm. An occasional small tumor is not grossly evident. Rarely, the tumor is predominantly or exclusively intratesticular (102). The tumor may infiltrate the adjacent spermatic cord, epididymis, or testis (fig. 7-37).

Microscopic Findings. Microscopic examination reveals patterns similar to those encountered in malignant mesotheliomas of the pleura and peritoneal cavity (figs. 7-39–7-49). Approximately 75 percent of the tumors are epithelial and 25 percent biphasic (fig. 7-44) (107). Purely sarcomatoid mesotheliomas, to the best of our knowledge, have not been described at this site. The epithelial tumors are typically papillary (figs. 7-39–7-41) or tubulopapillary (fig. 7-42). Papillary tumors may be predominantly exophytic and noninvasive, but at least focal infiltration of the wall of a hydrocele sac or the tunica occurs in most. The papillae often have thick fibrovascular cores (fig. 7-40), which are occasionally hyalinized, edematous (fig. 7-41), or even myxoid, and these are mostly lined by a single layer of cuboidal (fig. 7-40) to flat (fig. 7-41) neoplastic mesothelial cells. The infiltrating tubules vary from large and oval to small and round or slit-like (fig. 7-43). Rare tumors contain occasional psammoma bodies. When the tumor involves the testis proper, it usually effaces tubules but may infiltrate between them (fig. 7-47) and, rarely, exhibits a striking intratubular pattern of growth (fig. 7-48). Involvement of the skin of the scrotum, penis, or suprapubic area may occur, and pagetoid involvement of the skin has been described.

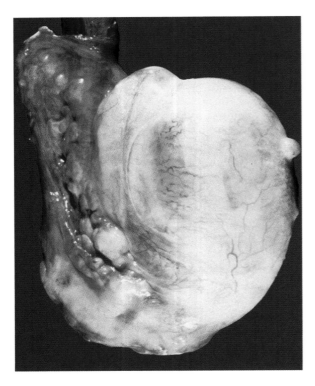

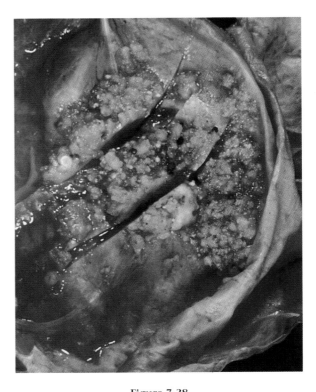

Figure 7-37

MALIGNANT MESOTHELIOMA

The tunica vaginalis is diffusely thickened by white tumor tissue which extends irregularly into the adjacent epididymis and surrounding soft tissue. (Fig. 14-18 from Ro JY, Grignon DJ, Amin MB, Ayala A. Atlas of surgical pathology of the male reproductive tract. Philadelphia: W.B. Saunders; 1997:177.)

Figure 7-38

MALIGNANT MESOTHELIOMA

The tunica vaginalis is studded by focally confluent papillary tumor tissue. (Fig. 8.7 from Young RH, Scully RE. Testicular tumors. Chicago: ASCP Press; 1990:172.)

Figure 7-39

MALIGNANT MESOTHELIOMA

A papillary neoplasm arises from the tunica vaginalis.

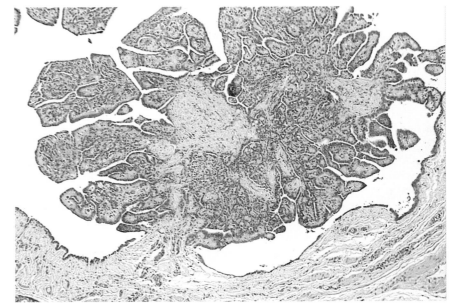

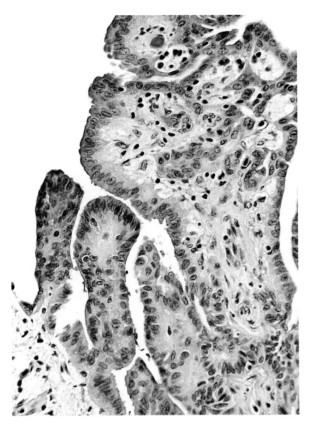

Figure 7-40

MALIGNANT MESOTHELIOMA

Papillae are lined by a single layer of cells with fairly bland cytologic features.

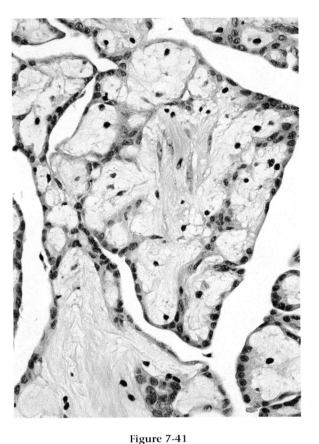

Figure 7-41

MALIGNANT MESOTHELIOMA

Broad, edematous papillae are lined by a single layer of flat, neoplastic mesothelial cells.

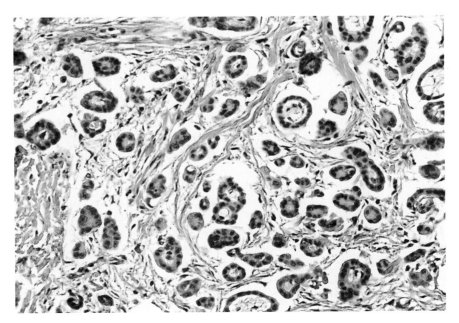

Figure 7-42

MALIGNANT MESOTHELIOMA

This tumor has a tubulo-papillary pattern.

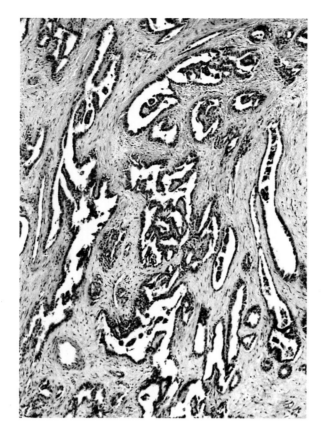

Figure 7-43

MALIGNANT MESOTHELIOMA

This slit-like pattern of glands is reminiscent of a carcinoma of the rete testis.

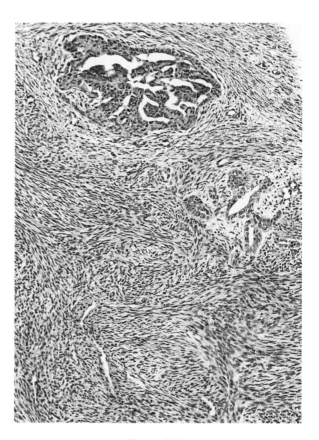

Figure 7-44

MALIGNANT MESOTHELIOMA

This tumor has a distinct biphasic pattern.

The neoplastic cells are typically cuboidal and uniform (fig. 7-40), with scant to moderate amounts of eosinophilic cytoplasm in well-differentiated tumors. Other cases are highly malignant appearing: they lack cilia and rarely show prominent cytoplasmic vacuoles and occasionally have abundant eosinophilic cytoplasm (fig. 7-45). The sarcomatous component of biphasic cases varies from relatively uniform spindle cells with tapered nuclei arranged in fascicles (fig. 7-44) to haphazard growth of plump, pleomorphic, stellate to epithelioid cells (fig. 7-45).

Immunohistochemical Findings. There is usually strong positivity for calretinin, EMA, thrombomodulin, and CK7. CK5/6 is also usually positive but frequently focally so (107,109). In one study, 2 of 18 cases showed focal (5 percent) cytoplasmic staining for Ber-EP4 (109). One case was positive for podoplanin (110) and

another for WT1 (111). CEA, TAG-72, CD15, PAX2, and PAX8 are negative (63,107,109).

Ultrastructural Findings. Ultrastructural examination shows long branching microvilli, cytoplasmic microfilaments, and desmosomes (112). The long microvilli are considered the most specific finding; they are found in the epithelioid cells but not the sarcomatous cells of biphasic tumors (113).

Differential Diagnosis. Malignant mesothelioma must be distinguished from florid mesothelial hyperplasia (114) and from other neoplasms that it may resemble. The clinical presentation is helpful in the distinction from hyperplasia, which is more common in hernia sacs than hydrocele sacs. Most hydroceles with mesothelial hyperplasia show fibrotic thickening of their walls secondary to recurrent exudates. The presence of a mass with the typical

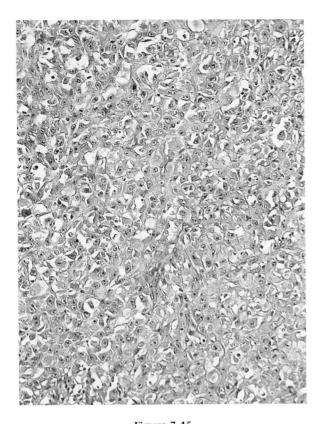

Figure 7-45

MALIGNANT MESOTHELIOMA

There is a sheet-like growth of cells with abundant eosinophilic cytoplasm.

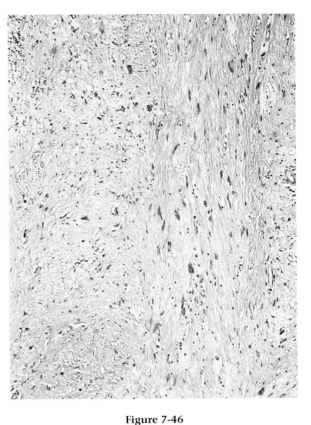

Figure 7-46

MALIGNANT MESOTHELIOMA

There is a sarcomatoid arrangement of highly atypical cells. An epithelioid component was present elsewhere.

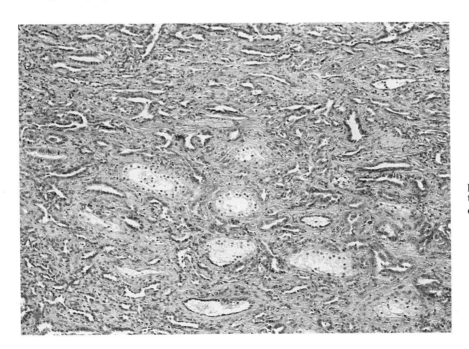

Figure 7-47

MALIGNANT MESOTHELIOMA

This tumor has a tubular pattern with prominent infiltration into the testicular parenchyma.

335

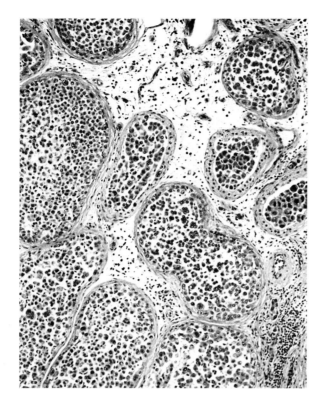

Figure 7-48

MALIGNANT MESOTHELIOMA

There is prominent growth within seminiferous tubules.

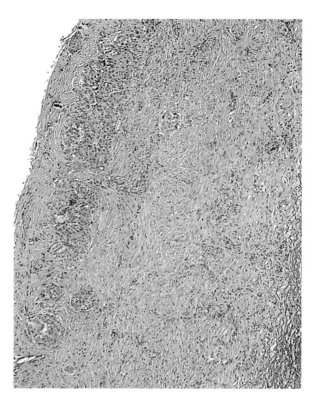

Figure 7-49

MALIGNANT MESOTHELIOMA

A tumor within a hydrocele sac specimen shows, at the left, a prominent, almost confluent band-like proliferation of atypical mesothelial cells, which focally infiltrate into the subjacent wall. On the basis of this field alone, establishing the diagnosis would be difficult.

studding of a hydrocele sac is incompatible with the diagnosis of mesothelial hyperplasia, which is almost invariably a microscopic finding only. Nonetheless, as noted above, some mesotheliomas have their gross features masked by inflammatory changes, and in such cases, microscopic findings are discriminatory. On microscopic examination, mesothelial hyperplasia does not exhibit the complex, arborizing, papillary fibrous stalks of papillary mesotheliomas. In mesothelial hyperplasia dominated by a tubular pattern, there is usually an intense inflammatory background, an organized "layered" arrangement of the tubules, and a lack of the overt invasion almost always appreciable in mesothelioma. In mesothelial hyperplasia, there is a zonation of cellularity from near the surface, where it is greatest, to the deeper aspect. Additionally, the hyperplastic mesothelial cells tend to "stop" along a fairly well-defined linear interface with the fibrous stroma of the hydrocele, whereas mesotheliomas show irregular penetration and lack the gradient

of cellularity (115). Deep penetration into muscle strongly correlates with mesothelioma (115).

The differential diagnosis with serous tumors is considered with those tumors.

The clinical features of carcinoma of the rete testis overlap with those of mesothelioma, and, in addition, both tumors may have papillary and tubular patterns. Rarely, mesothelioma also has slit-like tubules similar to those of carcinomas of the rete testis (47). Features that are helpful in the distinction of these two neoplasms have been previously discussed in the section dealing with rete testis carcinomas.

The grossly infiltrative growth of malignant mesothelioma helps distinguish it from the typically circumscribed adenomatoid tumor. Also, the round, oval, or slit-like tubules and characteristic intracytoplasmic vacuoles of adenomatoid tumor with bridging thread-like strands are rarely prominent features of malignant mesothelioma. Papillae are never prominent in adenomatoid tumor in contrast to mesothelioma. Cytologic atypia and mitotic activity are features of some mesotheliomas but are absent in almost all adenomatoid tumors.

Pleomorphic sarcomas with abundant eosinophilic cytoplasm, including pleomorphic rhabdomyosarcoma and malignant fibrous histiocytoma, as well as metastatic high-grade carcinomas, may mimic mesothelioma. Appropriate immunostains can resolve this differential and gross differences are helpful, with prominent plaque-like or nodular thickening of the tunica vaginalis favoring mesothelioma.

Spread and Metastasis. Tumor progression is most commonly manifest as local recurrence involving scrotal skin and perineum. Next in frequency is lymph node metastasis, including retroperitoneal, inguinal, and iliac; the usual visceral sites are lung/pleura and liver. Peritoneal implants are also frequent.

Treatment and Prognosis. In a comprehensive review, 53 percent of patients developed recurrences and 38 percent of patients died of disease after a median survival period of 24 months (102). More than 60 percent of recurrences occur in the first 2 years after surgery, but recurrence as late as 15 years has been reported (107). Even low-grade papillary tumors may be clinically malignant (107). They may be multifocal, predisposing to recurrence, and tumors that were initially noninvasive may later exhibit stromal invasion in recurrences.

The extent of disease at presentation has important prognostic implications. Six of 13 (46 percent) patients who had tumor confined to a hydrocele sac and who had at least a 2-year follow-up were disease free (107). In contrast, only 1 of 19 (5 percent) patients with either local invasion of the spermatic cord, skin, or testis, or distant metastasis at the time of diagnosis was without disease. The prognosis is more favorable in patients younger than 60 years (102).

Aggressive therapy is required; radical orchiectomy is recommended. In about 15 percent of the cases, involvement of the scrotal skin at presentation has necessitated hemiscrotectomy. Dissection of clinically or radiographically involved lymph nodes has been advocated (102). Various chemotherapeutic regimens and

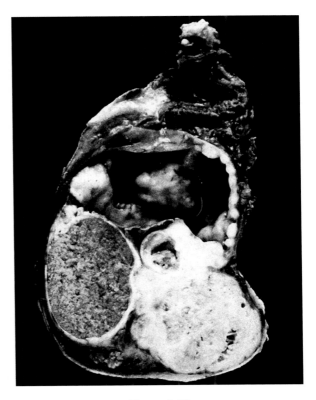

Figure 7-50

DESMOPLASTIC SMALL ROUND CELL TUMOR

The tunica vaginalis is distended and studded by multiple, variably sized gray-white tumor nodules. (Courtesy of Dr. J. Prat, Barcelona, Spain.)

radiation are used to treat metastatic disease, but their efficacy has not been proven to date.

DESMOPLASTIC SMALL ROUND CELL TUMOR

General and Clinical Features. Fewer than 20 cases of *desmoplastic small round cell tumor* have been described in the paratesticular region in the English language literature (116–125). The tumors usually present as scrotal masses in patients of the typical young age (17 to 43 years) for this malignant neoplasm. Although this is a highly malignant neoplasm, the prognosis of patients with paratesticular involvement is better than that of the most common intra-abdominal neoplasms, probably secondary to earlier discovery.

Gross Findings. The tumors usually range from 2.5 to 5.5 cm. They are typically bosselated or nodular, white to tan, firm masses that usually lack significant necrosis (fig. 7-50). Tumor

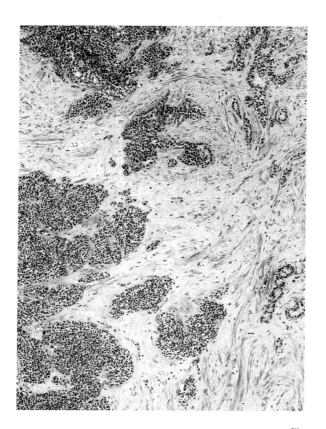
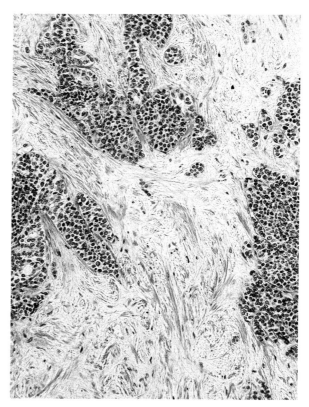

Figure 7-51

DESMOPLASTIC SMALL ROUND CELL TUMOR

Left: Solid nests of cells with scant cytoplasm lie in a desmoplastic stroma. Focal tubular differentiation is seen at the right.
Right: The cells have generally uniform oval nuclei.

studding of the tunics away from the dominant mass and extensive involvement of the epididymis are common.

Microscopic Findings. On microscopic examination the tumors are composed of multiple nodules that are typically made up of nests and islands of uniform-appearing small cells, which usually grow diffusely within the nests (fig. 7-51). Occasionally, short cords or small tubules (fig. 7-51, left) are evident. In some cases the nests have central zones of comedo-like necrosis (fig. 7-52). The intervening stroma has a typical desmoplastic appearance, as denoted by the name of this tumor. The tumor cells typically have scant cytoplasm, with round to oval nuclei having finely stippled chromatin and indistinct nucleoli. Some cells have appreciable eosinophilic cytoplasm. Mitotic figures are frequent. One reported tumor contained scattered psammoma bodies, and another had focal pseudorosettes.

Since the original description of this entity, a number of morphologic variants have become evident, including those with greater cellular pleomorphism, rhabdoid morphology, spindled configurations of the lesional cells, adenoid cystic-like architecture, and signet ring morphology (123). While not all have been seen in paratesticular cases, the potential remains.

Immunohistochemical Findings. One of the defining features of this tumor is its polyimmunophenotypic nature: it is usually positive for cytokeratin, desmin (fig. 7-53), EMA, neuron-specific enolase, and WT1 protein. CD99 and FLI1 protein, two markers of Ewing sarcoma/primitive neuroectodermal tumor, are usually negative. Myogenin and myoD1 are uniformly negative.

Ultrastructural Findings. These tumors frequently show juxtanuclear aggregates of intermediate filaments and, less commonly,

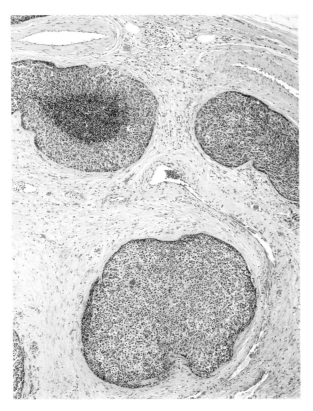

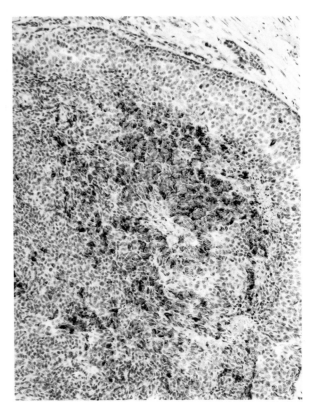

Figure 7-52

DESMOPLASTIC SMALL ROUND CELL TUMOR

There is conspicuous central necrosis within one of the tumor nests.

Figure 7-53

DESMOPLASTIC SMALL ROUND CELL TUMOR

There is patchy reactivity for desmin.

dendritic-like processes containing dense core neurosecretory-type granules (116,126). Glycogen may be present (116); thin, actin-like filaments and Z-bands are absent (126).

Cytologic Findings. There are sheets and cohesive clusters of densely packed cells with hyperchromatic nuclei having fine chromatin, irregular nuclear membranes, and usually inconspicuous nucleoli. The cytoplasm is scant (127–129). Some degree of nuclear molding may be seen (129). In some cases, a collagenous stromal component is apparent (129,130).

Special Techniques. This tumor has a distinctive cytogenetic anomaly involving a reciprocal translocation between portions of chromosomes 11 and 22, t(11;22)(p13;q12), which results in an EWS-WT1 gene fusion (131). The detection of the translocation by cytogenetic analysis or fluorescence in situ hybridization (FISH) provides confirmatory evidence of the diagnosis and may be of

crucial importance when the morphologic and immunohistochemical findings are atypical.

Differential Diagnosis. Desmoplastic small round cell tumor must be distinguished from three other "small blue cell" tumors that may be primary, or at least present, in the paratesticular area: embryonal rhabdomyosarcoma, malignant lymphoma, and retinal anlage tumor. Embryonal rhabdomyosarcoma occurs, with rare exceptions, at a much younger age (mean age, 6.6 years), and frequently has a myxoid to cellular stroma, unlike the uniformly desmoplastic stroma of this tumor. Occasional cells with striking eosinophilic cytoplasm or spindled cells point to rhabdomyoblastic differentiation. In conjunction with other features, their presence is helpful in establishing a diagnosis of rhabdomyosarcoma, and the demonstration of cytoplasmic cross striations is pathognomonic. Although cells with eosinophilic cytoplasm may be seen in

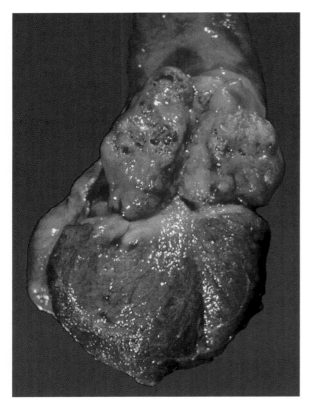

Figure 7-54
PAPILLARY CYSTADENOMA OF EPIDIDYMIS
The tumor is well circumscribed and yellow.

the desmoplastic tumor, they lack the densely eosinophilic quality of rhabdomyoblasts. Immunostains for desmin are not helpful in this differential diagnosis but those for cytokeratins, myogenin, and myoD1 are.

Malignant lymphomas may superficially appear similar to desmoplastic tumors but lack the characteristic nested pattern and desmoplastic stroma. In problematic cases, an appropriate panel of immunohistochemical stains (leukocyte common antigen, cytokeratin, desmin, and neuron-specific enolase) is helpful, especially in limited samples of small round cell tumors of this region.

As the morphologic spectrum of the desmoplastic small round cell tumor has expanded since its initial description, some unusual features, such as tubules and rosettes, may cause confusion. The differential diagnosis with retinal anlage tumor is discussed with the latter.

Treatment and Prognosis. For primary tumors, radical orchiectomy is usually performed. In some cases, desmoplastic round cell tumors involving the paratestis represent spread from an intraperitoneal tumor in the abdomen via a patent processus vaginalis. Unfortunately, the tumor has usually spread to abdominal peritoneal sites and is resistant to systemic treatment, although there are sporadic case reports of good responses to various regimens. About half of patients with paratesticular tumors are alive at least 2 years after diagnosis, which contrasts with the greater mortality seen in the abdominal cases (125).

PAPILLARY CYSTADENOMA OF THE EPIDIDYMIS

General and Clinical Features. *Papillary cystadenoma of the epididymis* is a benign neoplasm that is often associated with von Hippel-Lindau disease; one review found that 40 percent of patients had the syndrome (132), a figure that may be falsely high due to selection bias. In one study, all epididymides from patients with von Hippel-Lindau disease harbored at least microscopic foci of papillary cystadenoma (133). Clinical masses are found in one third to two thirds of patients upon careful examination (132). Bilateral papillary cystadenomas may be the initial manifestation of the disease (132,134). The neoplasms, both syndrome associated and sporadic, occur over a wide age range and are bilateral in about one third of the cases (135). Bilaterality occurs twice as frequently in those with von Hippel-Lindau disease (132). Although a scrotal mass is the usual presentation, some patients develop pain as the initial manifestation. Rarely, cystadenomas of this type are unassociated with the epididymis and occur high in the cord (136).

Gross Findings. The tumors are up to 5 cm in diameter and are centered in the head of the epididymis, consistent with a derivation from the efferent ductules (133). They may be cystic, solid, or cystic and solid; some are bright yellow (fig. 7-54) or tan.

Microscopic Findings. Tubules and cysts that often contain an eosinophilic colloid-like secretion are present. Variably prominent papillae often project into the cysts (fig. 7-55). The papillae are lined by a single layer of cytologically benign columnar cells that typically have clear glycogen and lipid-rich cytoplasm (fig. 7-56)

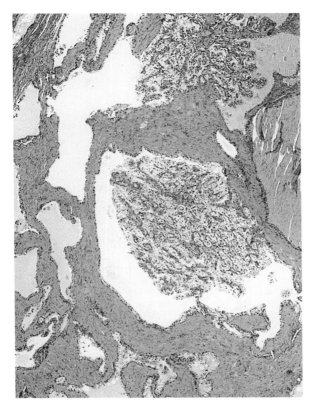

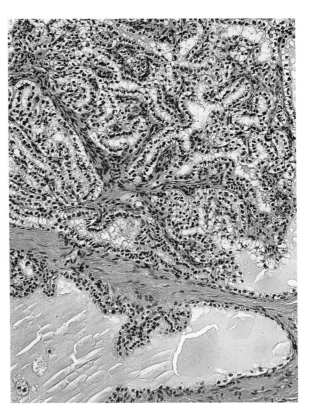

Figure 7-55

PAPILLARY CYSTADENOMA OF EPIDIDYMIS

Papillae project into several cysts.

Figure 7-56

PAPILLARY CYSTADENOMA OF EPIDIDYMIS

The clear cytoplasm and bland cytologic features are evident.

(137). One unique tumor we saw apparently underwent malignant degeneration.

Immunohistochemical Findings. Papillary cystadenomas are positive for several cytokeratins (CK7, CAM5.2, AE1/AE3) and EMA (138). PAX2 and RCC marker may also be positive (139), although RCC marker is more commonly negative (138). CD10 is negative in the epididymal cases but was positive in a mesosalpingeal example (138). CK20 is negative (138).

Ultrastructural Findings. The cells contain cytoplasmic aggregates of glycogen granules and lipid droplets (140). Microvilli and occasional cilia are present at the apex.

Special Techniques. In patients with von Hippel-Landau disease who have a germline mutation of the VHL gene, there is a somatic mutation in the second allele within the cells of the efferent ductules (133). Because of loss of VHL protein, hypoxia-inducible factor increases

and induces tumor formation by downstream signaling events (133).

Differential Diagnosis. The features of epididymal papillary cystadenoma are unlike those of any other entity at this site, and, accordingly, there are few realistic considerations in the differential diagnosis. Spermatocele with proliferative epithelium ("mural papilloma") is distinguished from epididymal papillary cystadenoma by its more focal nature, its more cuboidal or even flattened epithelium, and the association with degenerating spermatozoa (141). Metastatic renal cell carcinoma generally exhibits a more heterogeneous microscopic appearance, greater cytologic atypia, or a striking sinusoidal vascular pattern. Unlike papillary cystadenoma, clear cell renal carcinoma is negative for CK7 and positive for CD10 (138). We have seen a unique cystadenoma of the epididymis that formed long, villous-like processes

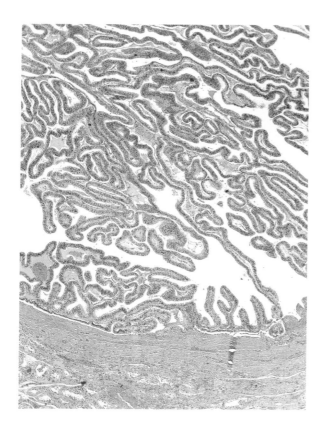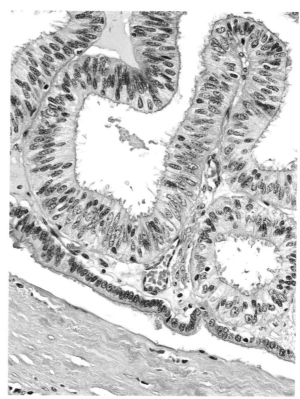

Figure 7-57

CYSTADENOMA OF EPIDIDYMIS

Left: There is an intracystic proliferation of long, villus-like processes adjacent to the testis.
Right: Cytologically bland, pseudostratified, columnar epithelium with apical cilia line the fibrovascular cores.

lined by ciliated columnar cells with eosinophilic cytoplasm rather than clear cytoplasm that, in our opinion, merited distinction from conventional papillary cystadenoma (fig. 7-57).

CARCINOMA OF THE EPIDIDYMIS

General, Clinical, and Gross Features. Only 10 epididymal carcinomas hold up to close scrutiny (figs. 7-58, 7-59) (142–145). The tumors occurred in adults who had no distinctive clinical features. Specifically, there was no evidence of von Hippel-Lindau disease in any patient. The gross characteristics were not distinctive (fig. 7-59).

Microscopic Findings. These tumors are usually characterized by tubular (fig. 7-58) or tubulopapillary structures lined by clear cells that at least focally contain glycogen. In one unpublished case that we saw, there was a component of a papillary cystadenoma that correlated

with a 40-year history of a small epididymal mass that underwent recent rapid growth (fig. 7-59). Rarely, the tumor has the features of a squamous cell carcinoma (135), a small cell carcinoma (144), or a basaloid carcinoma (145). The rare epididymal squamous metaplasia (see chapter 8) may provide the basis for squamous cell carcinoma at this site.

Differential Diagnosis. Adenocarcinoma of the epididymis may be confused with clear cell papillary cystadenoma or metastatic adenocarcinoma. Although there are some shared architectural and cytologic features with the cystadenoma, specifically the tubulocystic aspect and focal clear cells, the obviously invasive glandular pattern, focal necrosis, and cytologic features of adenocarcinoma are differentiating features. As with any carcinoma of the testicular and paratesticular regions, a metastasis should always be carefully excluded by appropriate microscopic

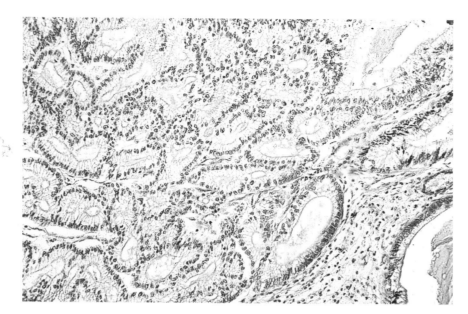

Figure 7-58

**ADENOCARCINOMA
OF EPIDIDYMIS**

There is a confluent growth of glands lined by columnar cells with abundant pale cytoplasm.

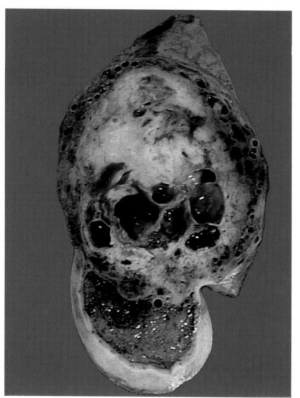

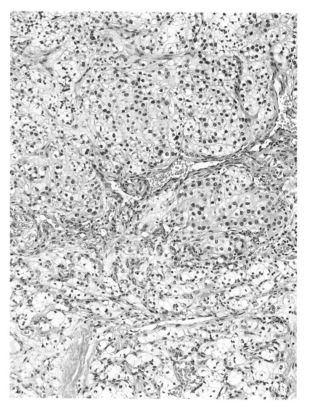

Figure 7-59

CLEAR CELL CARCINOMA OF THE EPIDIDYMIS ASSOCIATED WITH PAPILLARY CYSTADENOMA

Left: A yellow-gray mass with areas of hemorrhage and cystic degeneration abuts the testis. (Courtesy of Dr. N. Kanomata, Kurashiki, Okayama, Japan)

Right: A diffuse pattern of atypical clear cells (top) is contiguous with a tubular pattern of benign papillary cystadenoma (bottom).

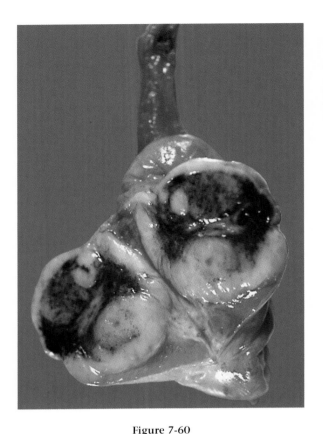

Figure 7-60

RETINAL ANLAGE TUMOR

There is prominent pigmentation of the neoplasm.

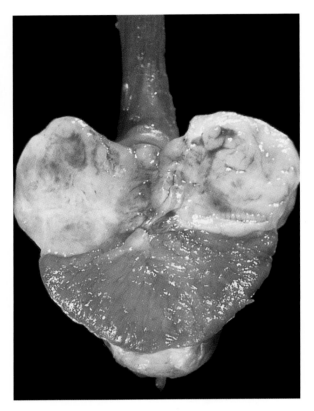

Figure 7-61

RETINAL ANLAGE TUMOR

Much of the sectioned surface of this neoplasm is gray-tan, with only focal pigmentation.

analysis and, if indicated, clinical investigation. Finally, it should be remembered that the epithelium of the normal epididymis often shows a cribriform pattern and occasionally contains atypical cells similar to those seen more commonly in the seminal vesicle (146,147).

RETINAL ANLAGE TUMOR

General and Clinical Features. The rare *retinal anlage tumor,* also called *melanotic neuroectodermal tumor, melanotic hamartoma,* and *melanotic progonoma,* occurs in the epididymis (148–154), usually in children 10 months of age or less. Three of 21 tumors of this type proved clinically malignant, with the development of lymphatic-based spread (149,154).

Gross Findings. Most of the tumors are well circumscribed and round to oval. They are usually 4 cm or less in diameter. The sectioned surface is typically brown or black, at least focally (fig. 7-60),

but may be predominantly or even exclusively cream colored (148) or gray (fig. 7-61).

Microscopic Findings. Microscopic examination reveals sheets, nests (figs. 7-62–7-64), cords, and spaces (fig. 7-65) composed of or lined by cells of two types: large columnar to cuboidal cells with vesicular nuclei and prominent nucleoli, often containing melanin pigment in their cytoplasm (figs. 7-63, 7-64), and a predominant population of smaller cells with round to oval, hyperchromatic nuclei and scanty cytoplasm (fig. 7-64). The latter cells may exhibit considerable mitotic activity, and, when prominent, individual fields may resemble neuroblastoma, but Homer-Wright rosettes are absent. The tumor cells may infiltrate between the epididymal tubules (fig. 7-66), a finding not indicative of a malignant nature, and usually lie in a fibrous, rarely desmoplastic, stroma (fig. 7-62).

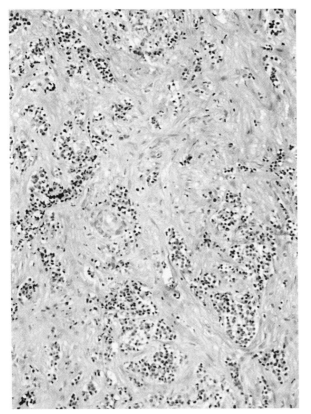

Figure 7-62

RETINAL ANLAGE TUMOR

Nests of cells lie in a fibrous stroma. At this magnification, melanin pigmentation is inconspicuous.

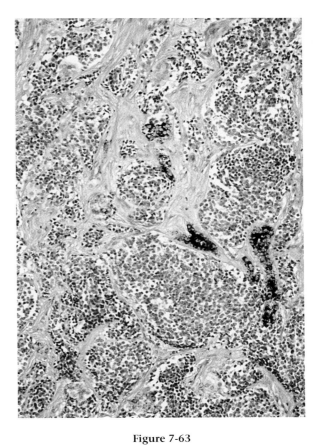

Figure 7-63

RETINAL ANLAGE TUMOR

Nests of nonpigmented cells are separated by stroma in which lie other cells that are overtly pigmented.

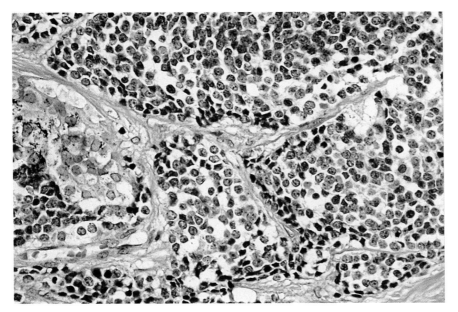

Figure 7-64

RETINAL ANLAGE TUMOR

Most of the cells in the nests are small, with scant cytoplasm, and resemble the cells of neuroblastoma, but occasional larger cells at the left have some melanin pigment in their cytoplasm.

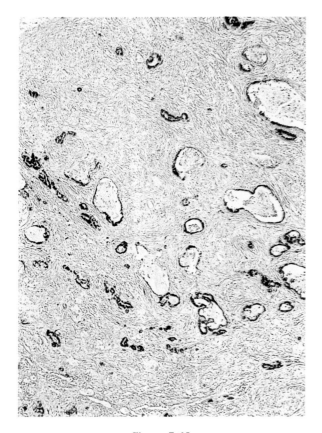

Figure 7-65

RETINAL ANLAGE TUMOR

Tubules and cysts are lined by cells with prominent melanin pigmentation.

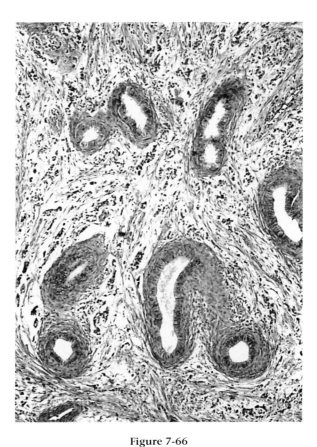

Figure 7-66

RETINAL ANLAGE TUMOR

The tumor infiltrates irregularly between epididymal tubules.

Masson-Fontana stains aid in the identification of melanin pigment, which establishes the diagnosis. Those cases that have followed a malignant course are not distinguishable from the benign ones, although in one there was an unusual single file pattern of growth in a desmoplastic stroma (149).

Immunohistochemical Findings. Both the large and small cells are positive immunohistochemically for neuron-specific enolase, synaptophysin, and HMB45 (151,152,155); S-100 protein may be identified in the large cells (152) but is often negative (151). There is less frequent, more variable reactivity for glial fibrillary acidic protein, desmin, EMA, and Leu-7 (CD57). Cytokeratin is usually restricted to the large cells (151,155).

Ultrastructural Findings. The small cells show neuroblastic features with neurosecretory granules and the large cells demonstrate melanosomes in various stages of development.

Cytologic Findings. Large and small tumor cells are seen, the former with abundant cytoplasm containing occasional melanotic granules and the latter with scant cytoplasm and high nuclear to cytoplasmic ratios (156,157).

Special Techniques. Molecular genetic studies of this tumor have been negative for MYCN amplification, chromosome 1p deletion, and 11:22 chromosomal translocations, supporting no relationship to neuroblastoma, Ewing sarcoma/primitive neuroectodermal tumor, and desmoplastic small round cell tumor (158). Flow cytometric studies have shown both diploid and aneuploid results that lacked correlation with clinical recurrences (159).

Differential Diagnosis. Because of its cellularity, mitotic activity, and small cells, retinal anlage tumor may resemble several small cell malignant tumors that occur in this location in children, particularly embryonal rhabdomyosarcoma, undifferentiated sarcoma (148), and metastatic or primary neuroblastoma (160,161). Desmoplastic small round cell tumor may also be a consideration when the two cell types and melanin pigment are inconspicuous. By definition, they must be present to establish the diagnosis of retinal anlage tumor and should be assiduously sought before making a more ominous, and erroneous, diagnosis (148). Differentiation from desmoplastic small round cell tumor is particularly problematic in the rare case in which the retinal anlage tumor has a desmoplastic stroma. Appropriate immunostains may help in this circumstance. Although both neuroblastoma and desmoplastic small round cell tumor may express neuroendocrine-type markers, neither is positive with HMB45, and neuroblastoma is cytokeratin negative. Malignant lymphoma may potentially enter the differential diagnosis but is unlikely to be a problem except perhaps in a biopsy specimen. The paratesticular location of the retinal anlage tumor and the absence of associated teratomatous elements distinguish it from the exceedingly rare melanotic neuroectodermal tumor of the testis (see chapter 4).

Treatment and Prognosis. As of 2006, there were 21 cases involving the epididymis and/or testis (154). Of these, 3 tumors (14 percent) metastasized, either to lymph nodes or adjacent lymphatics. All of the patients, however, were alive after treatment on follow-up from 28 to 48 months (154). Local excision is the usual treatment, with lymph node dissection reserved for those with clinical evidence of nodal involvement.

SOFT TISSUE TUMORS: BENIGN OR LOCALLY AGGRESSIVE

Benign soft tissue tumors are rare in the testis but more common in the spermatic cord and epididymis. *Lipomas* and *leiomyomas* are the most common benign tumors in this region (162), but essentially any soft tissue tumor may be seen in the paratesticular soft tissue or spermatic cord, and rarely in the testis itself (163,164). In one general hospital series, lipomas outnumbered leiomyomas about 4 to 1

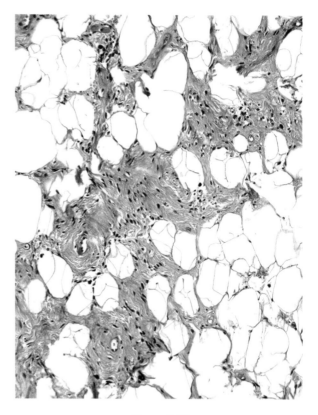

Figure 7-67

SPINDLE CELL LIPOMA OF PARATESTICULAR REGION

This neoplasm was diffusely positive for CD34. There is overlap with the features of mammary-type myofibroblastoma.

(163). It remains controversial whether most of the lipomas are true neoplasms or examples of lipomatous hyperplasia, and it may be difficult to distinguish those that develop from the cord from those that originate in the preperitoneal fat and invade the cord secondarily (165). Nonencapsulated accumulations of mature adipose tissue, scrotal lipomatosis, may mimic a lipoma and have been recorded to cause massive enlargement of the scrotum (166).

Variant morphologies of lipoma are seen, including the spindle cell type (fig. 7-67) (167) (the morphologic, immunohistochemical, and cytogenetic features of which overlap with those of mammary-type myofibroblastoma and cellular angiofibroma [168,168a]), as well as *angiolipoma* (164), *angiomyxolipoma* (169), and *myolipoma* (164). Occasionally, paratesticular leiomyomas have an epithelioid (170) or

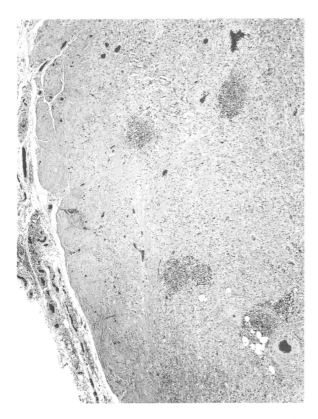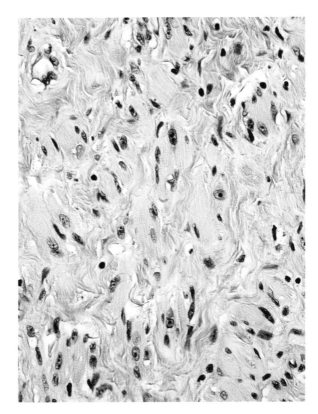

Figure 7-68

RHABDOMYOMA, GENITAL TYPE, OF PARATESTICULAR REGION

Left: A nodular proliferation of rhabdomyocytes is interspersed with collagen and occasional collections of lymphocytes.

Right: The elongated lesional cells are present in a collagenous stroma and show distinct cross striations.

plexiform morphology (171) or have an appearance similar to a leiomyoma of the uterus with bizarre nuclei (172). Paratesticular *rhabdomyomas* (fig. 7-68) (164,173), *perineuriomas* (174,175), *desmoid-type fibromatoses* (176–178), *hemangiomas* (179), *neurofibromas* (180), *granular cell tumors* (181), *ganglioneuromas* (182), *schwannomas* (183–185), *myxomas* (186), and *superficial angiomyxomas* (187) are rare, as are *lipoblastomas* in infants (188,189). A testicular *myofibroma* in a 3-month-old infant has been reported (190), as have a testicular *interdigitating dendritic cell tumor* and an *inflammatory myofibroblastic tumor* in a 37- and 33-year-old, respectively (191). The features of the various soft tissue tumors are as seen elsewhere. Only lesions of particular interest that cause significant diagnostic difficulty or are recently described are reviewed here.

Fibromatous Tumors

General and Clinical Features. A classification of the *fibromatous tumors* and tumor-like lesions is presented in Table 7-1. Fibromas of the testicular parenchyma are rare if those of gonadal stromal origin, which are histologically identical to the much more common ovarian fibromas, are excluded (192,193). These tumors and those of likely myofibroblastic derivation were considered together in chapter 6. One example we saw replaced almost the whole testis (fig. 7-69) and was extensively hyalinized (192). Another example grossly simulated a seminoma (194).

More common, although still rare, are fibromas of the testicular tunics (fig. 7-70). Some authors consider those tumors to be part of the spectrum of "fibrous pseudotumor" of "inflammatory sclerotic" subtype (195) but

Table 7-1

CLASSIFICATION OF BENIGN FIBROMATOUS TUMORS AND TUMOR-LIKE LESIONS OF TESTIS, ADNEXA, AND CORD

Tumors
  Parenchymal fibromas of gonadal stromal origin
  Fibromas of tunica albuginea[a]
  Paratesticular fibromas of soft tissue type[a]
  Angiomyofibroblastoma-like tumor (cellular angiofibroma)

Tumor-Like Lesions[b]
  Fibrous pseudotumor
  Proliferative funiculitis (inflammatory myofibro-blastic tumor)

[a]Some cases meet the criteria for "solitary fibrous tumor."
[b]Discussed in chapter 8.

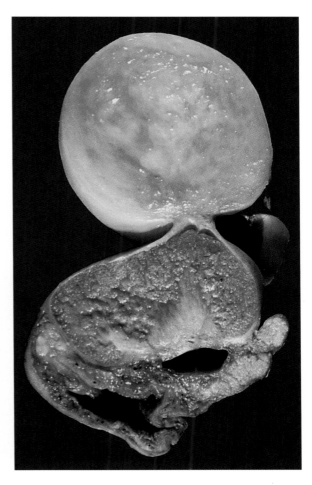

Figure 7-70

FIBROMA OF TUNICA ALBUGINEA

The pedunculated tumor is tethered to the tunica by a small stalk. The underlying testis is uninvolved. (Fig. 8.32 from Young RH, Scully RE. Testicular tumors. Chicago: ASCP Press; 1990:184.)

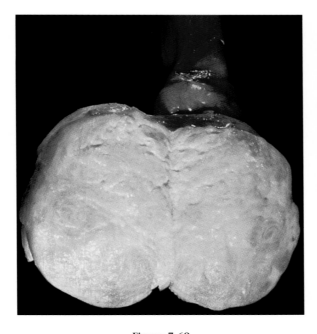

Figure 7-69

FIBROMA OF TESTIS

The testicular parenchyma is replaced by a large white mass that was firm.

we regard such cases as fibromas with features similar to solitary fibrous tumor. Fibromas of the tunics are seen over a wide age range, from the second to eighth decades (192,195). The patients present with scrotal masses.

Gross Findings. Most fibromas of the tunics are circumscribed, white, whorled nodules that may be pedunculated (fig. 7-70), although focal infiltration into the adjacent testis occurs in

some. Variable myxoid change may be present. Most are attached to the tunica albuginea, although they may also be separate from it with a covering of tunica vaginalis (192,195). Massive size is possible but uncommon.

Microscopic Findings. On microscopic examination, these neoplasms are typically mildly to moderately cellular, with bland, oval (fig. 7-71), spindle, or stellate cells lying in a myxoid or collagenous matrix (fig. 7-72) that is typically prominently vascular (fig. 7-73). Those tumors resembling the solitary fibrous tumor (fig. 7-73) frequently have thick bundles of eosinophilic collagen, a hemangiopericytomatous-type

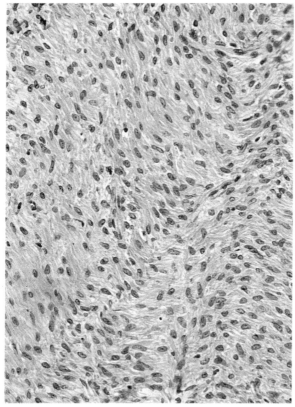

Figure 7-71

FIBROMA OF TUNICA ALBUGINEA

The tumor cells are regular without atypical cytologic features.

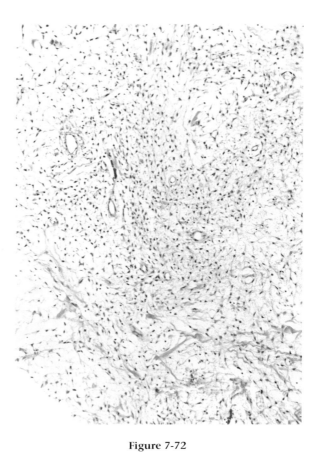

Figure 7-72

FIBROMA OF TUNICA ALBUGINEA

Round to stellate spindle cells lie within an edematous background.

Figure 7-73

FIBROMA OF TUNICA ALBUGINEA

This tumor is vascular and has features resembling those of the so-called solitary fibrous tumor.

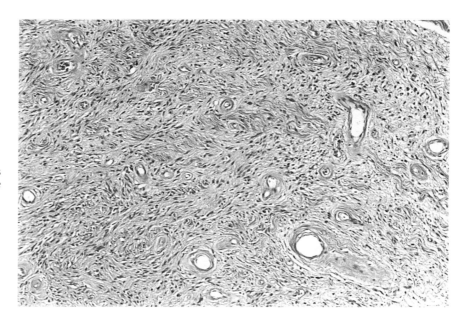

branching vasculature, and reactivity for CD34 (192,195).

Differential Diagnosis. True fibromas of the paratesticular region may be confused with the reactive fibrous proliferations referred to by a variety of terms such as fibrous pseudotumor. Fibromas, however, lack the association with a hydrocele, trauma, or conspicuous inflammation that is often present in non-neoplastic proliferations; the latter are usually multinodular or diffuse hypocellular fibroblastic proliferations with abundant, often hyalinized collagen that is frequently calcified and may exhibit prominent inflammation. Fibromas lack the granulation tissue-like pseudosarcomatous cellularity and infiltration of so-called proliferative funiculitis.

Cellular Angiofibroma/ Angiomyofibroblastoma-Like Tumor

General and Clinical Findings. *Cellular angiofibroma* (also known as *angiomyofibroblastoma-like tumor*) occurs most commonly in middle-aged to older men (median age, 60 years) as a scrotal or inguinal mass that clinically is usually felt to represent a hernia (196,197). Such masses may be of months' to years' duration, and are usually painless.

Gross and Microscopic Findings. On gross examination, they are usually circumscribed, with an approximate mean diameter of 8 cm. The cut surface is typically soft to rubbery and gray-white to yellow-tan or pink; sometimes they are mucoid (fig. 7-74) (197). Foci of necrosis are uncommon (196,197). A multilobular pattern is present in a minority of cases (196).

Although grossly circumscribed (fig. 7-74), infiltrative growth is appreciable at the periphery of about 15 percent of cases on microscopic examination (196). Entrapped adipocytes, especially at the tumor periphery, are seen in some cases (fig. 7-75). Spindle cells with tapered to ovoid nuclei are either randomly arranged or form short fascicles in an edematous to fibrous stroma, with numerous small to medium-sized thick-walled blood vessels that may demonstrate hyaline or fibrinoid change (fig. 7-75). The overall cellularity is generally moderate. Occasionally, degenerative-type nuclear atypia is seen. Mitotic activity is generally sparse but mitotic figures may number up to 10 per 10 high-power fields (196). Lymphocytes and mast cells are scattered

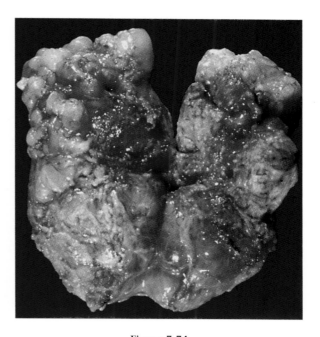

Figure 7-74

CELLULAR ANGIOFIBROMA

The tumor forms a lobulated, well-circumscribed, reddish tan mass. (Courtesy of Dr. W. Laskin, Chicago, IL.)

in the stroma in most cases. Exceptionally, there is sarcomatous transformation (198).

Immunohistochemical Findings. Immunoreactivity for CD34 occurs in about 75 percent of the cases whereas positivity for smooth muscle actin (25 percent), estrogen receptor (20 percent), progesterone receptor (20 percent), and desmin (8 percent) is less common (196). Stains for S-100 protein are negative.

Differential Diagnosis. The distinction of cellular angiofibroma from aggressive angiomyxoma is discussed with the latter. Other considerations include spindle cell lipoma, mammary-type myofibroblastoma, and solitary fibrous tumor. Spindle cell lipomas have thicker "ropey" collagen bundles, less prominent blood vessels, and usually a more conspicuous adipocytic component. In mammary-type myofibroblastoma, the lesional cells have a more fascicular pattern, the vessels are less conspicuous and there is frequent desmin positivity, features that contrast with those of cellular angiofibroma. Solitary fibrous tumor has more variable cellularity and a more consistent

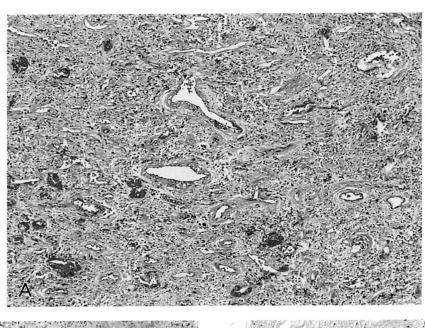

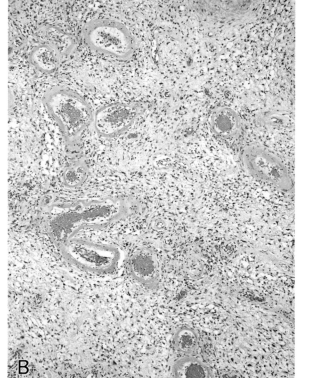
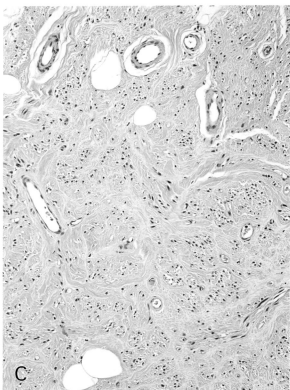

Figure 7-75

CELLULAR ANGIOFIBROMAS

A: Prominent vascularity and the cellular intervening stroma are seen. (Courtesy of Dr. J. Fetsch, Washington, DC.)

B: Vessels with fibrinoid change are especially prominent in this case.

C: This tumor, in addition to its prominent vascularity and bland-appearing lesional cells, incorporates fat at its periphery. It was diffusely CD34 reactive.

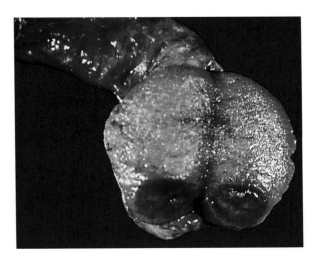

Figure 7-76

HEMANGIOMA OF TESTIS

The lesion is well circumscribed and red.

hemangiopericytomatous vascular pattern than cellular angiofibroma.

Treatment and Prognosis. These benign tumors are treated by conservative local excision. Focal recurrence is rare.

Vascular Tumors

Most subtypes of benign *vascular tumor* have been reported in the testis including capillary, cavernous, and epithelioid (histocytoid) hemangiomas (figs. 7-76–7-81) (85). Two "anastomosing" hemangiomas of the testis were recently documented (198a). A paratesticular location is less frequent, with reports of two cavernous hemangiomas involving the epididymis and spermatic cord (199,200).

Vascular tumors occur over a wide age range from infancy to the elderly (201). Most patients present with a mass that, on occasion, undergoes

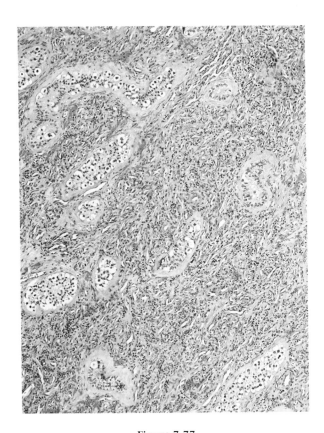

Figure 7-77

HEMANGIOMA OF TESTIS

The lesion infiltrates between the seminiferous tubules.

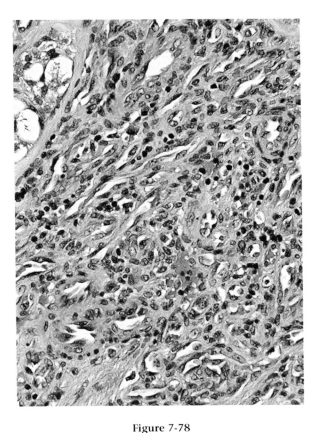

Figure 7-78

HEMANGIOMA OF TESTIS

High-power view of tumor in figure 7-77 shows a cellular neoplasm.

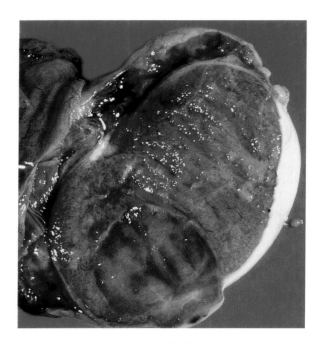

Figure 7-79

EPITHELIOID HEMANGIOMA OF TESTIS

Although the tumor is focally hemorrhagic, much of the sectioned surface has a fleshy tan appearance. (Courtesy of Dr. R. Archibald, San Jose, CA.)

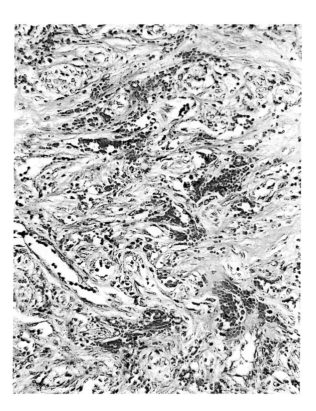

Figure 7-81

EPITHELIOID HEMANGIOMA OF TESTIS

Another area from the tumor in figure 7-80 shows abundant red blood cells within many of the lumens, which in this figure are more characteristic of vascular channels than in the prior figure.

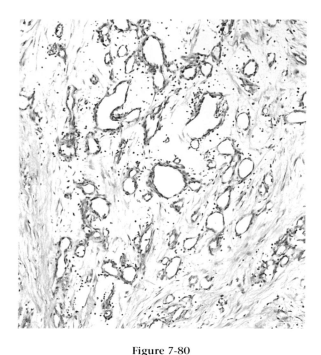

Figure 7-80

EPITHELIOID HEMANGIOMA OF TESTIS

Note the resemblance to an adenomatoid tumor.

rapid enlargement secondary to intraparenchymal and intratumoral hemorrhage.

The microscopic features are similar to those of hemangiomas at other sites. The cellular nature of some (202), especially in conjunction with an intertubular pattern of growth (fig. 7-77), may cause diagnostic confusion until the vascular nature of the channels is appreciated. They may also be mitotically active (fig. 7-78). One rare case had a multifocal growth pattern (203). The epithelioid examples have variably sized tubular channels lined by plump endothelial cells with eosinophilic cytoplasm (figs. 7-79–7-81). Cytoplasmic strands may bridge across the lumens in a manner similar to the adenomatoid tumor (85), which is a major differential diagnostic consideration. Since some epithelioid hemangiomas stain for cytokeratin, such positivity should not be taken as evidence

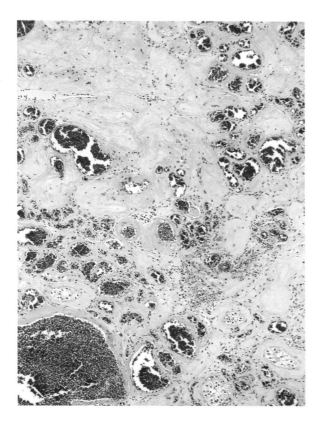

Figure 7-82

**MULTIPLE TELANGIECTASIAS OF TESTIS
IN KLIPPEL-TRENAUNAY-WEBER SYNDROME**

Dilated blood vessels interweave with seminiferous tubules.

against a vascular tumor, although the intense and diffuse staining in adenomatoid tumors contrasts with the usually more focal reactivity in epithelioid hemangiomas. Confirmation of the vascular nature of the lesion is obtained with the usual endothelial cell markers.

We have seen multiple dilated vascular channels throughout the testis of a patient with the Klippel-Trenaunay-Weber syndrome (fig. 7-82). These do not represent neoplasms but dilated arteriovenous anastomoses, perhaps caused by a developmental anomaly. Correlation with the clinical history is of obvious importance in the distinction from hemangioma.

The "anastomosing" hemangioma (198a) may be misinterpreted as angiosarcoma but, in contrast to angiosarcoma, it lacks multilayering, hyperchromasia, and conspicuous mitotic figures.

Myoid Gonadal Stromal Tumor

Myoid gonadal stromal tumor, an uncommon spindle cell tumor that is typically seen in the third or fourth decade of life, is hypothesized to arise from peritubular myoid cells (204). The patients present with either a mass or pain.

On gross examination, the tumors are typically circumscribed, nonencapsulated gray-white nodules. On microscopic examination, they form short, interwoven fascicles of bland spindle cells with tapered nuclei and intervening collagen (fig. 7-83). They are reactive for smooth muscle actin, smooth muscle myosin, S-100 protein, and, variably, desmin, similar to peritubular myoid cells (204). Some examples probably have been reported as leiomyomas but they lack the broad fascicular arrangements typical of leiomyoma, which are S-100 negative in contrast to the myoid gonadal stromal tumor. The behavior is benign.

Aggressive Angiomyxoma

General and Clinical Features. *Aggressive angiomyxomas,* originally described in the soft tissues of the pelvis and perineum of young women (205), also occur in the inguinal region, scrotum, and paratestis of children and men (206–208). In one survey, they were seven times less frequent in males than females (209). Male patients range from 1 to 82 years of age (mean, 46 years) (210) and present with masses.

Gross Findings. On gross examination, aggressive angiomyxomas are typically large (usually 5 to 15 cm) and occasionally massive, poorly circumscribed, nonencapsulated myxoid neoplasms (fig. 7-84) (208,211,212). The cut surface is generally solid, often gelatinous, and gray-white to yellow, and lacks necrosis.

Microscopic Findings. On microscopic examination, there are spindled to stellate cells loosely dispersed in a myxoid stroma containing fine collagen fibrils (fig. 7-85). The lesional cells have bland cytologic features with dense chromatin and inconspicuous mitotic activity (fig. 7-85). A characteristic feature is the distinct vascular component of the tumor, which is composed of randomly distributed, thin- to thick-walled vessels. Some of the vessel walls are prominently hyalinized. Small clusters of smooth muscle cells characteristically surround many vessels. A light infiltrate of scattered

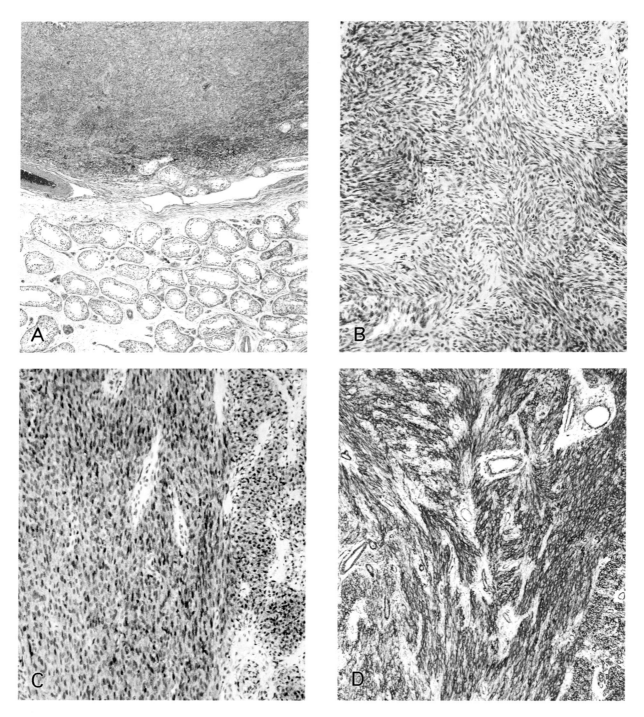

Figure 7-83

MYOID GONADAL STROMAL TUMORS

A: The tumor is circumscribed but not encapsulated, with incorporation of a few tubules at its periphery. (Courtesy of Dr. N. Weidner, San Diego, CA.)

B: Short, interwoven fascicles of spindled cells create a storiform pattern.

C: The lesional cells show nuclear and cytoplasmic reactivity for S-100 protein.

D: There is strong, diffuse immunoreactivity for smooth muscle myosin.

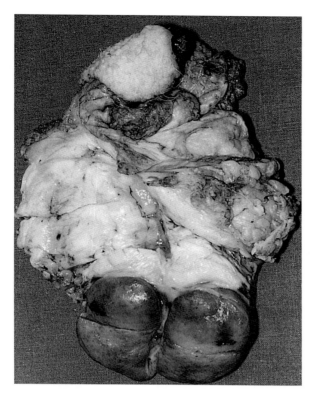

Figure 7-84

AGGRESSIVE ANGIOMYXOMA

An ill-defined mass of myxoid tissue fills the paratesticular region and extends to the scrotal skin (top). Testis is at the bottom. (Courtesy of Dr. J.C. Iezzoni, Charlottesville, VA.)

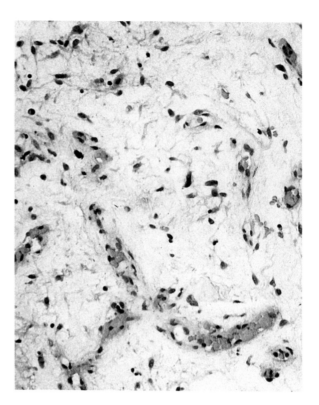

Figure 7-85

AGGRESSIVE ANGIOMYXOMA

Delicate blood vessels in a myxoid background are seen.

lymphocytes is seen in some cases, and many contain mast cells. Extravasation of erythrocytes is common. Peripheral infiltration of adipose tissue or other structures is usually found.

Immunohistochemical Findings. These neoplasms are positive for vimentin and CDK4, with variable results for CD34, desmin, smooth muscle actin, muscle-specific actin, and estrogen and progesterone receptors (210,213). MDM2 and S-100 protein are negative (213,214).

Ultrastructural Findings. Examination shows the fibroblastic features of the lesional cells, including numerous dilated cisternae of rough endoplasmic reticulum and frequent mitochondria. Actin-like filaments with focal densities suggest myofibroblastic differentiation (215).

Differential Diagnosis. Aggressive angiomyxoma is distinguished from angiomyofibroblastoma-like tumors (cellular angiofibroma) by its infiltrative nature, lesser cellularity, and the more attenuated nature of its cells. Aggressive angiomyxoma is more commonly desmin reactive than cellular angiofibroma. Myxoid neurofibroma lacks the prominent vascularity of aggressive angiomyxoma and shows S-100 protein positivity. Superficial angiomyxoma differs by its dermal or subcutaneous localization in the scrotum, frequently distinct multinodular growth pattern, occasional S-100 protein positivity, and negativity for desmin and estrogen and progesterone receptors (187).

Treatment and Prognosis. Because of their infiltrative growth, aggressive angiomyxomas are prone to local recurrence. Metastasis is rare. Wide excision is the preferred treatment whenever technically feasible.

Mammary-Type Myofibroblastoma

Mammary-type myofibroblastoma is a rare tumor of the paratestis but more commonly seen proximate to it in the inguinal region (168). Two paratesticular tumors occurred in a 60- and

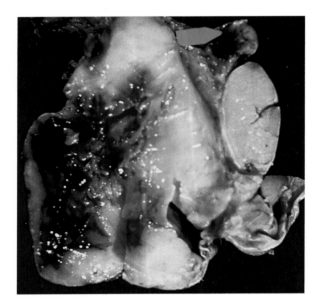

Figure 7-86

PARATESTICULAR EMBRYONAL RHABDOMYOSARCOMA

Extensive hemorrhage and an unremarkable testis (top).

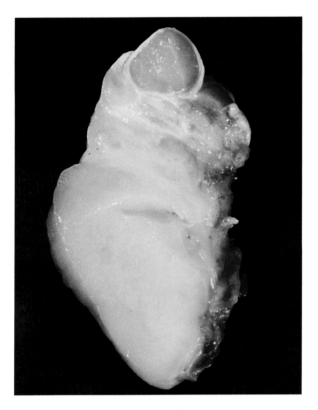

Figure 7-87

PARATESTICULAR EMBRYONAL RHABDOMYOSARCOMA, SPINDLE CELL TYPE

This tumor, which was fairly firm, has a focally whorled appearance in contrast to the tumor in figure 7-86.

85-year-old man and measured 7 and 13 cm in diameter (168,216). Both were well-circumscribed, unencapsulated, solid gray masses; one had a nodular cut surface and central myxoid change. On microscopic examination there were variably sized fascicles of spindle cells in a densely collagenous, sometimes prominently hyalinized, stroma, admixed with mast cells and occasional adipocytes. Mild nuclear atypia occurred in at least one tumor but mitotic activity was low, without atypical forms. There is usual immunoreactivity for both CD34 and desmin. Recurrences do not develop after marginal excision (168).

SOFT TISSUE TUMORS: MALIGNANT

In a review of paratesticular tumors, the 34 sarcomas consisted of 14 *rhabdomyosarcomas,* 9 *liposarcomas,* 7 *leiomyosarcomas,* and 4 malignant fibrous histiocytomas (currently termed *undifferentiated pleomorphic sarcoma*) (164). The most common sarcoma in adults is liposarcoma (217–219) and in children, rhabdomyosarcoma (220–223). Rarely, rhabdomyosarcomas, or even more exceptionally other sarcomas, originate in the testis of adults (224–228). Any malignant soft tissue tumor can be seen in the paratesticular tissues, as exemplified by reports of rhabdoid tumor of the spermatic cord (229), but most are rare and the features are

as seen elsewhere (227,228,230). Fibromatosis of the spermatic cord has also been described (176). Only the most frequent sarcomas in this location or those that are disproportionately represented are considered here in greater detail. The reader is referred to the numerous excellent sources concerning soft tissue pathology for information concerning other sarcomas that may be encountered in the paratestis.

Rhabdomyosarcoma

General and Clinical Features. In a large study of paratesticular *rhabdomyosarcomas* from the Intergroup Rhabdomyosarcoma Study Group, the mean age of the patients was 6.6 years (222). The presentation is almost always a painless mass. The tumors range from 1 to 18 cm in maximum dimension, with the majority from 4 to 6 cm. Most are of the embryonal subtype (figs. 7-86–7-91), including a higher proportion of the spindle-

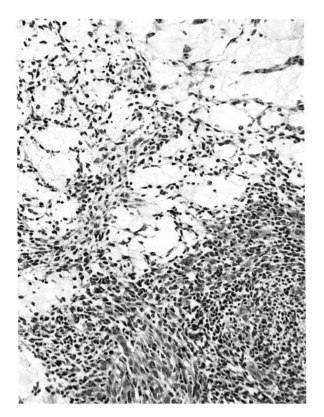

Figure 7-88

PARATESTICULAR EMBRYONAL RHABDOMYOSARCOMA

Variable cellularity is seen in this tumor. In the cellular areas, there are small hyperchromatic cells with scant cytoplasm and larger spindle-shaped cells with appreciable cytoplasm.

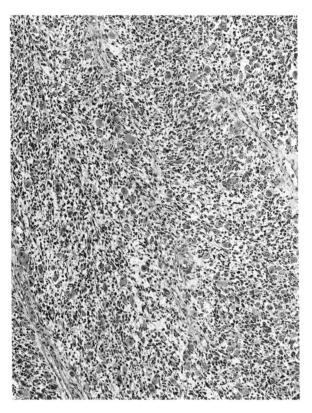

Figure 7-89

PARATESTICULAR EMBRYONAL RHABDOMYOSARCOMA

Differentiated rhabdomyoblastic cells with abundant eosinophilic cytoplasm are admixed with primitive small tumor cells.

cell variant (figs. 7-87, 7-90, 7-91) with its more favorable prognosis, than at other sites (222). In the Intergroup study, almost 70 percent of the embryonal rhabdomyosarcomas were "conventional," approximately 27 percent were of the spindle cell subtype, and the small remainder were mixed spindle and nonspindle types.

Gross Findings. On gross examination, conventional embryonal rhabdomyosarcomas are typically lobulated, gray-white to pink-tan, glistening, soft tumors that often show focal hemorrhage and necrosis (fig. 7-86). Spindle cell variants are firm, well demarcated, and nonencapsulated, and may have a whorled "leiomyomatous" appearance (fig. 7-87).

Microscopic Findings. On microscopic examination, embryonal rhabdomyosarcomas typically resemble their soft tissue and head and neck counterparts. They are characterized by primitive oval to elongated cells, often with uniform hyperchromatic nuclei and myxoid areas (fig. 7-88). Variation in cellularity is characteristic as are admixed differentiated rhabdomyoblasts with hyperchromatic nuclei and distinct eosinophilic cytoplasm that may have discernible cross striations (fig. 7-89).

The spindle cell type (222) is characterized by elongated fusiform cells sometimes arranged in fascicles (fig. 7-90), with a variably prominent stroma that may be markedly collagenized. Some have a prominent storiform pattern. The cytoplasm in these cases is fibrillar, in contrast to the more densely eosinophilic cytoplasm of typical embryonal rhabdomyosarcoma. Classic areas of typical embryonal neoplasia are almost always found, albeit focally in some cases, especially at the periphery of spindle cell variants. Necrosis is infrequent in this subtype.

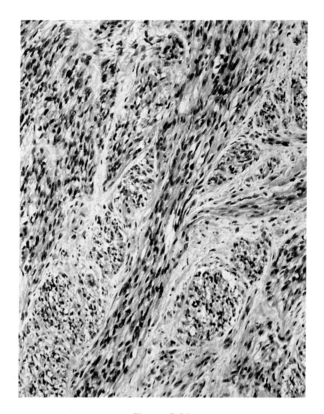

Figure 7-90

**PARATESTICULAR EMBRYONAL
RHABDOMYOSARCOMA, SPINDLE CELL TYPE**

There is a resemblance to leiomyosarcoma. (Courtesy of Dr. J.Y. Ro, Houston, TX.)

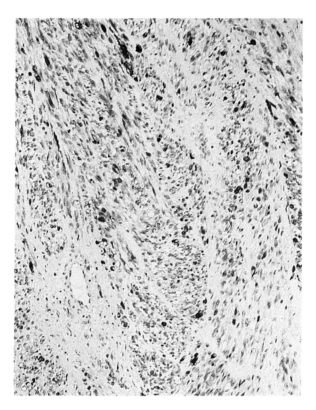

Figure 7-91

**PARATESTICULAR EMBRYONAL
RHABDOMYOSARCOMA, SPINDLE CELL TYPE**

An immunohistochemical stain for myoglobin is strongly positive.

About 6 percent of paratesticular rhabdomyosarcomas of childhood are of the alveolar subtype (222). This tumor has interlacing strands of fibrovascular stroma that create a honeycomb pattern of spaces containing solid or loose clusters of undifferentiated or slightly differentiated tumor cells with generally scant, eosinophilic cytoplasm (fig. 7-92). Tumors with solid clusters of cells form the "solid" variant. Distinct rhabdomyoblasts are less common than in the embryonal subtype and cross striations are rare. Occasional giant tumor cells are present in some cases (fig. 7-92), as in other sites. Rarely, pleomorphic rhabdomyosarcomas occur in the paratesticular soft tissues, usually in the elderly (231).

Immunohistochemical and Ultrastructural Findings. Although the diagnosis of rhabdomyosarcoma in the paratesticular region is usually based on routinely stained sections, immunohistochemical and ultrastructural studies may help in the distinction from other round cell and spindle cell tumors of this region. The neoplastic cells are positive for desmin, muscle-specific actin (clone HHF-35), myogenin (fig. 7-93), MyoD1, and less commonly, myoglobin (fig. 7-91). The spindle cell variant is positive for titin, a high molecular weight skeletal muscle protein that appears at a late stage of myogenesis, particularly in the postmitotic myoblasts and myotubules, with positive staining consistent with the differentiated nature of this subtype. The stellate and round cells of embryonal rhabdomyosarcoma are negative for titin. Myogenin reactivity is patchy in the embryonal subtype (fig. 7-93) and diffusely positive in the alveolar variant.

Ultrastructural examination shows thick and thin filaments in the cytoplasm of most tumor cells, mainly as haphazard tangles of filaments. Occasionally these are organized in the form of Z-bands (fig. 7-94).

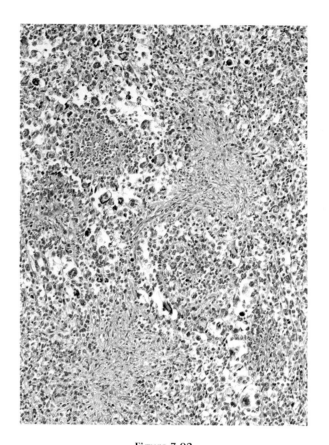

Figure 7-92

PARATESTICULAR ALVEOLAR RHABDOMYOSARCOMA

Discohesive nests of small tumor cells with admixed tumor giant cells are set in a fibrous stroma.

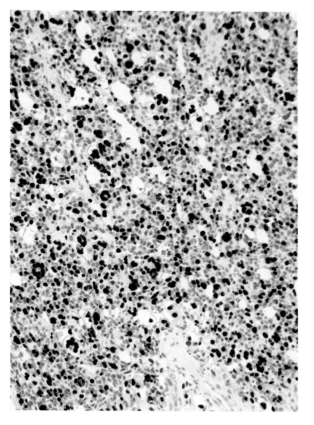

Figure 7-93

PARATESTICULAR EMBRYONAL RHABDOMYOSARCOMA

An immunohistochemical stain for myogenin stains a minority of the neoplastic nuclei.

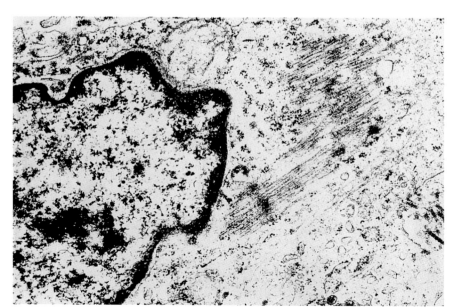

Figure 7-94

PARATESTICULAR EMBRYONAL RHABDOMYOSARCOMA, SPINDLE CELL TYPE

Ultrastructurally, the cytoplasm contains thick and thin filaments which occasionally are oriented and inserted into perpendicular densities (Z bands). (Courtesy of Dr. J.Y. Ro, Houston, TX.)

Special Techniques. Cytogenetic studies have verified that the alveolar subtype is associated with either a t(2;13)(q35;q14) or t(1;13)(p36;q14) translocation that results in either a PAX3-FOXO1 or PAX7-FOXO1 fusion, respectively.

Differential Diagnosis. The differential diagnosis of embryonal rhabdomyosarcoma of the conventional type includes malignant lymphoma, desmoplastic small round cell tumor, and retinal anlage tumor. Both malignant lymphoma and embryonal rhabdomyosarcoma have a fairly diffuse growth pattern, however, the presence of occasional cells with intensely eosinophilic cytoplasm and more variable cellularity with myxoid zones is indicative of embryonal rhabdomyosarcoma, as are the differing nuclear features. Appropriate immunostains, if necessary, easily resolve this problem.

The spindle cell variant of embryonal rhabdomyosarcoma should be differentiated from leiomyosarcoma and fibrosarcoma; a review of paratesticular sarcomas that had been included in the original study of the British Testicular Tumour Panel (232) verified that several cases of spindle cell rhabdomyosarcoma had been classified as either leiomyosarcoma or fibrosarcoma. If pleomorphism is prominent, malignant fibrous histiocytoma (undifferentiated pleomorphic sarcoma) is also a consideration. Although most errors regarding subclassification of spindle cell sarcomas, including undifferentiated pleomorphic sarcoma, leiomyosarcoma, and fibrosarcoma, are not therapeutically critical, this is not true for rhabdomyosarcoma, which has specific treatment. The three former tumors occur in a much older age group than the younger patients with spindle cell embryonal rhabdomyosarcoma. Leiomyosarcomas generally have a more consistent fascicular arrangement and are positive for smooth muscle actin, in addition to muscle-specific actin and desmin, which also stain rhabdomyosarcomas. They are negative for myogenin, however, in contrast to rhabdomyosarcoma. Spindle cell rhabdomyosarcomas, by definition, have a predominant spindle cell morphology, but there are often foci of conventional embryonal rhabdomyosarcoma and they retain the characteristic immunohistochemical profile.

Meconium periorchitis may surround atrophic skeletal muscle fibers, especially at the periphery, and may be misinterpreted as rhabdomyosarcoma. Unlike rhabdomyosarcoma, meconium periorchitis usually presents in neonates or infants, lacks the cytologic features of malignancy, and has a more variegated appearance, with myxoid zones, lymphocytes, pigmented macrophages, foreign body giant cells, extracellular bile pigment, desquamated keratinocytes, and calcifications (233).

Treatment and Prognosis. The treatment of paratesticular rhabdomyosarcoma includes radical orchiectomy, usually in conjunction with chemotherapy and sometimes with surgery (retroperitoneal lymphadenectomy) or radiation therapy. For patients with initially nonmetastatic tumors, the 5-year survival rate is 95 percent but only 22 percent if metastatic at presentation (234). The spindle cell variant is less commonly metastatic to the retroperitoneal lymph nodes at presentation compared to nonspindled variants, 16 percent and 36 percent, respectively, which likely accounts for the 96 percent overall survival rate at 5-years for these patients as opposed to an 80 percent 5-year survival rate for those with nonspindled paratesticular embryonal rhabdomyosarcoma (222). The alveolar subtype has not been associated with a worse outcome than the nonalveolar variants in some studies (235), although this may be secondary to its more intensive treatment. Apart from metastases at presentation, tumor size in excess of 5 cm and older age (10 years or older) are associated with a poorer outcome (236).

Liposarcoma

General and Clinical Features. Paratesticular *liposarcoma* usually presents as a painless mass in older patients (mean, 65 years), but it spans a wide age range from the teenage years (rarely) to the very elderly (164,217–219,237). Most of paratesticular liposarcomas arise from the spermatic cord (237). The occasional extension of a retroperitoneal liposarcoma through the inguinal canal and into the spermatic cord and paratestis must always be considered in cases of paratesticular liposarcoma and excluded by appropriate clinical and radiographic studies.

Gross and Findings. The well-differentiated tumors are usually lobulated, bulky, yellow masses often resembling a lipoma (fig. 7-95), although some show bands of gray-white fibrous tissue on cut surface to a greater extent

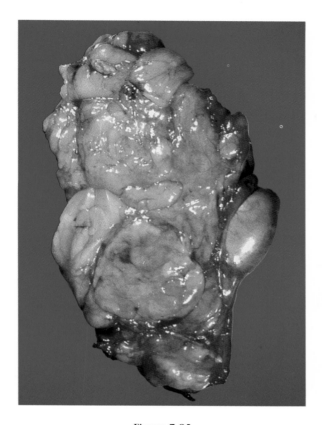

Figure 7-95

**WELL-DIFFERENTIATED
LIPOSARCOMA OF SPERMATIC CORD**

A well-circumscribed, large, golden yellow mass with a lobulated appearance is grossly suggestive of a fatty tumor (testis is at right). (Fig. 14-36 from Ro JY, Grignon DJ, Amin MB, Ayala A. Atlas of surgical pathology of the male reproductive tract. Philadelphia: W.B. Saunders; 1997:185.)

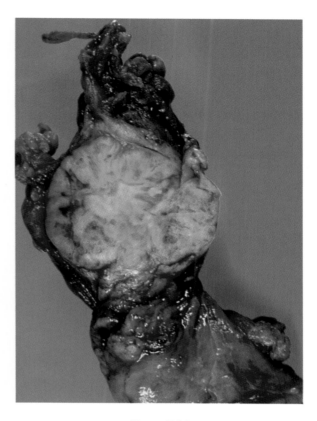

Figure 7-96

LIPOSARCOMA OF SPERMATIC CORD

A large yellow tumor that had the features of a pleomorphic liposarcoma on microscopic examination expands the cord. (Courtesy of Dr. J. Watts, Royal Oak, MI.)

than typically seen in conventional lipomas. In one series, the mean diameter was 12 cm (237). Pleomorphic liposarcomas or those with a prominent dedifferentiated component are gray and white, fleshy and firm (fig. 7-96). Invasion of the testicular parenchyma occurs rarely.

Microscopic Findings. On microscopic examination, liposarcomas of the paratesticular region display the spectrum observed elsewhere. The most common subtype is the *well-differentiated liposarcoma,* which can be lipoma-like, sclerosing, or inflammatory. These variants lack any clinically significant differences, and combinations of them may be seen. In the *lipoma-like variant,* most of the neoplasm may consist of mature-appearing adipocytic cells, with rare

cells showing distinct nuclear enlargement and hyperchromasia. Rare atypical lipoblasts and occasional fibrous bands containing widely spaced atypical cells may be seen; when these features are prominent, the tumor is classified as *sclerosing liposarcoma* (fig. 7-97). The *inflammatory variant* is common in the paratesticular region (238). Its features include a nodular infiltrate of lymphocytes and plasma cells with foci of plasma cell-rich stroma that often contains scattered atypical, frequently multinucleated cells (fig. 7-98).

Rarely, well-differentiated liposarcomas of the paratestis show foci of gradual transition to a low-grade smooth muscle component (*lipoleiomyosarcoma*) (239). Myxoid stromal change in some well-differentiated liposarcomas may lead to a misinterpretation of myxoid liposarcoma, an issue discussed with the differential diagnosis.

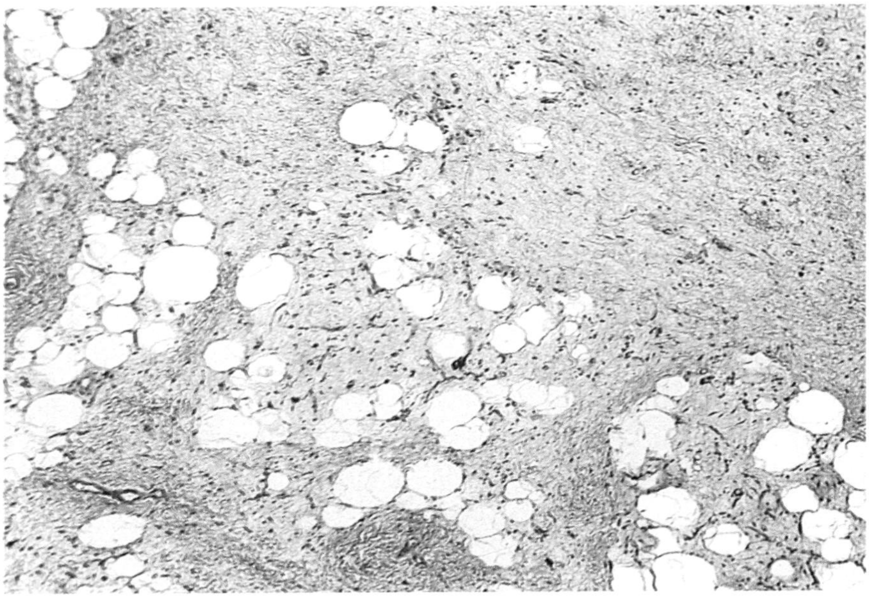

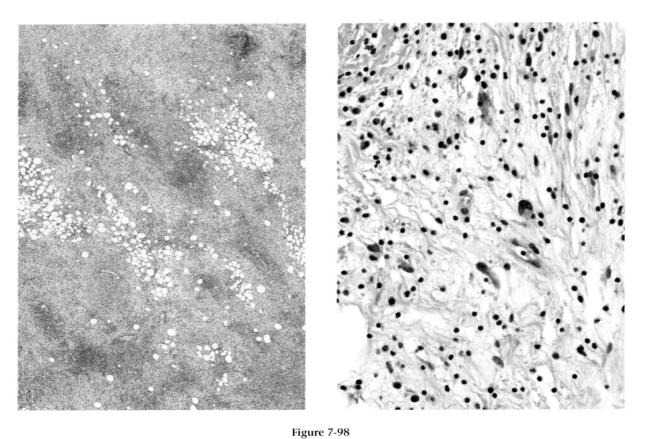

Figure 7-97

SCLEROSING LIPOSARCOMA OF SPERMATIC CORD

Atypical lipoblasts are visible.

Figure 7-98

INFLAMMATORY LIPOSARCOMA OF THE SPERMATIC CORD

Left: There is a diffuse lymphoplasmacytic infiltrate amid fatty and fibrous areas.
Right: Atypical spindle cells are widely scattered in the inflamed background.

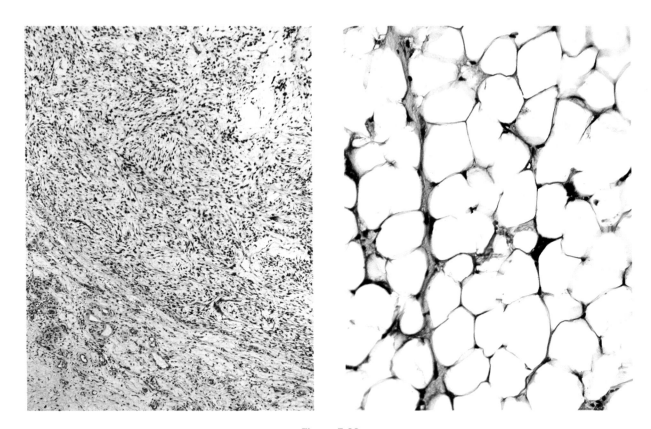

Figure 7-99

DEDIFFERENTIATED LIPOSARCOMA OF SPERMATIC CORD

Left: A spindle cell sarcoma showing no evident lipogenic differentiation has a storiform arrangement.
Right: Atypical adipocytes are identified in contiguous lipogenic foci.

Dedifferentiated liposarcoma is the next most frequent subtype (237). It consists of a well-differentiated component and a variably prominent second component that is usually high grade but occasionally low grade and that, in isolation, is not diagnostic of a fatty tumor (fig. 7-99). The high-grade component usually has the morphology of an undifferentiated pleomorphic sarcoma, whereas the low-grade one usually consists of a modestly cellular proliferation of generally uniform spindle cells in a dense, fibrous stroma with scant mitotic figures and no necrosis (237). The amount of the dedifferentiated component should be recorded.

Myxoid liposarcomas, with their characteristic prominent plexiform vascular network, are rare in the paratestis. They may have a round cell component (237). *Pleomorphic liposarcoma* is also rare (240) and necessitates the identification of unequivocal lipoblasts, sometimes requiring prolonged search, to distinguish it from high-grade pleomorphic sarcoma, not otherwise specified. *Spindle cell liposarcoma* is a very rare, low-grade form of paratesticular liposarcoma that is separated from either low-grade or dedifferentiated liposarcoma by its molecular biologic properties (241). It shows a parallel arrangement of slender spindle cells associated with atypical lipogenic cells and, in some cases, distinct lipoblasts (241).

Immunohistochemical and Molecular Findings. Immunohistochemical studies show frequent positivity for MDM2 and CDK4 in the lipoma-like, sclerosing, inflammatory, and dedifferentiated subtypes but not the myxoid/round cell or usually the spindle cell subtype (241,242). FISH for MDM2 amplification is a more sensitive and specific method of diagnosis than immunohistochemistry in needle biopsy specimens for these tumors (243). S-100 protein stains may facilitate identification of lipoblasts in the inflammatory variant and the spindle cell type (238,241), with the latter frequently showing reactivity for CD34.

Differential Diagnosis. The differential diagnosis of well-differentiated liposarcoma includes sclerosing lipogranuloma and large lipomas. Both of these lack atypical adipocytes and lipoblasts, and the former entity may be distinguished by its association with a histiocytic, including giant cell or granulomatous, reaction to exogenous lipid. Myxoid change in well-differentiated liposarcoma may cause confusion with myxoid liposarcoma, but the plexiform vascularity and negativity for MDM2 and CDK4 of the latter are helpful distinguishing features.

Dedifferentiated liposarcoma of the paratestis may have foci identical to inflammatory myofibroblastic tumor, desmoid-type fibromatosis, and nodular fasciitis (244). Distinction depends on the identification of a diagnostic low-grade component and MDM2 positivity. Myxoid lesions of the paratesticular region, including myxofibrosarcoma (myxoid malignant fibrous histiocytoma), embryonal rhabdomyosarcoma, and aggressive angiomyxoma may mimic a myxoid liposarcoma. Myxofibrosarcoma lacks lipoblasts or the typical vascular pattern of liposarcoma; embryonal rhabdomyosarcoma has a more variable cellularity comprised of undifferentiated small cells with occasional forms suggesting rhabdomyoblastic differentiation; and aggressive angiomyxoma lacks lipoblasts and, while having a prominent vascular component, lacks the plexiform vascular pattern of myxoid liposarcoma.

The differentiation of inflammatory well-differentiated liposarcoma from a reactive inflammatory condition hinges upon the diligent search for atypical cells, including lipoblasts, and the presence of a conventional component. The differential of inflammatory liposarcoma and inflammatory pseudotumor is discussed with the latter (see chapter 8). The distinction of pleomorphic liposarcoma from undifferentiated pleomorphic sarcoma depends upon the identification of lipoblasts in the former. Spindle cell liposarcoma may be confused with low-grade dedifferentiated liposarcoma; the presence in the latter of a component of conventional well-differentiated liposarcoma, its reactivity for MDM2 and CDK4, and its lack of adipocytic

differentiation in the spindle cell component are helpful distinguishing features.

Treatment and Prognosis. In the single largest series, 60 percent of well-differentiated liposarcomas (including pure subtypes and combinations of lipoma-like, sclerosing, and inflammatory morphologies) recurred locally one or more times, sometimes many years after initial excision, the longest documented interval being 21 years (237). None of these tumors, however, metastasized and all but 1 of 10 patients with follow-up were disease-free after re-excision. Dedifferentiation of well-differentiated liposarcoma confers metastatic potential on the tumor. One of five dedifferentiated liposarcomas with follow-up recurred, and a 30-cm tumor with high-grade dedifferentiation metastasized, causing death (237). Pleomorphic liposarcoma is a high-grade malignancy that frequently metastasizes, most commonly to the lungs (240). Although the experience is limited, spindle cell liposarcoma appears to behave similarly to well-differentiated liposarcoma, recurring locally but not metastasizing (241). Myxoid/round cell liposarcoma has metastatic potential (237).

The usual initial treatment for all forms of paratesticular liposarcoma is wide excision, which generally entails radical orchiectomy. Additional therapy is indicated in some cases if margins are positive, the tumor is high grade, or both, using the principles generally applicable to these tumors at other sites.

Leiomyosarcoma

General and Clinical Features. *Leiomyosarcoma* in the paratesticular region arises most often from the soft tissues of the spermatic cord or testicular tunics, but also from the epididymis (245,246). In the single largest series, there were 10 cases involving the spermatic cord; 11, the tunics; and 1, the epididymis (246). The reported age range is 17 to 92 years (247), but more than 80 percent occur in men over 40 years of age (164,232,248), with a median of 64 years (246). The presentation is a painless scrotal mass. One was associated with paraneoplastic human chorionic gonadotropin (hCG) production (249).

Gross and Microscopic Findings. Grossly, the tumors are solid, grayish white and may be whorled or, if high grade, hemorrhagic and necrotic (fig. 7-100). The typical microscopic

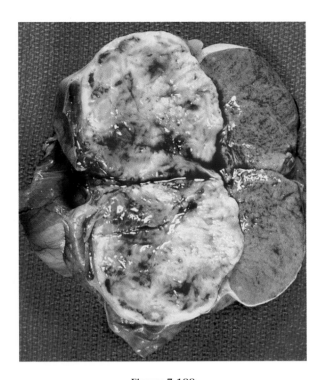

Figure 7-100

PARATESTICULAR LEIOMYOSARCOMA

There are foci of hemorrhage and necrosis.

features make the diagnosis usually straightforward: fascicles of spindled cells with eosinophilic cytoplasm that possess cigar-shaped nuclei. Nuclear pleomorphism and anaplasia vary in individual cases, and tumors cover the entire spectrum of differentiation, from low to high grade. In the largest series (246), there was prognostic value in separating the tumors into three grades based on the extent of necrosis, degree of pleomorphism, and amount of mitotic activity. Grade 1 tumors lacked necrosis, had less than 6 mitotic figures per 10 high-power fields, and had infrequent pleomorphic nuclei; grade 2 tumors had focal (less than 15 percent) necrosis, and/or more than 6 mitotic figures per 10 high-power fields, or had prominent nuclear pleomorphism; grade 3 tumors had over 15 percent necrosis. Occasional tumors may show well-described variant morphologies (246) as are more commonly seen at other sites, including inflammatory (250), myxoid (251), and epithelioid (246,252,253). One tumor had a component of osteoclast-like giant cells (254).

The tumors immunohistochemically and ultrastructurally show evidence of smooth muscle differentiation. CD34 positivity occurs in some.

Differential Diagnosis. The chief differential diagnostic consideration is the separation of low-grade leiomyosarcoma from leiomyoma. Some degree of nuclear pleomorphism, in conjunction with any mitotic activity, justifies a diagnosis of leiomyosarcoma, as does tumor cell necrosis. Rarely, a paratesticular leiomyoma may show the bizarre nuclei much more commonly seen in uterine tumors (255), but these cases lack mitotic activity and necrosis. Such cases are more common in the skin of the scrotum (256). The rare smooth muscle hyperplasia of the adnexa (see chapter 8) (257), because it may have an ill-defined gross appearance and pseudoinfiltrative growth around normal structures, may cause concern for leiomyosarcoma, but its lack of atypia, necrosis, and mitotic activity are distinct from leiomyosarcoma. The differential diagnosis also includes the spindle cell variant of embryonal rhabdomyosarcoma (discussed with the latter entity).

Treatment and Prognosis. The usual treatment is radical orchiectomy. The prognosis is grade dependent. In the largest series (246), 10 of 10 patients with either grade 1 or grade 2 tumors did not develop metastases (although local recurrences were seen in 2), whereas all 4 with grade 3 tumors died of metastatic leiomyosarcoma at 3.5 to 12.0 years. These data agree with analysis of individually reported cases, which shows that about one third of the patients die of metastatic sarcoma.

Other Sarcomas

Approximately 35 cases of *undifferentiated pleomorphic sarcoma* (*malignant fibrous histiocytoma*) of the spermatic cord have been described in the English and Japanese literature since 1967 (164,258–260). The mean age of these patients is 64 years (range, 15 to 84 years), with 80 percent being over 50 years old (260). Grossly, the neoplasms have a variegated gray-white appearance with necrosis, hemorrhage, and variable cystic change. The most frequent subtype is pleomorphic, not otherwise specified, although tumors with inflammatory and myxoid features also occur. The distinction from pleomorphic and

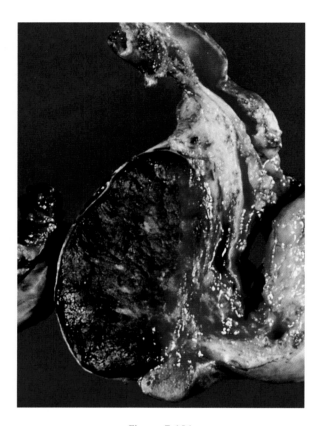

Figure 7-101

KAPOSI SARCOMA OF TESTIS

The testis is replaced by a hemorrhagic mass. (Courtesy of Dr. J. Henley, Indianapolis, IN.)

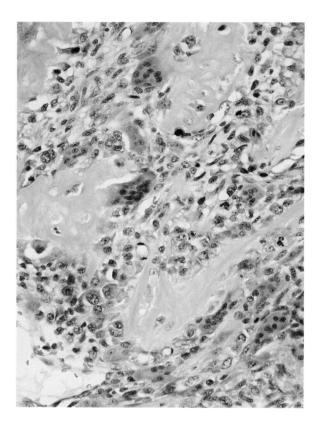

Figure 7-102

EXTRAOSSEOUS OSTEOSARCOMA OF THE PARATESTIS

Osteoid production and mitotic figures are seen.

inflammatory liposarcoma requires identification of lipoblasts. Dedifferentiated liposarcoma, in addition to having an identifiable low-grade component, is also characterized by amplification of 12q13-15, corresponding to the MDM2 and CDK4 genes, the proteins of which may be detected immunohistochemically; these changes are absent in undifferentiated pleomorphic sarcoma. The follow-up information is limited, but approximately one third of patients have adverse outcomes in the form of local recurrence or distant metastasis.

Fibrosarcomas of this region are rare. Of six cases of "fibrosarcoma" originally included in the British Testicular Tumour Panel and Registry, five were reclassified as other sarcomas using more modern criteria (232). One malignant example of solitary fibrous tumor occurring at this site had retroperitoneal metastases after 16 months (261). The primary tumor in that case

had a low mitotic rate and limited atypia but did exhibit necrosis.

At least two cases of *Kaposi sarcoma* of the testis have been reported (262,263), and we have seen another unpublished example (fig. 7-101). Angiosarcomas of the testis or its adnexa are equally rare (224), and we have seen an unpublished example of *extraosseous osteosarcoma* in the paratestis of an elderly man (fig. 7-102). One case of *Ewing sarcoma/peripheral primitive neuroectodermal tumor* has been reported in the testis of a 46-year-old man (264), with immunohistochemical and molecular confirmation, and we have seen a second case with similar findings, including the characteristic 11:22 translocation.

Differential Diagnosis of Testicular Sarcomas

The diagnosis of a pure sarcoma of any type in the testis should only be made after thorough sampling to exclude an underlying tumor from which the sarcoma may have arisen, such as a teratoma or spermatocytic seminoma. Occasionally, only the presence of IGCNU is a clue that a sarcoma arose from a germ cell tumor. As previously discussed (see chapter 4), the most common sarcoma of germ cell origin is rhabdomyosarcoma, with the embryonal subtype more frequent than either the alveolar or pleomorphic variants.

When the entire testis has been replaced by a sarcoma it may not be possible, based on conventional pathologic features alone, to determine whether a sarcoma arose from a prior germ cell tumor or de novo, although chromosome 12p amplification supports the former. Careful gross examination is required to exclude growth of a sarcoma from the paratestis into the testis. Unclassified sex cord–stromal tumors may have a prominent and atypical spindle cell component that mimics a sarcoma unless thorough sampling permits identification of its more distinctive epithelial features. Reticulum stains prove useful in the distinction of some sex cord–stromal tumors from sarcomas, since the former may show reticulum fibers surrounding nests of sex cord elements that are not apparent in routinely stained sections. Leydig cell tumors may undergo sarcomatous transformation that is only recognizable on the basis of an identifiable conventional component (265). This should not be confused with spindle cell growth of Leydig cell tumor wherein the spindle cells retain Leydig cell features and appropriate immunoreactivity. Ewing sarcoma should not be confused with the primitive neuroectodermal tumors that develop from germ cell tumors, as the latter are almost always of central type and lack the molecular and immunohistochemical findings characteristic of Ewing sarcoma/peripheral primitive neuroectodermal tumor (266).

OTHER RARE PRIMARY TUMORS

Wilms Tumor

There are three reported cases of primary extrarenal Wilms tumor in the testicular adnexa of children who were 6 months, 13 months, and 3.5 years of age (267–269). The tumors occurred within the spermatic cord and ranged from 0.5 to 5.0 cm. They consisted of varying admixtures of primitive blastema, tubules, and stroma. Nephrogenic rests occurred adjacent to two of the tumors (267,268). The largest tumor, from the 3.5-year-old, metastasized to the lung after 1 year but the patient was well 18 months later, having received radiation therapy and chemotherapy.

Despite its rarity, the diagnosis of extrarenal Wilms tumor should be made with ease because of its distinctive features, which are different from those of any other tumor in the testis or adnexa. It should also be distinguished from nephrogenic rests, which may be associated with it or stand alone (270,271) and the equally rare examples of apparently benign metanephric hamartoma (see chapter 8).

Wilms tumor may metastasize to the testis and paratestis (272–274); its distinction from primary extrarenal Wilms tumor largely depends upon clinical information, although the absence of nephrogenic rests is supportive. Occasional cases of Wilms tumor-like foci in immature teratomas of the testis (275) are distinguished from extrarenal Wilms tumor by their association with other teratomatous components. Rare pure testicular Wilms tumors of germ cell origin are also described and recognizable by an association with IGCNU and the presence of i(12p) (276).

Squamous Cell Carcinoma

Two primary *squamous cell carcinomas* of the testis were thought to originate from epidermoid cysts in a 51-year-old and a 64-year-old man (277,278). Such lesions should, of course, be distinguished from metastatic squamous cell carcinoma, enabled in these cases by a convincing origin from epidermoid cysts. If the latter were to be effaced by cancer, clinical studies to exclude metastasis would be indicated. Another squamous cell carcinoma developed from a teratoma in a 45-year-old man (279). One paratesticular squamous cell carcinoma arose in a hydrocele sac in an 85-year-old man (280); there was continuity between the invasive carcinoma and the highly dysplastic metaplastic squamous epithelium lining the hydrocele sac. A primary epididymal squamous cell carcinoma was described earlier in this chapter (see Carcinoma of the Epididymis).

Paraganglioma

We are aware of seven *paragangliomas* of the spermatic cord in the English language literature

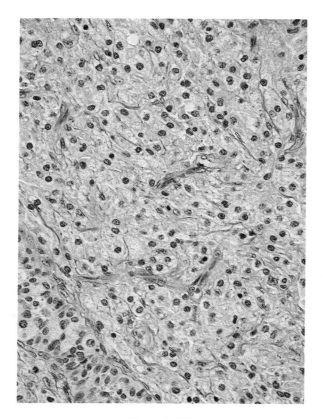

Figure 7-103

JUVENILE XANTHOGRANULOMA OF TESTIS

There is an infiltrate of cells with pale, eosinophilic cytoplasm and round to oval nuclei. Focal preservation of a seminiferous tubule (lower left) is seen.

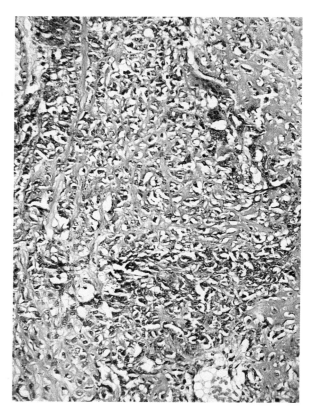

Figure 7-104

CARCINOSARCOMA OF TESTIS

The dark blue areas of carcinoma have prominent intervening foci of osteosarcoma with conspicuous osteoid.

(281–283). None was associated with convincing evidence of function. They measured up to 10 cm and had the typical pathologic features. In one, there was evident vascular space invasion (283). No case is known to have metastasized, although follow-up was not available or was limited in several.

Juvenile Xanthogranuloma

Five cases of *juvenile xanthogranuloma* of the testis or epididymis have been reported in infants from 2.5 to 13.0 months of age (284). In four of these cases, the lesion was solitary but one patient also had multiple skin nodules. Grossly, they formed masses that varied from yellow to tan-white. On microscopic examination, there were intertubular to confluent infiltrates of mononuclear cells that mimicked the patterns commonly encountered in leukemias and lym-

phomas. The cells were mostly round to oval but occasionally spindled, with uniform nuclei and moderate amounts of pale to eosinophilic cytoplasm (fig. 7-103). In contrast to the cutaneous lesions, Touton giant cells were usually absent. The cells stained for CD68 and factor XIIIa and were negative for S-100 protein and CD1a (284).

The follow-up in these cases has been benign. One that was incompletely excised developed local recurrence that underwent spontaneous regression (285).

Carcinosarcoma

We have seen one unpublished example of *carcinosarcoma* of the testis of an 84-year-old man. In this case, islands of poorly differentiated carcinoma were admixed with areas of osteosarcoma (fig. 7-104). This tumor did not have epithelium that was recognizably of müllerian

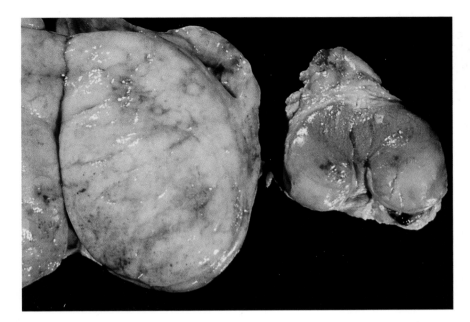

Figure 7-105

MALIGNANT LYMPHOMA OF TESTIS

Both testes are involved by tumor, with one being much larger than the other.

type, in which instance the tumor would be classified as a müllerian carcinosarcoma. It also did not have features diagnostic of a Sertoli nature, although that was not investigated by inhibin staining (see chapter 6).

Testicular Tumor of Uncertain Cell Type Associated with Cushing Syndrome

In one remarkable case, a 3-year-old boy with signs and symptoms of Cushing syndrome had a massive left testicular neoplasm that was considered responsible for the syndrome. The tumor, which was malignant and caused the death of the patient, could not be classified with certainty but had features suggestive of adrenal cortical type, consistent with the clinical findings (286). Potentially, the tumor may have arisen from adrenal cortical rests.

HEMATOPOIETIC AND LYMPHOID TUMORS

Malignant Lymphoma

General and Clinical Features. *Malignant lymphomas* account for 2 to 5 percent of all primary testicular neoplasms (287–307) and for about 50 percent of those in men over 60 years of age (287–293,308,309). Lymphomas are one of a triad of tumors, along with spermatocytic seminoma and metastatic tumors, which pathologists should particularly consider in older patients, assuming reasonably appropriate morphology.

The median patient age is 67 years (179), with only rare cases in children (301). Lymphoma is the most common bilateral testicular tumor (fig. 7-105); bilaterality has occurred in up to 38 percent of the cases, although the overall frequency is 12 to 18 percent. Bilateral involvement is usually metachronous, with the most common presentation being a unilateral mass. Approximately two thirds of patients have localized disease (Ann Arbor stage I or II), and the remainder have involvement of lymph nodes or extranodal sites, most commonly Waldeyer ring, central nervous system, bone, or skin; the latter are also common sites of relapse. Rare intrascrotal lymphomas are primary in the epididymis or cord, or at least present at those sites (291,299).

The most common type by far is *diffuse large B-cell lymphoma*, representing up to 90 percent of testicular lymphomas (179,291,310). *Follicular lymphomas* are more common in children than adults. Both in children and adults, they appear to be different from the usual nodal-based follicular lymphomas seen in older patients (311–313). They are more frequently localized, lack both Bcl-2 immunoreactivity and BCL2 translocations, and are grade 3, although with indolent behavior (311,313,314). Similar observations have recently been made in ovarian follicular lymphomas (315). Less common are *lymphoplasmacytoid, small lymphocytic,*

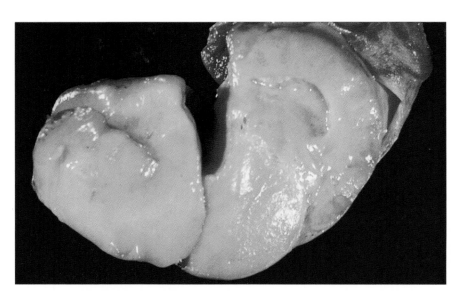

Figure 7-106

MALIGNANT LYMPHOMA OF TESTIS

The testis is effaced by creamy white tissue that extensively involves the epididymis. (Fig. 7.1 from Young RH, Scully RE. Testicular tumors. Chicago: ASCP Press; 1990:155.)

follicular (179,311), *Burkitt* (291), *lymphoblastic* (179), *mantle cell* (316), *plasmablastic* (317), and *peripheral T-cell* (179,302) *lymphomas.*

A rare form of lymphoma, *extranodal natural killer (NK)/T-cell lymphoma, nasal type,* which is most common in the midline facial region, appears to have some proclivity to occur in the testis, although its overall scarcity still makes this an infrequent event (318). This type of lymphoma tends to occur at a younger age (mean, 51 years) (318) than diffuse large B-cell lymphoma and is more common in Asian populations. Four cases of *anaplastic, CD30-positive lymphoma* involving the testis are reported (288,292,319,320), one of them of the neutrophil-rich variant. *Hodgkin disease* of the testis is extremely rare (321). Additional information on lymphomas is found within monographs devoted to the lymph nodes (322).

Gross Findings. Gross examination discloses partial or complete replacement of the testis by a fleshy to firm, often lobulated, cream-colored, tan, pale yellow, or slightly pink homogeneous mass (fig. 7-106). The median diameter is approximately 6 cm. There may be focal areas of necrosis. Epididymal involvement by lymphoma is present on gross inspection in half of the cases (fig. 7-106). The appearance closely resembles that of a seminoma, but seminoma involves the epididymis or spermatic cord much less often.

Microscopic Findings. In some cases, low-power microscopic examination shows pre-dominant intertubular infiltration by tumor cells (fig. 7-107), but in others, effacement of the tubules occurs, with the neoplastic cells invading and filling tubules within the tumor in as many as 80 percent of the cases (fig. 7-108). Staining for reticulum fibrils reveals separation of the fibrils in the walls of the tubules that have been invaded by lymphoma cells, in contrast to condensation of the fibrils in the walls of tubules invaded by seminoma cells. In 30 percent of the cases there is sclerosis that may be extensive (fig. 7-109). Testicular lymphoma involves the epididymis in 60 percent of the cases and the spermatic cord in 40 percent (291). Vascular invasion is seen in approximately 60 percent of the cases. The large B-cell lymphomas typically show diffuse, strong staining of pan-B-cell antigens (CD19, CD20, CD22, CD79a), with a preponderance of the activated, nongerminal center B-cell type rather than the germinal center B-cell type (323–325).

Extranodal NK/T-cell lymphomas, nasal type, are composed of small, medium-sized, or large cells and frequently show angiocentric, angiodestructive growth (289). They express a limited number of T-cell associated antigens, usually CD2 and cytoplasmic CD3, as well as the NK-cell–associated antigen CD56. Nearly all also contain Epstein-Barr virus genetic material.

CD30-positive anaplastic large cell lymphoma (figs. 7-110–7-113) often has a cohesive pattern of growth, forming nests and cords. Prominent intratubular growth is sometimes seen.

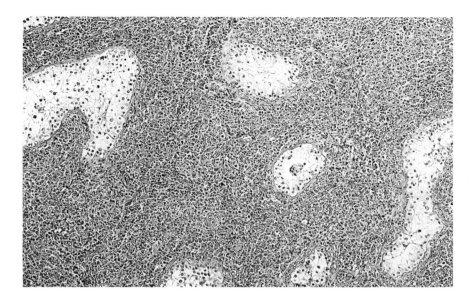

Figure 7-107

**MALIGNANT LYMPHOMA
OF TESTIS**

There is striking intertubular growth on low-power examination.

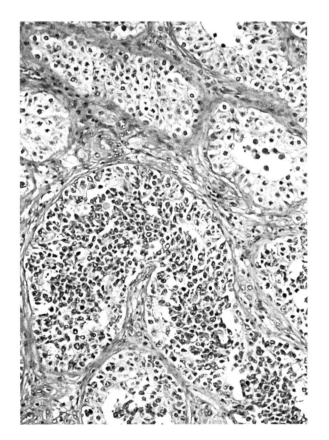

Figure 7-108

MALIGNANT LYMPHOMA

Several seminiferous tubules are filled by lymphoma cells, with scant involvement of the intertubular tissue in this area.

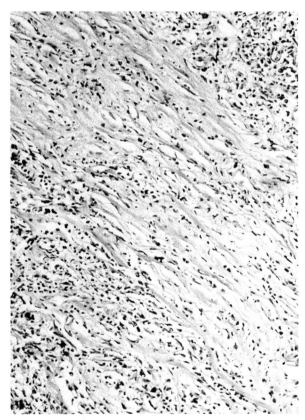

Figure 7-109

MALIGNANT LYMPHOMA

There is extensive sclerosis.

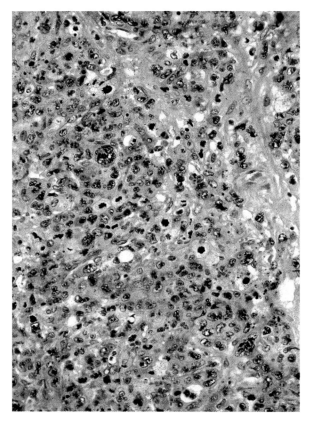

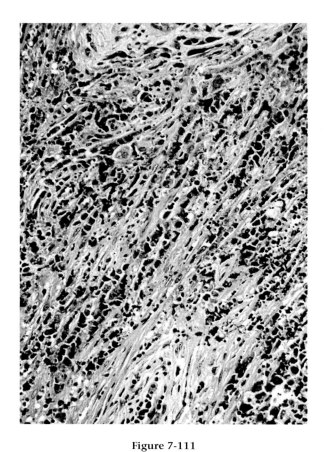

Figure 7-110

ANAPLASTIC LARGE CELL LYMPHOMA

There is a resemblance to a poorly differentiated carcinoma.

Figure 7-111

ANAPLASTIC LARGE CELL LYMPHOMA

The prominent growth in cords simulates an epithelial neoplasm.

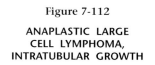

Figure 7-112

ANAPLASTIC LARGE CELL LYMPHOMA, INTRATUBULAR GROWTH

The pattern is reminiscent of that of intratubular embryonal carcinoma.

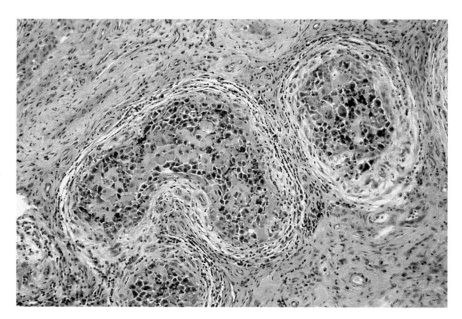

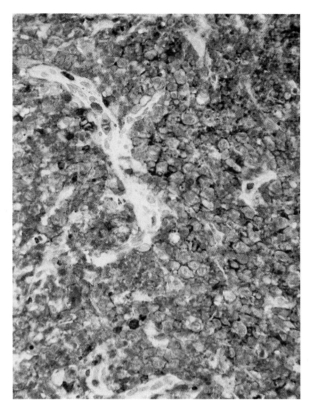

Figure 7-113

ANAPLASTIC LARGE CELL LYMPHOMA

The tumor cells are immunoreactive for CD43.

Differential Diagnosis. Testicular lymphomas are often confused with seminoma of the usual or spermatocytic type (326). In general, lymphomas occur at an older age than do usual seminomas. The characteristic intertubular pattern of growth of lymphoma is initially suggestive of the diagnosis in many cases but is not specific, and the diagnosis must be further supported by appreciation of the characteristic cytomorphologic features of lymphoma. Seminoma cells, unlike most lymphoma cells, have distinct cell membranes, abundant glycogen-rich cytoplasm, and rounded but focally flattened central nuclei with one or a few prominent nucleoli. Some seminomas show, at their periphery, the prominent intertubular growth that is so typical of lymphoma, and this may, rarely, be a predominant pattern in seminoma. The cells of spermatocytic seminomas are glycogen-free, polymorphous, and of three distinct types (see chapter 3).

Immunohistochemical staining for leukocyte common antigen and B-cell– (CD19, CD20, CD22) and T-cell– (CD3) associated antigens helps in problem cases, as does OCT3/4, which is uniformly negative in lymphoma and positive in usual seminoma. SALL4 is positive in spermatocytic seminoma and negative in lymphoma with the exception of B lymphoblastic lymphoma, which is unlikely to be mistaken for spermatocytic seminoma (327).

Viral and granulomatous orchitis may be confused with lymphoma, but the heterogeneous and benign-appearing inflammatory cellular infiltrates of these lesions contrast with the more homogeneous and malignant-appearing infiltrate of lymphoma. Viral orchitis, additionally, has a patchy rather than diffuse distribution, and often shows intratubular predominance (328).

Distinction of lymphoma from embryonal carcinoma is rarely a problem except in the exceptional case of involvement of the testis by an anaplastic large cell lymphoma. In one case, this differential diagnosis was difficult because of a striking presence in the lymphoma of epithelial-like formations which mimicked embryonal carcinoma (292). Further confusion was caused by the prominent intratubular growth of the tumor cells with necrosis, a picture similar to that of intratubular embryonal carcinoma. Absence of epithelial differentiation and IGCNU, and the presence of markedly irregular, twisted nuclei suggested lymphoma and prompted appropriate immunohistochemical confirmation (positive for CD45, T-cell markers [CD3, CD45RO, CD43], and CD30, and negative for B-cell markers, placental alkaline phosphatase, and cytokeratin). We have also encountered a case of NK/T-cell lymphoma with similarly striking intratubular growth.

Treatment and Prognosis. Treatment and prognosis are both subtype dependent and stage dependent. Most patients receive orchiectomy and polyagent chemotherapy. In a large population-based study that included 769 patients with diffuse large B-cell lymphoma who were diagnosed between 1980 and 2005, the disease-specific survival rates at 3, 5, and 15 years were 72, 62, and 43 percent, respectively. Patients with stage I and II disease have significantly longer overall survival periods compared to those with stage III or IV disease (329). In a single large series, two additionally identified favorable prognostic features were unilateral tumors and sclerosis (291). The 5-year survival rate for patients with unilateral disease was 40 percent compared to 0 percent for those with bilateral disease, and patients whose tumors had sclerosis had a 5-year disease-free survival rate of 72 percent compared to 16 percent for patients whose tumors lacked sclerosis. Follicular lymphomas, which are typically stage IE, have a favorable outcome in virtually all cases (311,313), to the extent that it has been suggested that those stage IE cases in children may be treated by orchiectomy alone without adjuvant chemotherapy (313). On the other hand, NK/T-cell lymphomas have a uniformly aggressive course with no known survivors (318).

Multiple Myeloma and Plasmacytoma

General and Clinical Findings. Two percent of patients with *multiple myeloma* have testicular involvement but usually it is not detected until autopsy. Rarely, the involvement is clinically evident, and in a few cases, testicular enlargement precedes recognition of the disease. Approximately 60 cases of testicular or epididymal *plasmacytoma* have now been reported in the English language literature (330–336). The patients ranged from 26 to 89 years of age (mean, 55 years). Almost half had a prior history of some form of plasma cell neoplasia. Of these, approximately 50 percent had multiple myeloma, while roughly equal numbers of the remainder had single osseous or extramedullary plasmacytomas, or both. Most have lesions at other sites when the testicular tumor is discovered, and most have progressive disease and die of myeloma. One patient with reported plasmacytoma had the acquired immunodeficiency syndrome (337), although we feel that plasmablastic lymphoma was not excluded as an alternative diagnosis. Rarely, patients have an apparently isolated testicular plasmacytoma, but the follow-up has been short in some of these cases. In others, long-term follow-up subsequently documented multiple myeloma, as in a patient who developed numerous osseous lesions 7 years after an apparently isolated testicular plasmacytoma (338). In one case, a patient with an epididymal plasmacytoma treated

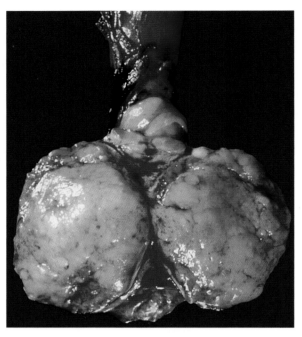

Figure 7-114

PLASMACYTOMA OF TESTIS

The testis is replaced by a creamy white mass.

only by orchiectomy was alive at 5 years (339). In one remarkable case, a patient had multiple extramedullary plasmacytomas, including a testicular tumor on one side, followed 8 years later by an epididymal plasmacytoma on the opposite side. At the time of last follow-up, 26 years after initial presentation, he was well and had been disease free for 9 years (331).

Gross Findings. Testicular plasmacytomas are usually firm to soft, tan to golden-tan to gray-white neoplasms (fig. 7-114). They measure up to 8 cm in greatest dimension and often replace most of the testicular parenchyma (331). They rarely have the characteristic fleshy white appearance and extratesticular involvement of lymphoma presenting in the testis. They may be extensively hemorrhagic (fig. 7-115). Bilateral involvement is rare (340).

Microscopic Findings. There is typically a central area of effacement of the underlying testicular tubules and a peripheral zone with intertubular growth of the neoplastic cells (fig. 7-116). Although in most cases a substantial number of tumor cells are plasma cells (fig. 7-117), it is not rare for many of the tumor cells

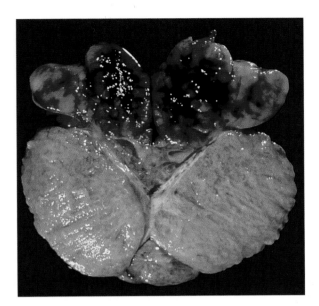

Figure 7-115

PLASMACYTOMA OF EPIDIDYMIS

The tumor is extensively hemorrhagic.

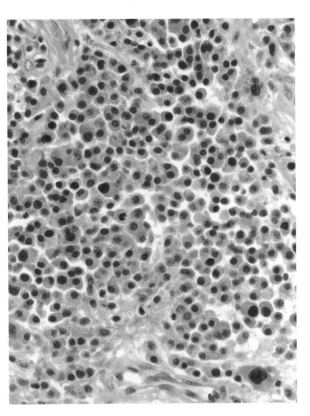

Figure 7-117

PLASMACYTOMA OF TESTIS

The plasmacytoid nature of the tumor cells is evident.

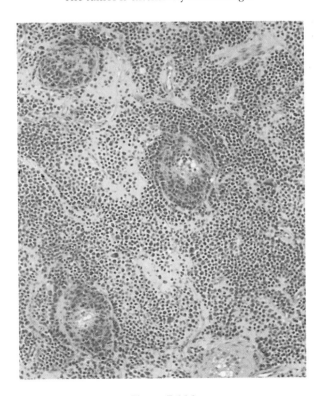

Figure 7-116

PLASMACYTOMA OF TESTIS

There is prominent intertubular growth but, in addition, several tubules are invaded by the neoplastic plasma cells.

to have features that are deceptive with respect to their plasma cell nature. For example, they often do not have the characteristic cartwheel chromatin of the mature plasma cell but rather have vesicular nuclei with small or large central nucleoli and less chromatin along the nuclear membrane than normal plasma cells. Binucleated and multinucleated cells are often scattered among the mononuclear tumor cells. Scattered anaplastic or bizarre cells may be present.

Immunohistochemical Findings. CD138 is positive in virtually all cases, as is cytoplasmic staining for either kappa or lambda light chains. Reactivity for leukocyte common antigen (CD45) and EMA occurs in approximately 60 percent of cases, whereas CD79a is positive in over 80 percent. CD20 and PAX5 are usually negative.

Differential Diagnosis. The most realistic considerations in the differential diagnosis are non-Hodgkin lymphoma and seminoma of both typical and spermatocytic types. In a series of seven testicular plasmacytomas, three were submitted with these provisional diagnoses (331). The tumor cells in lymphoma typically have less abundant cytoplasm than do plasma cells and lack a paranuclear hof, with the exception of plasmablastic lymphoma, which is exceptionally rare in the testis (341). In addition, sclerosis is common in testicular lymphoma but rarely, if ever, seen in plasmacytoma. Clinical and gross features provide some clues to the diagnosis. Most testicular lymphomas present with disease confined to the testis and paratestis whereas most testicular plasmacytomas are associated with widespread disease at diagnosis, although, as noted above, there are striking exceptions. Simultaneous involvement of both testes by a mass is much more common in lymphoma than in plasmacytoma. In problematic cases, immunohistochemical staining demonstrates that plasmacytomas do not express CD20, PAX5, or surface IgM, whereas these are commonly seen in large cell lymphomas of the testis. On the other hand, CD138 is positive in plasmacytoma and negative in large cell lymphoma. EMA positivity also favors plasmacytoma over large cell lymphoma, with the exception of the anaplastic large cell (Ki-1) variant. Plasmablastic lymphoma is rare and typically occurs in the setting of immunodeficiency, most often infection with the human immunodeficiency virus. Neoplastic cells are mostly large, with vesicular nuclei and prominent nucleoli. Mitotic figures are frequent. The immunophenotype is similar to that of plasmacytoma except that plasmablastic lymphoma has a higher proliferation index and usually is positive for Epstein-Barr virus early RNA.

The distinction from seminoma should be straightforward on routine light microscopic examination because of the marked difference in the cytologic features of these two tumors. In a rare problematic case, staining of seminoma for glycogen and differences in immunohistochemical staining of these tumors are diagnostic.

A more realistic problem is differentiation from spermatocytic seminoma because various cell types of that neoplasm are mimicked, to some extent, by the variations in cell size and shape seen in some cases of plasmacytoma. For example, the granular chromatin of some cells in plasmacytoma may suggest the "spi-

reme"-type chromatin seen in some cells of spermatocytic seminoma. Careful high-power scrutiny in such cases should show many cells with the characteristic features of immature plasma cells: eccentric nuclei and amphophilic cytoplasm with a paranuclear hof. Immunostaining for SALL4 is positive in spermatocytic seminoma and negative in plasmacytoma/myeloma (327,342).

Leydig cell tumor may enter the differential diagnosis because, like plasmacytoma, it has cells with appreciable eosinophilic cytoplasm. However, Leydig cell tumors are usually well-circumscribed, dark brown to tan tumors in which the neoplastic cells have more granular cytoplasm, lack a paranuclear hof, and have different nuclear characteristics. Appropriate immunostains resolve this and additional diagnostic issues if the light microscopy is equivocal and the potential for alternative interpretations is appreciated.

Leukemia, Including Myeloid Sarcoma

General and Clinical Features. Microscopic evaluation at autopsy shows that the testis is involved in 64 percent of patients with *acute leukemia* and 22 percent of those with *chronic leukemia* (309). The testis is enlarged in 5 to 10 percent of these cases. Testicular swelling is evident during life in only 5 percent of patients with leukemia, and testicular enlargement as a presenting manifestation of the disease is exceptionally rare. Clinically evident testicular involvement at presentation occurs in 2.3 percent of cases (343), a figure that is similar to the frequency of occult testicular involvement in biopsy specimens after chemotherapy to detect early relapse in patients with acute lymphoblastic leukemia (344).

Microscopic Findings. On microscopic examination, the pattern of leukemic infiltration is usually similar to that of lymphoma, predominantly intertubular, with tubular invasion and effacement of the tubules in some cases. Growth in cords may be conspicuous and confusing. In one exceptional case, there was mostly intratubular growth of immature myeloid cells (345). We are aware of fewer than 30 cases of myeloid sarcoma (tumors composed of immature myeloid cells, previously known as chloroma or granulocytic sarcoma) of the testis that have

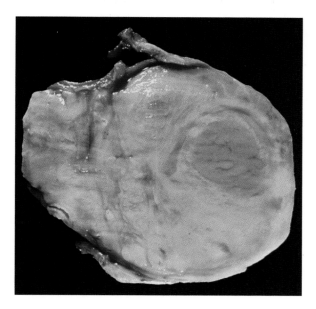

Figure 7-118

MYELOID SARCOMA OF TESTIS

The compressed testis (yellow-orange tissue) is surrounded by a creamy tumor that extensively obliterates the paratesticular soft tissues.

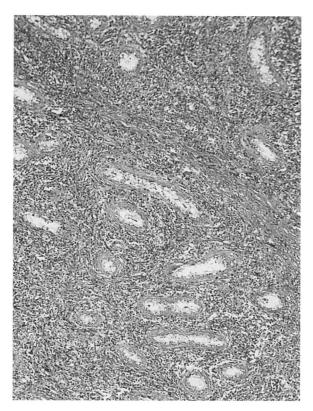

Figure 7-119

MYELOID SARCOMA OF TESTIS

There is prominent intertubular growth of tumor cells.

been reported in the English language literature, most in the form of individual case reports with only a few small series (346,347). In approximately 70 percent of those cases, the testis either represented a site of relapse in patients with established myeloid neoplasia or was the site of presentation for patients who had simultaneous occult leukemia or who subsequently developed it. In eight cases, however, the testis was an apparently isolated site of myeloid sarcoma and the patient did not develop subsequent leukemia, although follow-up was limited in some or the patient received treatment (345–349). In two cases, the patients received no treatment other than orchiectomy and remained disease-free at 7 years of follow-up (350,351). Myeloid sarcoma may also involve the epididymis.

Differential Diagnosis. Myeloid sarcomas are essentially indistinguishable from malignant lymphoma on gross examination, although, potentially, a green color may be suggestive of myeloid sarcoma based on the experience with extratesticular cases; we are unaware, however, that this has been documented in a testicular example. The testicular myeloid sarcomas we have seen were associated with

particularly prominent extratesticular extension (fig. 7-118). Microscopic evaluation of myeloid sarcomas (fig. 7-119) may cause major diagnostic problems: several cases have been misinterpreted as malignant lymphoma (fig. 7-120) or plasmacytoma (fig. 7-121). Features favoring the diagnosis of myeloid sarcoma rather than lymphoma include a slightly smaller cell size, more evenly dispersed chromatin, and less prominent nucleoli than found in most large cell lymphomas. The nuclei of myeloid sarcoma cells may be round or indented but usually lack the sharp angulation of cleaved lymphoid cells. If immature cells with recognizable myeloid differentiation, such as eosinophilic myelocytes, are found, myeloid sarcoma is strongly suggested. Enzyme histochemical stains for chloroacetate esterase (Leder stain) (fig. 7-122) or immunohistochemical stains for lysozyme, myeloperoxidase, CD34, and CD117 should facilitate the diagnosis. CD20 is not expressed

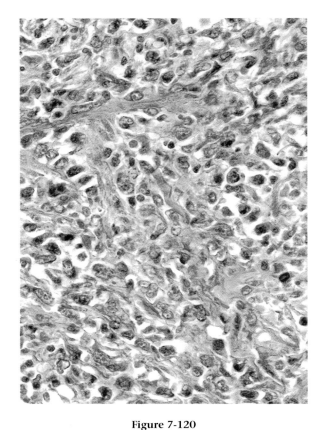

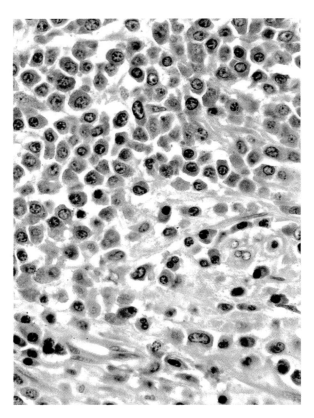

Figure 7-120

MYELOID SARCOMA OF TESTIS

The tumor cells have prominently cleaved nuclei. Note the resemblance to a large cell lymphoma.

Figure 7-121

MYELOID SARCOMA OF TESTIS

Most of the tumor cells have eccentric nuclei and abundant eosinophilic cytoplasm, and simulate plasma cells.

Figure 7-122

MYELOID SARCOMA OF TESTIS

The tumor cells are positive when stained for chloroacetate esterase.

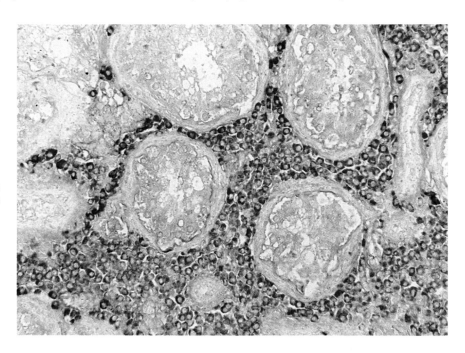

in myeloid sarcoma, whereas most lymphomas of the testis are CD20-positive, diffuse large B-cell lymphomas.

Plasmacytoma may be suggested because of a large number of myelocytes with eccentric nuclei and moderate amounts of pink cytoplasm (fig. 7-121). An associated chronic inflammatory cell infiltrate, with small lymphocytes and mature plasma cells, may further complicate the interpretation. However, the predominant population in myeloid sarcoma lacks the coarsely clumped chromatin, paranuclear hof, and more abundant nongranular cytoplasm characteristic of plasma cells. In addition, testicular myeloid sarcomas often exhibit prominent intrascrotal, extratesticular spread, whereas testicular plasmacytomas are almost always confined to the testis. Both myeloperoxidase and lysozyme immunostains are also helpful in this differential diagnosis.

SECONDARY TUMORS

General and Clinical Features. Although there were no nonhematopoietic metastases in over 600 autopsies of males dying of cancer at one center (352), metastases accounted for 3.6 percent of testicular tumors at another institution (353). The tumors are found most often in men over 50 years of age, but approximately one third of patients are under 40 years (354,355). They usually occur in patients with a known primary elsewhere, but the testicular mass is the presenting manifestation in 6 percent of cases (353) and, in a series of nonincidental cases that were received in consultation, there was no known history of a prior tumor in 62 percent (53). Carcinomas of the prostate gland (figs. 7-123–7-128) and lung most commonly metastasize to the testis, with the former accounting for about 45 percent and the latter 20 percent of metastatic carcinomas to the testis in the literature (53). Metastatic prostate cancer is found in 6 percent of therapeutic orchidectomy specimens (356). The next most frequent sources of metastatic carcinomas derive from the kidney (13 percent) (fig. 7-129), colorectum (9 percent), and urinary bladder (fig. 7-130) or renal pelvis (4 percent) (53). Metastatic melanoma is also a frequent finding among metastatic solid tumors to the testis (figs. 7-131–7-133). Melanospermia may be present in cases of melanoma (357–359).

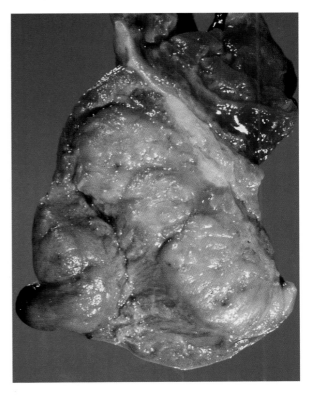

Figure 7-123

METASTATIC ADENOCARCINOMA OF PROSTATE TO TESTIS

Much of the testis is replaced by a lobulated yellow-brown tumor.

Occasional carcinoid tumors have metastasized to the testis (360). In one case (361), pressure on a probable testicular metastasis produced clinical manifestations of the carcinoid syndrome. Almost 4 percent of males with neuroblastoma had testicular metastases in one report (362). Testicular spread of many other tumors have been reported, including carcinomas of the pancreas, bile duct, liver, thyroid gland, and penis; retinoblastoma; pleural mesothelioma; adenoid cystic carcinoma; Wilms tumor; Merkel cell tumor (fig. 7-134); and occasional sarcomas (fig. 7-135) (363–371).

The routes of spread include the vas deferens for prostatic carcinoma, spermatic veins for renal cell carcinoma, lymphatics for intestinal carcinoma, and blood vessels for lung carcinoma. The diagnostic problems posed by testicular metastases are enhanced when the tumor presents clinically and there is concern

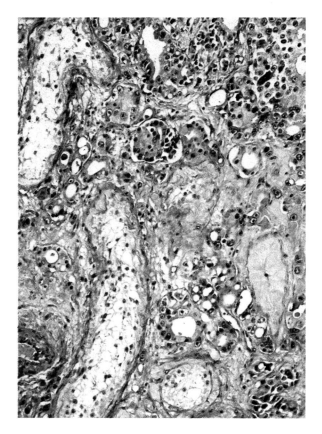

Figure 7-124

**METASTATIC ADENOCARCINOMA
OF PROSTATE TO TESTIS**

Clusters of tumor cells and a few neoplastic glands are present in the intertubular region.

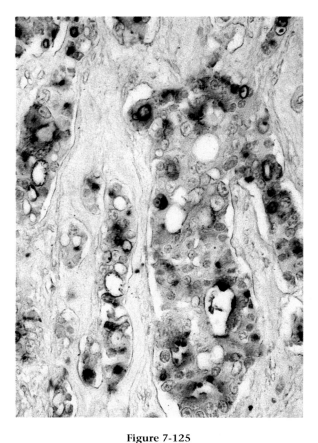

Figure 7-125

**METASTATIC ADENOCARCINOMA
OF PROSTATE TO TESTIS**

The tumor in figure 7-124 exhibits a strong immuno-histochemical reaction for prostate-specific antigen.

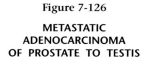

Figure 7-126

**METASTATIC
ADENOCARCINOMA
OF PROSTATE TO TESTIS**

The appearance in this case caused confusion initially with a Leydig cell tumor.

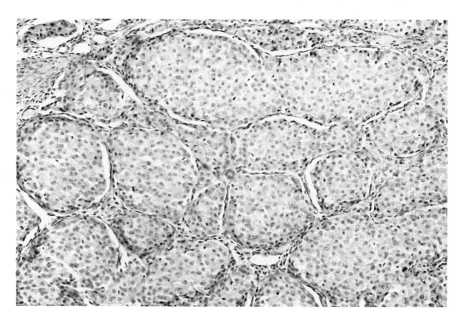

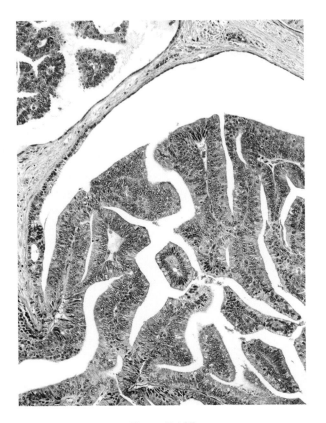

Figure 7-127

**METASTATIC ADENOCARCINOMA
OF PROSTATE TO TESTIS**

This tumor, which has the appearance of a ductal type of prostatic adenocarcinoma, grows within dilated channels of the rete testis and partially replaces the rete epithelium (left).

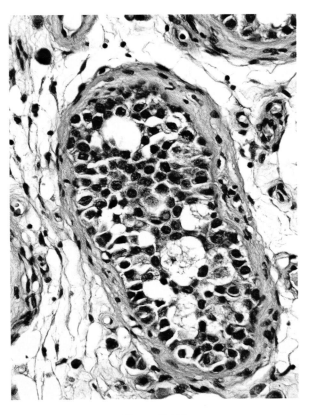

Figure 7-128

**METASTATIC ADENOCARCINOMA
OF PROSTATE TO TESTIS**

Extensive intratubular growth in this case caused initial confusion with seminoma.

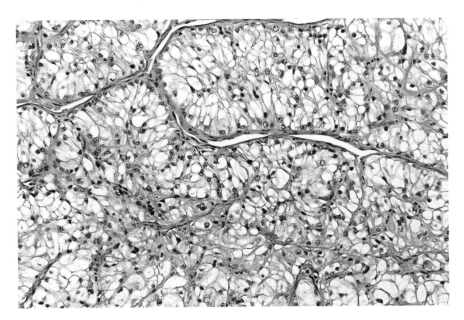

Figure 7-129

**METASTATIC RENAL CELL
CARCINOMA TO THE TESTIS**

The tubular growth pattern and clear cell morphology led to a misinterpretation as Sertoli cell tumor.

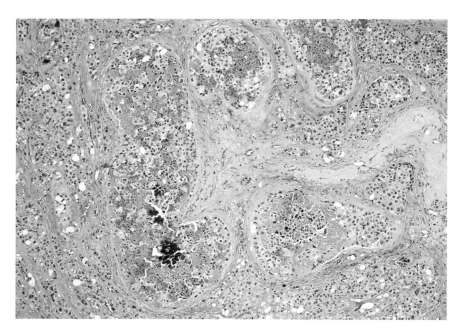

Figure 130

METASTATIC TRANSITIONAL CELL CARCINOMA OF THE BLADDER TO THE TESTIS

Prominent intratubular growth with comedo-type necrosis may result in confusion with embryonal carcinoma.

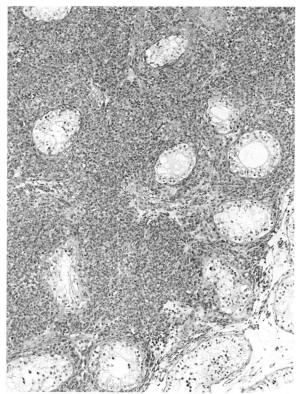

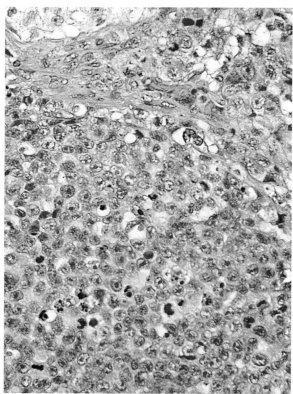

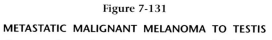

Figure 7-131

METASTATIC MALIGNANT MELANOMA TO TESTIS

Because of prominent intertubular growth, the initial impression is lymphoma.

Figure 7-132

METASTATIC MALIGNANT MELANOMA TO TESTIS

The tumor cells are highly malignant, with prominent mitotic activity. A portion of a seminiferous tubule is seen at the top.

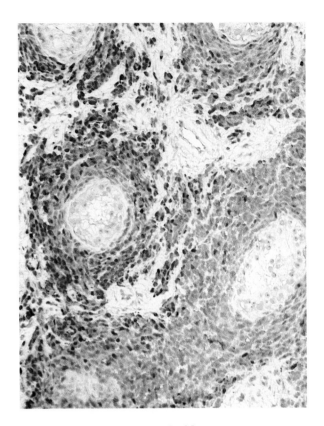

Figure 7-133

METASTATIC MALIGNANT MELANOMA TO TESTIS

The prominent intertubular growth in this case is highlighted by an immunohistochemical stain for S-100 protein.

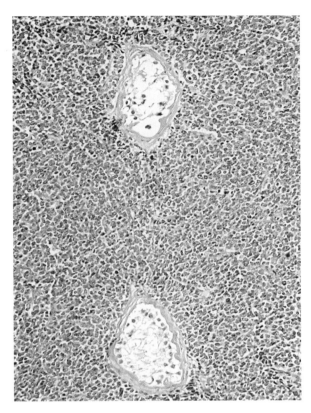

Figure 7-134

METASTATIC MERKEL CELL TUMOR TO TESTIS

There is a prominent intertubular pattern of growth, and at this magnification, the picture is indistinguishable from that of malignant lymphoma or certain other metastatic tumors such as melanoma.

for a primary neoplasm. In this circumstance, bilateral involvement, a feature that normally favors metastasis, is seen in only 8 percent of cases (53), whereas its overall frequency is approximately 20 percent when considering all cases of testicular metastases. In our experience with metastatic tumors to the testis that were received in consultation, prostatic carcinoma remained the most common single entity, followed by renal carcinoma (372), colonic carcinoma, and urothelial carcinoma.

Gross Findings. Sectioning usually reveals single or multiple nodules that may be confluent (fig. 7-123), but diffuse involvement is also seen. The presence of multiple nodules should raise the possibility of metastasis, particularly in a patient over 50 years of age, but nodules were identified grossly in only 8 percent of nonincidentally presenting cases (53).

Microscopic Findings and Differential Diagnosis. On microscopic examination, the tumor is usually predominantly in the interstitium (fig. 7-124), but the neoplastic cells may also invade the tubules (figs. 7-128, 7-130). There may be prominent involvement of blood vessels in the testis, epididymis, and cord, which should suggest the diagnosis, assuming the morphology is inconsistent with a primary testicular neoplasm. Lymphatic involvement was found in 69 percent of a series of 26 metastatic carcinomas (53).

The microscopic features of most metastatic tumors are incompatible with a primary testicular tumor, but nonetheless, occasionally significant errors in interpretation occur. Prostatic carcinoma of ductal type has a tendency to grow within the rete testis (fig. 7-127), possibly

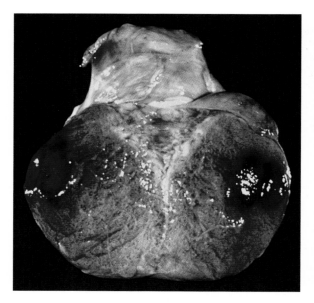

Figure 7-135

METASTATIC ANGIOSARCOMA TO TESTIS
A hemorrhagic nodule is present.

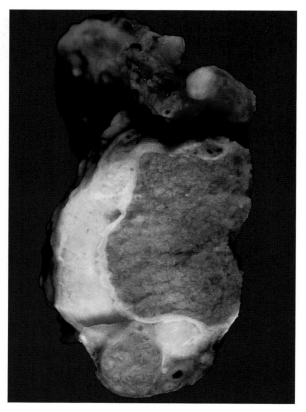

Figure 7-136

**METASTATIC ADENOCARCINOMA FROM
PANCREAS ENCASING EPIDIDYMIS**

A plaque-like growth of yellow-white tumor is seen.
(Courtesy of Dr. J. Eble, Indianapolis, IN.)

causing confusion with a primary carcinoma of the rete testis (53). Almost any tumor type may demonstrate prominent intratubular growth; some cases of metastatic prostatic carcinoma with this feature may mimic, to a limited degree, seminoma with an intratubular component (fig. 7-128). Examples of urothelial carcinoma with necrosis of intratubular tumor may be confused with embryonal carcinoma showing the characteristic comedo pattern of its intratubular component (fig. 7-130) (53). Metastatic melanoma may be misdiagnosed as seminoma (359) or, when there is prominent intertubular growth (fig. 7-131), large cell lymphoma. We have also seen metastatic renal cell carcinoma of the clear cell type misinterpreted as Sertoli cell tumor and seminoma (fig. 7-129) (372). In occasional difficult cases, special stains, particularly for mucin, argyrophil granules, and melanin, and immunoperoxidase studies, particularly for prostatic carcinoma (fig. 7-125), malignant melanoma (fig. 7-133), or specific markers of germ cell tumors and sex cord-stromal tumors that are in the differential diagnosis, may provide significant aid.

Metastases to the epididymis (fig. 7-136) (373) and cord (163) are occasionally challenging, both clinically and pathologically, when the tumor presents at these metastatic sites. Twenty-three metastatic tumors have presented as epididymal masses, with primary sites in the colon (7 cases), stomach (5 cases), pancreas (3 cases), prostate and kidney (2 cases each), ileum (carcinoid) (3 cases), and liver (1 case) (163,374). The morphologic differences from any primary tumor of the epididymis should suggest the possibility of a metastasis in most cases. Prominent vascular space invasion may also be helpful. In a series of malignant paratesticular and spermatic cord tumors from a general hospital, 10 tumors were primary and 9 metastatic (163). Six of the metastases involved the spermatic cord, and four of these presented prior to the identification of the primary tumor.

REFERENCES

1. De Nictolis M, Tommasoni S, Fabris G, Prat J. Intratesticular serous cystadenoma of borderline malignancy. A pathological, histochemical and DNA content study of a case with long-term follow-up. Virchows Arch A Pathol Anat Histol 1993;423:221-5.

2. Kernohan NM, Coutts AG, Best PV. Cystadeno-carcinoma of the appendix testis. Histopathology 1990;17:147-54.

3. Remmele W, Kaiserling E, Zerban U, et al. Serous papillary cystic tumor of borderline malignancy with focal carcinoma arising in testis: case report with immunohistochemical and ultrastructural observations. Hum Pathol 1992;23:75-9.

4. Walker AN, Mills SE, Stanley CM. Borderline serous cystadenoma of the tunica vaginalis testis. Surg Pathol 1988;1:431-6.

5. Young RH, Scully RE. Testicular and paratesticular tumors and tumor-like lesions of ovarian common epithelial and mullerian types. A report of four cases and review of the literature. Am J Clin Pathol 1986;86:146-52.

6. McClure RF, Keeney GL, Sebo TJ, Cheville JC. Serous borderline tumor of the paratestis: a report of seven cases. Am J Surg Pathol 2001;25:373-8.

7. Axiotis CA. Intratesticular serous papillary cystadenoma of low malignant potential: an ultrastructural and immunohistochemical study suggesting mullerian differentiation. Am J Surg Pathol 1988;12:56-63.

8. Jones MA, Young RH, Srigley JR, Scully RE. Paratesticular serous papillary carcinoma. A report of six cases. Am J Surg Pathol 1995;19:1359-65.

9. Becerra P, Isaac MA, Marquez B, Garcia-Puche JL, Zuluaga A, Nogales FF. Papillary serous carcinoma of the tunica vaginalis testis. Pathol Res Pract 2000;196:781-2.

10. Blumberg HM, Hendrix LE. Serous papillary adenocarcinoma of the tunica vaginalis of the testis with metastasis. Cancer 1991;67:1450-3.

11. Elbadawi A, Batchvarov MM, Linke CA. Intratesticular papillary mucinous cystadenocarcinoma. Urology 1979;14:280-4.

12. Ulbright TM, Young RH. Primary mucinous tumors of the testis and paratestis: a report of nine cases. Am J Surg Pathol 2003;27:1221-8.

13. Shimbo M, Araki K, Kaibuchi T, Kuramochi H, Mori I. Mucinous cystadenoma of the testis. J Urol 2004;172:146-7.

14. Uschuplich V, Hilsenbeck JR, Velasco CR. Paratesticular mucinous cystadenoma arising from an oviduct-like mullerian remnant: a case report

and review of the literature. Arch Pathol Lab Med 2006;130:1715-7.

15. Mesia L, Georgsson S, Zuretti A. Ossified intratesticular mucinous tumor. Arch Pathol Lab Med 1999;123:244-6.

16. Nistal M, Revestido R, Paniagua R. Bilateral mucinous cystadenocarcinoma of the testis and epididymis. Arch Pathol Lab Med 1992;116:1360-3.

17. Teo CH, Chua WJ, Consigliere DT, Raju GC. Primary intratesticular mucinous cystadenocarcinoma. Pathology 2005;37:92-4.

18. Iuga AC, Mull J, Batra R, Miller W. Mucinous cystadenocarcinoma of the testis: a case report. Hum Pathol 2011;42:1343-7.

19. Nochomovitz LE, Orenstein JM. Adenocarcinoma of the rete testis. Review and regrouping of reported cases and a consideration of miscellaneous entities. J Urogenit Pathol 1991;1:11-40.

20. Brennan MK, Srigley JR. Brenner tumor of the testis: case report and review of other intrascrotal examples. J Urol Pathol 1999;10:219-28.

21. Caccamo D, Socias M, Truchet C. Malignant Brenner tumor of the testis and epididymis. Arch Pathol Lab Med 1991;115:524-7.

22. Goldman RL. A Brenner tumor of the testis. Cancer 1970;26:853-6.

23. Nogales FF, Jr., Matilla A, Ortega I, Alvarez T. Mixed Brenner and adenomatoid tumor of the testis: an ultrastructural study and histogenetic considerations. Cancer 1979;43:539-43.

24. Uzoaru I, Ray VH, Nadimpalli V. Brenner tumor of the testis. Immunohistochemical comparison with its ovarian counterpart. J Urol Pathol 1995;3:249-53.

25. Ross L. Paratesticular Brenner-like tumor. Cancer 1968;21:722-6.

26. Tulunay O, Gogus C, Baltaci S, Bulut S. Clear cell adenocarcinoma of the tunica vaginalis of the testis with an adjacent uterus-like tissue. Pathol Int 2004;54:641-7.

27. Fleshman RL, Wasman JK, Bodner DG, Young RH, MacLennan GT. Mesodermal adenosarcoma of the testis. Am J Surg Pathol 2005;29:420-3.

28. Walker AN, Mills SE. Glandular inclusions in inguinal hernial sacs and spermatic cords. Müllerian-like remnants confused with functional reproductive structures. Am J Clin Pathol 1984;82:85-9.

29. Sundarasivarao D. The mullerian vestiges and benign epithelial tumors of the epididymis. J Pathol Bacteriol 1953;66:417-31.

30. Kellert E. An ovarian type pseudomucinous cystadenoma in the scrotum. Cancer 1959;12:187-90.

31. Scully RE, Young RH, Clement PB. Tumors of the ovary, maldeveloped gonads, fallopian tube and broad ligament. AFIP Atlas of Tumor Pathology. 3rd Series, Fascicle 23. Washington DC: American Registry of Pathology; 1998.

32. Guarch R, Rivas A, Puras A, Pesce C. Papillary serous carcinoma of ovarian type of the testis with borderline differentiation. Histopathology 2005;46:588-90.

33. Brito CG, Bloch T, Foster RS, Bihrle R. Testicular papillary cystadenomatous tumor of low malignant potential: a case report and discussion of the literature. J Urol 1988;139:378-9.

34. McCluggage WG, Shah V, Nott C, Clements B, Wilson B, Hill CM. Cystadenoma of spermatic cord resembling ovarian serous epithelial tumour of low malignant potential: immunohistochemical study suggesting mullerian differentiation. Histopathology 1996;28:77-80.

35. Vaughn DJ, Rizzo TA, Malkowicz SB. Chemosensitivity of malignant ovarian-type surface epithelial tumor of testis. Urology 2005;66:658.

36. Altaffer LF 3rd, Dufour DR, Castleberry GM, Steele SM Jr. Coexisting rete testis adenoma and gonadoblastoma. J Urol 1982;127:332-5.

37. Jones MA, Young RH. Sertoliform rete cystadenoma: a report of two cases. J Urol Pathol 1997;7:47-53.

38. Murao T, Tanahashi T. Adenofibroma of the rete testis. A case report with electron microscopic findings. Acta Pathol Jpn 1988;38:105-12.

39. Sinclair AM, Gunendran T, Napier-Hemy RD, Lee S, Denley H. Sertoliform cystadenoma of the rete testis. Pathol Int 2006;56:568-9.

40. Jones EC, Murray SK, Young RH. Cysts and epithelial proliferations of the testicular collecting system (including rete testis). Semin Diagn Pathol 2000;17:270-93.

41. Janane A, Ghadouane M, Alami M, Abbar M. Paratesticular adenofibroma. Scand J Urol Nephrol 2003;37:179-80.

42. Fridman E, Skarda J, Ofek-Moravsky E, Cordoba M. Complex multilocular cystic lesion of rete testis, accompanied by smooth muscle hyperplasia, mimicking intratesticular Leydig cell neoplasm. Virchows Arch 2005;447:768-71.

43. Kacar A, Senel E, Caliskan D, Demirel F, Tiryaki T. Sertoliform cystadenoma: a case with overlapping features. Pediatr Dev Pathol 2011;14:138-43.

44. Hartwick RW, Ro JY, Srigley JR, Ordoñez NG, Ayala AG. Adenomatous hyperplasia of the rete testis. A clinicopathologic study of nine cases. Am J Surg Pathol 1991;15:350-7.

45. Nistal M, Paniagua R. Adenomatous hyperplasia of the rete testis. J Pathol 1988;154:343-6.

46. Nistal M, Castillo MC, Regadera J, Garcia-Cabezas MA. Adenomatous hyperplasia of the rete testis. A review and report of new cases. Histol Histopathol 2003;18:741-52.

47. Amin MB. Selected other problematic testicular and paratesticular lesions: rete testis neoplasms and pseudotumors, mesothelial lesions and secondary tumors. Mod Pathol 2005;18 Suppl 2:S131-S145.

48. Ulbright TM, Gersell DJ. Rete testis hyperplasia with hyaline globule formation. A lesion simulating yolk sac tumor. Am J Surg Pathol 1991;15:66-74.

49. Sanchez-Chapado M, Angulo JC, Haas GP. Adenocarcinoma of the rete testis. Urology 1995;46:468-75.

50. Nakagawa T, Hiraoka N, Ihara F, Komiyama M, Kanai Y, Matsuno Y. Primary adenocarcinoma of the rete testis with preceding diagnosis of pulmonary metastases. Int J Urol 2006;13:1532-5.

51. Rubegni P, Poggiali S, De Santi M, et al. Cutaneous metastases from adenocarcinoma of the rete testis. J Cutan Pathol 2006;33:181-4.

52. Nochomovitz LE, Orenstein JM. Adenocarcinoma of the rete testis: consolidation and analysis of 31 reported cases with a review of miscellaneous entities. J Urol Pathol 1994;2:1-37.

53. Ulbright TM, Young RH. Metastatic carcinoma to the testis: a clinicopathologic analysis of 26 non-incidental cases with emphasis on deceptive features. Am J Surg Pathol 2008;32:1683-93.

54. Watson PH, Jacob VC. Adenocarcinoma of the rete testis with sertoliform differentiation. Arch Pathol Lab Med 1989;113:1169-71.

55. Crisp-Lindgren N, Travers H, Wells MM, Cawley LP. Papillary adenocarcinoma of the rete testis: autopsy findings, histochemistry, immunohistochemistry, ultrastructure, and clinical correlations. Am J Surg Pathol 1988;12:492-501.

56. Visscher DW, Talerman A, Rivera LR, Mazur MT. Adenocarcinoma of the rete testis with a spindle cell component. A possible metaplastic carcinoma. Cancer 1989;64:770-5.

57. Samaratunga H, Kanowski P, Gloughlin B, Walker N, Searle J. Adenocarcinoma of the rete testis with intratubular invasion of the testis. J Urol Pathol 1994;2:291-300.

58. Perimenis P, Athanasopoulos A, Speakman M. Primary adenocarcinoma of the rete testis. Int Urol Nephrol 2003;35:373-4.

59. Okada H, Hanioka K, Fujisawa M, Arakawa S, Kamidono S, Ohbayashi C. Primary adenocarcinoma of the rete testis. Br J Urol 1997;79:300-2.

60. Skailes GE, Menasce L, Banerjee SS, Shanks JH, Logue JP. Adenocarcinoma of the rete testis. Clin Oncol (R Coll Radiol) 1998;10:401-3.

61. Glazier DB, Vates TS, Cummings KB, Antoun S. Adenocarcinoma of the rete testis. World J Urol 1996;14:397-400.

62. Perry BB, Outman JE, Olsen LT, Damjanov I, Langenstroer P, Thrasher JB. Adenocarcinoma of the rete testis presenting in an undescended testicle. J Urol 2003;170:1304.

63. Tong GX, Memeo L, Colarossi C, et al. PAX8 and PAX2 immunostaining facilitates the diagnosis of primary epithelial neoplasms of the male genital tract. Am J Surg Pathol 2011;35:1473-83.

64. Chitale SV, Waterfall NB, Blackshaw AJ. Adenocarcinoma of rete testis masquerading as epididymal cysts. Br J Urol 1998;81:922-3.

65. Menon PK, Vasudevarao, Sabhiki A, Kudesia S, Joshi DP, Mathur UB. A case of carcinoma rete testis: histomorphological, immunohistochemical and ultrastructural findings and review of literature. Ind J Cancer 2002;39:106-11.

66. Burns MW, Chandler WL, Krieger JN. Adenocarcinoma of rete testis. Role of inguinal orchiectomy plus retroperitoneal lymph node dissection. Urology 1991;37:571-3.

67. Mrak RE, Husain MM, Schaefer RF. Ultrastructure of metastatic rete testis adenocarcinoma. Arch Pathol Lab Med 1990;114:84-8.

68. Black WC, Benitez RE, Buesing OR, Hojnoski W. Bizarre adenomatoid tumor of testicular tunics. Cancer 1964;17:1472-6.

69. Wachter DL, Wunsch PH, Hartmann A, Agaimy A. Adenomatoid tumors of the female and male genital tract. A comparative clinicopathologic and immunohistochemical analysis of 47 cases emphasizing their site-specific morphologic diversity. Virchows Arch 2011;458:593-602.

70. Kiely EA, Flanagan A, Williams G. Intrascrotal adenomatoid tumours. Br J Urol 1987;60:255-7.

71. Miller F, Lieberman MK. Local invasion in adenomatoid tumors. Cancer 1968;21:933-9.

72. Golden A, Ash JE. Adenomatoid tumors of the genital tract. Am J Pathol 1945;21:63-79.

73. Barwick KW, Madri JA. An immunohistochemical study of adenomatoid tumors utilizing keratin and factor VIII antibodies. Evidence for a mesothelial origin. Lab Invest 1982;47:276-80.

74. Broth G, Bullock WK, Morrow J. Epididymal tumors. 1. Report of 15 new cases including review of literature. 2. Histochemical study of the so-called adenomatoid tumor. J Urol 1968;100:530-6.

75. Davy CL, Tang CK. Are all adenomatoid tumors adenomatoid mesotheliomas? Hum Pathol 1981;12:360-9.

76. De Klerk DP, Nime F. Adenomatoid tumors (mesothelioma) of testicular and paratesticular tissue. Urology 1975;6:635-41.

77. Glantz GM. Adenomatoid tumors of the epididymis: a review of 5 new cases, including a case report associated with hydrocele. J Urol 1966;95:227-33.

78. Jackson JR. The histogenesis of the "adenomatoid" tumor of the genital tract. Cancer 1958;11:337-50.

79. Longo VJ, McDonald JR, Thompson GJ. Primary neoplasms of the epididymis. Special reference to adenomatoid tumors. JAMA 1951;147:937-41.

80. Mackay B, Bennington JL, Skoglund RW. The adenomatoid tumor: fine structural evidence for a mesothelial origin. Cancer 1971;27:109-15.

81. Stavrides A, Hutcheson JB. Benign mesotheliomas of testicular appendages: a morphologic and histochemical study of seven cases and review of theories of histogenesis. J Urol 1960;83:448-53.

82. Taxy JB, Battifora H, Oyasu R. Adenomatoid tumors: a light microscopic, histochemical, and ultrastructural study. Cancer 1974;34:306-16.

83. Yasuma T, Saito S. Adenomatoid tumor of the male genital tract—a pathological study of eight cases and review of the literature. Acta Pathol Jpn 1980;30:883-906.

84. Hes O, Perez-Montiel DM, Alvarado C, et al. Thread-like bridging strands: a morphologic feature present in all adenomatoid tumors. Ann Diagn Pathol 2003;7:273-7.

85. Banks ER, Mills SE. Histiocytoid (epithelioid) hemangioma of the testis. The so-called vascular variant of "adenomatoid tumor". Am J Surg Pathol 1990;14:584-9.

86. Kausch I, Galle J, Buttner H, Bohle A, Jocham D. Leiomyo-adenomatoid tumor of the epididymis. J Urol 2002;168:636.

87. Sangoi AR, McKenney JK, Schwartz EJ, Rouse RV, Longacre TA. Adenomatoid tumors of the female and male genital tracts: a clinicopathological and immunohistochemical study of 44 cases. Mod Pathol 2009;22:1228-35.

88. Williams SB, Han M, Jones R, Andrawis R. Adenomatoid tumor of the testes. Urology 2004;63:779-81.

89. Skinnider BF, Young RH. Infarcted adenomatoid tumor: a report of five cases of a facet of a benign neoplasm that may cause diagnostic difficulty. Am J Surg Pathol 2004;28:77-83.

90. Delahunt B, Eble JN, King D, Bethwaite PB, Nacey JN, Thornton A. Immunohistochemical evidence for mesothelial origin of paratesticular adenomatoid tumour. Histopathology 2000;36:109-15.

91. Detassis C, Pusiol T, Piscioli F, Luciani L. Adenomatoid tumor of the epididymis: immunohistochemical study of 8 cases. Urol Int 1986;41:232-4.

92. Kommoss F, Oliva E, Bittinger F, et al. Inhibin-alpha CD99, HEA125, PLAP, and chromogranin immunoreactivity in testicular neoplasms and the androgen insensitivity syndrome. Hum Pathol 2000;31:1055-61.

93. Moch H, Ohnacker H, Epper R, Gudat F, Mihatsch MJ. A new case of malignant mesothelioma of the tunica vaginalis testis. Immunohistochemistry in comparison with an adenomatoid tumor of the testis. Pathol Res Pract 1994;190:400-4.

94. Said JW, Nash G, Lee M. Immunoperoxidase localization of keratin proteins, carcinoembryonic antigen, and factor VIII in adenomatoid tumors: evidence for a mesothelial derivation. Hum Pathol 1982;13:1106-8.

95. Sakai T, Nakada T, Kono T, Katayama T, Masuda S. Adenomatoid tumor of the epididymis with special reference to immunohistochemical study of 3 cases. Hinyokika Kiyo 1989;35:1537-42.

96. Ferenczy A, Fenoglio J, Richart RM. Observations on benign mesothelioma of the genital tract (adenomatoid tumor): a comparative ultrastructural study. Cancer 1972;30:244-60.

97. Rege JD, Amarapurkar AD, Phatak AM. Fine needle aspiration cytology of adenomatoid tumor. A case report. Acta Cytol 1999;43:495-7.

98. Monappa V, Rao AC, Krishnanand G, Mathew M, Garg S. Adenomatoid tumor of tunica albuginea mimicking seminoma on fine needle aspiration cytology: a case report. Acta Cytol 2009;53:349-52.

99. Tewari R, Mishra MN, Salopal TK. The role of fine needle aspiration cytology in evaluation of epididymal nodular lesions. Acta Cytol 2007;51:168-70.

100. Bisceglia M, Dor DB, Carosi I, Vairo M, Pasquinelli G. Paratesticular mesothelioma. Report of a case with comprehensive review of literature. Adv Anat Pathol 2010;17:53-70.

101. Attanoos RL, Gibbs AR. Primary malignant gonadal mesotheliomas and asbestos. Histopathology 2000;37:150-9.

102. Plas E, Riedl CR, Pfluger H. Malignant mesothelioma of the tunica vaginalis testis: review of the literature and assessment of prognostic parameters. Cancer 1998;83:2437-46.

103. de Lima GR, de Oliveira VP, Reis PH, Pinheiro FG, Lima MV, Gonzaga-Silva LF. A rare case of malignant hydrocele in a young patient. J Pediatr Urol 2009;5:243-5.

104. Khan MA, Puri P, Devaney D. Mesothelioma of tunica vaginalis testis in a child. J Urol 1997;158:198-9.

105. Grove A, Jensen ML, Donna A. Mesotheliomas of the tunica vaginalis testis and hernial sacs. Virchows Arch A Pathol Anat Histopathol 1989;415:283-92.

106. Kasdon EJ. Malignant mesothelioma of the tunica vaginalis propria testis. Report of two cases. Cancer 1969;23:1144-50.

107. Jones MA, Young RH, Scully RE. Malignant mesothelioma of the tunica vaginalis: a clinicopathologic analysis of 11 cases with review of the literature. Am J Surg Pathol 1995;19:815-25.

108. Daya D, McCaughey WT. Well-differentiated papillary mesothelioma of the peritoneum. A clinicopathologic study of 22 cases. Cancer 1990;65:292-6.

109. Winstanley AM, Landon G, Berney D, Minhas S, Fisher C, Parkinson MC. The immunohistochemical profile of malignant mesotheliomas of the tunica vaginalis: a study of 20 cases. Am J Surg Pathol 2006;30:1-6.

110. Fukunaga M. Well-differentiated papillary mesothelioma of the tunica vaginalis: a case report with aspirate cytologic, immunohistochemical, and ultrastructural studies. Pathol Res Pract 2010;206:105-9.

111. Al-Salam S, Hammad FT, Salman MA, AlAshari M. Expression of Wilms tumor-1 protein and CD 138 in malignant mesothelioma of the tunica vaginalis. Pathol Res Pract 2009;205:797-800.

112. Mikuz G, Höpfel-Kreiner I. Papillary mesothelioma of the tunica vaginalis propria testis. Case report and ultrastructural study. Virchows Arch A Pathol Anat Histol 1982;396:231-8.

113. Shimada S, Ono K, Suzuki Y, Mori N. Malignant mesothelioma of the tunica vaginalis testis: a case with a predominant sarcomatous component. Pathol Int 2004;54:930-4.

114. Rosai J, Dehner LP. Nodular mesothelial hyperplasia in hernia sacs: a benign reactive condition simulating a neoplastic process. Cancer 1975;35:165-75.

115. Churg A. Paratesticular mesothelial proliferations. Semin Diagn Pathol 2003;20:272-8.

116. Gerald WL, Miller HK, Battifora H, Miettinen M, Silva EG, Rosai J. Intra-abdominal desmoplastic small round-cell tumor: report of 19 cases of a distinctive type of high-grade polyphenotypic malignancy affecting young individuals. Am J Surg Pathol 1991;15:499-513.

117. Cummings OW, Ulbright TM, Young RH, Del Tos AP, Fletcher CD, Hull MT. Desmoplastic small round cell tumors of the paratesticular region. A report of six cases. Am J Surg Pathol 1997;21:219-25.

118. Ordonez NG, El-Naggar AK, Ro JY, Silva EG, Mackay B. Intra-abdominal desmoplastic small cell tumor: a light microscopic, immunocytochemical, ultrastructural, and flow cytometric study. Hum Pathol 1993;24:850-65.

119. Prat J, Matias-Guiu X, Algaba F. Desmoplastic small round-cell tumor. Am J Surg Pathol 1992;16:306-7.

120. Furman J, Murphy WM, Wajsman Z, Berry AD 3rd. Urogenital involvement by desmoplastic small round-cell tumor. J Urol 1997;158:1506-9.

121. Garcia-Gonzalez J, Villanueva C, Fernandez-Acenero MJ, Paniagua P. Paratesticular desmoplastic small round cell tumor: case report. Urol Oncol 2005;23:132-4.

122. Kawano N, Inayama Y, Nagashima Y, et al. Desmoplastic small round-cell tumor of the paratesticular region: report of an adult case with demonstration of EWS and WT1 gene fusion using paraffin-embedded tissue. Mod Pathol 1999;12:729-34.

123. Ordonez NG. Desmoplastic small round cell tumor: I: a histopathologic study of 39 cases with emphasis on unusual histological patterns. Am J Surg Pathol 1998;22:1303-13.

124. Roganovich J, Bisogno G, Cecchetto G, d'Amore ES, Carli M. Paratesticular desmoplastic small round cell tumor: case report and review of the literature. J Surg Oncol 1999;71:269-72.

125. Thuret R, Renaudin K, Leclere J, Battisti S, Bouchot O, Theodore C. Uncommon malignancies: case 3. Paratesticular desmoplastic small round-cell tumor. J Clin Oncol 2005;23:6253-5.

126. Ordonez NG. Desmoplastic small round cell tumor: II: an ultrastructural and immunohistochemical study with emphasis on new immunohistochemical markers. Am J Surg Pathol 1998;22:1314-27.

127. Waugh MS, Dash RC, Turner KC, Dodd LG. Desmoplastic small round cell tumor: using FISH as an ancillary technique to support cytologic diagnosis in an unusual case. Diagn Cytopathol 2007;35:516-20.

128. Insabato L, Di Vzio D, Lambertini M, Bucci L, Pettinato G. Fine needle aspiration cytology of desmoplastic small round cell tumor. A case report. Acta Cytol 1999;43:641-6.

129. Ali SZ, Nicol TL, Port J, Ford G. Intraabdominal desmoplastic small round cell tumor: cytopathologic findings in two cases. Diagn Cytopathol 1998;18:449-52.

130. Ferlicot S, Coue O, Gilbert E, et al. Intraabdominal desmoplastic small round cell tumor: report of a case with fine needle aspiration, cytologic diagnosis and molecular confirmation. Acta Cytol 2001;45:617-21.

131. Gerald WL, Ladanyi M, de Alava E, et al. Clinical, pathologic, and molecular spectrum of tumors associated with t(11;22)(p13;q12): desmoplastic small round-cell tumor and its variants. J Clin Oncol 1998;16:3028-36.

132. Odrzywolski KJ, Mukhopadhyay S. Papillary cystadenoma of the epididymis. Arch Pathol Lab Med 2010;134:630-3.

133. Glasker S, Tran MG, Shively SB, et al. Epididymal cystadenomas and epithelial tumourlets: effects of VHL deficiency on the human epididymis. J Pathol 2006;210:32-41.

134. Lamiell JM, Salazar FG, Hsia YE. von Hippel-Lindau disease affecting 43 members of a single kindred. Medicine (Baltimore) 1989;68:1-29.

135. Price EB Jr. Papillary cystadenoma of the epididymis. A clinicopathologic analysis of 20 cases. Arch Pathol 1971;91:456-70.

136. Ben-Izhak O. Solitary papillary cystadenoma of the spermatic cord presenting as an inguinal mass. J Urol Pathol 1997;7:55-61.

137. Meyer JS, Roth LM, Silverman JL. Papillary cystadenomas of the epididymis and spermatic cord. Cancer 1964;17:1241-7.

138. Aydin H, Young RH, Ronnett BM, Epstein JI. Clear cell papillary cystadenoma of the epididymis and mesosalpinx: immunohistochemical differentiation from metastatic clear cell renal cell carcinoma. Am J Surg Pathol 2005;29:520-3.

139. Gokden N, Gokden M, Phan DC, McKenney JK. The utility of PAX-2 in distinguishing metastatic clear cell renal cell carcinoma from its morphologic mimics: an immunohistochemical study with comparison to renal cell carcinoma marker. Am J Surg Pathol 2008;32:1462-7.

140. Torikata C. Papillary cystadenoma of the epididymis. An ultrastructural and immunohistochemical study. J Submicro Cytol Pathol 1994;26:387-93.

141. Manivel JC. Pseudoneoplastic lesions of the male genitals. In: Wick MR, Humphrey PA, Ritter JH, eds. Pathology of pseudoneoplastic lesions. New York: Lippincott-Raven Press; 1997:247-63.

142. Jones MA, Young RH, Scully RE. Adenocarcinoma of the epididymis: a report of four cases and review of the literature. Am J Surg Pathol 1997;21:1474-80.

143. Salm R. Papillary carcinoma of the epididymis. J Pathol 1969;97:253-9.

144. Lima GC, Varkarakis IM, Allaf ME, Fine SW, Kavoussi LR. Small cell carcinoma of epididymis: multimodal therapy. Urology 2005;66:432.

145. Kamal BA. Basaloid carcinoma of epididymis. Urology 2005;65:1227.

146. Kuo T, Gomez LG. Monstrous epithelial cells in human epididymis and seminal vesicles. A pseudomalignant change. Am J Surg Pathol 1981;5:483-90.

147. Shah VI, Ro JY, Amin MB, Mullick S, Nazeer T, Ayala AG. Histologic variations in the epididymis: findings in 167 orchiectomy specimens. Am J Surg Pathol 1998;22:990-6.

148. Diamond DA, Breitfeld PP, Bur M, Gang D. Melanotic neuroectodermal tumor of infancy: an important mimicker of paratesticular rhabdomyosarcoma. J Urol 1992;147:673-5.

149. Johnson RE, Scheithauer BW, Dahlin DC. Melanotic neuroectodermal tumor of infancy: a review of seven cases. Cancer 1983;52:661-6.

150. Murayama T, Fujita K, Ohashi T, Matsushita T. Melanotic neuroectodermal tumor of the epididymis in infancy: a case report. J Urol 1989;141:105-6.

151. Pettinato G, Manivel JC, d'Amore ES, Jaszcz W, Gorlin RJ. Melanotic neuroectodermal tumor of infancy. A reexamination of a histogenetic problem based on immunohistochemical, flow cytometric, and ultrastructural study of 10 cases. Am J Surg Pathol 1991;15:233-45.

152. Raju U, Zarbo RJ, Regezi JA, Krutchkoff DJ, Perrin EV. Melanotic neuroectodermal tumors of infancy: intermediate filament-, neuroendocrine-, and melanoma-associated antigen profiles. Appl Immunohistochem 1993;1:69-76.

153. Ricketts RR, Majmudarr B. Epididymal melanotic neuroectodermal tumor of infancy. Hum Pathol 1985;16:416-20.

154. Kruse-Losler B, Gaertner C, Burger H, Seper L, Joos U, Kleinheinz J. Melanotic neuroectodermal tumor of infancy: systematic review of the literature and presentation of a case. Oral Surg Oral Med Oral Pathol Oral Radiol Endod 2006;102:204-16.

155. Jurincic-Winkler C, Metz KA, Klippel KF. Melanotic neuroectodermal tumor of infancy (MNTI) in the epididymis. A case report with immunohistological studies and special consideration of malignant features. Zentralbl Pathol 1994;140:181-5.

156. Toda T, Sadi AM, Kiyuna M, Egawa H, Tamamoto T, Toyoda Z. Pigmented neuroectodermal tumor of infancy in the epididymis. A case report. Acta Cytol 1998;42:775-80.

157. Pantanowitz L, Galan A, Gang DL, Crisi GM, LaPolice P, Goulart RA. Diagnostic cytologic features of an epididymal melanotic neuroectodermal tumor of infancy present in scrotal fluid: a case report. Acta Cytol 2006;50:460-5.

158. Khoddami M, Squire J, Zielenska M, Thorner P. Melanotic neuroectodermal tumor of infancy: a molecular genetic study. Pediatr Dev Pathol 1998;1:295-9.

159. Kapadia SB, Frisman DM, Hitchcock CL, Ellis GL, Popek EJ. Melanotic neuroectodermal tumor of infancy. Clinicopathological, immunohistochemical, and flow cytometric study. Am J Surg Pathol 1993;17:566-73.

160. Calonge WM, Heitor F, Castro LP, et al. Neonatal paratesticular neuroblastoma misdiagnosed as in utero torsion of testis. J Pediatr Hematol Oncol 2004;26:693-5.

161. Matsunaga T, Takahashi H, Ohnuma N, et al. Paratesticular neuroblastoma with N-myc activation. J Pediatr Surg 1993;28:1612-4.

162. Spark RP. Leiomyoma of epididymis. Arch Pathol Lab Med 1972;93:18-21.

163. Lioe TF, Biggart JD. Tumours of the spermatic cord and paratesticular tissue. A clinicopathological study. Br J Urol 1993;71:600-6.

164. Srigley JR, Hartwick RW. Tumors and cysts of the paratesticular region. Pathol Annu 1990;25(Pt 2):51-108.

165. Cecil AB. Intrascrotal lipomata. J Urol 1927;17:557-66.

166. Lander EB, Lee I. Giant scrotal lipomatosis. J Urol 1996;156:1773.

167. Al Rashid M, Soundra Pandyan GV. Spindle cell lipoma of the spermatic cord. Saudi Med J 2004;25:667-8.

168. McMenamin ME, Fletcher CD. Mammary-type myofibroblastoma of soft tissue: a tumor closely related to spindle cell lipoma. Am J Surg Pathol 2001;25:1022-9.

168a. Chen BJ, Mariño-Enriquez A, Fletcher CD, Hornick JL. Loss of retinoblastoma protein expression in spindle cell/pleomorphic lipomas and cytogenetically related tumors: an immunohistochemical study with diagnostic implications. Am J Surg Pathol 2012;36:1119-28.

169. Mai KT, Yazdi HM, Collins JP. Vascular myxolipoma ("angiomyxolipoma") of the spermatic cord. Am J Surg Pathol 1996;20:1145-8.

170. Tokunaka S, Taniguchi N, Hashimoto H, Yachiku S, Fujita M. Leiomyoblastoma of the epididymis in a child. J Urol 1990;143:991-3.

171. Busmanis I. Paratesticular plexiform tumour of myofibroblastic origin. Histopathology 1991;18:178-80.

172. Nistal M, Paniagua R. Primary neuroectodermal tumour of the testis. Histopathology 1985;9:1351-9.

173. Tanda F, Rocca PC, Bosincu L, Massarelli G, Cossu A, Manca A. Rhabdomyoma of the tunica vaginalis of the testis: a histologic, immunohistochemical, and ultrastructural study. Mod Pathol 1997;10:608-11.

174. Hornick JL, Fletcher CD. Soft tissue perineurioma: clinicopathologic analysis of 81 cases including those with atypical histologic features. Am J Surg Pathol 2005;29:845-58.

175. Fagerli JC, Hasegawa SL, Schneck FX. Paratesticular perineurioma: initial description. J Urol 1999;162:881-2.

176. Lai FM, Allen PW, Chan LW, Chan PS, Cooper JE, Mackenzie TM. Aggressive fibromatosis of the spermatic cord. A typical lesion in a "new" location. Am J Clin Pathol 1995;104:403-7.

177. Sumi Y, Shindoh N, Komura S et al. Paratesticular aggressive fibromatosis: CT findings. Abdom Imaging 2000;25:210-2.

178. Gluck RW, Bloiso G, Glasser J. Paratesticular desmoid tumor. Urology 1987;29:648-9.

179. Chetty R, Bandid S, Freedman D. Cavernous haemangioma of the epididymis mimicking a testicular malignancy. Aust N Z J Surg 1993;63:235-7.

180. Turkyilmaz Z, Sonmez K, Karabulut R, et al. A childhood case of intrascrotal neurofibroma with a brief review of the literature. J Pediatr Surg 2004;39:1261-3.

181. Chung H. Granular cell tumor of the spermatic cord: a case report with light and electron microscopic study. J Urol 1978;120:379-82.

182. Pardalidis NP, Grigoriadis K, Papatsoris AG, Kosmaoglou EV, Horti M. Primary paratesticular adult ganglioneuroma. Urology 2004;63:584-5.

183. Chan PT, Tripathi S, Low SE, Robinson LQ. Case report—ancient schwannoma of the scrotum. BMC Urol 2007;7:1.

184. Jiang R, Chen JH, Chen M, Li QM. Male genital schwannoma, review of 5 cases. Asian J Androl 2003;5:251-4.

185. Montgomery JS, Hollenbeck BK, Fisher PC, Murphy HS, Underwood W 3rd. Benign paratesticular schwannoma. Can J Urol 2004;11:2393-5.

186. Schiff SF, Lachman MF, Hammers L. Paratesticular myxoma: case report and review. J Urol 1993;149:132-3.

187. Fetsch JF, Laskin WB, Tavassoli FA. Superficial angiomyxoma (cutaneous myxoma): a clinicopathologic study of 17 cases arising in the genital region. Int J Gynecol Pathol 1997;16:325-34.

188. Turner DT, Shah SM, Jones R. Intrascrotal lipoblastoma. Br J Urol 1998;81:166-7.

189. Del Sordo R, Cavaliere A, Sidoni A, Colella R, Bellezza G. Intrascrotal lipoblastoma: a case report and review of the literature. J Pediatr Surg 2007;42:E9-11.

190. Fine SW, Davis NJ, Lykins LE, Montgomery E. Solitary testicular myofibroma: a case report and review of the literature. Arch Pathol Lab Med 2005;129:1322-5.

191. Nistal M, Gonzalez-Peramato P, Serrano A, Reyes-Mugica M, Cajaiba MM. Primary intratesticular spindle cell tumors: interdigitating dendritic cell tumor and inflammatory myofibroblastic tumor. Int J Surg Pathol 2011;19:104-9.

192. Jones MA, Young RH, Scully RE. Benign fibromatous tumors of the testis and paratesticular region: a report of 9 cases with a proposed classification of fibromatous tumors and tumor-like lesions. Am J Surg Pathol 1997;21:296-305.

193. Parveen T, Fleischmann J, Petrelli M. Benign fibrous tumor of the tunica vaginalis testis. Report of a case with light, electron microscopic, and immunocytochemical study, and review of the literature. Arch Pathol Lab Med 1992;116:277-80.

194. Belville WD, Insalaco SJ, Dresner ML, Buck AS. Benign testis tumors. J Urol 1982;128:1198-200.

195. Miyamoto H, Montgomery EA, Epstein JI. Paratesticular fibrous pseudotumor: a morphologic and immunohistochemical study of 13 cases. Am J Surg Pathol 2010;34:569-74.

196. Iwasa Y, Fletcher CD. Cellular angiofibroma: clinicopathologic and immunohistochemical analysis of 51 cases. Am J Surg Pathol 2004;28: 1426-35.

197. Laskin WB, Fetsch JF, Mostofi FK. Angiomyofibroblastoma-like tumor of the male genital tract: analysis of 11 cases with comparison to female angiomyofibroblastoma and spindle cell lipoma. Am J Surg Pathol 1998;22:6-16.

198. Chen E, Fletcher CD. Cellular angiofibroma with atypia or sarcomatous transformation: clinicopathologic analysis of 13 cases. Am J Surg Pathol 2010;34:707-714.

198a. Montgomery E, Epstein JI. Anastomosing hemangioma of the genitourinary tract: a lesion mimicking angiosarcoma. Am J Surg Pathol 2009;33:1364-9.

199. Chetty R. Epididymal cavernous haemangiomas. Histopathology 1993;22:396-8.

200. Liokumovich P, Herbert M, Sandbank J, Schvimer M, Dolberg L. Cavernous hemangioma of spermatic cord: report of a case with immunohistochemical study. Arch Pathol Lab Med 2002;126:357-8.

201. Suriawinata A, Talerman A, Vapnek JM, Unger P. Hemangioma of the testis: report of unusual occurrences of cavernous hemangioma in a fetus and capillary hemangioma in an older man. Ann Diagn Pathol 2001;5:80-3.

202. Hargreaves HK, Scully RE, Richie JP. Benign hemangioendothelioma of the testis: case report with electron microscopic documentation and review of the literature. Am J Clin Pathol 1982;77:637-42.

203. Iczkowski KA, Kiviat J, Cheville JC, Bostwick DG. Multifocal capillary microangioma of the testis. J Urol Pathol 1997;7:113-9.

204. Du S, Powell J, Hii A, Weidner N. Myoid gonadal stromal tumor: a distinct testicular tumor with peritubular myoid cell differentiation. Hum Pathol 2012;43:144-9.

205. Steeper TA, Rosai J. Aggressive angiomyxoma of the female pelvis and perineum. Report of nine cases of a distinctive type of gynecologic soft-tissue neoplasm. Am J Surg Pathol 1983;7:463-75.

206. Carlinfante G, De Marco L, Mori M, Ferretti S, Crafa P. Aggressive angiomyxoma of the spermatic cord. Two unusual cases occurring in childhood. Pathol Res Pract 2001;197:139-44.

207. Idrees MT, Hoch BL, Wang BY, Unger PD. Aggressive angiomyxoma of male genital region. Report of 4 cases with immunohistochemical evaluation including hormone receptor status. Ann Diagn Pathol 2006;10:197-204.

208. Tsang WY, Chan JK, Lee KC, Fisher C, Fletcher CD. Aggressive angiomyxoma: a report of four cases occurring in men. Am J Surg Pathol 1992;16:1059-65.

209. Jingping Z, Chunfu Z. Clinical experiences on aggressive angiomyxoma in China (report of 93 cases). Int J Gynecol Cancer 2010;20:303-7.

210. Kidric DM, MacLennan GT. Aggressive angiomyxoma of the male genital region. J Urol 2008;180:1506.

211. Clatch RJ, Drake WK, Gonzalez JG. Aggressive angiomyxoma in men: a report of two cases associated with inguinal hernias. Arch Pathol Lab Med 1993;117:911-3.

212. Iezzoni JC, Fechner RE, Wong LS, Rosai J. Aggressive angiomyxoma in males: a report of four cases. Am J Clin Pathol 1995;104:391-6.

213. van Roggen JF, van Unnik JA, Briaire-de Brujin IH, Hogendoorn PC. Aggressive angiomyxoma: a clinicopathological and immunohistochemical study of 11 cases with long-term follow-up. Virchows Arch 2005;446:157-63.

214. Hastak MS, Raghuvanshi SR, Sahu S, Vyankatesh A, Ramraje SN, Ranjan A. Aggressive angiomyxoma in men. J Assoc Physicians India 2008;56:373-5.

215. Durdov MG, Tomic S, Pisac VP, Spoljar MS. Aggressive angiomyxoma of scrotum. Scand J Urol Nephrol 1998;32:299-302.

216. Mukonoweshuro P, McCormick F, Rachapalli V, Natale S, Smith ME. Paratesticular mammary-type myofibroblastoma. Histopathology 2007;50:396-7.

217. Bellinger MF, Gibbons MD, Koontz WW Jr, Graff M. Paratesticular liposarcoma. Urology 1978;11:285-8.

218. Johnson DE, Harris JD, Ayala AG. Liposarcoma of spermatic cord. Urology 1978;11:190-2.

219. Schwartz SL, Swierzewski SJ 3rd, Sondak VK, Grossman HB. Liposarcoma of the spermatic cord: report of 6 cases and review of the literature. J Urol 1995;153:154-7.

220. Cecchetto G, Grotto P, De Bernardi B, Indolfi P, Perilongo G, Carli M. Paratesticular rhabdomyo-sarcoma in childhood: experience of the Italian Cooperative Study. Tumori 1988;74:645-7.

221. Horn RC, Enterline HT. Rhabdomyosarcoma: a clinicopathologic study and classification of 39 cases. Cancer 1958;11:181-99.

222. Leuschner I, Newton WA Jr, Schmidt D, et al. Spindle cell variants of embryonal rhabdomyo-sarcoma in the paratesticular region. A report of the Intergroup Rhabdomyosarcoma Study. Am J Surg Pathol 1993;17:221-30.

223. Loughlin KR, Retik AB, Weinstein HJ, et al. Genitourinary rhabdomyosarcoma in children. Cancer 1989;63:1600-6.

224. Masera A, Ovcak Z, Mikuz G. Angiosarcoma of the testis. Virchows Archiv 1999;434:351-3.

225. Prince CL. Rhabdomyosarcoma of the testicle. J Urol 1942;48:187-95.

226. Ravich L, Lerman PH, Drabkin JW, Foltin E. Pure testicular rhabdomyosarcoma. J Urol 1965;94:596-9.

227. Yachia D, Auslaender L. Primary leiomyosar-coma of the testis. J Urol 1989;141:955-6.

228. Zukerberg LR, Young RH. Primary testicular sarcoma: a report of two cases. Hum Pathol 1990;21:932-5.

229. Kawanishi Y, Tamura M, Akiyama K, et al. Rhabdoid tumours of the spermatic cord. Br J Urol 1989;63:439-40.

230. Algaba F, Trias I, Castro C. Inflammatory malignant fibrous histiocytoma of the spermatic cord with eosinophilia. Histopathology 1989;14:319-21.

231. Lanzafame S, Fragetta F, Emmanuele C, et al. Paratesticular pleomorphic rhabdomyosarcoma in the elderly. Int J Surg Pathol 1999;7:27-32.

232. Soosay GN, Parkinson MC, Paradinas J, Fisher C. Paratesticular sarcomas revisited: a review of cases in the British Testicular Tumour Panel and Registry. Br J Urol 1996;77:143-6.

233. Dehner LP, Scott D, Stocker JT. Meconium peri-orchitis: a clinicopathologic study of four cases with a review of the literature. Hum Pathol 1986;17:807-12.

234. Ferrari A, Bisogno G, Casanova M, et al. Paratesticular rhabdomyosarcoma: report from the Italian and German Cooperative Group. J Clin Oncol 2002;20:449-55.

235. Ferrari A, Bisogno G, Casanova M, et al. Is alveolar histotype a prognostic factor in paratesticular rhabdomyosarcoma? The experience of Italian and German Soft Tissue Sarcoma Cooperative Group. Pediatr Blood Cancer 2004;42:134-8.

236. Crist WM, Anderson JR, Meza JL, et al. Intergroup rhabdomyosarcoma study-IV: results for patients with nonmetastatic disease. J Clin Oncol 2001;19:3091-102.

237. Montgomery E, Fisher C. Paratesticular liposarcoma: a clinicopathologic study. Am J Surg Pathol 2003;27:40-7.

238. Kraus MD, Guillou L, Fletcher CD. Well-differentiated inflammatory liposarcoma: an uncommon and easily overlooked variant of a common sarcoma. Am J Surg Pathol 1997;21:518-27.

239. Folpe AL, Weiss SW. Lipoleiomyosarcoma (well-differentiated liposarcoma with leiomyosarcomatous differentiation): a clinicopathologic study of nine cases including one with dedifferentiation. Am J Surg Pathol 2002;26:742-9.

240. Downes KA, Goldblum JR, Montgomery EA, Fisher C. Pleomorphic liposarcoma: a clinicopathologic analysis of 19 cases. Mod Pathol 2001;14:179-84.

241. Mentzel T, Palmedo G, Kuhnen C. Well-differentiated spindle cell liposarcoma ('atypical spindle cell lipomatous tumor') does not belong to the spectrum of atypical lipomatous tumor but has a close relationship to spindle cell lipoma: clinicopathologic, immunohistochemical, and molecular analysis of six cases. Mod Pathol 2010;23:729-36.

242. Binh MB, Sastre-Garau X, Guillou L, et al. MDM2 and CDK4 immunostainings are useful adjuncts in diagnosing well-differentiated and dedifferentiated liposarcoma subtypes: a comparative analysis of 559 soft tissue neoplasms with genetic data. Am J Surg Pathol 2005;29:1340-7.

243. Weaver J, Rao P, Goldblum JR, et al. Can MDM2 analytical tests performed on core needle biopsy be relied upon to diagnose well-differentiated liposarcoma? Mod Pathol 2010;23:1301-6.

244. Lucas DR, Shukla A, Thomas DG, Patel RM, Kubat AJ, McHugh JB. Dedifferentiated liposarcoma with inflammatory myofibroblastic tumor-like features. Am J Surg Pathol 2010;34: 844-51.

245. Farrell MA, Donnelly BJ. Malignant smooth muscle tumors of the epididymis. J Urol 1980; 124:151-3.

246. Fisher C, Goldblum JR, Epstein JI, Montgomery E. Leiomyosarcoma of the paratesticular region: a clinicopathologic study. Am J Surg Pathol 2001;25:1143-9.

247. Varzaneh FE, Verghese M, Shmookler BM. Paratesticular leiomyosarcoma in an elderly man. Urology 2002;60:1112.

248. Grey LF, Sorial RF, Shaw WH. Spermatic cord sarcoma. Leiomyosarcoma and retroperitoneal lymph node dissection. Urology 1986;27:28-31.

249. Seidl C, Lippert C, Grouls V, Jellinghaus W. [Leiomyosarcoma of the spermatic cord with paraneoplastic beta-hCG production]. Pathologe 1998;19:146-50. [German]

250. Merchant W, Calonje E, Fletcher CD. Inflammatory leiomyosarcoma: a morphological subgroup within the heterogeneous family of so-called inflammatory malignant fibrous histiocytoma. Histopathology 1995;27:525-32.

251. Rubin BP, Fletcher CD. Myxoid leiomyosarcoma of soft tissue, an underrecognized variant. Am J Surg Pathol 2000;24:927-36.

252. Ptochos A, Iosifidis N, Papazafiriou G, Kehagia-Koutoufari T, Karagiannopoulou G. Primary paratesticular epithelioid leiomyosarcoma. Urol Int 2003;70:321-3.

253. Suster S. Epithelioid leiomyosarcoma of the skin and subcutaneous tissue. Clinicopathologic, immunohistochemical, and ultrastructural study of five cases. Am J Surg Pathol 1994;18:232-40.

254. Konety BR, Singh J, Lyne JC, Salup RR. Leiomyosarcoma with osteoclast-like giant cells of the spermatic cord. A case report and review of the literature. Urol Int 1996;56:259-62.

255. Borri A, Nesi G, Bencini L, Pernice LM. Bizarre leiomyoma of the epididymis. A case report. Minerva Urol Nefrol 2000;52:29-31.

256. Slone S, O'Connor D. Scrotal leiomyomas with bizarre nuclei: a report of three cases. Mod Pathol 1998;11:282-7.

257. Barton JH, Davis CJ Jr, Sesterhenn IA, Mostofi FK. Smooth muscle hyperplasia of the testicular adnexa clinically mimicking neoplasia: clinicopathologic study of sixteen cases. Am J Surg Pathol 1999;23:903-9.

258. Eltorky M, O'Brien TF, Walzer Y. Primary paratesticular maignant fibrous histiocytoma: case report and review of the literature. J Urol Pathol 1994;1:425-9.

259. Sclama AO, Berger BW, Cherry JM, Young JD Jr. Malignant fibrous histiocytoma of the spermatic cord: the role of retroperitoneal lymphadenectomy in management. J Urol 1983;130: 577-9.

260. Lin BT, Harvey DA, Medeiros LJ. Malignant fibrous histiocytoma of the spermatic cord: report of two cases and review of the literature. Mod Pathol 2002;15:59-65.

261. Vallat-Decouvelaere AV, Dry SM, Fletcher CD. Atypical and malignant solitary fibrous tumors in extrathoracic locations: evidence of their comparability to intra-thoracic tumors. Am J Surg Pathol 1998;22:1501-11.

262. Kneale BJ, Bishop NL, Britton JP. Kaposi's sarcoma of the testis. Br J Urol 1993;72:116-7.

263. Weil DA, Ruckle HC, Lui PD, Saukel W. Kaposi's sarcoma of the testicle. AIDS Read 1999;9:455-6, 461.

264. Heikaus S, Schaefer KL, Eucker J, et al. Primary peripheral primitive neuroectodermal tumor/Ewing's tumor of the testis in a 46-year-old man-differential diagnosis and review of the literature. Hum Pathol 2009;40:893-7.

265. Ulbright TM, Srigley JR, Hatzianastassiou DK, Young RH. Leydig cell tumors of the testis with unusual features. Adipose differentiation, calcification with ossification, and spindle-shaped tumor cells. Am J Surg Pathol 2002;26:1424-33.

266. Ulbright TM, Hattab EM, Zhang S, et al. Primitive neuroectodermal tumors in patients with testicular germ cell tumors usually resemble pediatric-type central nervous system embryonal neoplasms and lack chromosome 22 rearrangements. Mod Pathol 2010;23:972-80.

267. Cooke A, Deshpande AV, La Hei ER, Kellie S, Arbuckle S, Cummins G. Ectopic nephrogenic rests in children: the clinicosurgical implications. J Pediatr Surg 2009;44:e13-6.

268. Orlowski JP, Levin HS, Dyment PG. Intrascrotal Wilms' tumor developing in a heterotopic renal anlage of probable mesonephric origin. J Pediatr Surg 1980;15:679-82.

269. Taylor WF, Myers M, Taylor WR. Extrarenal Wilms' tumour in an infant exposed to intrauterine phenytoin. Lancet 1980;2:481-2.

270. Goldberg J, Drut R. Ectopic immature renal tissue. Report of two cases. Pathol Res Pract 1984;179:115-23.

271. Oottamasathien S, Wills ML, Brock JW 3rd, Pope JC 4th. Primary extrarenal nephroblastomatosis. Urology 2007;69:184.

272. Aydin GB, Ciftci AO, Yalcin B, et al. Paratesticular metastasis from Wilms tumor associated with a hydrocele. Pediatr Blood Cancer 2006;47:97-9.

273. Trobs RB, Friedrich T, Lotz I, Bennek J. Wilms' tumour metastasis to the testis: long-term survival. Pediatr Surg Int 2002;18:541-2.

274. Sauter ER, Schorin MA, Farr GH Jr, Falterman KW, Arensman RM. Wilms' tumor with metastasis to the left testis. Am Surg 1990;56:260-2.

275. Emerson RE, Ulbright TM, Zhang S, Foster RS, Eble JN, Cheng L. Nephroblastoma arising in a germ cell tumor of testicular origin. Am J Surg Pathol 2004;28:687-92.

276. Gillis AJ, Oosterhuis JW, Schipper ME, et al. Origin and biology of a testicular Wilms' tumor. Genes Chromosomes Cancer 1994;11:126-35.

277. Shih DF, Wang JS, Tseng HH. Primary squamous cell carcinoma of the testis. J Urol 1996;156:1772.

278. Kim NR, Cho HY, Yoon SJ, Park JH, Ha SY. Primary squamous cell carcinoma in the testis: a case report. J Korean Med Sci 2010;25:634-7.

279. Cimic J, Oosterhof GO, Koot RA, Debruyne FM. Testicular teratoma with malignant transformation, presenting as squamous cell carcinoma with metastatic localization in the penile corpus cavernosum. Br J Urol 1997;79:142-3.

280. Bryan RL, Liu S, Newman J, O'Brien JM, Considine J. Squamous cell carcinoma arising in a chronic hydrocoele. Histopathology 1990;17:178-80.

281. Dharkar D, Kraft JR. Paraganglioma of the spermatic cord. An incidental finding. J Urol Pathol 1994;2:89-93.

282. Mashat F, Meccawi A, Garg S, Christian E. Paraganglioma of the spermatic cord. Ann Saudi Med 1993;13:208-10.

283. Gupta R, Howell RS, Amin MB. Paratesticular paraganglioma: a rare cause of an intrascrotal mass. Arch Pathol Lab Med 2009;133:811-3.

284. Suson K, Mathews R, Goldstein JD, Dehner LP. Juvenile xanthogranuloma presenting as a testicular mass in infancy: a clinical and pathologic study of three cases. Pediatr Dev Pathol 2010;13:39-45.

285. Ruiz E, Pozo P, Toselli L, Fernandez M, Christiansen S, Lambertini R. Unusual benign paratesticular tumor in an infant mimicking rhabdomyosarcoma. Urology 2008;71:1067-9.

286. Engel FL, McPherson HT, Fetter BF, et al. Clinical, morphological and biochemical studies on a malignant testicular tumor. J Clin Endocrinol Metab 1964;24:528-42.

287. Abell MR, Holtz F. Testicular and paratesticular neoplasms in patients 60 years of age and older. Cancer 1968;21:852-70.

288. Akhtar M, Al-Dayel F, Siegrist K, Ezzat A. Neutrophil-rich Ki-1-positive anaplastic large cell lymphoma presenting as a testicular mass. Mod Pathol 1996;9:812-5.

289. Chan JK, Tsang WY, Lau WH, et al. Aggressive T/natural killer cell lymphoma presenting as testicular tumor. Cancer 1996;77:1198-205.

290. Doll DC, Weiss RB. Malignant lymphoma of the testis. Am J Med 1986;81:515-24.

291. Ferry JA, Harris NL, Young RH, Coen J, Zietman A, Scully RE. Malignant lymphoma of the testis, epididymis, and spermatic cord. A clinicopathologic study of 69 cases with immunophenotypic analysis. Am J Surg Pathol 1994;18:376-90.

292. Ferry JA, Ulbright TM, Young RH. Anaplastic large cell lymphoma presenting in the testis. J Urol Pathol 1997;5:139-47.

293. Gowing NF. Malignant lymphoma of the testis. Br J Urol 1964;36:85-94.

294. Haddy TB, Sandlund JT, Magrath IT. Testicular involvement in young patients with non-Hodgkin's lymphoma. Am J Pediat Hematol Oncol 1988;10:224-9.

295. Hayes MM, Sacks MI, King HS. Testicular lymphoma. A retrospective review of 17 cases. S Afr Med J 1983;64:1014-6.

296. Hsueh C, Gonzalez-Crussi F, Murphy SB. Testicular angiocentric lymphoma of postthymic T-cell type in a child with T-cell acute lymphoblastic leukemia in remission. Cancer 1993;72:1801-5.

297. Jackson SM, Montessori GA. Malignant lymphoma of the testis: review of 17 cases in British Columbia with survival related to pathological subclassification. J Urol 1980;123:881-3.

298. Martenson JA Jr, Buskirk SJ, Ilstrup DM, et al. Patterns of failure in primary testicular non-Hodgkin's lymphoma. J Clin Oncol 1988;6:297-302.

299. McDermott MB, O'Briain DS, Shiels OM, Daly PA. Malignant lymphoma of the epididymis. A case report of bilateral involvement by a follicular large cell lymphoma. Cancer 1995;75:2174-9.

300. Mehrotra RR, Wahal KM, Agarwal PK. Testicular lymphoma: a clinicopathologic study of 22 cases. Indian J Pathol Microbiol 1978;21:91-6.

301. Moertel CL, Watterson J, McCormick SR, Simonton SC. Follicular large cell lymphoma of the testis in a child. Cancer 1995;75:1182-6.

302. Moller MB, d'Amore F, Christensen BE. Testicular lymphoma: a population-based study of incidence, clinicopathological correlations and prognosis. The Danish Lymphoma Study Group, LYFO. Eur J Cancer 1994;30A:1760-4.

303. Nonomura N, Aozasa K, Ueda T, et al. Malignant lymphoma of the testis: histological and immunohistological study of 28 cases. J Urol 1989;141:1368-71.

304. Sussman EB, Hajdu SI, Lieberman PH, Whitmore WF. Malignant lymphoma of the testis: a clinicopathologic study of 37 cases. J Urol 1977;118:1004-7.

305. Talerman A. Primary malignant lymphoma of the testis. J Urol 1977;118:783-6.

306. Turner RR, Colby TV, MacKintosh FR. Testicular lymphomas: a clinicopathologic study of 35 cases. Cancer 1981;48:2095-102.

307. Wilkins BS, Williamson JM, O'Brien CJ. Morphological and immunohistological study of testicular lymphomas. Histopathology 1989;15:147-56.

308. Froberg MK, Hamati H, Kant JA, Addya K, Salhany KE. Primary low-grade T-helper cell testicular lymphoma. Arch Pathol Lab Med 1997;121:1096-9.

309. Givler RL. Testicular involvement in leukemia and lymphoma. Cancer 1969;23:1290-5.

310. Ferry JA. Lymphomas of the male genital tract. In: Ferry JA, ed. Extranodal lymphomas. Philadelphia: Elsevier/Saunders; 2011:238-58.

311. Bacon CM, Ye H, Diss TC, et al. Primary follicular lymphoma of the testis and epididymis in adults. Am J Surg Pathol 2007;31:1050-8.

312. Pileri SA, Sabattini E, Rosito P, et al. Primary follicular lymphoma of the testis in childhood: an entity with peculiar clinical and molecular characteristics. J Clin Pathol 2002;55:684-8.

313. Heller KN, Teruya-Feldstein J, La Quaglia MP, Wexler LH. Primary follicular lymphoma of the testis: excellent outcome following surgical resection without adjuvant chemotherapy. J Pediatr Hematol Oncol 2004;26:104-7.

314. Swerdlow SH. Pediatric follicular lymphomas, marginal zone lymphomas, and marginal zone hyperplasia. Am J Clin Pathol 2004;122:S98-109.

315. Õzsan N, Bedke BJ, Law ME, et al. Clinicopathologic and genetic characterization of follicular lymphomas presenting in the ovary reveals 2 distinct subgroups. Am J Surg Pathol 2011;35:1691-9.

316. Licci S, Morelli L, Covello R. Primary mantle cell lymphoma of the testis. Ann Hematol 2011; 90:483-4.

317. Sugimoto K, Koike H, Esa A. Plasmablastic lymphoma of the right testis. Int J Urol 2011;18:85-6.

318. Ornstein DL, Bifulco CB, Braddock DT, Howe JG. Histopathologic and molecular aspects of CD56+ natural killer/ T-cell lymphoma of the testis. Int J Surg Pathol 2008;16:291-300.

319. Azua-Romeo J, Alvarez-Alegret R, Serrano P, Mayayo E. Primary anaplastic large cell lymphoma of the testis. Int Urol Nephrol 2004;36:393-6.

320. Lagmay J, Termuhlen A, Fung B, Ranalli M. Primary testicular presentation of ALK-1-negative anaplastic large cell lymphoma in a pediatric patient. J Pediatr Hematol Oncol 2009;31:330-2.

321. Seliem RM, Chikwava K, Swerdlow SH, Young RH, Ferry JA. Classical Hodgkin's lymphoma presenting as a testicular mass: report of a case. Int J Surg Pathol 2007;15:207-12.

322. Swerdlow SH, Campo E, Harris NL, et al, eds. WHO classification of tumours of haematopoietic and lymphoid tissues. Lyon: International Agency for Research on Cancer; 2008.

323. Al-Abbadi MA, Hattab EM, Tarawneh MS, Amr SS, Orazi A, Ulbright TM. Primary testicular diffuse large B-cell lymphoma belongs to the nongerminal center B-cell-like subgroup: A study of 18 cases. Mod Pathol 2006;19:1521-7.

324. Kemmerling R, Stintzing S, Muhlmann J, Dietze O, Neureiter D. Primary testicular lymphoma: a strictly homogeneous hematological disease? Oncol Rep 2010;23:1261-7.

325. Booman M, Douwes J, Glas AM, de Jong D, Schuuring E, Kluin PM. Primary testicular diffuse large B-cell lymphomas have activated B-cell-like subtype characteristics. J Pathol 2006;210:163-71.

326. Melicow MM. Classification of tumors of the testis: a clinical and pathological study based on 105 primary and 13 secondary cases in adults, and 3 primary and 4 secondary cases in children. J Urol 1955;73:547-74.

327. Cao D, Li J, Guo CC, Allan RW, Humphrey PA. SALL4 is a novel diagnostic marker for testicular germ cell tumors. Am J Surg Pathol 2009;33:1065-77.

328. Braaten KM, Young RH, Ferry JA. Viral-type orchitis: a potential mimic of testicular neoplasia. Am J Surg Pathol 2009;33:1477-84.

329. Mazloom A, Fowler N, Medeiros LJ, Iyengar P, Horace P, Dabaja BS. Outcome of patients with diffuse large B-cell lymphoma of the testis by era of treatment: the M. D. Anderson Cancer Center experience. Leuk Lymphoma 2010;51:1217-24.

330. Dolin S, Dewar JP. Extramedullary plasmacytoma. Am J Pathol 1956;32:83-103.

331. Ferry JA, Young RH, Scully RE. Testicular and epididymal plasmacytoma: a report of 7 cases, including three that were the initial manifestation of plasma cell myeloma. Am J Surg Pathol 1997;21:590-8.

332. Hayes DW, Bennett WA, Heck FJ. Extramedullary lesions in multiple myeloma. Review of literature and pathologic studies. AMA Arch Pathol 1952;53:262-72.

333. Avitable AM, Gansler TS, Tomaszewski JE, Hanno P, Goldwein MI. Testicular plasmacytoma. Urology 1989;34:51-4.

334. Levin HS, Mostofi FK. Symptomatic plasmacytoma of the testis. Cancer 1970;25:1193-203.

335. Melicow MM, Cahill GF. Plasmacytoma (multiple myeloma) of testis: a report of four cases and review of the literature. J Urol 1954;71:103-13.

336. Unger PD, Strauchen JA, Greenberg M, Kirschenbaum A, Rabinowitz A, Parsons RB. Testicular plasmacytoma: a report of a case and a review of the literature. J Urol Pathol 1998;7:207-14.

337. Ramadan A, Naab T, Frederick W, Green W. Testicular plasmacytoma in a patient with the acquired immunodeficiency syndrome. Tumori 2000;86:480-2.

338. Hou TY, Dai MS, Kao WY. Testicular plasmacytoma with bone dissemination without medullary plasmacytosis. Ann Hematol 2003;82:518-20.

339. Gowing NF. Malignant lymphoma of the testis. In: Pugh RC, ed. Pathology of the testis. Oxford: Blackwell Scientific; 1976:334-55.

340. Pham TH, Shetty SD, Stone CH, De Peralta-Venturina M, Menon M. Bilateral synchronous testicular plasmacytoma. J Urol 2000;164(Pt 1):781.

341. Schichman SA, McClure R, Schaefer RF, Mehta P. HIV and plasmablastic lymphoma manifesting in sinus, testicles, and bones: a further expansion of the disease spectrum. Am J Hematol 2004;77:291-5.

342. Cui W, Kong NR, Ma Y, Amin HM, Lai R, Chai L. Differential expression of the novel oncogene, SALL4, in lymphoma, plasma cell myeloma, and acute lymphoblastic leukemia. Mod Pathol 2006;19:1585-92.

343. Hijiya N, Liu W, Sandlund JT, et al. Overt testicular disease at diagnosis of childhood acute lymphoblastic leukemia: lack of therapeutic role of local irradiation. Leukemia 2005;19:1399-403.

344. Arya LS, Kotikanyadanam SP, Bhargava M, et al. Pattern of relapse in childhood ALL: challenges and lessons from a uniform treatment protocol. J Pediatr Hematol Oncol 2010;32:370-5.

345. Rawal A, Keeler TC, Milano MA. Testicular extramedullary myeloid cell tumor: report of a case with unique clinicopathologic features and a brief review of the literature. Arch Pathol Lab Med 2004;128:332-4.

346. Valbuena JR, Admirand JH, Lin P, Medeiros LJ. Myeloid sarcoma involving the testis. Am J Clin Pathol 2005;124:445-52.

347. Ferry JA, Srigley JR, Young RH. Granulocytic sarcoma of the testis: a report of two cases of a neoplasm prone to misinterpretation. Mod Pathol 1997;10:320-5.

348. Eggener SE, Abrahams A, Keeler TC. Granulocytic sarcoma of the testis. Urology 2004;63:584-5.

349. Armstrong MB, Nafiu OO, Valdez R, Park JM, Williams JA, Wechsler DS. Testicular chloroma in a nonleukemic infant. J Pediatr Hematol Oncol 2005;27:393-6.

350. Lagerveld BW, Wauters CA, Karthaus HF. Testicular granulocytic sarcoma without systemic leukemia. Urol Int 2005;75:94-6.

351. Constantinou J, Nitkunan T, Al-Izzi M, Mc-Nicholas TA. Testicular granulocytic sarcoma, a source of diagnostic confusion. Urology 2004;64:807-9.

352. Tiltman AJ. Metastatic tumours in the testis. Histopathology 1979;3:31-7.

353. Patel SR, Richardson RL, Kvols L. Metastatic cancer to the testes: a report of 20 cases and review of the literature. J Urol 1989;142:1003-5.

354. Hanash KA, Carney JA, Kelalis PP. Metastatic tumors to testicles: routes of metastasis. J Urol 1969;102:465-8.

355. Price EB Jr, Mostofi FK. Secondary carcinoma of the testis. Cancer 1957;10:592-5.

356. Johansson JE, Lannes P. Metastases to the spermatic cord, epididymis and testicles from carcinoma of the prostate—five cases. Scand J Urol Nephrol 1983;17:249-51.

357. Dasgupta TD, Grabstald H. Melanoma of the genitourinary tract. J Urol 1965;93:607-14.

358. Lowell DM, Lewis EL. Melanospermia: a hitherto undescribed entity. J Urol 1966;95:407-11.

359. Richardson PG, Millward MJ, Shrimankar JJ, Cantwell BM. Metastatic melanoma to the testis simulating primary seminoma. Br J Urol 1992;69:663-5.

360. Berdjis CC, Mostofi FK. Carcinoid tumors of the testis. J Urol 1977;118:777-82.

361. Dockerty MB, Scheifley CH. Metastasizing carcinoid tumor: report of an unusual case with episodic cyanosis. Am J Clin Pathol 1955;25:770-4.

362. Kushner BH, Vogel R, Hajdu SI, Helson L. Metastatic neuroblastoma and testicular involvement. Cancer 1985;56:1730-2.

363. Bouvier DP, Fox CW Jr, Frishberg DP, Kozakowski M, Cobos E. A solitary testicular relapse of a rhabdomyosarcoma in an adult. Cancer 1990;65:2611-4.

364. Cho KR, Olson JL, Epstein JI. Primitive rhabdomyosarcoma presenting with diffuse bone marrow involvement: an immunohistochemical and ultrastructural study. Mod Pathol 1988;1:23-8.

365. Grignon DJ, Shum DT, Hayman WP. Metastatic tumours of the testes. Can J Surg 1986;29:359-61.

366. Hanash KA. Metastatic tumors to the testicles. Prog Clin Biol Res 1985;203:61-7.

367. Johnson DE, Jackson L, Ayala AG. Secondary carcinoma of the testis. South Med J 1971;64:1128-30.

368. Pienkos EJ, Jablokow VR. Secondary testicular tumors. Cancer 1972;30:481-5.

369. Ro JY, Ayala AG, Têtu B, et al. Merkel cell carcinoma metastatic to the testis. Am J Clin Pathol 1990;94:384-9.

370. Ro JY, Sahin AA, Ayala AG, Ordonez NG, Grignon DJ, Popok SM. Lung carcinoma with metastasis to testicular seminoma. Cancer 1990;66:347-53.

371. Young RH, Van Patter HT, Scully RE. Hepatocellular carcinoma metastatic to the testis. Am J Clin Pathol 1987;87:117-20.

372. Datta MW, Ulbright TM, Young RH. Renal cell carcinoma metastatic to the testis and its adnexa: a report of five cases including three that accounted for the initial clinical presentation. Int J Surg Pathol 2001;9:49-56.

373. Smallman LA, Odedra JK. Primary carcinoma of sigmoid colon metastasizing to epididymis. Urology 1984;23:598-9.

374. Kanomata N, Eble JN. Adenocarcinoma of the pancreas presenting as an epididymal mass. A case report and literature review. J Urol Pathol 1997;6:159-70.

8 TUMOR-LIKE LESIONS

Although most masses within the scrotal sac are neoplasms, a few are due to diverse non-neoplastic processes (1,2). Additionally, some microscopic findings of these processes may cause concern for an incidentally discovered neoplasm. The proportion of non-neoplastic mimics of neoplasia varies widely in the literature: one comprehensive review from the British Testicular Tumour Panel (3) reported a frequency of 6 percent, a lower figure, likely due to selection bias, than that reported in another series from a large general hospital in the United States (4), which found that almost 30 percent of processes in over 200 explorations performed for the suspicion of testicular or paratesticular cancer were non-neoplastic (Table 8-1). The proportion of non-neoplastic lesions is even higher in children, with one study reporting a frequency of 54 percent (5).

This chapter focuses primarily on lesions that may be misinterpreted by the pathologist; certain non-neoplastic processes that are not prone to misinterpretation as preneoplastic or neoplastic are not covered, and excellent reviews of these topics are available (6). Lesions of an infectious nature (7) are generally clinically recognized as such, although a few are mentioned here.

LEYDIG CELL HYPERPLASIA AND EXTRAPARENCHYMAL LEYDIG CELLS

General Features. *Leydig cell hyperplasia* occurs whenever the testis is exposed to elevated levels of luteinizing hormone, as in cases of central precocity and the androgen insensitivity syndrome, or chorionic gonadotropin, which is secreted by several types of neoplasm (Table 8-2) (8–15). Rarely, Leydig cells mature morphologically and physiologically independently of pituitary stimulation (gonadotropin-independent sexual precocity) but caused by constitutive activating mutations in the luteinizing hormone receptor (testotoxicosis) or by acquired mutations in the G-protein signaling pathway (McCune-Albright syndrome) (8,16).

In testes with marked tubular atrophy and sclerosis, Leydig cells may appear hyperplastic, forming nodular aggregates or growing diffusely and occupying much of the parenchyma. Although it is often uncertain whether such prominence of Leydig cells reflects pseudohyperplasia secondary to tubular atrophy or true hyperplasia, it may be sufficiently striking to lead to a misdiagnosis of a neoplasm, especially in cases of Klinefelter syndrome and related disorders.

Gross and Microscopic Findings. Leydig cell hyperplasia is rarely grossly visible but can

Table 8-1

NON-NEOPLASTIC DISORDERS SIMULATING NEOPLASMS

Disorder[a]	Series A[b]	Series B[c]
Idiopathic granulomatous orchitis	16	8
Nonspecific epididymoorchitis	5	–
Sperm granuloma	4	–
Hydrocele with marked fibrosis[d]	4	19
Fibrous pseudotumor	3	–
Malakoplakia	1	–
Syphilitic gumma	1	–
Tuberculous epididymoorchitis	1	9
Inflammatory pseudotumor	1	–
Organized hematoma	1	–
Cysts	1	22
Torsion	–	3
Sarcoidosis	–	2
Cholesterol granuloma, xanthogranuloma, foreign body granuloma	–	4
TOTAL	38	67

[a]Some lesions have been reclassified according to currently used terminology.
[b]Series A: Non-neoplastic lesions of testis and paratestis simulating malignancy: British Testicular Tumour Panel, 1964 (5).
[c]Series B: Non-neoplastic lesions suspicious of cancer. Henry Ford Hospital, 1965-1985 (3).
[d]One case was associated with mesothelial hyperplasia, another may possibly have represented resolved meconium periorchitis.

produce multiple, small, yellow-brown spots or, rarely, larger nodules (fig. 8-1). Microscopic examination shows small aggregates or nodules of Leydig cells (fig. 8-2), without effacement of underlying tubules, although tubular atrophy may suggest effacement. These features and the clinical background generally facilitate the

distinction from a neoplasm. In atrophic testes, Leydig cells may be present within the seminiferous tubules (fig. 8-3, left) (17).

Differential Diagnosis. In some cases Leydig cells outside the testicular parenchyma may cause confusion for those who are unaware that they are often present in the tunica albuginea and beyond it. In an autopsy study of almost 300 patients (11), Leydig cells were found in the tunica albuginea in 66 percent (fig. 8-3, right), and in the paratesticular and spermatic cord soft tissue in 3 percent (fig. 8-4). A study of orchiectomy specimens demonstrated extraparenchymal Leydig cells in over 90 percent of the cases, most commonly in the testicular tunics but also in the spermatic cord in almost 15 percent (18). These cells frequently involve nerves (fig. 8-4), which should not be misinterpreted as indicating that they are neoplastic (17).

Table 8-2
CAUSES OF LEYDIG CELL HYPERPLASIA
Central sexual precocity
Gonadotropin-independent sexual precocity ("testotoxicosis")
Germ cell tumor, testicular or extratesticular, with human chorionic gonadotropin (hCG) production
Paraneoplastic hCG production by nongerm cell tumors
Klinefelter and related syndromes
Androgen insensitivity syndrome

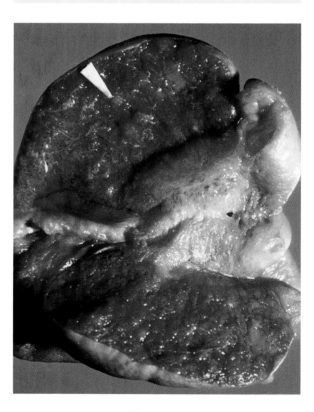

Figure 8-1

LEYDIG CELL HYPERPLASIA

Multiple, small, light tan nodules are visible within the testicular parenchyma (arrow indicates one).

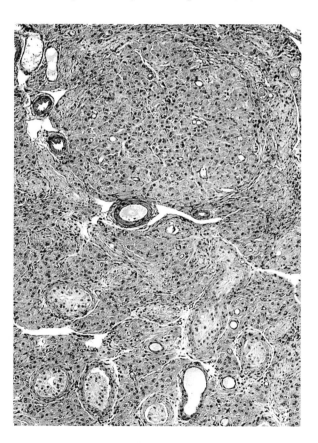

Figure 8-2

LEYDIG CELL HYPERPLASIA

Residual seminiferous tubules are seen at the bottom.

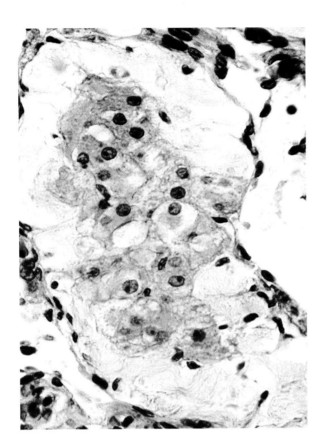
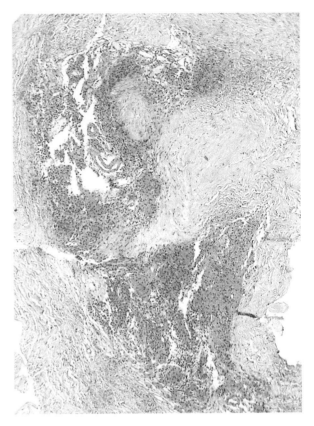

Figure 8-3

UNUSUAL LOCATIONS OF LEYDIG CELLS

Left: Leydig cells are within an atrophic testicular tubule.
Right: Hyperplastic Leydig cells are present within the tunica albuginea.

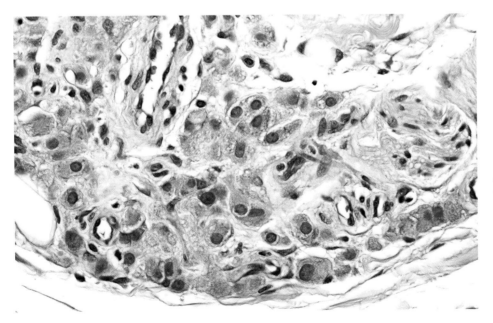

Figure 8-4

EXTRATESTICULAR LEYDIG CELLS

In the spermatic cord, aggregates of Leydig cells are associated with nerves and blood vessels.

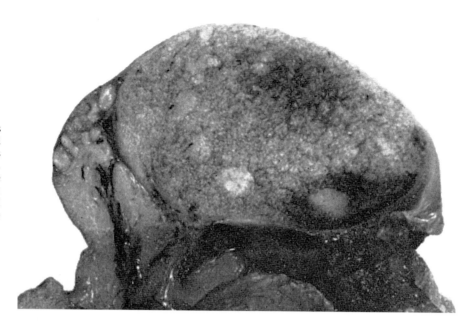

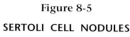

Figure 8-5

SERTOLI CELL NODULES

Several small white nodules are visible on the sectioned surface of a cryptorchid testis from a 33-year-old patient. (Fig. 8 from Halley JB. The growth of Sertoli cell tumors: a possible index of differential gonadotropin activity in the male. J Urol 1963;90:225.)

SERTOLI CELL NODULES

Definition and General Features. *Sertoli cell nodules* are usually small clusters of immature tubules that are typically an incidental finding on microscopic examination but which infrequently are grossly visible as small, white nodules (fig. 8-5) (19). These lesions are often encountered in cryptorchid testes, but 22 percent of descended testes in one study also harbored them (20). Rarely, they attain sufficient size to be clinically palpable or detected as a discrete mass on ultrasonographic examination (21,22). In this circumstance, they are more apt to be misinterpreted as a neoplasm, usually as a Sertoli cell tumor.

Microscopic Findings. On microscopic examination, aggregates of tubules lined by immature Sertoli cells typically contain central, round deposits of basement membrane (figs. 8-6, 8-7) that may exhibit laminated calcifications. Frequently, the tubular diameters are larger than the normal seminiferous tubules. The lining Sertoli cells are associated with scattered spermatogonia in some cases (fig. 8-8), and Leydig cells may be present between the tubules (fig. 8-7). In some large lesions, the intratubular nature of the process is less clear and there is a nodule showing a confluent growth of cords, trabeculae, and tubules composed of immature Sertoli cells and spermatogonia interspersed with globules and trabeculae of basement mem-

brane (fig. 8-9). Large nodules consisting almost entirely of basement membrane are rare.

Differential Diagnosis. Although Sertoli cell nodules have often been referred to in the literature as tubular adenoma, Pick adenoma, or Sertoli cell adenoma, they are almost certainly non-neoplastic. Their characteristic morphology and usual microscopic size permit their distinction from true Sertoli or Sertoli-Leydig cell tumors, which do not have an integral germ cell component, unlike many Sertoli cell nodules, and which generally lack conspicuous deposits of basement membrane. In patients with germ cell tumors, Sertoli cell nodules may be colonized by intratubular germ cell neoplasia, unclassified type (IGCNU) and thereby resemble gonadoblastoma (see fig. 5-36).

TESTICULAR "TUMOR" OF THE ADRENOGENITAL SYNDROME

General and Clinical Features. Masses composed of steroid-type cells develop in and adjacent to the testes of a significant number of males with untreated or inadequately treated adrenogenital syndrome (23–28). Although some have referred to these lesions as "testicular adrenal rest tumors," it is unlikely that they develop from adrenal cortical rests, which are exclusively extratesticular and often some distance from the testis. For this reason, we prefer

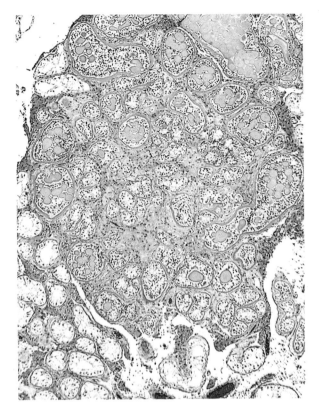

Figure 8-6

SERTOLI CELL NODULE

The periphery of the lesion is well circumscribed but somewhat irregular. Leydig cells are present in the stroma.

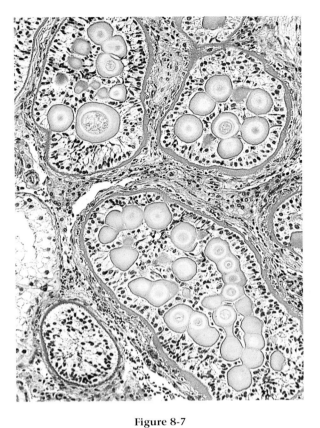

Figure 8-7

SERTOLI CELL NODULE

The annular hyaline foci, which are sometimes calcified, may suggest Call-Exner bodies or a sex cord tumor with annular tubules.

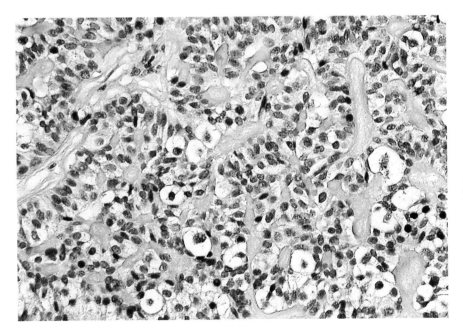

Figure 8-8

SERTOLI CELL NODULE

Occasional spermatogonia intermingle with immature Sertoli cells and eosinophilic deposits of basement membrane.

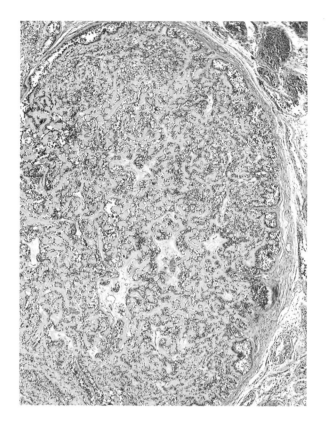

Figure 8-9

SERTOLI CELL NODULE

Confluent growth of the cellular components and basement membrane is seen in a large lesion.

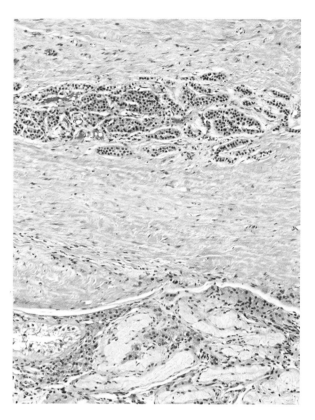

Figure 8-10

STEROID CELL REST

Nests and trabeculae of eosinophilic steroid cells are present within the tunica albuginea.

the term, *testicular "tumor" of the adrenogenital syndrome.* It has been hypothesized that these "tumors" represent nodular hyperplasias of generally inconspicuous nests of steroid cells that are occasionally appreciated as an incidental finding near the testicular hilum (fig. 8-10) (29).

These masses, which may become evident in childhood or adult life, occur most often in patients with the salt-losing form of the adrenogenital syndrome (21-hydroxylase deficiency). Clues to the diagnosis include clinical evidence of the adrenogenital syndrome or a family history of it, and bilateral involvement. Laboratory examination shows the features of the underlying adrenogenital syndrome, including elevated plasma levels of adrenocorticotropic hormone (ACTH), androstenedione, and 17-hydroxyprogesterone, and increases in urinary 17-ketosteroids and pregnanetriol. A persistent elevation of 17-ketosteroids in the absence of

detectable metastatic disease after the removal of a "Leydig cell tumor" suggests the possibility of an underlying adrenogenital syndrome.

The tumors synthesize what are considered adrenal-specific steroids and transcribe mRNA for the ACTH and angiotensin II receptors (30,31), supporting a close relationship to adrenal cortical cells. Other characteristic features are their enlargement and enhanced hormonal secretion after the administration of ACTH (26) and a decrease in their size and hormone output after suppression of ACTH by the administration of corticosteroids. Since they respond to ACTH suppression, surgical excision is generally considered unnecessary except for cosmetic reasons or pain. Nonetheless, the report of one patient with the adrenogenital syndrome who developed a malignant tumor interpreted as a Leydig cell tumor (crystals of Reinke were not identified) (32) provides a cautionary note

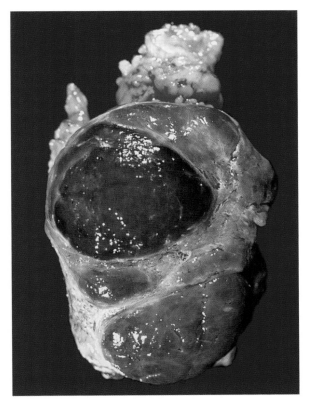

Figure 8-11

**TESTICULAR "TUMOR" OF
THE ADRENOGENITAL SYNDROME**

The mass is composed of multiple brown-green to almost black nodules intersected by fibrous septa. (Fig. 9.5 from Young RH, Scully RE. Testicular tumors, Chicago: ASCP Press; 1990:201.)

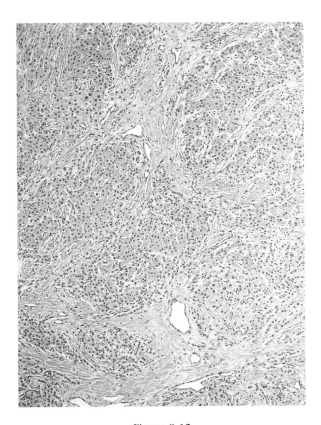

Figure 8-12

**TESTICULAR "TUMOR" OF
THE ADRENOGENITAL SYNDROME**

Eosinophilic cells are arranged in anastomosing nests that are separated by a prominent fibrous stroma.

against considering all steroid cell tumors in these patients as invariably benign. One reported case occurred in a cryptorchid testis and was admixed with a myelolipoma and had an adjacent seminoma (33).

Gross Findings. The masses measure up to 10 cm in diameter, appear to originate in the hilar region, and extend peripherally into the parenchyma. Sectioning typically reveals multiple dark brown nodules or a single lobulated mass traversed by fibrous septa (fig. 8-11).

Microscopic Findings. Large cells resembling Leydig cells typically grow in nodules that often have a conspicuous, sometimes hyalinized, stroma that segregates the cells into variably sized islands (fig. 8-12). Seminiferous tubules may be encountered within the lesion. The cells

have abundant eosinophilic cytoplasm which may contain a large amount of lipochrome pigment (fig. 8-13) but lacks crystals of Reinke. The nuclei may be atypical in a spotty manner (fig. 8-14), but mitotic activity is rare. Foci of adipose metaplasia occurred in 5 of 9 cases (56 percent) in one study (34).

Immunohistochemical Findings. Most lesions are positive for alpha-inhibin, CD56, and synaptophysin (fig. 8-15) and usually negative for cytokeratins, chromogranin, S-100 protein, and the estrogen, progesterone, and androgen receptors (34,35).

Differential Diagnosis. A report of three boys with precocious puberty due to the adrenogenital syndrome, each of whom had bilateral testicular tumors, emphasizes the potential for misdiagnosis, even today, as two of the cases were initially interpreted as Leydig cell tumors

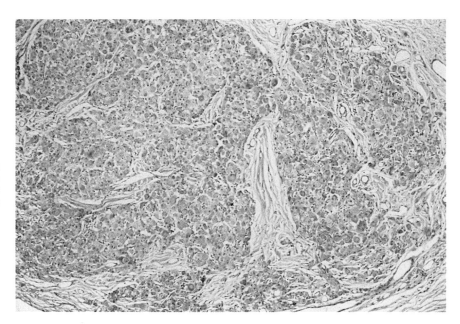

Figure 8-13

TESTICULAR "TUMOR" OF THE ADRENOGENITAL SYNDROME

The lesional cells grow in nodular aggregates. Their cytoplasm contains large amounts of brown-yellow lipochrome pigment.

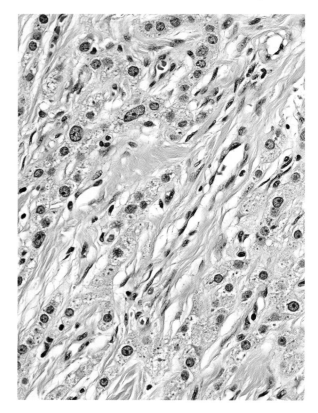

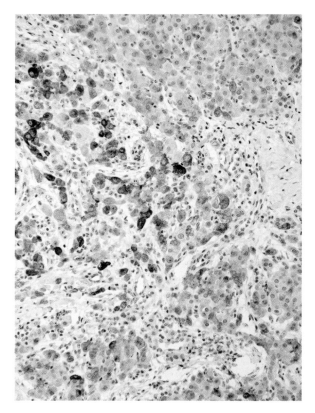

Figure 8-14

TESTICULAR "TUMOR" OF THE ADRENOGENITAL SYNDROME

There is random nuclear atypia.

Figure 8-15

TESTICULAR "TUMOR" OF THE ADRENOGENITAL SYNDROME

There is patchy cytoplasmic reactivity for synaptophysin (antisynaptophysin immunostain).

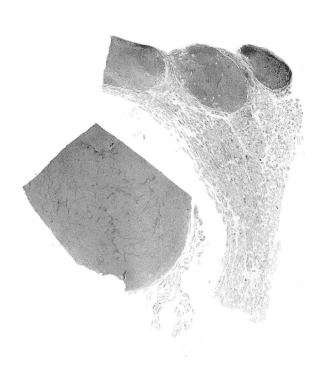
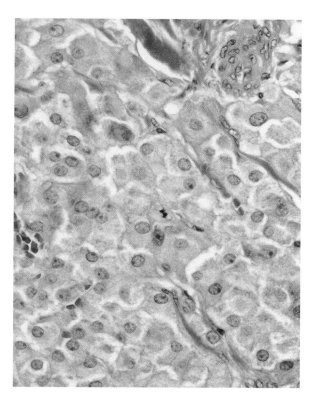

Figure 8-16

TESTICULAR "TUMOR" OF NELSON SYNDROME

Left: Multiple nodules of different sizes are present in the testis.

Right: The cells in the nodules have pale, eosinophilic cytoplasm and abundant lipochrome. There are occasional mitotic figures (center). (Courtesy of Dr. H. Levin, Cleveland, OH.)

(36). The usual bilaterality and frequent multifocality of these masses contrasts with the usual solitary nature of Leydig cell tumors. They are typically dark brown, whereas Leydig cell tumors are more often yellow or yellow-tan. Preserved seminiferous tubules may be present within them but are found only rarely within a Leydig cell tumor. The cells tend to be larger and to have more abundant cytoplasm than those of Leydig cell tumors and contain lipochrome pigment more frequently and in greater amounts. Crystals of Reinke have not been identified within the cells but are found in at least one third of Leydig cell tumors. Additional features that favor adrenogenital nodules are prominent fibrous bands, more common adipose metaplasia, spotty nuclear pleomorphism, and absence of mitotic activity (34). Positivity for synaptophysin and CD56 and negativity for androgen receptor contrast with the findings in Leydig cell tumor (34,35).

STEROID CELL NODULES
WITH OTHER ADRENAL DISEASES

Testicular or paratesticular nodules of steroid cells may be seen in patients with *Nelson syndrome* (the rapid growth of an ACTH-secreting pituitary adenoma after bilateral adrenalectomy for Cushing syndrome) (37,38). These lesions have biologic, biochemical, and pathologic similarities to the lesions of the adrenogenital syndrome, they develop in the setting of elevated ACTH levels, and they may produce cortisol with the resultant recurrence of the Cushing syndrome. The gross and microscopic features are as described above for the adrenogenital syndrome (fig. 8-16).

Testicular steroid cell nodules also develop in patients who have features of the syndrome described by Carney as "the complex of myxomas, spotty pigmentation, and endocrine overactivity" (39). Patients with *Carney complex* usually

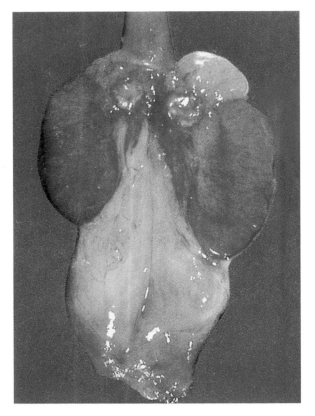

Figure 8-17

ADRENAL CORTICAL REST

A discrete, small, round, orange-yellow nodule lies between the testis and epididymis. (Fig. 9.1 from Young RH, Scully RE. Testicular tumors, Chicago: ASCP Press; 1990:199.)

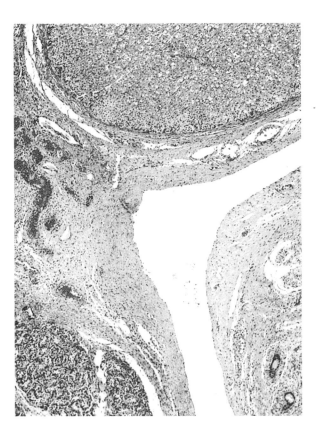

Figure 8-18

ADRENAL CORTICAL REST

A portion of the well-encapsulated nodule of adrenal cortical tissue is seen at the top, with fetal testis and epididymis at the bottom. (Courtesy of Dr. E. Lack, Washington, DC.)

have normal or low ACTH levels and primary pigmented nodular adrenocortical hyperplasia or a pituitary adenoma that secretes growth hormone. The steroid cell nodules are usually found incidentally when the patients are discovered to have a large cell calcifying Sertoli cell tumor, the most common testicular manifestation of this unusual syndrome. Although crystals of Reinke have been identified in the steroid cell nodules in at least one of these cases, indicating a Leydig cell nature, they have not been found in the majority of them. The steroid cell nodules may be located in the hilus and may be associated with cells that appear to be mature adipocytes.

Small steroid cell nodules may be seen in the testicular hilum of boys with *Cushing syndrome and adrenal nodular hyperplasia*, outside of the context of the adrenogenital syndrome, Nelson syndrome, or Carney complex (28,40). These lesions, except for their microscopic size, are similar to those of the adrenogenital syndrome.

ADRENAL CORTICAL RESTS

Yellow-orange nodules of *ectopic adrenocortical tissue*, usually under 0.5 cm in diameter, are found in the spermatic cord, epididymis, rete testis, and tunica albuginea, and between the epididymis and testis, in approximately 10 percent of infants (fig. 8-17); they are also seen occasionally in older males (41–43). Microscopic examination reveals encapsulated nodules (fig. 8-18) that typically exhibit the zonation of the normal adrenal cortex (fig. 8-19); occasionally, the rests are unencapsulated. These lesions lack a component comparable to the adrenal medulla.

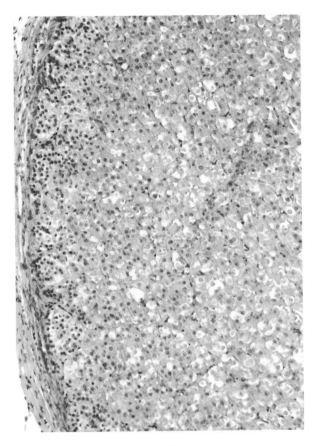

Figure 8-19

ADRENAL CORTICAL REST

Most of the cells are of the fetal cortical type. A thin layer of definitive cortex is present just beneath the capsule. (Courtesy of Dr. E. Lack, Washington, DC.)

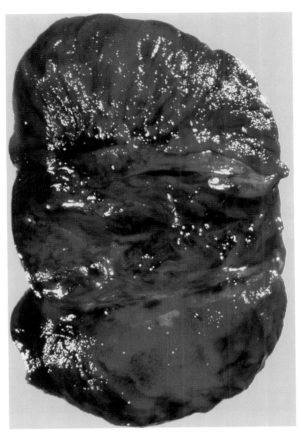

Figure 8-20

HEMORRHAGIC INFARCTION OF TESTIS

Diffuse blood fills the parenchyma.

TORSION, INFARCTS, AND HEMATOMAS OF TESTIS

A *testicular infarct* may be caused by thrombotic vascular occlusion or torsion (44). Conditions predisposing to thrombosis include polycythemia, infection (45), trauma, vasculitis (46), inherited coagulation disorders, and sickle cell disease (47). Occasionally, a testicular infarct clinically simulates a neoplasm, particularly when the infarct is remote (48), although it has been suggested that high frequency ultrasound may aid in this distinction (49). The sectioned surfaces of an infarct may be hemorrhagic (fig. 8-20) or pale (fig. 8-21). Microscopic examination shows necrotic tubules and, in most cases, varying degrees of hemorrhage (fig. 8-22). Care should be taken to exclude a necrotic tumor such as a seminoma that may possibly be mistaken for an infarct. The underlying pattern of a neoplasm, with ghost outlines of tumor cells, is still visible in such cases, and there are usually some residual, non-necrotic seminiferous tubules that may demonstrate IGCNU. Additionally, the numerous outlines of necrotic seminiferous tubules that are characteristic of acute and subacute infarcts are absent. Remote infarcts may be associated with marked fibrosis, cholesterol clefts, and calcification.

Testicular torsion may induce prominent reactive changes in the paratesticular soft tissues that simulate an inflammatory pseudotumor (50). We have seen a number of cases of *hemorrhagic infarcts* that were clinically mistaken for neoplasms when the intratesticular vessels showed, in addition to recent thrombi, marked intimal thickening, fibrinoid change, and

411

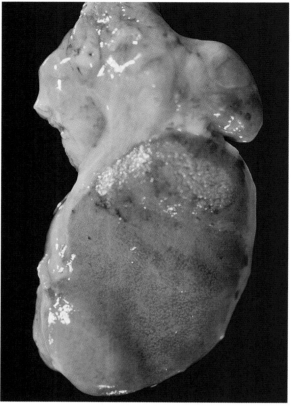

Figure 8-21

TESTICULAR INFARCT, REMOTE

The granular yellow lesion in the upper pole of the testis was clinically thought to be a neoplasm.

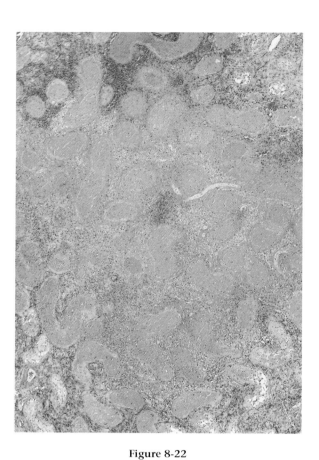

Figure 8-22

TESTICULAR INFARCT

Outlines of necrotic seminiferous tubules are focally surrounded by blood (top).

Figure 8-23

TESTICULAR VASCULOPATHY

There is marked intimal proliferation with luminal narrowing and fibrin deposits in a vessel close to a parenchymal infarct.

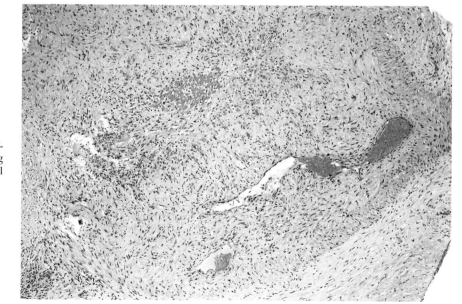

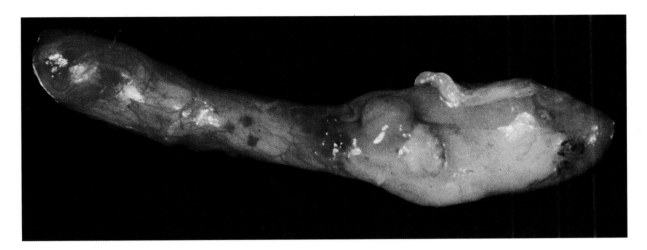

Figure 8-24

INFARCTION OF TESTIS IN UTERO

The spermatic cord terminates in a fibrous "nubbin" that represents the infarcted testis. (Courtesy of Dr. A.R. Schned, Lebanon, NH.)

fibrous obliteration (fig. 8-23) unassociated with any major vasculitic component. It is our hypothesis that these infarcts and vasculopathic changes are related to chronic intermittent torsion.

In utero infarction of the testis, designated as either the *vanishing testis syndrome* (51) or the *testicular regression syndrome* (52), results in a small, fibrotic nodule that may not be readily identifiable as a testis. Patients typically present in infancy with an impalpable testis, and scrotal exploration identifies a "fibrous nubbin," usually attached to an identifiable vas deferens (fig. 8-24) (51). The epididymis is less consistently present; in one study of 77 cases, it was identified in 36 percent (52). When unilateral, the left testis is predominantly affected in a 2-3:1 ratio. Bilateral involvement occurs in about 20 percent of the cases (51,53). On microscopic examination, there are calcifications, often with a ring-like configuration, in a variably dense fibrous stroma with hemosiderin deposits (figs. 8-25, 8-26) and, sometimes, multinucleated giant cells. Prominent veins, representing remnants of the pampiniform plexus, are seen in most cases (54). Atrophic fibers from the cremasteric muscle may mimic Leydig cells (51). Seminiferous tubule remnants are often not apparent (51,52). This constellation of features should allow for the diagnosis, otherwise there is clinical concern for ectopy, which may induce unnecessary surgery.

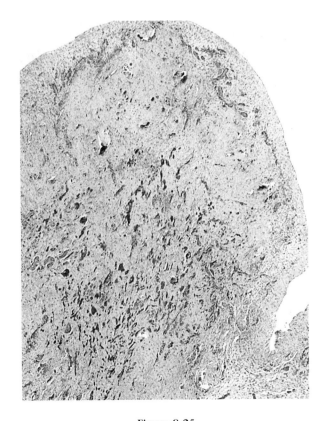

Figure 8-25

INFARCTION OF TESTIS IN UTERO

The shape of a fetal testis is recognizable, but the entire organ is infarcted with secondary fibrosis and prominent siderophages.

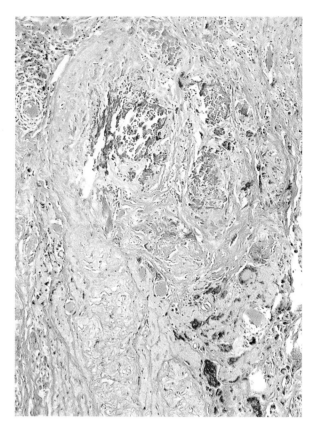

Figure 8-26

INFARCTION OF TESTIS IN UTERO

There is prominent calcification and hemosiderin deposition in a dense fibrous stroma.

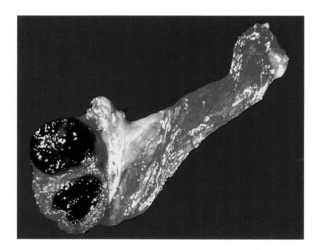

Figure 8-27

HEMATOMA OF TESTIS

The large, sharply circumscribed hematoma is secondary to localized necrotizing arteritis with rupture. (Fig. 9.42 from Young RH, Scully RE. Testicular tumors, Chicago: ASCP Press; 1990:219.)

Although *testicular hemorrhage* is usually related to infarction or a malignant neoplasm, trauma or rupture of an artery secondary to arteritis (55,56) may lead to the formation of a large *hematoma* (fig. 8-27), which on gross examination may be confused with a choriocarcinoma (57). Sometimes the inflammation and edema of testicular and paratesticular vasculitis, in the absence of a hematoma, result in a mass that clinically mimics a neoplasm (58,59).

Testicular and *epididymal vasculitis* may be accompanied or followed by evidence of systemic vasculitis, but it also occurs as an isolated phenomenon (46,60). In cases of periarteritis nodosa, there is commonly paratesticular and testicular involvement, with secondary infarcts (55). Granulomatous vasculitis may also involve either the testis or paratestis, causing a tumor-like mass (58). We have seen such a case associated with Crohn disease (61).

TESTICULAR APPENDAGES AND WALTHARD NESTS

There are five *testicular appendages*: the appendix testis (hydatid of Morgagni), the appendix epididymis, the paradidymis (organ of Giraldes), and the inferior and superior aberrant ducts (vas aberrans of Haller) (62,63). The latter two are infrequently present and not a source of concern for surgical pathologists. In most instances, the paradidymis is not as striking grossly as it is in the accompanying illustration (fig. 8-28), in which it is seen as the most superior of the three visible appendages, that in the middle being the appendix epididymis and the inferior the appendix testis with its characteristic attachment to the anterosuperior aspect of the upper pole of the testis (see also figs. 1-4, 1-5). Because the latter two structures are those that are usually grossly visible and often are pedunculated, they may undergo torsion and infarction (figs. 8-29, 8-30) with accompanying significant symptoms (64,65). Identifying the characteristic structure and epithelium of the appendages is often difficult but may be important for establishing the correct clinicopathologic correlation. Confusion

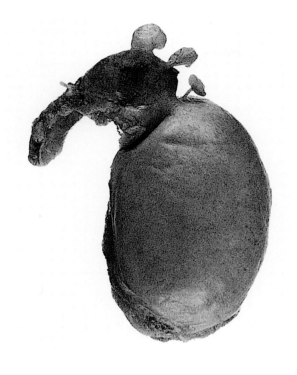

Figure 8-28

MAJOR TESTICULAR APPENDAGES

From left to right: the paradidymis (organ of Giraldes), appendix epididymis, and appendix testis. (Fig. 104A from Algaba F. Atlas de patologia de los tumores urogenitales. Barcelona: Fundacion Puigvert; 1991:253.)

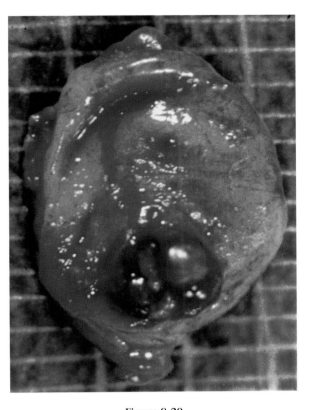

Figure 8-29

INFARCTED APPENDIX TESTIS

There is a discrete hemorrhagic nodule.

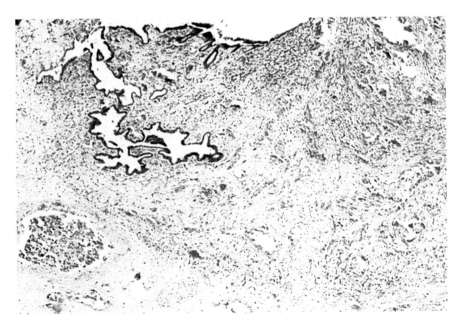

Figure 8-30

INFARCTED APPENDIX TESTIS

Some viable epithelium is visible, but the remaining tissue is infarcted with focal calcification.

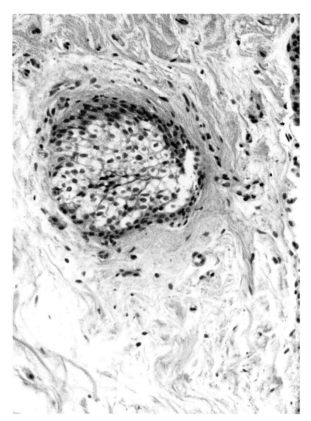

Figure 8-31

WALTHARD NEST

A discrete nest of transitional cells is present in the lining of the tunica vaginalis.

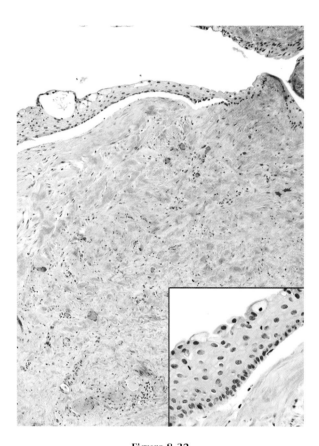

Figure 8-32

CYSTIC WALTHARD NEST

A nest of transitional cells in the tunica vaginalis has undergone cystic change. The inset shows the lining of transitional-type epithelium with occasional mucous cells.

with a neoplasm is unlikely. The classic study of Sundarasivarao (63) provides detailed information on the testicular appendages, but a brief summary follows.

The appendix testis is found in about 80 percent of carefully examined testes (63). It typically measures from 2 to 4 mm but is occasionally larger. It contains a fibrovascular core of loose connective tissue covered by simple cuboidal to low columnar müllerian-type epithelium that merges with the mesothelium of the tunica vaginalis lateral to its base. The epithelium typically invaginates into the underlying stroma, but isolated müllerian duct remnants may be seen in the stroma, which is occasionally calcified.

The usually cystic appendix epididymis is less frequently present (about 25 percent of the cases) and arises from the anterosuperior pole of the head of the epididymis. It is lined by cuboidal to low columnar epithelium, which may be ciliated, and shows some secretory activity. Rarely, marked cystic change of the appendix epididymis presents as a paratesticular mass (66).

The mesothelium of the tunica vaginalis undergoes transitional metaplasia in about 12 percent of cases (63). This results in epithelial nests (fig. 8-31) similar to the Walthard nests that commonly occur on the serosa of the fallopian tube in females, and, like them, may undergo cystic change (fig. 8-32). Their possible role in giving rise to the rare testicular Brenner tumor has been previously mentioned (see chapter 7).

ORCHITIS AND EPIDIDYMITIS

In most cases of *orchitis* and *epididymitis*, the diagnosis is made clinically and pathologic

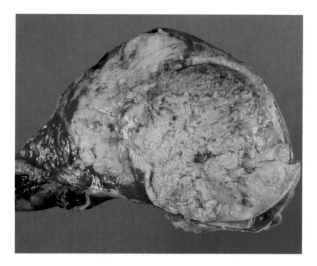

Figure 8-33

ACUTE EPIDIDYMOORCHITIS

Both the testis and epididymis are involved, with evident liquefactive necrosis in the testis.

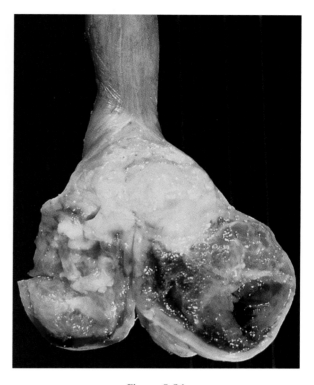

Figure 8-34

CHRONIC EPIDIDYMOORCHITIS

There is prominent destruction of the testicular parenchyma with cyst formation and extensive involvement of the epididymis and paratesticular soft tissues by fibrosis.

examination of specimens does not occur. It is typically only when an inflammatory mass persists following conservative treatment or because of intractable pain that excision is performed.

Bacterial Orchitis

General Features. The testis is usually involved by bacterial spread from the epididymis, and most cases originate as an ascending infection from the lower genitourinary tract, with *Escherichia coli* and other gram-negative organisms the most common pathogens. In sexually active individuals, *Neisseria gonorrhea and Chlamydia trachomatis* are frequently implicated. In endemic areas, epididymoorchitis may be a manifestation of brucellosis (67). Rare cases due to *Nocardia asteroides* occur in the context of immunosuppression (68).

Gross and Microscopic Findings. The gross appearance is variable. The testis may contain abscesses (fig. 8-33) or be fibrotic and adherent to adjacent tissues (fig. 8-34), which are also fibrotic. Occasionally, a neoplasm is suggested in longstanding cases (2,69). Isolated abscesses of the epididymis and testis are less frequently encountered; in chronic cases of the former, ill-defined, fibrotic paratesticular "masses" may be striking (fig. 8-35).

Microscopic examination discloses varying amounts of acute and chronic inflammation, abscess formation, granulation tissue, and fibrosis, depending on the duration of the process. In some cases there is focal infarction, which may be the result of venous occlusion (45).

Differential Diagnosis. Longstanding cases of bacterial orchitis may result in the morphologic picture of xanthogranulomatous orchitis, analogous to the much more commonly occurring xanthogranulomatous pyelonephritis. Conditions associated with its development include urinary outflow obstruction, diabetes, spinal cord injury, and urethral instrumentation (70). Implicated organisms include *E. coli*, *Pseudomonas aeruginosa*, and *Actinomyces* species (71). Patients commonly present with a solid and cystic inflammatory mass with areas of red, brown, and yellow friable tissue. Adhesions of the testis to the tunica vaginalis and beyond to the scrotal skin may occur. The characteristic

417

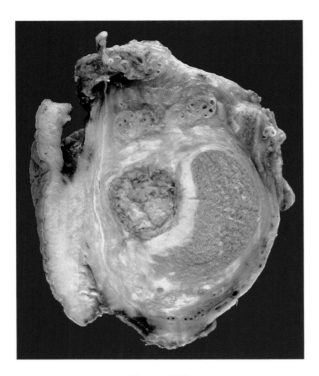

Figure 8-35

EPIDIDYMAL ABSCESS

An abscess centered in the epididymis is associated with marked fibrosis in the surrounding tissues but lacks significant extension into the testicular parenchyma.

microscopic features include varying proportions of foamy macrophages, lymphoplasmacytic infiltrates, neutrophilic microabscesses, fibrosis, and necrotic tissue. Confusion with the equally rare Rosai-Dorfman disease of the testis (72) may occur, but the inflammatory component in xanthogranulomatous orchitis is more varied and the histiocytes lack the conspicuous lymphocytic emperipolesis of Rosai-Dorfman disease.

Viral Orchitis

General Features. A number of viruses cause orchitis: mumps virus (the most common viral pathogen to produce orchitis), Coxsackie B virus, Epstein-Barr virus (infectious mononucleosis), varicella virus (chickenpox), variola virus (smallpox), dengue virus, and bunyavirus (sandfly fever) (73). The diagnosis of these infections is almost always made clinically and, with the exception of mumps orchitis, little is known concerning the pathologic findings in the testis.

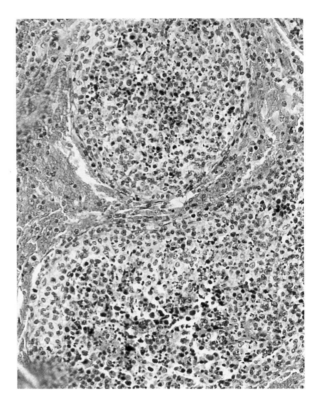

Figure 8-36

MUMPS ORCHITIS

The tubules are filled with mononuclear cells, polymorphonuclear leukocytes, degenerating cells, and nuclear debris.

Clinical Features. The testis is involved in approximately one quarter of adult males with mumps, but in fewer than 1 percent of children with this disease. Testicular involvement is bilateral in almost one fifth of the cases and is accompanied by epididymitis in 85 percent (74). The testis is swollen and tender, and incision of the tunica albuginea reveals edema and, in some cases, hemorrhage.

Microscopic Findings. Microscopic examination discloses interstitial edema early in the disease course, followed by vascular dilatation and interstitial lymphocytic infiltration, sometimes accompanied by neutrophils and macrophages (74). Subsequently, interstitial hemorrhage occurs, along with inflammatory cell infiltration of the seminiferous tubules and degeneration of the germinal epithelium (fig. 8-36). Healing results in patchy hyalinization of tubules and interstitial fibrosis, with intervening unaffected areas.

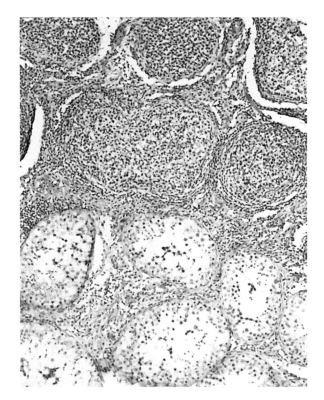

Figure 8-37

VIRAL ORCHITIS

The tubules at the top are distended by a prominent mononuclear cell infiltrate which also involves the interstitial tissue. (Fig. 9.16 from Young RH, Scully RE. Testicular tumors. Chicago: ASCP Press; 1990:206.)

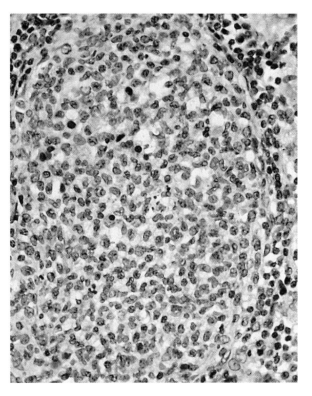

Figure 8-38

VIRAL ORCHITIS

A tubule is distended by mononuclear cells and surrounded by lymphocytes. (Fig. 9.17 from Young RH, Scully RE. Testicular tumors. Chicago: ASCP Press; 1990:207.)

The microscopic features of other rarely described forms of viral orchitis, many of which are due to Coxsackie B (75), resemble those of mumps orchitis. In the exceptional cases in which mumps orchitis precedes parotitis or is the only evidence of the infection, or cases in which orchitis is the exclusive or major manifestation of another viral illness, the clinical and ultrasonographic findings may suggest a neoplasm (76). In our experience with 10 such cases in patients 18 to 37 years old, all presented with testicular enlargement, pain, or both (76). On gross examination of orchiectomy specimens, most did not demonstrate a discrete mass but had areas of hemorrhage and induration, although in one a lobulated, golden mass was identified. Microscopic features included patchy intratubular and intertubular lymphohistiocytic infiltrates (figs. 8-37, 8-38), as well as foci of hemorrhage and edema.

Differential Diagnosis. The distension of tubules by inflammatory cells in viral orchitis mimics, at low magnification, the pattern of intratubular seminoma, although the cytological features are diagnostic of an inflammatory process if care is taken not to mistake activated lymphocytes for neoplastic cells. In additional contrast to most seminomas is the preservation of tubular architecture.

Autoimmune Orchitis/Vasculitis

A number of diseases of an autoimmune nature, or at least a presumed autoimmune nature, manifest in the testis and cause clinical concern for a neoplasm because of associated testicular swelling or pain. In many cases, the primary focus of involvement is the testicular vascular system with the production of vasculitis. *Polyarteritis nodosa* may present in the testis

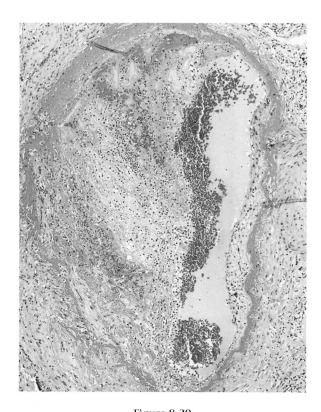

Figure 8-39

**POLYARTERITIS NODOSA-LIKE
VASCULITIS OF THE TESTIS**

Fibrinoid necrosis of the wall of a muscular arteriole.

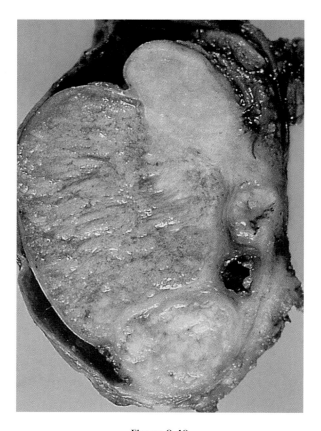

Figure 8-40

TUBERCULOUS EPIDIDYMOORCHITIS

There is extensive nodular involvement of the entire epididymis and secondary involvement of the testis. (Fig. 9.18 from Young RH, Scully RE. Testicular tumors. Chicago: ASCP Press; 1990:207.)

and mimic a neoplasm because of palpable firmness or mass and testicular pain (56,59,77). On microscopic examination, the characteristic fibrinoid necrosis of medium-sized muscular arteries is seen (fig. 8-39), often in conjunction with infarcts. Presentation in the epididymis or spermatic cord may also occur (56,60,78). Although characteristically a systemic process, a number of cases of polyarteritis of the testis and paratesticular structures have been apparently isolated phenomena, with no evidence of systemic vasculitis.

Small vessel vasculitis of the testis occurs in patients with *Henoch-Schönlein purpura*, which is associated with orchitis in 14 percent of male patients but rarely is a presenting manifestation (79). Epididymoorchitis is seen in about 10 percent of patients with *Behçet disease* (80), and orchitis in occasional patients with *relapsing polychondritis* (81). Testicular vasculitis may also be a manifestation of *rheumatoid arthritis,*

Goodpasture syndrome, systemic lupus erythematosus (SLE) (82,83), and *SLE/scleroderma overlap syndrome* (84). One case of *giant cell arteritis,* which clinically mimicked a neoplasm, occurred in the testis of a patient who had systemic involvement (85).

Granulomatous Orchitis, Infectious

Many infectious organisms that involve the testis result in *granulomatous orchitis*. The potential infections include tuberculosis, syphilis, brucellosis, and leprosy, as well as organisms such as fungi, parasites, and rickettsia. In tuberculosis the epididymis is the primary site of genital tract involvement (fig. 8-40), and the testis is usually affected only in the late stages (fig. 8-41) (86,87). Epididymal involvement usually reflects prostatic infection which, in turn, is

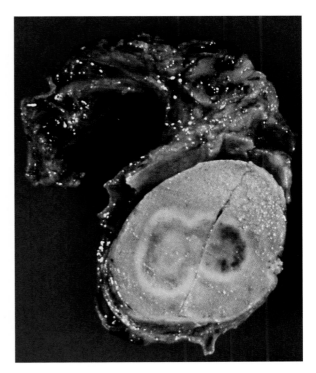

Figure 8-42

SYPHILITIC GUMMA OF TESTIS

A large area of necrotic tissue is surrounded by a thick rim of white tissue.

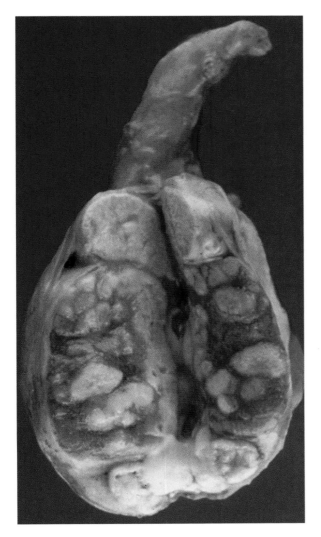

Figure 8-41

TUBERCULOSIS OF THE TESTIS

Multiple white nodules extensively involve the testicular parenchyma in this autopsy case. Epididymal involvement is prominent. (Fig. 9.19 from Young RH, Scully RE. Testicular tumors. Chicago: ASCP Press; 190:207.)

associated with renal and pulmonary tuberculosis. This sequence of involvement, the 30 percent frequency of bilaterality, and the 50 percent frequency of an abscess or sinus tract formation are important clues to the infectious nature of the process. The microscopic findings are as seen elsewhere and may be duplicated by iatrogenic infection secondary to bacillus Calmette-Guérin instilled in the urinary bladder for the treatment of urothelial carcinoma (88).

Histoplasmosis (89) and *coccidioidomycosis* (90) may selectively involve the epididymis. In cases of *syphilis*, a gumma may mimic a neoplasm on clinical and gross evaluation (fig. 8-42), but the microscopic features, consisting of a central necrotic area with retention of tubular outlines surrounded by a variably prominent epithelioid and giant cell reaction and a usually conspicuous peripheral zone of fibrous and granulation tissue (fig. 8-43), are unlike those of any neoplasm (91). In cases of *leprosy*, the testes are usually normal or decreased in size but are occasionally enlarged. The microscopic findings in the three stages of this disease (vascular, interstitial, and obliterative) are unlikely to cause confusion with a neoplasm (92).

Granulomatous Orchitis, Idiopathic

General and Clinical Features. *Idiopathic granulomatous orchitis* accounts for 0.2 percent of testicular masses and, in the experience of the British Testicular Tumour Panel (2), is the

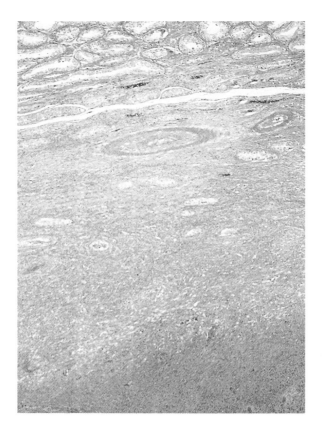

Figure 8-43

SYPHILITIC GUMMA OF TESTIS

Gummatous necrosis is bordered by a zone of fibrous tissue containing chronic inflammatory cells. (Fig. 9.21 from Young RH, Scully RE. Testicular tumors. Chicago: ASCP Press; 1990:209.)

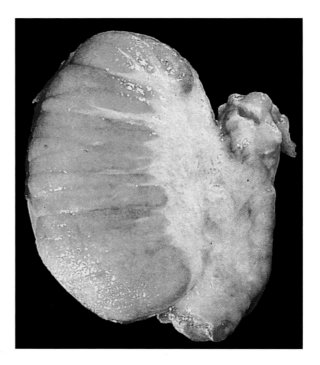

Figure 8-44

GRANULOMATOUS ORCHITIS, IDIOPATHIC

The parenchyma is replaced by lobulated, pale yellow tissue, with fibrosis in the rete and epididymis. (Fig. 9.22 from Young RH, Scully RE. Testicular tumors. Chicago: ASCP Press; 1990:209.)

most common non-neoplastic lesion to mimic a malignant neoplasm (Table 8-1). It usually occurs during the fifth or sixth decade (2,93), and follows a urinary tract infection with gram-negative bacilli in about two thirds of the cases. Additional cases are associated with a preceding viral-like illness or trauma (94). Although some cases of granulomatous orchitis are clinically indistinguishable from a neoplasm, others have a history of a flu-like illness, the sudden onset of testicular swelling, and the usual associated pain or tenderness suggesting an inflammatory process. The testis enlarges, sometimes with pain or tenderness, which may disappear, leaving a painless mass (2). The contralateral testis is occasionally affected metachronously. Although the pathogenesis is not entirely clear, one hypothesis is that some form of testicular insult (e.g., bacte-

rial or viral infection, trauma) results in tubular injury and loss of the blood-testis barrier with the exposure of the antigens on spermatozoa and spermatogenic cells to a cellular immune reaction that goes on to induce additional tubular damage in a self-sustaining cycle.

Gross Findings. Typically, there is thickening of the tunica albuginea and replacement of the testicular parenchyma by homogeneous, sometimes lobulated, tan-yellow, gray, or white tissue (fig. 8-44). The process is usually diffuse but there is sometimes a localized, well-circumscribed nodule. The involved foci are often firm and rubbery and have a reduced tendency to bulge on sectioning compared to many neoplasms. The epididymis and spermatic cord are involved in about half the cases, and an exudate is often present on the tunica vaginalis, which may show fibrous adhesions. Rarely, the epididymis is the site of predominant (fig. 8-45) or exclusive (95) involvement by an idiopathic granulomatous or xanthogranulomatous process (see below).

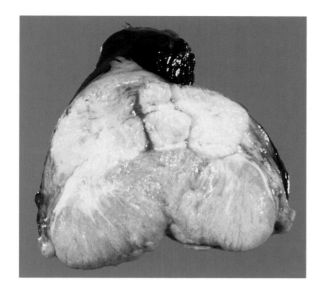

Figure 8-45

GRANULOMATOUS EPIDIDYMITIS, IDIOPATHIC

There is extensive involvement of the epididymis by an ill-defined, yellow-white mass, with lesser involvement of the testis.

Microscopic Findings. Microscopic examination of the testis shows filling of the seminiferous tubules by inflammatory cells, with a predominance of epithelioid histiocytes (fig. 8-46), but also intermixed lymphocytes and plasma cells; Langhans-type giant cells are seen in one third of the cases (fig. 8-47). In most cases, the interstitial tissue contains numerous chronic inflammatory cells, including eosinophils, and also may exhibit granulomatous inflammation in the form of infiltrates of epithelioid histiocytes. The process may extend to involve the epididymis.

Differential Diagnosis. The primarily intratubular location of the granulomatous process is helpful in differentiating the lesion from granulomatous orchitis of infectious origin and from sarcoidosis, in both of which the granulomas are predominantly interstitial. Necrosis within

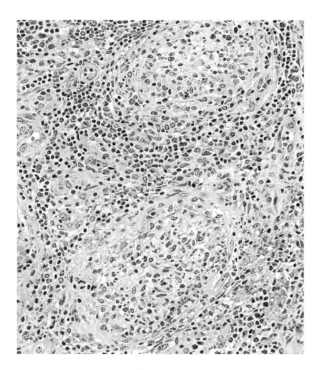

Figure 8-46

GRANULOMATOUS ORCHITIS, IDIOPATHIC

Two tubules are filled with epithelioid histiocytes and chronic inflammatory cells. The interstitium is also involved by the infiltrate.

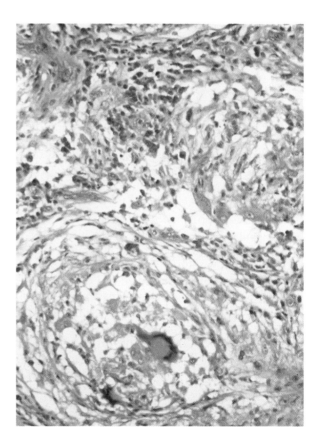

Figure 8-47

GRANULOMATOUS ORCHITIS, IDIOPATHIC

A high-power view shows epithelioid histiocytes and two giant cells.

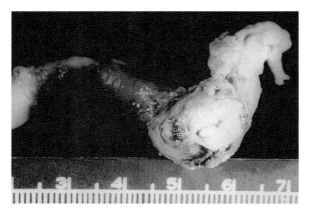

Figure 8-48

GRANULOMATOUS EPIDIDYMITIS

There is nodular thickening of the epididymis.

the granulomas may be seen in the infectious lesions, but is rarely, if ever, identified in idiopathic granulomatous orchitis. Identification of organisms by smear, culture, or histochemical study of paraffin-embedded material is indicated to exclude specific forms of infectious granulomatous orchitis. A potential pitfall in interpretation is the fact that remnants of sperm may be acid-fast positive in cases of idiopathic granulomatous orchitis. The granulomatous reaction of seminoma may cause confusion with idiopathic granulomatous orchitis but tends to have a greater interstitial rather than intratubular distribution, and seminoma cells, even if rare, can be identified, although occasional use of seminoma-highlighting immunostains is helpful. Viral orchitis may have a similar appearance but the intratubular infiltrates of macrophages more frequently have admixed neutrophils and lack the giant cells seen in many cases of idiopathic granulomatous orchitis. The prominent foamy macrophages that characterize xanthogranulomatous orchitis are rarely found in idiopathic granulomatous orchitis.

Granulomatous Epididymitis

Granulomatous epididymitis is usually a rare incidental finding at autopsy or in surgical specimens obtained for other indications, but in one personally observed case formed a mass that required exploration and removal to exclude a neoplasm (fig. 8-48) (96). The patients may have a history of vascular disease, prior surgery in

the region such as herniorrhaphy, or bacterial epididymitis. The reported age range is 30 to 62 years (97). The process is unilateral. Findings on gross examination may be inconspicuous.

Microscopically, zones of necrosis center on the efferent ducts, with a surrounding zone of granulomatous inflammation (fig. 8-49, left). Peripheral to this, and near adjacent intact ducts, a lymphocytic infiltrate occurs, but neutrophils are often inconspicuous (although in the case we have seen there was a significant intraductal neutrophilic component). Secondary changes may include sperm granulomas, ceroid granulomas, macrophage accumulation in the duct lumens, and regenerative changes of the efferent ductal epithelium including squamous metaplasia (fig. 8-49, right).

An ischemic origin is hypothesized for at least some of the cases (97); this appears more likely for those cases localized to the caput. Others may represent an obstructive phenomenon with duct rupture and secondary granulomatous inflammation to extravasated duct contents, including spermatozoa. It is important to exclude an infectious etiology by appropriate stains and culture.

Sarcoidosis

Sarcoidosis may affect the epididymis and, rarely, the testis (98); exceptional cases with prominent testicular enlargement have provoked orchiectomy. In a review in 1993, 28 mainly black patients had epididymal involvement, with testicular involvement in 6 (98). The epididymal disease is usually unilateral, nodular (fig. 8-50), and painless, but epididymitis may be mimicked. For testicular cases, the differential diagnosis includes seminoma with massive granulomatous inflammation, but the granulomas in seminoma are typically less organized and discrete, and, although markedly obscured in some cases, seminoma cells or IGCNU is always found on close scrutiny. In contrast to idiopathic granulomatous orchitis, the granulomas in sarcoidosis are interstitial.

Malakoplakia

General and Clinical Features. *Malakoplakia* involves the testis alone in about two thirds of the cases, and both the epididymis and testis in most of the remainder (99,100). The right testis is more

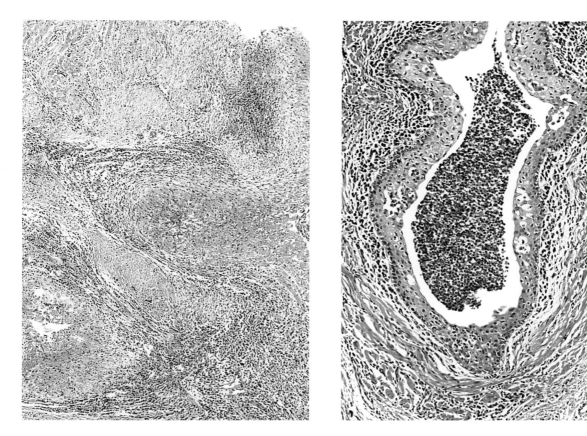

Figure 8-49

GRANULOMATOUS EPIDIDYMITIS

Left: Zones of necrosis are centered on the efferent ducts of the epididymis, with a surrounding mononuclear infiltrate.
Right: Squamous metaplasia of the epithelium of an efferent duct, with intraluminal inflammatory cells. (Both illustrations are from the case depicted in figure 8-48.)

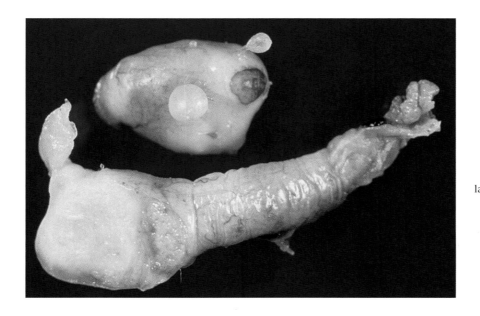

Figure 8-50

SARCOIDOSIS OF THE EPIDIDYMIS

The yellow-white mass simulates a neoplasm.

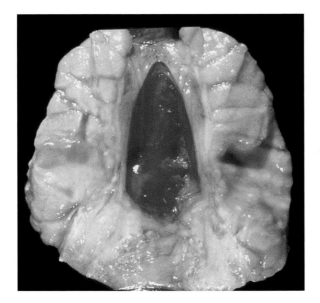 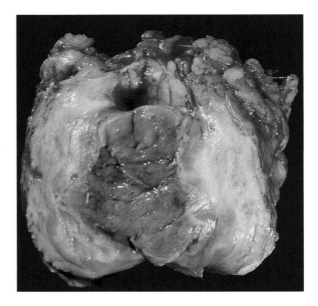

Figure 8-51

MALAKOPLAKIA OF TESTIS

Left: The testis is replaced by a lobulated yellow mass that simulates a neoplasm. There is, however, a small area of abscess formation. (Fig. 9.25 from Young RH, Scully RE. Testicular tumors. Chicago: ASCP Press; 1990:211.)

Right: There is conspicuous abscess formation, with necrotic tissue and fibrosis, more obviously indicative of an inflammatory process than the specimen on the left.

often affected than the left. Rarely, there is isolated epididymal involvement. The symptoms are non-specific; occasionally, there is a history of a prior urinary tract infection, often with *Escherichia coli*, or immunosuppression (101). The testis is usually enlarged and may be difficult to remove because of fibrous adhesions to surrounding tissues. In all the reported cases, testicular enlargement was unilateral and occurred in adults.

Gross Findings. Sectioning shows replacement of all or part of the testicular parenchyma by yellow (fig. 8-51, left), tan, or brown tissue, which is often divided into lobules by bands of fibrous tissue. The consistency is usually soft, but may be firm if there is prominent fibrosis. One or more abscesses and the presence of epididymal involvement and reactive inflammatory changes in the tunics are clues to the diagnosis (fig. 8-51, right).

Microscopic Findings. The tubules and interstitial tissue are replaced by large histiocytes with abundant, granular, eosinophilic cytoplasm (von Hansemann cells), some of which contain solid and targetoid, calcific, basophilic cytoplasmic inclusions of varying sizes (Michaelis-Gutmann bodies) (fig. 8-52). In occasional cases, the von Hansemann cells have a spindled configuration (fig. 8-53). Acute and chronic inflammatory cells, granulation tissue, fibrosis, and abscesses are also usually present and may obscure the characteristic features of the process, especially if Michaelis-Gutmann bodies are inconspicuous. These structures are accentuated by periodic acid-Schiff, von Kossa, and iron stains (fig. 8-54), which are positive in almost all cases. Ultrastructural studies have shown that the Michaelis-Gutmann bodies are phagolysosomes that ingest the breakdown products of bacteria of various types, most often *E. coli* (100).

Differential Diagnosis. Malakoplakia is sometimes confused with a Leydig cell tumor, but the latter does not involve the tubules and its cells lack the characteristic features of von Hansemann cells, including Michaelis-Gutmann bodies. Antibodies directed against histiocytic markers (CD68, KP1, CD163) (fig. 8-53) and inhibin resolve this differential diagnosis, with expected positive and negative results, respectively, in malakoplakia, and the opposite pattern in Leydig cell tumor.

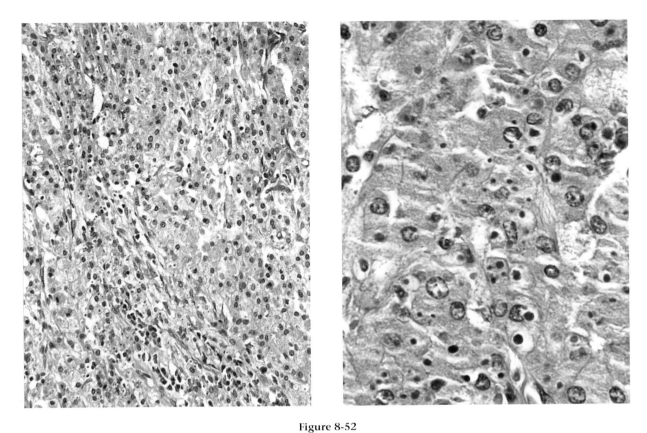

Figure 8-52

MALAKOPLAKIA OF TESTIS

Left: There is sheet-like growth of histiocytes with eosinophilic cytoplasm (von Hansemann cells).
Right: Many eosinophilic histiocytes (von Hansemann cells) contain targetoid basophilic inclusions (Michaelis-Gutmann bodies).

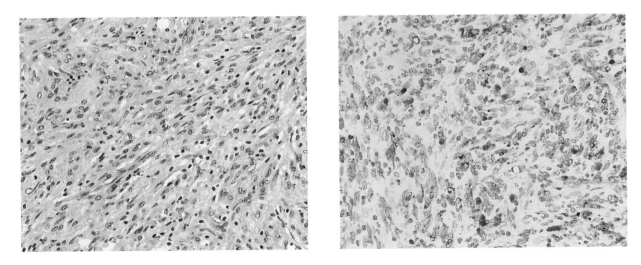

Figure 8-53

MALAKOPLAKIA OF TESTIS

The spindle-shaped cells (left) stain for the histiocytic marker KP1 (right).

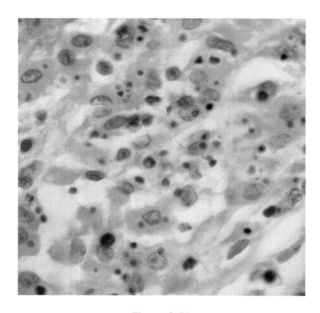

Figure 8-54

MALAKOPLAKIA OF TESTIS

Michaelis-Guttman bodies are positive with an iron stain.

ROSAI-DORFMAN DISEASE (SINUS HISTIOCYTOSIS WITH MASSIVE LYMPHADENOPATHY)

Idiopathic *Rosai-Dorfman disease* exceptionally involves the testis and epididymis and may be clinically confused with a neoplasm (72,102–104). Children and adults are affected; there is typically involvement at other sites, most notably lymph nodes; and patients may have polyclonal hypergammaglobulinemia. Testicular involvement may be bilateral (synchronous or metachronous) or unilateral. Patterns of involvement include a distinct testicular or epididymal nodule; a soft, discolored focus; or diffuse testicular replacement, with homogeneous involvement producing symmetric, firm and rubbery enlargement (fig. 8-55).

On microscopic examination, the typical pale eosinophilic histiocytes, some containing lymphocytes within their cytoplasm (so called emperipolesis), are distributed in the testicular interstitium (fig. 8-55) (102). The histiocytic cells are positive for S-100 protein and CD68 and negative for CD1a. The clinical course is variable, largely depending on the extent of involvement at other sites. This process must be distinguished from true neoplastic infiltrates of a histiocytic nature.

HYDROCELE-RELATED CHANGES AND MISCELLANEOUS OTHER ABNORMALITIES OF THE TUNICA VAGINALIS

In cases of simple, uncomplicated *hydrocele*, clinical and pathologic evaluation is straightforward, but in some longstanding hydroceles there may be marked chronic inflammation and fibrosis, with tethering of the testis to the tunica vaginalis such that a neoplasm is mimicked on clinical examination (fig. 8-56) (2,69). On microscopic examination, distinction from a neoplasm is straightforward. Squamous metaplasia is rarely seen (105), providing a histogenesis for the rare squamous cell carcinomas that complicate hydroceles (see chapter 7). When there is extensive hemorrhage into a hydrocele (hematocele) (fig. 8-57), thorough sectioning may be needed to exclude an underlying neoplasm. Calcification (106) and cholesterol granulomas (fig. 8-58) (107) may involve the tunica vaginalis in some cases.

A feature of chronic hydrocele is the development of conspicuous foci of mesothelial hyperplasia with extension into zones of reactive fibrosis (fig. 8-59). This is a common complication of inflamed hydroceles; it was identified in 14 of 18 cases in the series of the British Testicular Tumour Panel (73). Thus, nests, tubules, and strands of reactively atypical mesothelial cells with pseudoinvasive growth may suggest malignant mesothelioma. In some cases, there is also papillary mesothelial hyperplasia involving the surface. In contrast with most mesotheliomas, these reactive mesothelial proliferations do not form a grossly evident lesion. Their microscopic distinction from mesothelioma is discussed in chapter 7 and depends largely on decreasing mesothelial cellularity from the superficial to the deep zones of the hydrocele sac, a rather abrupt linear interface with noninvolved deeper tissues (108), and the characteristic inflammatory background.

Hydroceles or spermatoceles may rarely contain highly cellular clusters of small, hyperchromatic cells showing nuclear molding, raising concern for small cell carcinoma (109). The absence of mitotic activity and apoptosis, and immunohistochemical staining similar to that of the non-neoplastic rete testis, are evidence that these cellular clusters represent sloughed, non-neoplastic rete epithelium. In support, no small cell carcinoma was identified on follow-up in five such cases (109).

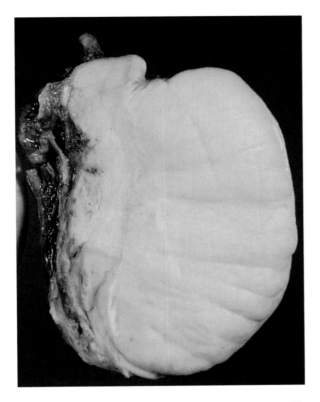

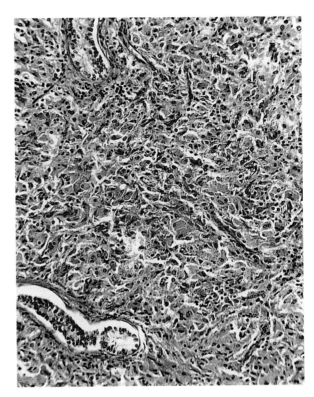

Figure 8-55

ROSAI-DORFMAN DISEASE

Left: The cut surface is homogeneous and bulging.

Right: Plump cells with abundant eosinophilic cytoplasm grow between seminiferous tubules. There are also scattered chronic inflammatory cells. (Figs. 1 and 2 from Azoury FJ, Reed RJ. Histiocytosis: report of an unusual case. N Engl J Med 1966;274:928-929.)

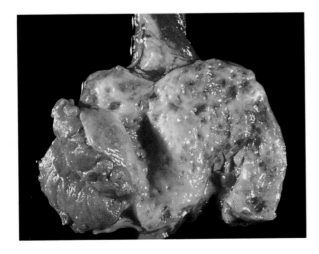

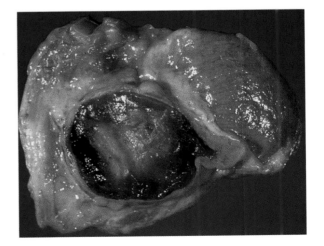

Figure 8-56

HYDROCELE SAC

There is marked, irregular thickening of the tunica vaginalis.

Figure 8-57

HEMATOCELE

A hydrocele sac contains an old blood clot within its lumen.

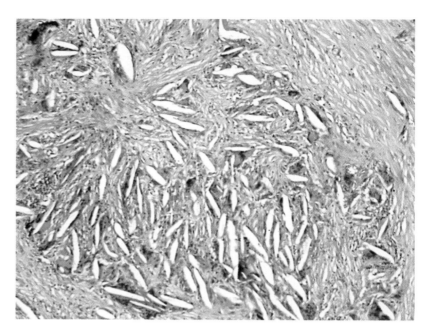

Figure 8-58

CHOLESTEROL GRANULOMA

Many cholesterol clefts are present within a fibrotic tunica vaginalis. (Courtesy of Dr. F. Algaba, Barcelona, Spain.)

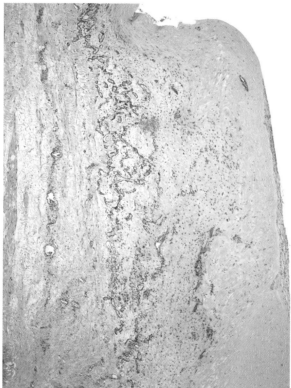

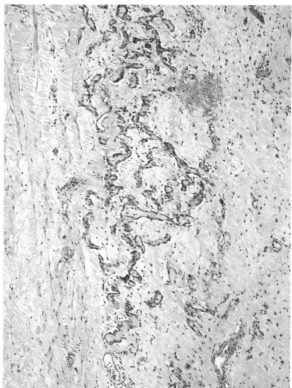

Figure 8-59

MESOTHELIAL HYPERPLASIA IN A CHRONIC HYDROCELE

Left: The fibrotically thickened wall of a chronic hydrocele contains a band of entrapped, hyperplastic mesothelium. Granulation tissue is superficial (right) to the mesothelium.

Right: The mesothelium forms tubules and has an abrupt interface with the deep stroma (left).

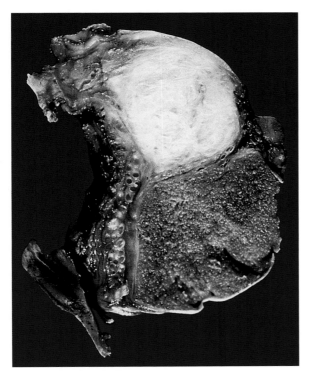

Figure 8-60

PROLIFERATIVE FUNICULITIS

A solid white mass replaces much of the lower portion of the spermatic cord.

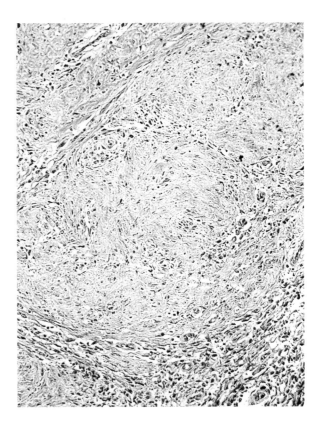

Figure 8-61

PROLIFERATIVE FUNICULITIS

The lesion is characterized by myofibroblasts and inflammatory cells with marked fibrosis. (Courtesy of Dr. C.D.M. Fletcher, Boston, MA.)

PROLIFERATIVE FUNICULITIS (PSEUDOSARCOMATOUS MYOFIBROBLASTIC PROLIFERATION; INFLAMMATORY PSEUDOTUMOR)

General and Clinical Features. The spermatic cord is the most common site in the male genital tract for the lesions that are variously reported under the above and other diverse designations (2,50,110–115). They are usually incidental findings noted at operation for inguinal hernia repair in middle-aged to older men, but occasionally the patient notes a mass (116). In some cases involving the epididymis the proliferation is a reaction to testicular torsion (50) and is usually noted as an incidental microscopic finding. If not completely excised, the possibility of recurrence exists, but, by definition, these lesions are nonmetastasizing. In two cases of *epididymal inflammatory pseudotumor* that presented as mass lesions, in situ hybridization studies failed to detect Epstein-Barr virus RNA, unlike some inflammatory pseudotumors at other sites (117).

Gross Findings. Typically, there is an ill-defined, gray-white mass with a firm or gelatinous consistency (fig. 8-60); rarely, cystic change and hemorrhage are seen or the lesion is well circumscribed. Most lesions do not exceed 3 cm in maximum dimension, but at least one measured 7 cm. Rare cases are centered on the rete testis or epididymis (111,112).

Microscopic Findings. The features of proliferative funiculitis are similar to those of nodular fasciitis. There is characteristically a moderately cellular, irregular, spindle cell proliferation in a loose collagenous stroma that may be focally or conspicuously myxoid. The process is typically heterogeneous in appearance, with the cellularity differing from area to area (fig. 8-61). The overall picture varies according to the degree of associated inflammation and the nature of the stroma. In at least some cases, the cellularity is more pronounced centrally (113), and there is often a focal fascicular arrangement. Infiltrative margins are typical. The lesional mesenchymal cells (fig. 8-62) usually have plump, oval to fusiform, vesicular nuclei, and some have conspicuous, tapering eosinophilic cytoplasm and mimic, to some degree, rhabdomyoblasts. In some cases, the presence of stellate cells in a myxoid background imparts a "tissue culture" appearance. Occasional cells have prominent eosinophilic nucleoli. Larger cells, resembling the "ganglion-like" cells of proliferative fasciitis of the soft tissues, may be encountered (fig. 8-62). The mitotic rate usually does not exceed 1 per 10 high-power fields, although in two cases associated with torsion there were 3 to 10 mitotic figures per 10 high-power fields (50). Abnormal mitotic figures are absent. The lesions are prominently vascular and there may be circumferential hyaline fibrosis of the blood vessel walls. In some cases, nests and tubules of reactive mesothelial cells are entrapped in the lesion, particularly at the periphery (118).

Immunohistochemistry is positive for actin and vimentin, less strongly for desmin, and rarely for cytokeratin. This is consistent with a myofibroblastic lineage, but has no great diagnostic value.

Differential Diagnosis. Potentially such lesions, like nodular fasciitis and similar processes elsewhere, may be confused with a malignant neoplasm, but awareness that they also occur in the paratestis should avoid this pitfall. In general, proliferative funiculitis appears, at least focally, similar to exuberant granulation tissue, and the inflammatory, reactive appearance suggests a non-neoplastic process. Nonetheless, the consideration of a sarcoma is not unreasonable in occasional instances. We have seen a case of inflammatory liposarcoma (119) of the spermatic cord that closely resembled proliferative funiculitis. The absence of a fascicular pattern and the presence of intermixed noncompressed fat, hyperchromatic atypical nuclei, and atypical adipocytes are distinguishing features of inflammatory liposarcoma (119). Inflammatory fibrosarcoma has not been described in this location, to our knowledge, but is a potential pitfall if the cytologic atypia of the lesional cells

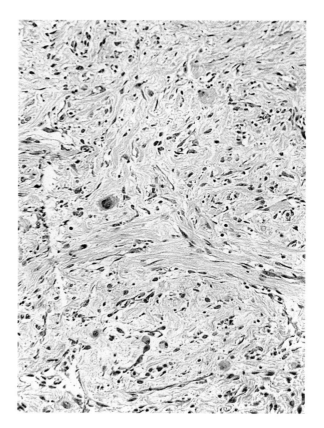

Figure 8-62

PROLIFERATIVE FUNICULITIS

A high-power view shows the characteristic myofibroblastic features of the majority of the lesional cells. Occasional larger, "ganglion-like" cells are seen.

is not appreciated (120,121). Nevertheless, a diagnosis of sarcoma should only be made after the possibility of a reactive process is carefully evaluated by noting the inflammatory nature of the lesion, lack of other than reactive cytologic atypia, usual lack of brisk mitotic activity, and absence, in most cases, of a gross appearance suggestive of a malignant tumor.

FIBROUS PSEUDOTUMOR, FIBROMATOUS PERIORCHITIS, NODULAR PERIORCHITIS

General and Clinical Features. The existence of fibromatous masses of the testicular tunics (114,122-130) and adjacent tissues has been long known, one of the earliest documented cases being referred to by Sir Astley Cooper in 1830 (131). In the first half of the twentieth century, Meyer (125) and Goodwin

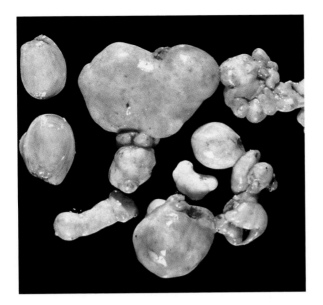

Figure 8-63

FIBROUS PSEUDOTUMOR

Multiple, discrete, free-lying masses were present in the tunica vaginalis ("corpora libera").

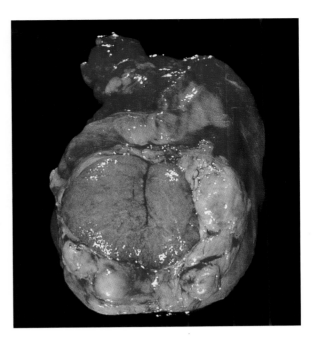

Figure 8-64

FIBROMATOUS PERIORCHITIS

This lesion forms an ill-defined mass encasing the testis.

(124) focused on the likely non-neoplastic reactive nature of such lesions, a viewpoint widely supported in the early 1960s when three cases of *nodular periorchitis* were included in the pseudotumors of the British Testicular Tumour Panel (114). Mostofi and Price, in the 1973 edition of the fascicle that considered the testis (132), introduced the term *fibrous pseudotumor*, which is now preferred for those cases that present as one or more discrete masses. When the process is ill-defined, sometimes forming a plaque-like lesion coating the testis, the term *fibromatous periorchitis* is perhaps preferable. Although usually adjacent to the testis, occasional lesions are present in the spermatic cord.

These lesions, which are seen at any age (128,130), usually present as a mass; there may be an associated hydrocele and history of trauma or infection (133,134). A rare patient had retroperitoneal fibrosis (73), leading to the speculation that lymphatic obstruction may play a role in the genesis of the testicular lesion (126). One patient had the nevoid basal cell carcinoma syndrome (135).

Gross Findings. In the more common, localized form, single or disseminated nodules (fig. 8-63) or, less frequently, plaques may be pres-

ent. They may be confluent and exceptionally encase the testis (fig. 8-64), or free and numerous, lying in the tunica vaginalis (fig. 8-63). Massive examples resulting in grotesque scrotal enlargement have been described (123). In the diffuse form of this disorder, dense fibrous tissue involves the tunica vaginalis (fig. 8-65). We have seen one case that was bilateral and extended into the testes (fig. 8-66). Sectioning reveals firm, sometimes stony hard, white tissue.

Microscopic Findings. Typically, hyalinized collagen (fig. 8-67), which may be focally (fig. 8-68) or massively calcified, is seen. Calcified examples are termed *calcifying fibrous pseudotumor* and, like their more common counterpart at a variety of soft tissue sites, are usually seen in children and young adults (136,137). Five calcifying fibrous pseudotumors located in the "scrotum," paratestis, and spermatic cord were identified in patients 19 to 55 years old (median, 21 years) who presented with masses (136,137). On gross examination, circumscribed but nonencapsulated, firm, gray-white, and occasionally lobulated masses, commonly measuring 2.5 to 4.0 cm are seen. Microscopic examination shows hyalinized fibrosclerotic tissue with a variable inflammatory component of lymphocytes and plasma cells and, with very rare exceptions, calcification of either psammomatous or dystrophic type. Widely spaced spindle-shaped cells with elongated to ovoid nuclei as well as numerous blood vessels are embedded within the dense collagenous background. Although recurrences of calcifying fibrous pseudotumor are documented at other sites, we are not aware of such an occurrence in the paratestis and proximate locations. In some cases, which presumably represent an earlier manifestation of the more fibrotic lesion, there is greater cellularity (128), with inflammation and granulation tissue (fig. 8-69).

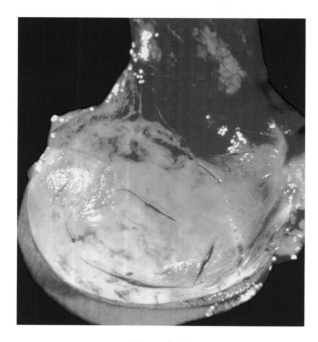

Figure 8-65

FIBROMATOUS PERIORCHITIS

A plaque-like lesion coats the testis.

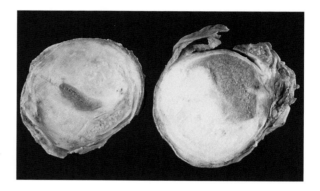

Figure 8-66

FIBROMATOUS PERIORCHITIS

The lesion is bilateral and extensively involves the testes. (Courtesy of Dr. A. Dorado, Panama.)

Figure 8-67

FIBROMATOUS PERIORCHITIS

Three discrete nodules are present on the tunica vaginalis.

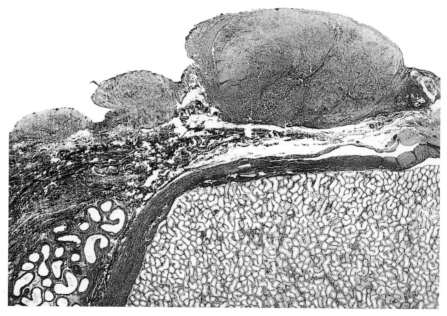

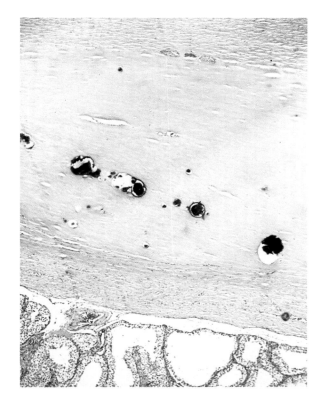

Figure 8-68

FIBROMATOUS PERIORCHITIS

A hyalinized plaque with focal calcification covers the testis.

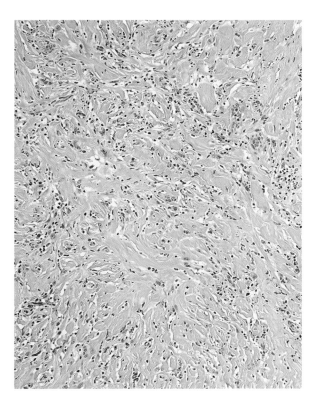

Figure 8-69

FIBROMATOUS PERIORCHITIS

This case shows greater cellularity than that of figure 8-68, with a combination of dense fibrosis, chronic inflammation, and myofibroblastic and vascular proliferation.

In one study of 13 cases of fibrous pseudotumor, the lesions were divided into three morphologic categories: hyalinized plaques without inflammation; inflammatory sclerotic, showing a combination of dense fibrosis in association with lymphocytes, plasma cells, and a capillary network; and myofibroblastic, with a cellular proliferation of "tissue culture-like" spindle cells and scant inflammation (133). Because of this latter pattern, it has been suggested that some cases of fibrous pseudotumor represent "matured" examples of pseudosarcomatous myofibroblastic proliferation (122), but the proclivity of the latter lesion for the spermatic cord and absence of staining for ALK-1 in fibrous pseudotumors (133,137) are contrary observations. A lesion possibly related to fibrous pseudotumor, with which we have no personal experience, is "constrictive albuginitis" (138).

Differential Diagnosis. Fibrous pseudotumor is distinguished from the rare fibroma of the tunics by its paucicellular nature in established cases and inflammatory appearance in earlier stages. The rare fibromatosis of the paratestis is more cellular than the typical case of fibrous pseudotumor, is overtly infiltrative, and stains for nuclear β-catenin, in contrast to the latter.

MECONIUM PERIORCHITIS

General and Clinical Features. *Meconium periorchitis* results from perforation of the bowel wall in utero, with the subsequent passage of meconium into the tunica vaginalis through a patent processus vaginalis. The usual presentation is a unilateral scrotal mass in the first few months of life, often clinically felt to be a neoplasm (139). Bilateral involvement is less common. Occasional cases present as an "acute scrotum" in the neonatal period (140). Delayed diagnosis may result in presentation in childhood as palpable scrotal nodules (141). Characteristic peritesticular calcifications on

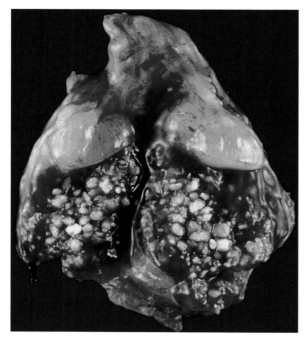

Figure 8-70

MECONIUM PERIORCHITIS
Multiple yellow nodules stud the tunica vaginalis.

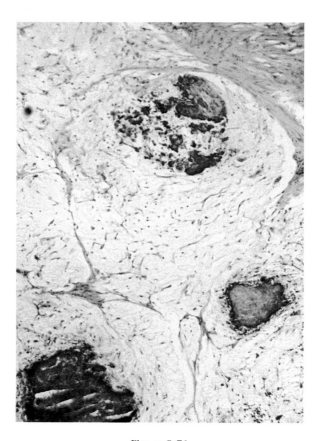

Figure 8-71

MECONIUM PERIORCHITIS
Lobules of myxoid tissue contain calcific deposits.

ultrasound examination in conjunction with abdominal calcifications on radiographs may allow for nonsurgical diagnosis, even prenatally, and conservative management. Meconium periorchitis is associated with cystic fibrosis in about 10 percent of cases (142).

Gross and Microscopic Findings. The typical gross manifestation is studding of the tunica vaginalis by yellowish to green gritty tissue (fig. 8-70). On microscopic examination, lobules of myxoid tissue containing spindle cells and scattered foci of calcification are seen (fig. 8-71). Scattered macrophages, some of which are pigmented, nucleated and anucleated squamous cells (fig. 8-72), and rare lanugo hairs may also be seen, as may mesothelial hyperplasia. Other than the macrophages, an inflammatory component is generally not striking.

Differential Diagnosis. The overall clinical background and distinctive gross appearance of meconium periorchitis enable its recognition, provided the observer is familiar with it. Confusion with a neoplasm is unlikely if it is remembered that testicular and paratesticular tumors in neonates are rare, with the majority

of cases representing testicular juvenile granulosa cell tumors that have a distinctly different morphology (see chapter 6). In utero testicular infarction results in atrophy (81), with scattered calcifications, but shares none of the other features of meconium periorchitis.

HISTIOCYTIC/MESOTHELIAL PROLIFERATIONS

General and Clinical Features. This common form of pseudotumor occurs in hydrocele sacs, hernia sacs (143), and specimens from other testicular and adnexal areas. In contrast to many pseudotumors, it is almost invariably an incidental finding on microscopic examination (144) and has no distinct gross features. It is seen at essentially all ages, but is more commonly identified in older patients who more frequently undergo hydrocelectomy. In a series describing the phenomenon in hernia sacs, however, 9 of the 13 patients were children (143). Similar

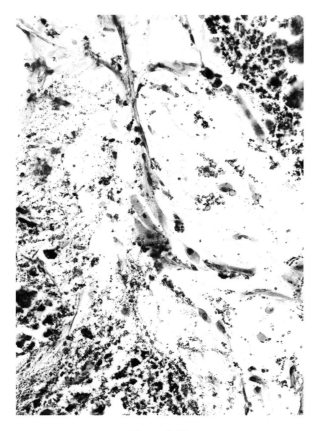

Figure 8-72

MECONIUM PERIORCHITIS

A higher power view of figure 8-71 shows granular calcifications, pigmented macrophages, and occasional squames in a myxoid stroma.

lesions have been identified in specimens originating from the pericardium and known as mesothelial/monocytic incidental cardiac excrescences (MICE).

Microscopic Findings. Aggregates of histiocytes and mesothelial cells, often in a fibrin-rich exudate, involve the serosal surface (fig. 8-73). The aggregates generally do not invade into underlying tissues to any appreciable extent. There may be mild nuclear pleomorphism, but the overall nuclear features are bland, and mitotic figures are rare. Most cells are histiocytic, as confirmed by positivity for markers such as CD68 and CD163 and negativity for cytokeratin (145).

Differential Diagnosis. The main entity in the differential diagnosis is malignant mesothelioma. Histiocytic/mesothelial lesions, however, lack the true papillae of well-differentiated pap-

illary mesothelioma and the invasive growth of other forms of mesothelioma (see chapter 7). Their histiocyte-rich nature is also in contrast to mesothelioma.

SCLEROSING LIPOGRANULOMA

General and Clinical Features. A granulomatous mass may result from the injection of lipids to enhance the size of the genitalia (*secondary sclerosing lipogranuloma*) (146) or develop as an idiopathic phenomenon (*primary sclerosing lipogranuloma*) (147). The mass usually involves the scrotum or penis but occasionally involves the spermatic cord (fig. 8-74), epididymis, or testis. In one review of 23 cases of secondary sclerosing lipogranuloma (146), 2 involved the cord and another 2 the testis, with bilateral testicular involvement in 1 case. Scrotal involvement is more common in primary cases and penile in secondary (148). Most patients are under 40 years of age and present with either a mass or pain. The primary form is more apt to be painless and spontaneously resolve than the secondary form (147,148).

Gross and Microscopic Findings. On gross examination, there is a firm, ill-defined, gray-white to yellow mass that may have multiple small cysts (fig. 8-74). The mass typically is a few centimeters in size but may be massive. On microscopic examination, lipid vacuoles of variable size are frequently surrounded by foreign body giant cells and embedded in a densely fibrotic stroma (fig. 8-75). A variable inflammatory infiltrate, consisting of histiocytes, lymphocytes, and eosinophils, is seen in the stroma in addition to the foreign body giant cells. The eosinophilic component is characteristically most prominent in the primary form (147,148). Oil red O stains on frozen sections confirm the lipid nature of the vacuoles, but are not necessary for diagnosis.

Differential Diagnosis. There are few differential diagnostic considerations. A metastasis of signet ring cell adenocarcinoma may be suggested but this does not provoke a foreign body reaction and the vacuoles contain mucin rather than lipid. Similarly, sclerosing liposarcoma lacks a foreign body giant cell reaction and the lesional cells are cytologically atypical, unlike the cellular components of sclerosing lipogranuloma.

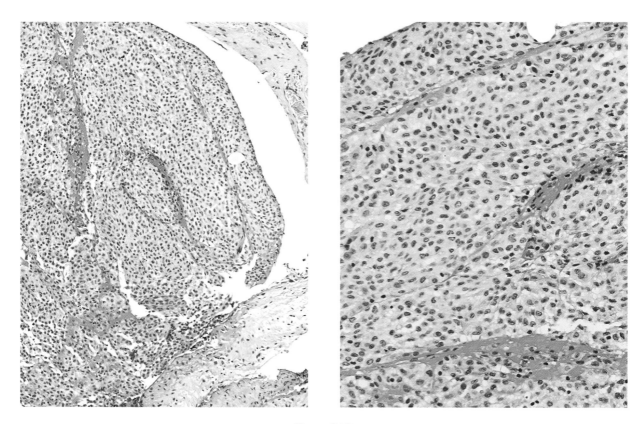

Figure 8-73

HISTIOCYTIC/MESOTHELIAL PROLIFERATION

Left: A hydrocele sac contains a nodular aggregate of cells on its surface.
Right: Most of the cells have the features of histiocytes, and there are admixed bands of fibrin.

Figure 8-74

LIPOGRANULOMA OF THE SPERMATIC CORD

The yellow mass is punctuated by small cysts and chalky foci of fat necrosis.

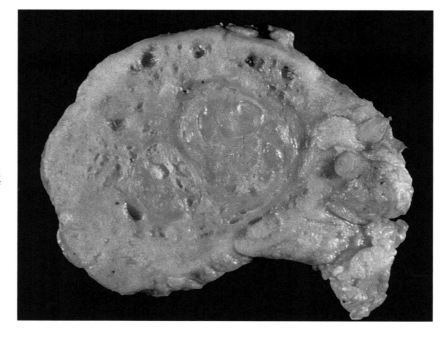

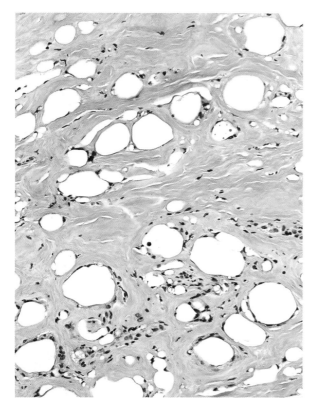

Figure 8-75

**SECONDARY SCLEROSING LIPOGRANULOMA
OF THE SPERMATIC CORD**

Multiple large lipid vacuoles in a dense stroma are surrounded by foreign body giant cells.

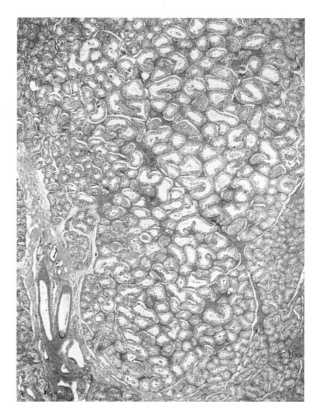

Figure 8-76

NODULAR PRECOCIOUS MATURATION

A nodule of mature testicular tissue contrasts with the normal prepubertal appearance elsewhere. This boy had an extratesticular, human chorionic gonadotropin (hCG)-secreting germ cell tumor.

ABNORMALITIES RELATED TO SEXUAL PRECOCITY/IDIOPATHIC HYPERTROPHY

Two lesions associated with sexual precocity can be confused with testicular tumors. The more common of these, the *testicular "tumor" of the adrenogenital syndrome*, has already been discussed earlier in this chapter. A rarer lesion is the so-called *nodular precocious maturation of the testis* in which gonadotropin-induced or gonadotropin-independent stimulation of the testis causes focal rather than diffuse stimulation of Leydig cells and tubules. In the gonadotropin-induced examples, which are most commonly due to a human chorionic gonadotropin (hCG)-secreting extragonadal germ cell tumor, this asymmetric development may result in a nodule that is visible on ultrasound examination. In such cases, microscopic examination shows variable degrees of maturation of tubules and Leydig cells within

the ill-defined nodule (fig. 8-76) and little or no maturation in the adjacent testis (149). In the rare gonadotropin-independent sexual precocity ("testotoxicosis"), similar focal maturation may be seen but a detectable mass has not been reported (150,151). Rarely, *idiopathic testicular hypertrophy* has been reported (152), and *macroorchidism*, without distinct nodule formation, may also be seen in patients with fragile X syndrome, prepubertal hypothyroidism, and follicle–stimulating hormone (FSH)–secreting pituitary adenomas.

HYPERPLASIA AND MISCELLANEOUS OTHER BENIGN LESIONS OF THE RETE TESTIS

True *hyperplasia of the rete testis* is rare (153, 154). In atrophic testes, a relative prominence of the rete may suggest hyperplasia (fig. 8-77) or even carcinoma. In many cases, the decision

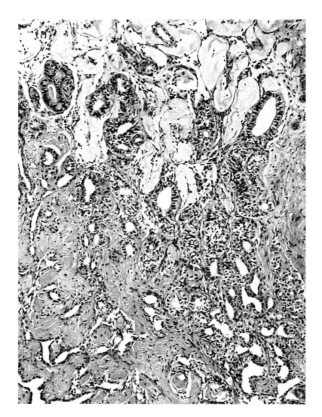

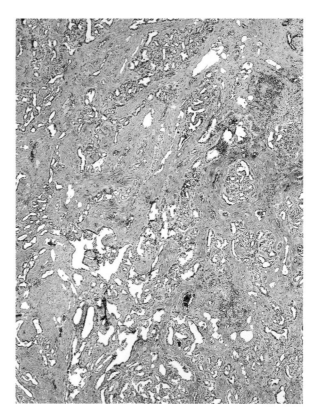

Figure 8-77

**RELATIVE HYPERPLASIA OF RETE
TESTIS AND EFFERENT DUCTULES**

The rete testis is prominent because the parenchyma is atrophic.

Figure 8-78

ADENOMATOUS HYPERPLASIA OF THE RETE TESTIS

The rete testis is greatly expanded but retains a branching and lobular pattern.

as to whether the rete is hyperplastic or not is subjective. What has been designated as adenomatous hyperplasia of the rete generally represents an incidental finding in cryptorchid testes or those examined at autopsy, but it may present as a mass (153,155). For those cases in which the lesion is nonincidental, a solid or cystic mass involves the hilum (153). At low magnification, there is expansion of the rete testis, up to one third of the size of the testis, with retention of its branching architecture (fig. 8-78). Its lining epithelium is frequently columnar but has bland cytologic features with frequently grooved nuclei. Mitotic figures are inconspicuous.

A different, *secondary form of rete hyperplasia* occurs when it is invaded by a germ cell neoplasm or other tumor (fig. 8-79) (156). The proliferation in these cases may exhibit solid, papillary, and microcystic patterns, with as-

sociated intracellular hyaline globules, leading to potential confusion with yolk sac tumor. In a study of 48 cases, hyperplastic epithelium with hyaline globules was found in the rete or tubuli recti in 16 of 27 cases of germ cell tumor, 1 of 5 other testicular tumors, and none of 16 non-neoplastic lesions (156). The hyperplastic epithelium of the rete in these cases is cytologically bland, and mitoses are absent or rare. In addition, the arborizing nature of the rete is apparent, unlike the diffuse or nodular growth of yolk sac tumor involving the rete.

Cystic dysplasia of the testis represents dilatation of the luminal spaces of the rete testis with secondary compression of the parenchyma. It is rare, presents mostly in infants and children, and is characterized by multiple anastomosing cysts of varying sizes and shapes separated by fibrous septa (157–160). It is associated with

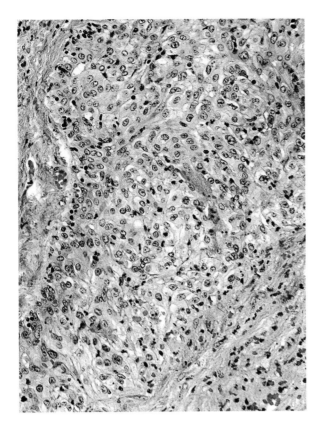 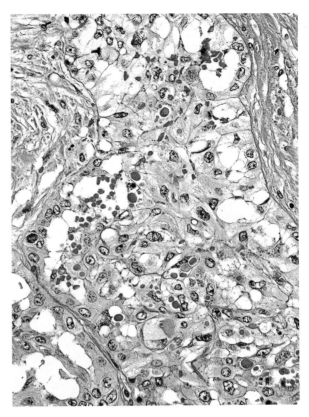

Figure 8-79

SECONDARY HYPERPLASIA OF THE RETE TESTIS WITH HYALINE GLOBULE PRODUCTION

Left: The lumen of the rete is expanded by a proliferation of bland rete epithelial cells.
Right: The benign cytologic features and hyaline globules are better seen in this high-power view from a different case. Microcysts are present.

ipsilateral renal agenesis and renal dysplasia and, rarely, with bilateral renal dysplasia (161–163). In one third of cases there is bilateral testicular involvement. Gross examination reveals a multicystic mass replacing much of the testis (fig. 8-80) or a more localized lesion based in the hilum. The process begins in the region of the rete testis and extends into the parenchyma, which may be compressed to a thin rim. The cysts are lined by a single layer of flat or cuboidal epithelial cells, similar to those of the rete testis (fig. 8-81).

A similar lesion, termed *acquired cystic transformation of the rete testis*, is seen in some patients on renal dialysis. There is expansion of the luminal spaces of the rete testis, which are lined by columnar to pseudostratified epithelium and contain proteinaceous fluid, spermatozoa, and calcium oxalate crystals (fig. 8-82, left) (164).

Cystic change of the rete (fig. 8-82, right) may also be seen in patients with obstructive lesions in the epididymis or compression of the efferent ductules by a varicocele.

Additional non-neoplastic lesions of the rete testis include a *hamartoma* in a 3-year-old that consisted of a disorganized collection of branching rete tubules in a fibrous stroma (66); *multilocular cystic change* in conjunction with prominent smooth muscle hyperplasia of the septa (165); and *epididymal-like metaplasia* of intratesticular portions of the rete testis/tubuli recti in older men with vascular disease and testicular atrophy (166). Rarely, microscopic proliferations of nodular to pedunculated connective tissue with focal calcification occur within the rete channels. These *nodular proliferations of calcifying connective tissue* are thought possibly to be related to organized blood (167).

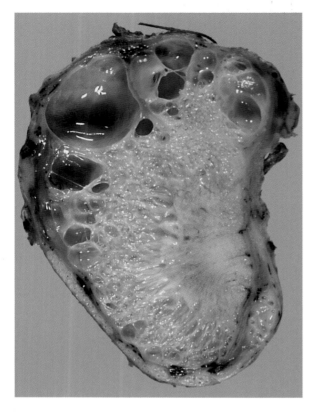

Figure 8-80

CYSTIC DYSPLASIA

Multiple cysts of varying sizes are visible. (Courtesy of Professor W. Wegmann, Liestal, Switzerland.)

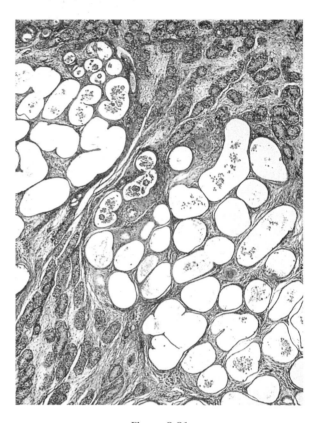

Figure 8-81

CYSTIC DYSPLASIA

Most of the cysts are dilated and lined by flattened epithelium. (Courtesy of Professor W. Wegmann, Liestal, Switzerland.)

CYSTS

General and Clinical Features. Whether some or all *epidermoid cysts* are neoplasms *(monodermal teratomas)* is a matter of controversy. In one study, 3 of 8 cases demonstrated loss of heterozygosity, lending some support for a neoplastic process (167a). Nonetheless, they are discussed here for the sake of convenience and their uniformly benign and possibly nonneoplastic nature. Epidermoid cysts account for approximately 1 percent of testicular parenchymal masses (168,169). Less commonly, they involve the tunica albuginea or the epididymis (66). In the testis, they are most common during the second to fourth decades but may be seen at any age. They average 2 cm in diameter, are round to oval, and are composed of yellow-white laminated cheesy material surrounded by a fibrous wall (fig. 8-83).

Microscopic Findings. Microscopic examination shows that at least part of the cyst wall is lined by keratinizing squamous epithelium (fig. 8-84), although the lining may be denuded over large areas, with ulceration, adjacent fibrosis (fig. 8-85), and a foreign body giant cell reaction. It is important to sample epidermoid cysts extensively to exclude other elements that indicate a teratomatous nature, although their unilocular nature and conspicuous laminated material on gross examination are exceedingly suggestive of the diagnosis. Extensive sampling of adjacent nonlesional tissue is also indicated because an association with IGCNU confirms the diagnosis of teratoma. IGCNU is not identified in cases of true epidermoid cyst (170,171), and the exclusion of IGCNU by examination of two or more biopsy specimens of the adjacent testis permits conservative local excision

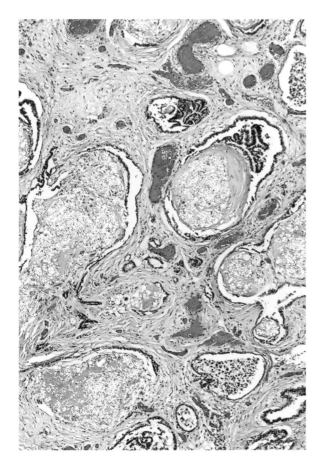 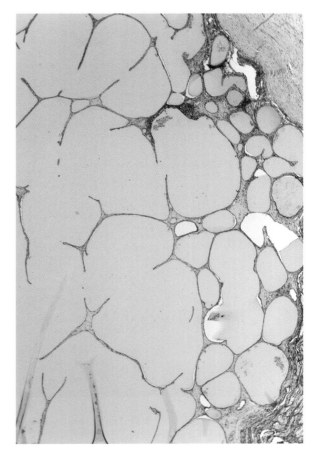

Figure 8-82

CYSTIC CHANGE OF RETE TESTIS

Left: The rete testis is dilated and contains polarizable calcium oxalate crystals admixed with proteinaceous, eosinophilic secretion. This autopsy specimen is from a patient on chronic renal dialysis, and the lesion is referred to as "acquired cystic transformation." (Photographed under polarized light.)

Right: There is marked cystic dilatation of the rete testis, which is filled with edema fluid secondary to compression by a mixed germ cell tumor.

(172,173). Additionally, epidermoid cysts lack abnormalities involving chromosome 12p, as detected by fluorescence in situ hybridization, which contrasts with 88 percent in teratomas of the usual type (174).

Other testicular and paratesticular cysts include those of the *tunica albuginea* (figs. 8-86, 8-87) (175,176), *isolated rete cysts* (fig. 8-88) (177, 178), *cystic Walthard nests, epididymal cysts* (fig. 8-89), *multilocular cysts of paradidymal origin* (179), *mesothelial cysts*, and *paratesticular dermoid cysts* (fig. 8-90) (66,180–182). A case of "multicystic mesothelioma" of the spermatic cord has been reported (177), but it is controversial whether this is a low-grade neoplasm (183) or a reactive, cystic mesothelial proliferation (184). All of these entities are uncommon. Cysts of the tunica albuginea usually do not exceed 4 cm, may be multiple, can be unilocular or multilocular, and usually contain serous fluid (176,185). Their lining consists of cuboidal or flat epithelial cells.

True hermaphrodites who are phenotypic males may have ovotestes or rarely, an ovary in the scrotum (186). The ovarian tissue may contain cystic follicles and corpora lutea, and on occasion, ovulation causes the sudden onset of hemorrhage with pain and a mass in the scrotum, simulating a testicular tumor (fig. 8-91).

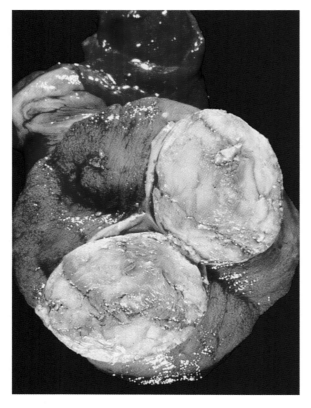

Figure 8-83

EPIDERMOID CYST OF TESTIS

The intratesticular cyst contains yellow-white material.

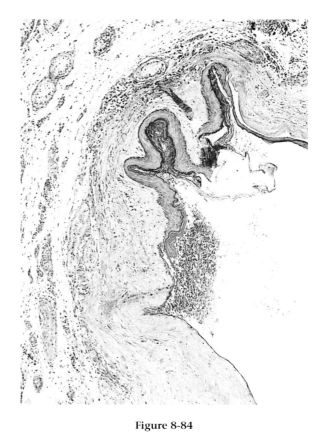

Figure 8-84

EPIDERMOID CYST OF TESTIS

A pure squamous cyst lining without other elements beneath.

Figure 8-85

EPIDERMOID CYST OF TUNICA VAGINALIS

The cyst ruptured and was associated with a prominent fibrotic response.

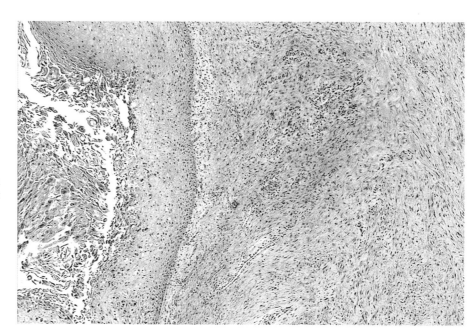

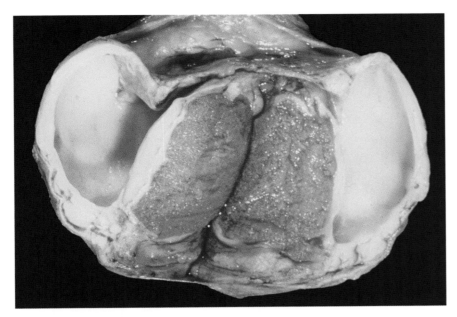

Figure 8-86

CYST OF TUNICA ALBUGINEA

A thickened, white tunica surrounds a large cystic space. (Courtesy of Dr. F. Askin, Baltimore, MD.)

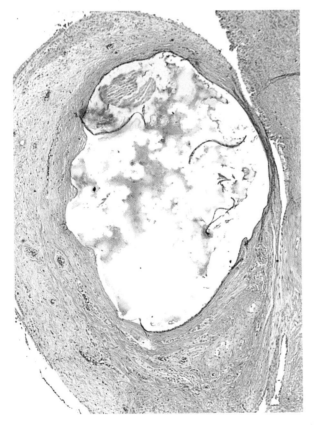

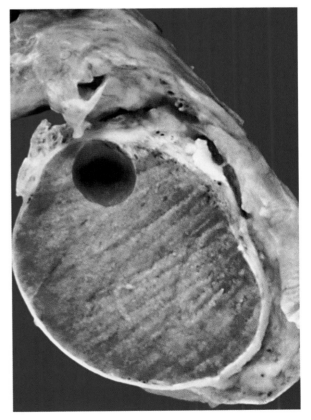

Figure 8-87

CYST OF TUNICA ALBUGINEA

A thin epithelial lining is barely discernible at this magnification.

Figure 8-88

CYST OF RETE TESTIS

The lesion is at the hilum. (Courtesy of Dr. J. Eble, Indianapolis, IN.)

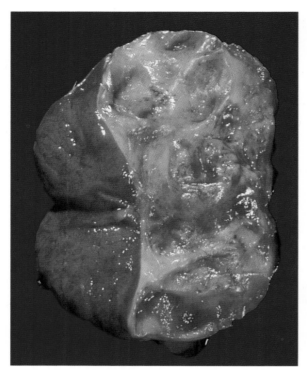

Figure 8-89

EPIDIDYMAL CYST

The multilocular cyst contained clear fluid.

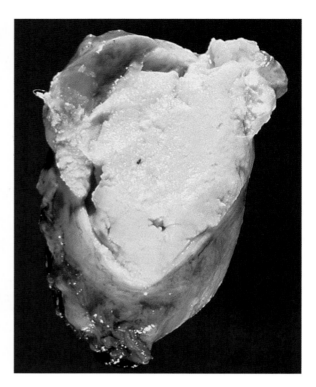

Figure 8-90

DERMOID CYST OF SPERMATIC CORD

Grumous material protrudes from the opened cyst.

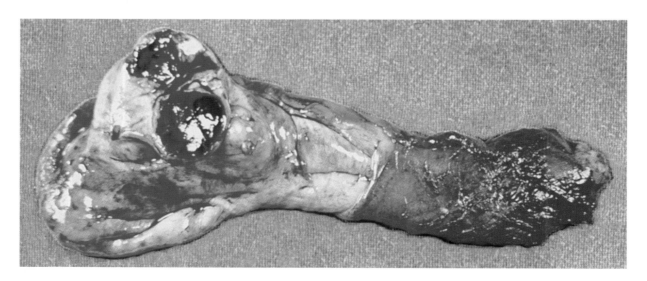

Figure 8-91

RUPTURED CORPUS LUTEUM IN A HERMAPHRODITE

A hemorrhagic corpus luteum is present in the upper pole of an ovotestis of a true hermaphrodite. This patient, a 14-year-old boy, presented with "testicular" pain and gynecomastia. Examination of the gonad led to the diagnosis of true hermaphroditism. (Courtesy of Dr. F. Vellios, Atlanta, GA and Dr. J. Albores-Saavedra, Dallas, TX.)

MICROLITHIASIS

Microlithiasis is found in patients without any underlying abnormality but also is associated with infertility, and, in at least one case, there was pulmonary alveolar microlithiasis (187–192). It often is initially appreciated on radiographic examination. Although two forms of microlithiasis have been described (191), we believe that this term should be restricted to cases having round, psammomatous calcifications within seminiferous tubules (fig. 8-92), as the "amorphous" type, representing dystrophic calcification that occurs in foci of regressed intratubular embryonal carcinoma (see chapter 5), has different clinical behavior. So defined, microlithiasis occurs with germ cell tumors in about 40 percent of cases, but also is seen in 1 to 5 percent of apparently normal men (193,194).

Follow-up studies show a statistically increased incidence of germ cell tumors in men with microlithiasis, but it is not frequent enough to justify routine ultrasonographic screening. More recently, microlithiasis has been identified at increased prevalence in men with familial testicular cancer and their relatives (195).

SPERMATOCELE

Spermatocele is an acquired, cystic lesion containing sperm that is usually caused by cystic dilatation of the efferent ductules of the head of the epididymis (196). Less commonly, the

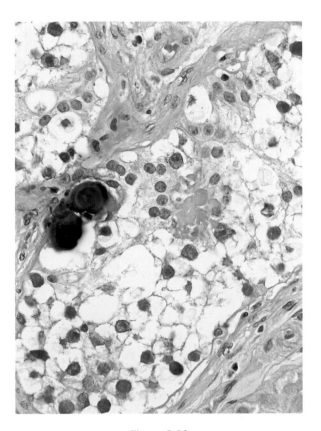

Figure 8-92

MICROLITHIASIS

Two psammomatous calcifications are seen in a tubule that also contains intratubular germ cell neoplasia, unclassified type (IGCNU).

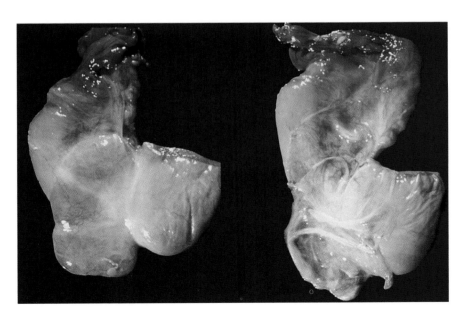

Figure 8-93

SPERMATOCELE

The thin, translucent wall of a spermatocele is apparent (left: unopened; right: opened).

lesion results from dilatation of the tubules of the rete testis or the aberrant ducts.

Spermatoceles appear at any age after puberty but have a peak incidence in the fourth and fifth decades, and a right-sided predominance (197). The cysts may be unilocular or multilocular, and may attain a large size (fig. 8-93). They have a thin translucent wall and contain cloudy fluid reflecting the contents of sperm.

Histologically, the fibromuscular wall is lined by a cuboidal to, rarely, pseudostratified epithelium. Rarely, spermatoceles contain mural papillary proliferations (papillomas) composed of small papillae with fibrovascular cores lined by bland columnar epithelium. The luminal contents consist of an eosinophilic secretion containing degenerated spermatozoa. Occasionally, they contain degenerated, sloughed cells of apparent rete epithelial origin that may resemble those in "small blue cell tumors" but these have no clinical significance (198). Occasionally, large spermatoceles undergo torsion (199,200).

SPERM GRANULOMA

General and Clinical Features. *Sperm granuloma* is a granulomatous reaction to extravasated sperm. A nodule is produced that is usually painful and may be clinically mistaken for a tumor (2,201–204). In one study of 60 cases, 8 were felt to represent a tumor of the epididymis or testis on clinical examination (203). In two large series, 1 to 5 percent of men undergoing vasectomy developed sperm granulomas (205,206), with vasitis nodosa also a significant complication of this procedure. Sperm granulomas are currently related to a prior vasectomy in over 40 percent of the cases. Other etiologies include trauma, infection, urinary tract obstruction, and prior surgery. About 80 percent of the patients are under 40 years of age (203). Approximately 90 percent of granulomas that follow vasectomy are in the vas deferens and the remainder in the epididymis.

Gross Findings. Sperm granulomas can measure up to 4 cm but average about 0.7 cm (203). They are typically firm nodules but may have small, soft, yellow to white foci on sectioning (fig. 8-94). They may be focally cystic due to secondary obstruction and dilatation of the epididymal ducts associated with the lesion.

Microscopic Findings. The appearance varies according to the stage of the process. In the

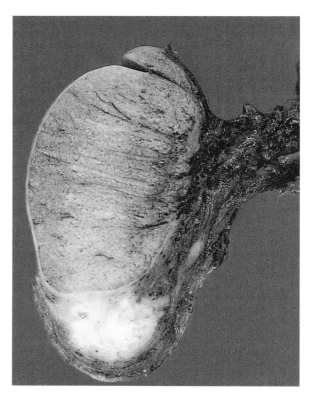

Figure 8-94

SPERM GRANULOMA

A firm, white nodule with foci of necrosis involves the lower pole of the epididymis. (Fig. 1 from Glassy FJ, Mostofi FK. Spermatic granulomas of the epididymis. Am J Clin Pathol 1956;26:1305.)

initial phase, there is an infiltrate of neutrophils, which is gradually replaced by epithelioid histiocytes. The histiocytes and occasional giant cells surround the sperm, resulting in the most characteristic appearance of the lesion (figs. 8-95, 8-96); calcification is occasionally seen. In the later stages, there is progressive fibrosis and hyalinization, and deposition of lipochrome pigment may be prominent. Sperm granulomas occurring in the vas deferens are associated with vasitis nodosa in approximately one third of the cases.

Differential Diagnosis. There are limited considerations. Some cases reported under the heading of "sperm granuloma" appear more typical of idiopathic granulomatous orchitis because of an absence or paucity of associated sperm and a history of a febrile illness.

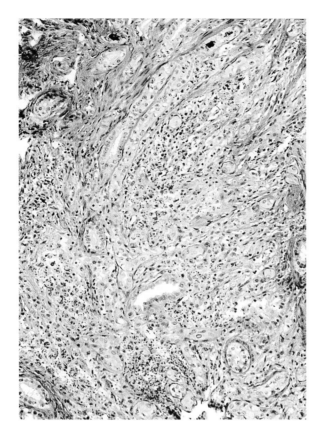

Figure 8-95

SPERM GRANULOMA

Darkly staining sperm are associated with epithelioid histiocytes. Several small tubules representing associated vasitis nodosa are visible.

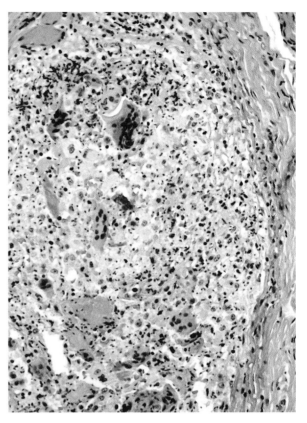

Figure 8-96

SPERM GRANULOMA

Langhans-type giant cells are conspicuous.

VASITIS NODOSA

General and Clinical Features. Benjamin et al. (207) coined the term *vasitis nodosa* because of similarity to salpingitis isthmica nodosa. It is usually encountered at the time of a vasovasostomy, and therefore typically occurs in young men of a mean age of 36 years and an interval from vasectomy to vasovasostomy of 1 to 15 (mean, 7) years (208). There may be associated pain, but most patients are asymptomatic. An analogous epididymal lesion, *epididymitis nodosa* (209), also occurs. Stout (210) described possibly similar pseudoneoplastic proliferations of the epididymis in response to inflammation.

Gross Findings. The lesions are typically firm nodules in the scrotal portion of the vas deferens, 5 to 6 cm above the testis (fig. 8-97),

corresponding to the frequent site of vasectomy (211). They usually measure up to just over 1 cm and typically have a white cut surface that may exude milky fluid.

Microscopic Findings. Microscopic examination reveals small, gland-like structures lined by cuboidal epithelium in the wall of the vas deferens and the surrounding adventitia (figs. 8-98, 8-99). The tubules have an irregular distribution, and perineural invasion may be observed (figs. 8-100, 8-101) (212–214). There are coexistent sperm granulomas in many cases, 70 percent in one series (208). The tubules may also contain histiocytes, some with ceroid pigment. Pagetoid spread of IGCNU may be seen within the proliferating tubules in patients with germ cell tumors (215).

Differential Diagnosis. The usual presence of sperm in the tubal lumens is important in

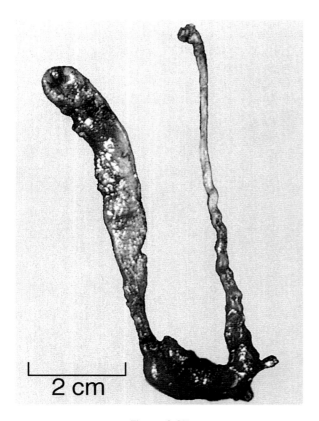

Figure 8-97

VASITIS NODOSA

Nodular thickening is apparent in the mid-portion (bottom) of the vas deferens. (Fig. 12-9A from Bostwick DG. Spermatic cord and testicular adnexa. In: Bostwick DG, Eble JN, eds. Urologic surgical pathology. St. Louis: Mosby; 1997:656.)

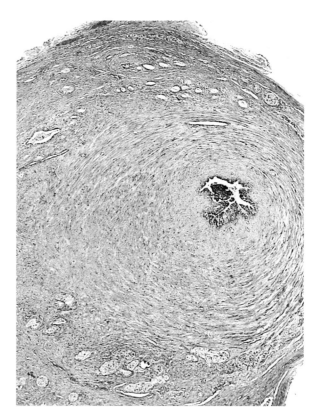

Figure 8-98

VASITIS NODOSA

Tubules involve the outer aspect of the wall of the vas deferens.

Figure 8-99

VASITIS NODOSA

The small tubules are irregularly disposed causing potential confusion with adenocarcinoma.

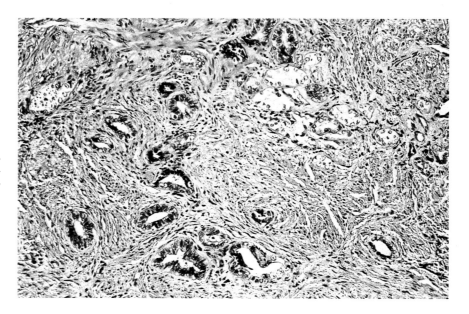

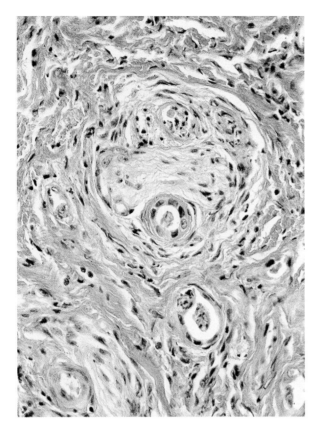

Figure 8-100

VASITIS NODOSA

The small tubules show perineural invasion. (Courtesy of Dr. K. Balogh, Boston, MA.)

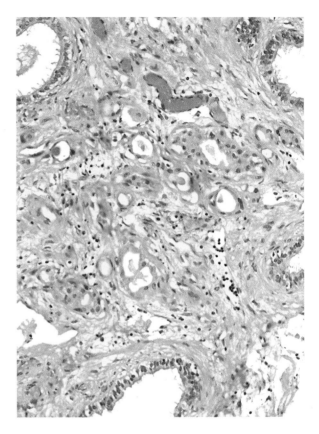

Figure 8-101

EPIDIDYMITIS NODOSA

A cluster of small tubules, resembling those of vasitis nodosa, is present between epididymal tubules.

distinguishing the tubules from the glands of adenocarcinoma, as is the lack of any significant cytologic atypia or mitotic activity, although nucleoli may be prominent.

SPLENIC-GONADAL FUSION

Splenic-gonadal fusion, in which splenic and gonadal tissues become adherent and fuse during early intrauterine development, is seen in both sexes but has a strong male predilection (216,217). The left side is almost invariably involved. The abnormality occurs in two forms, continuous and discontinuous. In the former, a cord connects the normal splenic tissue to the testis, while in the latter, no connection to the normally positioned spleen is present. In the continuous type, small aggregates of splenic tissue are found in the fibrous cord as it traverses the peritoneal cavity, or the cord is composed entirely of splenic tissue. Almost one third of the patients with the continuous form have severe defects of the extremities (peromelia), sometimes associated with micrognathia. In patients without associated congenital abnormalities, the clinical presentation is as a scrotal or inguinal mass, typically discovered during an operation for either an inguinal hernia (which is present in over one third of patients) or an undescended testis (present in one sixth). Two patients had scrotal pain during attacks of malaria.

The splenic tissue typically forms a discrete mass that is almost always fused to the upper pole of the testis or the head of the epididymis, but occasionally is attached to the lower pole and rarely is intratesticular. It is usually small but may be over 10 cm and has the characteristic gross (fig. 8-102) and microscopic features (fig. 8-103) of normal spleen.

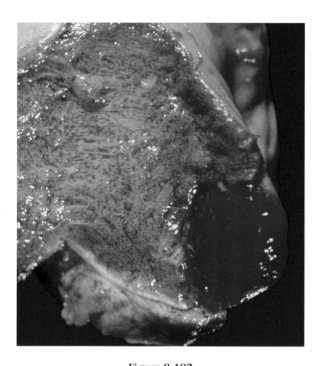

Figure 8-102

SPLENIC-GONADAL FUSION

Beefy red tissue consistent with spleen is located within the lower pole of the testis. (Fig. 9.37 from Young RH, Scully RE. Testicular tumors. Chicago: ASCP Press; 1990:217.)

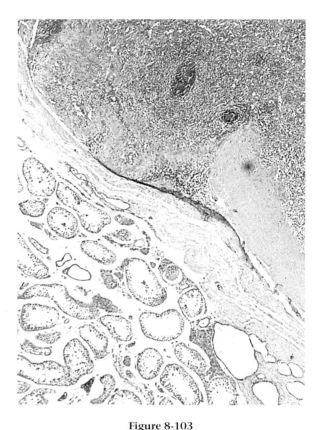

Figure 8-103

SPLENIC-GONADAL FUSION

Splenic tissue is separated from testicular tissue by a fibrous band.

SMOOTH MUSCLE HYPERPLASIA OF THE ADNEXA

This benign process usually occurs in middle-aged to older men (mean, 63 years) who present with a palpable mass, most commonly involving the epididymis (218). It consists of a frequently ill-defined, nodular, sometimes fusiform or cord-like growth of gray-white to tan tissue involving paratesticular structures. On microscopic examination, there are increased fascicles of smooth muscle that grow in a periductal, perivascular, or interstitial pattern around pre-existing structures. It differs from leiomyoma by its ill-defined gross appearance and loose arrangement of smooth muscle bundles that contrast with the circumscribed and cohesive fascicular arrangement of leiomyoma (218).

TUMOR-LIKE ASPECTS OF NORMAL HISTOLOGY

There are two normal histologic features of the epididymis that occasionally cause confusion with a dysplastic or neoplastic process (219). The first is a *prominent cribriform pattern of the epididymal tubules* that is occasionally seen (fig. 8-104). The lack of invasion, absence of neoplastic-type cytologic atypia of the epithelial cells, and awareness of the phenomenon should help avoid a misdiagnosis of carcinoma. Rarely, a similar cribriform process involves the efferent ductules, sometimes showing the cytoplasmic lipofuscin characteristic of those structures (fig. 8-105).

In the second normal variant, *bizarre nuclear atypicality*, similar to that more commonly identified in the seminal vesicle, may be seen in the efferent ductules and, to a lesser extent, in the epididymis proper (fig. 8-106). It was found in 28 percent of epididymal specimens in one study (220), apparently caused by fusion of several nuclei to form single, large, bizarre nuclei. The degenerative appearance of the nuclei, the focality of the process, and the lack of mitotic activity should facilitate its recognition.

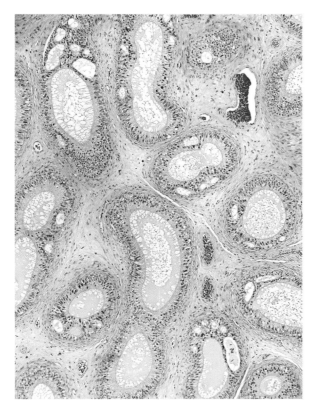

Figure 8-104

NORMAL EPIDIDYMIS

The cribriform appearance of the tubules may cause confusion with adenocarcinoma.

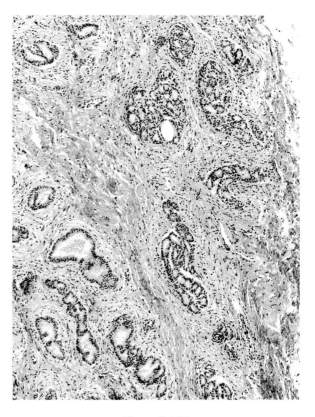

Figure 8-105

CRIBRIFORM HYPERPLASIA OF EFFERENT DUCTULES

There is a vaguely lobular arrangement of cribriform structures adjacent to identifiable efferent ductules.

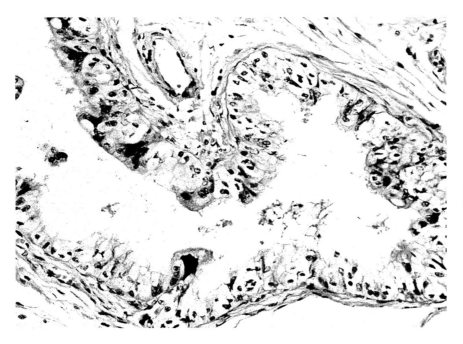

Figure 8-106

NORMAL EPIDIDYMIS

Degenerative nuclear features similar to those often seen in the seminal vesicles are present.

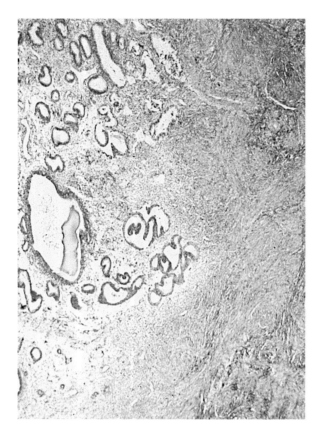

Figure 8-107

ENDOMETRIOSIS ADJACENT TO EPIDIDYMIS

Endometrial-type glands and stroma (left) are adjacent to smooth muscle (right) (trichrome stain).

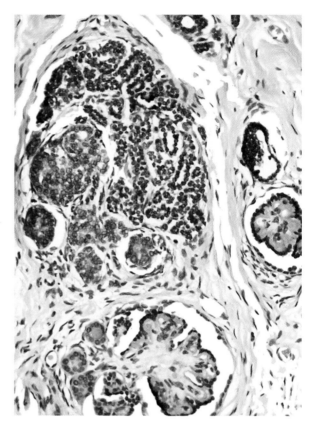

Figure 8-108

METANEPHRIC DYSPLASTIC HAMARTOMA OF EPIDIDYMIS

Immature tissue of renal type formed an epididymal mass.

MISCELLANEOUS OTHER LESIONS

Rare *uterus-like structures* occur in the paratesticular region of phenotypically normal men. They are composed of endometrial-type glands and stroma surrounded by bundles of smooth muscle (fig. 8-107) (221). One lesion arose in an 82-year-old man who had received diethylstilbestrol for carcinoma of the prostate gland and another was associated with clear cell carcinoma (222). Additional rare lesions include: *prostatic glands in the epididymis (223), osseous metaplasia of the epididymis (66),* several cases of a *spermatic cord mass* caused by a necrotic, granulomatous reaction induced by the injection of a sclerosing agent ("alparene no. 2") for the treatment of inguinal hernia (224), at least one case each of an *ossified calcific nodule (225)* and *fatty metaplasia (226), talc or*

starch granulomas causing masses (227,228), *congenital testicular lymphangiectasia* (229), *secondary oxalosis* associated with a sperm granuloma that formed a mass (230), *testicular amyloidosis* (231,232), and a *granulomatous nodule* in the vas deferens with stromal and epithelial atypia attributed to contrast medium (233). Examination of unexplained granulomatous lesions, particularly of the paratesticular region, by polarized light is crucial in elucidating the nature of those due to foreign material.

We have seen one example of *metanephric dysplastic hamartoma* (234) that occurred as an epididymal mass discovered at the time of surgery for a hernia repair in an 18-month-old boy. Microscopic examination showed scattered blastema with papillae, glomeruloid formations, and dysplastic tubules (fig. 8-108). Our personal experience with this process is limited to this

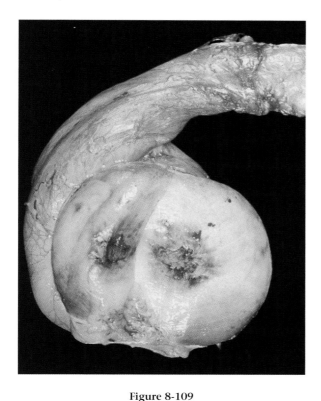

Figure 8-109

RADIATION FIBROSIS

Most of the testis is firm and white, potentially simulating a neoplasm.

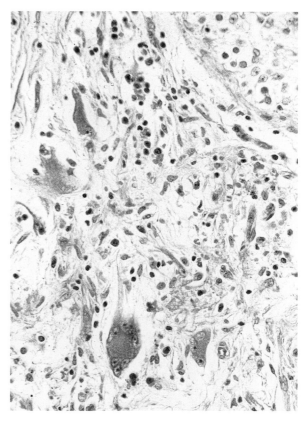

Figure 8-110

ATYPICAL STROMAL CELLS

Some cells are mononucleated and others are multinucleated. The nucleoli are conspicuous. A portion of a seminiferous tubule is seen at the top right.

one case, which was seen in consultation by Dr. Louis P. Dehner (Washington University School of Medicine, St. Louis, MO). Although the exact nature of this process is uncertain, its small size and the scattered presence of the immature elements without the usual confluence of a Wilms tumor are features that favor a peculiar, apparently benign process, rather than an extrarenal Wilms tumor.

We have seen a case of *radiation injury* to the testis that imparted a white, fibrotic tumor-like aspect (fig. 8-109) and also a case of *testicular edema* that mimicked a neoplasm on clinical examination, prompting orchiectomy. The edema was probably related to a coexistent hydrocele. Finally, *atypical mononucleated or multinucleated stromal cells of fibroblastic or myofibroblastic nature* may be seen in the testis (fig. 8-110) (235,236). In one series these were found in about 40 percent of cases at autopsy, with no clear etiology (235). In the most striking case we have seen, they were associated with idiopathic granulomatous orchitis (fig. 8-110).

REFERENCES

1. Mikuz G, Damjanov I. Inflammation of the testis, epididymis, peritesticular membranes, and scrotum. Pathol Annu 1982;17(Pt 1):101-28.
2. Morgan AD. Inflammatory lesions simulating malignancy. Br J Urol 1964;36(Suppl):95-102.
3. Collins DH, Pugh RC. Classification and frequency of testicular tumours. Br J Urol 1964;36(Suppl):1-11.
4. Haas GP, Shumaker BP, Cerny JC. The high incidence of benign testicular tumors. J Urol 1986;136:1219-20.
5. Aragona F, Pescatori E, Talenti E, Toma P, Malena S, Glazel GP. Painless scrotal masses in the pediatric population: prevalence and age distribution of different pathological conditions—A 10 year retrospective multicenter study. J Urol 1996;155:1424-6.
6. Nistal M, Paniagua R. Non-neoplastic diseases of the testis. In: Bostwick DG, Cheng L, eds. Urologic surgical pathology. 2nd ed. Philadelphia: Mosby Elsevier; 2008:614-755.
7. Connor DH, Chandler FW, Schwartz DA, Manz HJ, Lack EE. Pathology of infectious diseases. Stamford, CT: Appleton Lange; 1997.
8. Gondos B, Egli CA, Rosenthal SM, Grumbach MM. Testicular changes in gonadotropin-independent familial male sexual precocity. Familial testotoxicosis. Arch Pathol Lab Med 1985;109:990-5.
9. Jemerin EE. Hyperplasia and neoplasia of the interstitial cells of the testicle. Arch Surg 1937;35:967-8.
10. Mark GJ, Hedinger C. Changes in remaining tumor-free testicular tissue in cases of seminoma and teratoma. Virchows Arch Pathol Anat Physiol Klin Med 1965;340:84-92.
11. McDonald JH, Calams JA. A histological study of extraparenchymal Leydig-like cells. J Urol 1958;79:850-8.
12. Nelson AA. Giant interstitial cells and extraparenchymal interstitial cells of the human testis. Am J Pathol 1938;14:831-41.
13. Schedewie HK, Reiter EO, Beitins IZ, et al. Testicular leydig cell hyperplasia as a cause of familial sexual precocity. J Clin Endocrinol Metab 1981;52:271-8.
14. Umiker W. Interstitial cell hyperplasia in association with testicular tumors: a study of its relationship to urinary gonadotrophins, testicular atrophy and histological type of tumor. J Urol 1954;72:895-903.
15. Warren S, Olshausen KW. Interstitial cell growths of the testicle. Am J Pathol 1943;19:307-31.
16. Wierman ME, Beardsworth DE, Mansfield MJ, et al. Puberty without gonadotropins. A unique mechanism of sexual development. N Engl J Med 1985;312:65-72.
17. Halley JB. The infiltrative activity of Leydig cells. J Pathol Bacteriol 1961;81:347-53.
18. Jun SY, Ro JY, Park YW, Kim KR, Ayala AG. Ectopic Leydig cells of testis. An immunohistochemical study on tissue microarray. Ann Diagn Pathol 2008;12:29-32.
19. Halley JB. The growth of sertoli cell tumors: A possible index of differential gonadotrophin activity in the male. J Urol 1963;90:220-9.
20. Hedinger CE, Huber R, Weber E. Frequency of so-called hypoplastic or dysgenetic zones in scrotal and otherwise normal human testes. Virchows Arch Pathol Anat Physiol Klin Med 1967;342:165-8.
21. Vallangeon BD, Eble JN, Ulbright TM. Macroscopic sertoli cell nodule: a study of 6 cases that presented as testicular masses. Am J Surg Pathol 2010;34:1874-80.
22. Barghorn A, Alioth HR, Hailemariam S, Bannwart F, Ulbright TM. Giant Sertoli cell nodule of the testis: distinction from other Sertoli cell lesions. J Clin Pathol 2006;59:1223-5.
23. Carpenter PC, Wahner HW, Salassa RM, Duick DS. Demonstration of steroid-producing gonadal tumors by external scanning with the use of NP-59. Mayo Clin Proc 1979;54:332-4.
24. Chrousos GP, Loriaux DL, Sherins RJ, Cutler GB Jr. Unilateral testicular enlargement resulting from inapparent 21-hydroxylase deficiency. J Urol 1981;126:127-8.
25. Franco-Saenz R, Antonipillai I, Tan SY, McCorquodale M, Kropp K, Mulrow PJ. Cortisol production by testicular tumors in a patient with congenital adrenal hyperplasia (21-hydroxylase deficiency). J Clin Endocrinol Metab 1981;53:85-90.
26. Hamwi GJ, Gwinup G, Mostow JH, Besch PK. Activation of testicular adrenal rest tissue by prolonged excessive ACTH production. J Clin Endocrinol Metab 1963;23:861-9.
27. Miller EC Jr, Murray HL. Congenital adrenocortical hyperplasia: case previously reported as "bilateral interstitial cell tumor of the testicle." J Clin Endocrinol Metab 1962;22:655-7.
28. Rutgers JL, Young RH, Scully RE. The testicular "tumor" of the adrenogenital syndrome. A report of six cases and review of the literature on testicular masses in patients with adrenocortical disorders. Am J Surg Pathol 1988;12:503-13.

29. Paner GP, Kristiansen G, McKenney JK, Amin MB. Rete testis-associated nodular steroid cell nests: Description of putative pluripotential testicular hilus steroid cells. Am J Surg Pathol 2011;35:505-11.

30. Claahsen-van der Grinten HL, Otten BJ, Stikkelbroeck MM, Sweep FC, Hermus AR. Testicular adrenal rest tumours in congenital adrenal hyperplasia. Best Pract Res Clin Endocrinol Metab 2009;23:209-20.

31. Claahsen-van der Grinten HL, Otten BJ, Sweep FC, et al. Testicular tumors in patients with congenital adrenal hyperplasia due to 21-hydroxylase deficiency show functional features of adrenocortical tissue. J Clin Endocrinol Metab 2007;92:3674-80.

32. Davis JM, Woodroof J, Sadasivan R, Stephens R. Case report: congenital adrenal hyperplasia and malignant Leydig cell tumor. Am J Med Sci 1995;309:63-5.

33. Adesokan A, Adegboyega PA, Cowan DF, Kocurek J, Neal DE Jr. Testicular "tumor" of the adrenogenital syndrome: a case report of an unusual association with myelolipoma and seminoma in cryptorchidism. Cancer 1997;80:2120-7.

34. Ashley RA, McGee SM, Isotaolo PA, Kramer SA, Cheville JC. Clinical and pathological features associated with the testicular tumor of the adrenogenital syndrome. J Urol 2007;177:546-9.

35. Wang Z, Yang S, Shi H, et al. Histopathological and immunophenotypic features of testicular tumour of the adrenogenital syndrome. Histopathology 2011;58:1013-8.

36. Rich MA, Keating MA. Leydig cell tumors and tumors associated with congenital adrenal hyperplasia. Urol Clin North Am 2000;27:519-28.

37. Johnson RE, Scheithauer B. Massive hyperplasia of testicular adrenal rests in a patient with Nelson's syndrome. Am J Clin Pathol 1982;77:501-7.

38. Krieger DT, Samojlik E, Bardin CW. Cortisol and androgen secretion in a case of Nelson's syndrome with paratesticular tumors: response to cyproheptadine therapy. J Clin Endocrinol Metab 1978;47:837-44.

39. Carney JA, Gordon H, Carpenter PC, Shenoy BV, Go VL. The complex of myxomas, spotty pigmentation, and endocrine overactivity. Medicine 1985;64:270-83.

40. Rose EK, Enterline HT, Rhoads JE, Rose E. Adrenal cortical hyperfunction in childhood; report of a case with adrenocortical hyperplasia and testicular adrenal rests. Pediatrics 1952;9:475-84.

41. Dahl EV, Bahn RC. Aberrant adrenal cortical tissue near the testis in human infants. Am J Pathol 1962;40:587-98.

42. Delmas V, Dauge MC. [Accessory adrenals in the spermatic cord. Apropos of 2 cases.] Ann Urol 1986;20:261-4. [French]

43. Nelson AA. Accessory adrenal cortical tissue. Arch Pathol 1939;27:955-65.

44. Skoglund RW, McRoberts JW, Ragde H. Torsion of the spermatic cord: a review of the literature and an analysis of 70 new cases. J Urol 1970;104:604-7.

45. Hourihane DO. Infected infarcts of the testis: a study of 18 cases preceded by pyogenic epididymoorchitis. J Clin Pathol 1970;23:668-75.

46. Levine TS. Testicular and epididymal vasculitides. Is morphology a help in classification and prognosis? J Urol Pathol 1994;2:81-8.

47. Gofrit ON, Rund D, Shapiro A, Pappo O, Landau EH, Pode D. Segmental testicular infarction due to sickle cell disease. J Urol 1998;160:835-6.

48. Nayal W, Brassett C, Singh L, Boyd PJ. Segmental testicular ischaemia mimicking testicular tumour. Br J Urol 1996;78:318-9.

49. Sriprisad S, Kooiman GG, Muir GH, Sidhu PS. Acute segmental testicular infarction: differentiation from tumour using high frequency colour Doppler ultrasound. Br J Radiol 2001;74:965-7.

50. Yamashina M, Honma T, Uchijima Y. Myofibroblastic pseudotumor mimicking epididymal sarcoma. A clinicopathologic study of three cases. Pathol Res Pract 1992;188:1054-9.

51. Schned AR, Cendron M. Pathologic findings in the vanishing testis syndrome. J Urol Pathol 1997;6:95-107.

52. Smith NM, Byard RW, Bourne AJ. Testicular regression syndrome—a pathological study of 77 cases. Histopathology 1991;19:269-72.

53. Fan R, Ulbright TM. Does intratubular germ cell neoplasia, unclassified type exist in prepubertal, cryptorchid testes? Fetal Pediatr Pathol 2012;31:21-4.

54. Spires SE, Woolums CS, Pulito AR, Spires SM. Testicular regression syndrome: a clinical and pathologic study of 11 cases. Arch Pathol Lab Med 2000;124:694-8.

55. Dahl EV, Baggenstoss AH, DeWeerd JH. Testicular lesions of periarteritis nodosa with special reference to diagnosis. Am J Med 1960;28:222-8.

56. Shurbaji MS, Epstein JI. Testicular vasculitis: implications for systemic disease. Hum Pathol 1988;19:186-9.

57. Belville WD, Insalaco SJ, Dresner ML, Buck AS. Benign testis tumors. J Urol 1982;128:1198-200.

58. Corless CL, Daut D, Burke R. Localized giant cell vasculitis of the spermatic cord presenting as a mass lesion. J Urol Pathol 1997;6:235-42.

59. Dotan ZA, Laufer M, Heldenberg E, et al. Isolated testicular polyarteritis nodosa mimicking testicular neoplasm-long-term follow-up. Urology 2003;62:352.

60. Womack C, Ansell ID. Isolated arteritis of the epididymis. J Clin Pathol 1985;38:797-800.

61. Palmer-Toy DE, McGovern F, Young RH. Granulomatous orchitis and vasculitis with testicular infarction complicating Crohn's disease: a hitherto undescribed tumor-like lesion of the testis. J Urol Pathol 1999;11:143-50.

62. Rolnick D, Kawanoue S, Szanto P, Bush IM. Anatomical incidence of testicular appendages. J Urol 1968;100:755-6.

63. Sundarasivarao D. The müllerian vestiges and benign epithelial tumors of the epididymis. J Pathol Bacteriol 1953;66:417-32.

64. Arcadi JA. Torsion of the appendix epididymis: an unusual urological entity. J Urol 1963;89:467-9.

65. Nöske HD, Kraus SW, Altinkilic BM, Weidner W. Historical milestones regarding torsion of the scrotal organs. J Urol 1998;159:13-6.

66. Srigley JR, Hartwick RW. Tumors and cysts of the paratesticular region. Pathol Annu 1990;25(Pt 2):51-108.

67. Celen MK, Ulug M, Ayaz C, Geyik MF, Hosoglu S. Brucellar epididymo-orchitis in southeastern part of Turkey: an 8 year experience. Braz J Infect Dis 2010;14:109-15.

68. Routh JC, Lischer GH, Leibovich BC. Epididymo-orchitis and testicular abscess due to Nocardia asteroides complex. Urology 2005;65:591.

69. Honore LH. Nonspecific peritesticular fibrosis manifested as testicular enlargement. Arch Surg 1978;113:814-6.

70. Hill JR, Gorgon G, Wahl SJ, Armenakas NA, Fracchia JA. Xanthogranulomatous orchitis in a patient with a history of instrumentation and bacillus Calmette-Guerin therapy. Urology 2008;72:461-3.

71. Al-Said S, Ali A, Alobaidy AK, Mojeeb E, Al-Naimi A, Shokeir AA. Xanthogranulomatous orchitis: review of the published work and report of one case. Int J Urol 2007;14:452-4.

72. Fernandopulle SM, Hwang JS, Kuick CH, et al. Rosai-Dorfman disease of the testis: an unusual entity that mimics testicular malignancy. J Clin Pathol 2006;59:325-7.

73. Morgan AD. Inflammation and infestation of the testis and paratesticular structures. In: Pugh RC, ed. Pathology of the testis. Oxford: Blackwell Scientific; 1976:79-138.

74. Gall EA. The histopathology of acute mumps orchitis. Am J Pathol 1947;23:637-51.

75. Craighead JE, Mahoney EM, Carver DH, Naficy K, Fremont-Smith P. Orchitis due to Coxsackie virus group B, type 5. Report of a case with isolation of virus from the testis. N Engl J Med 1962;267:498-500.

76. Braaten KM, Young RH, Ferry JA. Viral-type orchitis: a potential mimic of testicular neoplasia. Am J Surg Pathol 2009;33:1477-84.

77. Mukamel E, Abarbanel J, Savion M, Konichezky M, Yachia D, Auslaender L. Testicular mass as a presenting symptom of isolated polyarteritis nodosa. Am J Clin Pathol 1995;103:215-7.

78. Kameyama K, Kuramochi S, Kamio N, Akasaka Y, Higa I, Hata J. Isolated periarteritis nodosa of the spermatic cord presenting as a scrotal mass: report of a case. Heart Ves 1998;13:152-4.

79. Jauhola O, Ronkainen J, Koskimies O, et al. Clinical course of extrarenal symptoms in Henoch-Schonlein purpura: a 6-month prospective study. Arch Dis Child 2010;95:871-6.

80. Pannek J, Haupt G. Orchitis due to vasculitis in autoimmune diseases. Scand J Rheumatol 1997;26:151-4.

81. Maillefert JF, De Wazieres B, Meignan F. Orchitis: an unusual feature in relapsing polychondritis. J Rheumatol 1994;21:1378-9.

82. MacIver H, Hordon L. An unusual case of testicular pain. Clin Rheumatol 2009;28:351-2.

83. Kuehn MW, Oellinger R, Kustin G, Merkel KH. Primary testicular manifestation of systemic lupus erythematosus. Eur Urol 1989;16:72-3.

84. Boulis ER, Majithia V. Orchitis in lupus/scleroderma overlap syndrome: a case report and literature review. Can J Urol 2010;17:5306-8.

85. Sundaram S, Smith DH. Giant cell arteritis mimicking a testicular tumour. Rheumatol Int 2001;20:215-6.

86. Ferrie BG, Rundle JS. Tuberculous epididymo-orchitis. A review of 20 cases. Br J Urol 1983;55:437-9.

87. Wechsler H, Westfall M, Lattimer JK. The earliest signs and symptoms in 127 male patients with genitourinary tuberculosis. J Urol 1960;83:801-3.

88. Harada H, Seki M, Shinojima H, Miura M, Hirano T, Togashi M. Epididymo-orchitis caused by intravesically instilled bacillus Calmette-Guerin: genetically proven using a multiplex polymerase chain reaction method. Int J Urol 2006;13:183-5.

89. Kanomata N, Eble JN. Fungal epididymitis caused by Histoplasm caspulatum. J Urol Pathol 1997;5:229-34.

90. Haddad FS. Coccidioidomycosis of the genitourinary tract with special emphasis on the epididymis and the prostate. J Urol Pathol 1996;4:205-11.

91. Menninger WC. Congenital syphilis of the testicle. With report of twelve autopsied cases. Am J Syphilis 1928;12:221-34.

92. Grabstald H, Swan LL. Genitourinary lesions in leprosy, with special reference to the problem of atrophy of the testes. J Am Med Assoc 1952;119;1287-91.

93. Spjut HJ, Thorpe JD. Granulomatous orchitis. Am J Clin Pathol 1956;26:136-45.

94. Perimenis P, Athanasopoulos A, Venetsanou-Petrochilou C, Barbalias G. Idiopathic granulomatous orchitis. Eur Urol 1991;19:118-20.

95. Wiener LB, Riehl PA, Baum N. Xanthogranulomatous epididymitis: a case report. J Urol 1987;138:621-2.

96. Yantiss RK, Young RH. Idiopathic granulomatous epidiymitis: report of a case and review of the literature. J Urol Pathol 1998;8:171-9.

97. Nistal M, Mate A, Paniagua R. Granulomatous epididymal lesion of possible ischemic origin. Am J Surg Pathol 1997;21:951-6.

98. Ryan DM, Lesser BA, Crumley LA, et al. Epididymal sarcoidosis. J Urol 1993;149:134-6.

99. McClure J. Malakoplakia. J Pathol 1983;140:275-330.

100. McClure J. Malakoplakia of the testis and its relationship to granulomatous orchitis. J Clin Pathol 1980;33:670-8.

101. Stevens SA. Malakoplakia of the testis. Br J Urol 1995;75:111-2.

102. Azoury FJ, Reed RJ. Histiocytosis. Report of an unusual case. N Engl J Med 1966;274:928-30.

103. Foucar E, Rosai J, Dorfman R. Sinus histiocytosis with massive lymphadenopathy (Rosai-Dorfman disease): review of the entity. Semin Diagn Pathol 1990;7:19-73.

104. Lossos IS, Okon E, Bogomolski-Yahalom V, Ron N, Polliack A. Sinus histiocytosis with massive lymphadenopathy (Rosai-Dorfman disease): report of a patient with isolated renotesticular involvement after cure of non-Hodgkin's lymphoma. Ann Hematol 1997;74:41-4.

105. King ES. Squamous epithelium in encysted hydrocele of the cord. A note on squamous epithelium of peritoneal origin. Aust N Z J Surg 1951;20:265-71.

106. Kokotas N, Kontogeorgos L, Kyriakidis A. Calcification of the tunica vaginalis. Br J Urol 1983;55:128.

107. Lowenthal SB, Goldstein AM, Terry R. Cholesterol granuloma of tunica vaginalis simulating testicular tumor. Urology 1981;18:89-90.

108. Churg A. Paratesticular mesothelial proliferations. Semin Diagn Pathol 2003;20:272-8.

109. Lane Z, Epstein JI. Small blue cells mimicking small cell carcinoma in spermatocele and hydrocele specimens: a report of 5 cases. Hum Pathol 2010;41:88-93.

110. Hollowood K, Fletcher CD. Pseudosarcomatous myofibroblastic proliferations of the spermatic cord ("prolifertive funiculitis"): histologic and immunohistochemical analysis of a distinctive entity. Am J Surg Pathol 1992;16:448-54.

111. Khalil KH, Ball RY, Eardley I, Ashken MH. Inflammatory pseudotumor of the rete testis. J Urol Pathol 1996;5:39-43.

112. Lam KY, Chan KW, Ho MH. Inflammatory pseudotumour of the epididymis. Br J Urol 1995;75:255-7.

113. Melamed MR, Farrow GM. Case of fibromyxomatous pseudotumor of the spermatic cord. In: Urologic neoplasms: based on the proceedings of the 50th Annual Anatomic Pathology Slide Seminar of the American Society of Clinical Pathologists. Chicago: ASCP Press; 1987:124-7.

114. Nishimura T, Akimoto M, Kawai H, Ohba S, Ohto S. Peritesticular xanthogranuloma. Urology 1981;18:189-90.

115. Piscioli F, Polla E, Pusiol T, Failoni G, Luciani L. Pseudomalignant cytologic presentation of spermatic hydrocele fluid. Acta Cytol 1983;27:666-70.

116. Milanezi MF, Schmitt F. Pseudosarcomatous myofibroblastic proliferation of the spermatic cord (proliferative funiculitis). Histopathology 1997;31:387-8.

117. Chan KW, Chan KL, Lam KY. Inflammatory pseudotumor of epididymis and Epstein-Barr virus: a study of two cases. Pathology 1997;29:100-1.

118. Michal M, Hes O, Kazakov DV. Mesothelial glandular structures within pseudosarcomatous proliferative funiculitis—a diagnostic pitfall: report of 17 cases. Int J Surg Pathol 2008;16:48-56.

119. Kraus MD, Guillou L, Fletcher CD. Well-differentiated inflammatory liposarcoma: an uncommon and easily overlooked variant of a common sarcoma. Am J Surg Pathol 1997;21:518-27.

120. Hollowood K, Fletcher CD. Soft tissue sarcomas that mimic benign lesions. Semin Diagn Pathol 1995;12:87-97.

121. Meis JM, Enzinger FM. Inflammatory fibrosarcoma of the mesentery and retroperitoneum. A tumor closely simulating inflammatory pseudotumor. Am J Surg Pathol 1991;15:1146-56.

122. Bëgin LR, Frail D, Brzezinski A. Myofibroblastoma of the tunica testis: evolving phase of so- called fibrous pseudotumor? Hum Pathol 1990;21:866-8.

123. Elem B, Patil PS, Lambert TK. Giant fibrous pseudotumor of the testicular tunics in association with Schistosoma haematobium infection. J Urol 1989;141:376-7.

124. Goodwin WE. Multiple, benign, fibrous tumors of tunica vaginalis testis. J Urol 1946;56:438-47.

125. Meyer AW. Corpora libera in the tunica vaginalis testis. Am J Pathol 1928;4:445-56.

126. Nistal M, Paniagua R, Torres A, Hidalgo L, Regadera J. Idiopathic peritesticular fibrosis associated with retroperitoneal fibrosis. Eur Urol 1986;12:64-8.

127. Parveen T, Fleischmann J, Petrelli M. Benign fibrous tumor of the tunica vaginalis testis. Report of a case with light, electron microscopic, and immunocytochemical study, and review of the literature. Arch Pathol Lab Med 1992;116:277-80.

128. Sen S, Patterson DE, Sandoval O Jr, Wold L. Testicular adnexal fibrous pseudotumors. Urology 1984;23:594-7.

129. Thompson JE, van der Walt JD. Nodular fibrous proliferation (fibrous pseudotumour) of the tunica vaginalis testis. A light, electron microscopic and immunocytochemical study of a case and review of the literature. Histopathology 1986;10:741-8.

130. Vates TS, Ruemmler-Fisch C, Smilow PC, Fleisher MH. Benign fibrous testicular pseudotumors in children. J Urol 1993;150:1886-8.

131. Cooper A. Observations on the structure and diseases of the testis. London, Longman, Rees, Orme, Brown, & Green; 1830.

132. Mostofi FK, Price EB Jr. Tumors of the male genital system. Atlas of Tumor Pathology, 2nd Series, Fascicle 8. Washington D.C.: Armed Forces Institute of Pathology; 1973.

133. Miyamoto H, Montgomery EA, Epstein JI. Paratesticular fibrous pseudotumor: a morphologic and immunohistochemical study of 13 cases. Am J Surg Pathol 2010;34:569-74.

134. Seethala RR, Tirkes AT, Weinstein S, Tomaszewski JE, Malkowicz SB, Genega EM. Diffuse fibrous pseudotumor of the testicular tunics associated with an inflamed hydrocele. Arch Pathol Lab Med 2003;127:742-4.

135. Watson RA, Harper BN. Paratesticular fibrous pseudotumor in a patient with Gorlin's syndrome: nevoid basal cell carcinoma syndrome. J Urol 1992;148:1254-5.

136. Fetsch JF, Montgomery EA, Meis JM. Calcifying fibrous pseudotumor. Am J Surg Pathol 1993;17:502-8.

137. Nascimento AF, Ruiz R, Hornick JL, Fletcher CD. Calcifying fibrous 'pseudotumor': clinicopathologic study of 15 cases and analysis of its relationship to inflammatory myofibroblastic tumor. Int J Surg Pathol 2002;10:189-96.

138. Shafik A. Constrictive albuginitis: report of 3 cases. J Urol 1979;122:269-71.

139. Dehner LP, Scott D, Stocker JT. Meconium periorchitis: a clinicopathologic study of four cases with a review of the literature. Hum Pathol 1986;17:807-12.

140. Stokes S 3rd, Flom S. Meconium filled hydrocele sacs as a cause of acute scrotum in a newborn. J Urol 1997;158:1960-1.

141. Mene M, Rosenberg HK, Ginsberg PC. Meconium periorchitis presenting as scrotal nodules in a five year old boy. J Ultrasound Med 1994;13:491-4.

142. Jeanty C, Bircher A, Turner C. Prenatal diagnosis of meconium periorchitis and review of the literature. J Ultrasound Med 2009;28:1729-34.

143. Rosai J, Dehner LP. Nodular mesothelial hyperplasia in hernia sacs: a benign reactive condition simulating a neoplastic process. Cancer 1975;35:165-75.

144. McCaughey WT, Al-Jabi M. Differentiation of serosal hyperplasia and neoplasia in biopsies. Pathol Annu 1986;21(Pt 1):271-93.

145. Ordonez NG, Ro JY, Ayala AG. Lesions described as nodular mesothelial hyperplasia are primarily composed of histiocytes. Am J Surg Pathol 1998;22:285-92.

146. Oertel YC, Johnson FB. Sclerosing lipogranuloma of male genitalia. Review of 23 cases. Arch Pathol Lab Med 1977;101:321-6.

147. Watanabe K, Hoshi N, Baba K, Fukuda T, Hakozaki H, Suzuki T. Immunohistochemical profile of primary sclerosing lipogranuloma of the scrotum: report of five cases. Pathol Int 1995;45:854-9.

148. Bussey LA, Norman RW, Gupta R. Sclerosing lipogranuloma: an unusual scrotal mass. Can J Urol 2002;9:1464-9.

149. Young RH, Scully RE. Testicular tumors. Chicago: ASCP Press; 1990.

150. Rosenthal SM, Grumbach MM, Kaplan SL. Gonadotropin-independent familial sexual precocity with premature Leydig and germinal cell maturation (familial testotoxicosis): effects of a potent luteinizing hormone-releasing factor agonist and medroxyprogesterone acetate therapy in four cases. J Clin Endocrinol Metab 1983;57:571-9.

151. Wierman ME, Beardsworth DE, Mansfield MJ, et al. Puberty without gonadotropins. A unique mechanism of sexual development. N Engl J Med 1985;312:65-72.

152. Nisula BC, Loriaux DL, Sherins RJ, Kulin HE. Benign bilateral testicular enlargement. J Clin Endocrinol Metab 1974;38:440-5.

153. Hartwick RW, Ro JY, Srigley JR, Ordoñez NG, Ayala AG. Adenomatous hyperplasia of the rete testis. A clinicopathologic study of nine cases. Am J Surg Pathol 1991;15:350-7.

154. Nistal M, Paniagua R. Adenomatous hyperplasia of the rete testis. J Pathol 1988;154:343-6.

155. Rosenberg R, Williamson MR. Lipomas of the spermatic cord and testis: report of two cases. J Clin Ultrasound 1989;17:670-4.

156. Ulbright TM, Gersell DJ. Rete testis hyperplasia with hyaline globule formation. A lesion simulating yolk sac tumor. Am J Surg Pathol 1991;15:66-74.

157. Nistal M, Regadera J, Paniagua R. Cystic dysplasia of the testis: light and electron microscopic study of three cases. Arch Pathol Lab Med 1984;108:579-83.

158. Tesluk H, Blankenberg TA. Cystic dysplasia of testis. Urology 1987;29:47-9.

159. Wegmann W, Illi O, Kummer-Vago M. [Cystic testis dysplasia with ipsilateral kidney agenesis]. Schweiz Med Wochenschr 1984;114:144-8. [German]

160. Wojcik LJ, Hansen K, Diamond DA, et al. Cystic dysplasia of the rete testis: a benign congenital lesion associated with ipsilateral urological anomalies. J Urol 1997;158:600-4.

161. Loo CK, Yung T. Cystic dysplasia of the testis: a report of three cases and review of the literature. Pediatr Pathol Lab Med 1995;15:885-93.

162. Camassei FD, Francalanci P, Ferro F, Capozza N, Boldrini R. Cystic dysplasia of the rete testis: report of two cases and review of the literature. Pediatr Dev Pathol 2002;5:206-10.

163. Eberli D, Gretener H, Dommann-Scherrer C, Pestalozzi D, Fehr JL. Cystic dysplasia of the testis: a very rare paediatric tumor of the testis. Urol Int 2002;69:1-6.

164. Nistal M, Santamaria L, Paniagua R. Acquired cystic transformation of the rete testis secondary to renal failure. Hum Pathol 1989;20:1065-70.

165. Fridman E, Skarda J, Ofek-Moravsky E, Cordoba M. Complex multilocular cystic lesion of rete testis, accompanied by smooth muscle hyperplasia, mimicking intratesticular Leydig cell neoplasm. Virchows Arch 2005;447:768-71.

166. Nistal M, Garcia-Cabezas MA, Castello MC, et al. Age-related epididymis-like intratesticular structures: benign lesions of Wolffian origin that can be misdiagnosed as testicular tumors. J Androl 2006;27:79-85.

167. Nistal M, Paniagua R. Nodular proliferation of calcifying connective tissue in the rete testis: a study of three cases. Hum Pathol 1989;20:58-61.

167a. Younger C, Ulbright TM, Zhang S, et al. Molecular evidence supporting the neoplastic nature of some epidermoid cysts of the testis. Arch Pathol Lab Med 2003;127:858-60.

168. Price EB Jr. Epidermoid cysts of the testis: a clinical and pathologic analysis of 69 cases from the testicular tumor registry. J Urol 1969;102:708-13.

169. Shah KH, Maxted WC, Chun B. Epidermoid cysts of the testis: a report of three cases and an analysis of 141 cases from the world literature. Cancer 1981;47:577-82.

170. Manivel JC, Reinberg Y, Niehans GA, Fraley EE. Intratubular germ cell neoplasia in testicular teratomas and epidermoid cysts. Correlation with prognosis and possible biologic significance. Cancer 1989;64:715-20.

171. Dieckmann KP, Loy V. Epidermoid cyst of the testis: a review of clinical and histogenetic considerations. Br J Urol 1994;73:436-41.

172. Reinberg Y, Manivel JC, Llerena J, Niehans G, Fraley EE. Epidermoid cyst (monodermal teratoma) of the testis. Br J Urol 1990;66:648-51.

173. Heidenreich A, Zumbe J, Vorreuther R, Klotz T, Vietsch H, Engelmann UH. [Testicular epidermoid cyst: orchiectomy or enucleation resection?]. Urologe A 1996;35:1-5. [German]

174. Cheng L, Zhang S, MacLennan GT, et al. Interphase fluorescence in situ hybridization analysis of chromosome 12p abnormalities is useful for distinguishing epidermoid cysts of the testis from pure mature teratoma. Clin Cancer Res 2006;12:5668-72.

175. Chou SJ, Liu HY, Fu YT, Shyu JS, Sun GH. Cysts of the tunica albuginea. Arch Androl 2004;50:89-92.

176. Nistal M, Iniguez L, Paniagua R. Cysts of the testicular parenchyma and tunica albuginea. Arch Pathol Lab Med 1989;113:902-6.

177. Tejada E, Eble JN. Simple cyst of the rete testis. J Urol 1988;139:376-7.

178. Davis RS. Intratesticular spermatocele. Urology 1998;51:167-9.

179. Schned AR, Seremetis GM, Rous SN. Paratesticular multicystic mass of Wolffian, probably paradidymal, origin. Am J Clin Pathol 1994;101:543-6.

180. Eason AA, Spaulding JT. Dermoid cyst arising in testicular tunics. J Urol 1977;117:539.

181. Ford J Jr, Singh S. Paratesticular dermoid cyst in 6-month-old infant. J Urol 1988;139:89-90.

182. Perez-Ordonez B, Srigley JR. Mesothelial lesions of the paratesticular region. Semin Diagn Pathol 2000;17:294-306.

183. Weiss SW, Tavassoli FA. Multicystic mesothelioma. An analysis of pathologic findings and biologic behavior in 37 cases. Am J Surg Pathol 1988;12:737-46.

184. McFadden DE, Clement PB. Peritoneal inclusion cysts with mural mesothelial proliferation. A clinicopathological analysis of six cases. Am J Surg Pathol 1986;10:844-54.

185. Warner KE, Noyes DT, Ross JS. Cysts of the tunica albuginea testis: a report of 3 cases with review of the literature. J Urol 1984;132:131-2.

186. Van Niekerk WA. True hermaphroditism. Pediatr Adolesc Endocrinol 1981;8:80-99.

187. Coetzee T. Pulmonary alveolar microlithiasis with involvement of the sympathetic nervous system and gonads. Thorax 1970;25:637-42.

188. Priebe CJ Jr, Garret R. Testicular calcification in a 4-year-old boy. Pediatrics 1970;46:785-8.

189. Furness PD, Husmann DA, Brock JW, et al. Multi-institutional study of testicular microlithiasis in childhood: a benign or premalignant condition? J Urol 1998;160:1151-4.

190. Mullins TL, Sant GR, Ucci AA Jr, Doherty FJ. Testicular microlithiasis occurring in postorchiopexy testis. Urology 1986;27:144-6.

191. Renshaw AA. Testicular calcifications: incidence, histology and proposed pathological criteria for testicular microlithiasis. J Urol 1998;160:1625-8.

192. Weinberg AG, Currarino G, Stone IC Jr. Testicular microlithiasis. Arch Pathol 1973;95:312-4.

193. Ahmad I, Krishna NS, Clark R, Nairn R, Al-Saffar N. Testicular microlithiasis: prevalence and risk of concurrent and interval development of testicular tumor in a referred population. Int Urol Nephrol 2007;39:1177-81.

194. DeCastro BJ, Peterson AC, Costabile RA, DeCastro BJ, Peterson AC, Costabile RA. A 5-year followup study of asymptomatic men with testicular microlithiasis. J Urol 2008;179:1420-3.

195. Korde LA, Premkumar A, Mueller C, et al. Increased prevalence of testicular microlithiasis in men with familial testicular cancer and their relatives. Br J Cancer 2008;99:1748-53.

196. Wakely CP. Cysts of the epididymis, the so-called spermatocele. Br J Surg 1943;31:165-71.

197. Walsh TJ, Seeger KT, Turek PJ. Spermatoceles in adults: when does size matter? Arch Androl 2007;53:345-8.

198. Humphrey PA, Kaleem Z, Swanson PE, Vollmer RT. Pseudohyperplastic prostatic adenocarcinoma. Am J Surg Pathol 1998;22:1239-46.

199. Jassie MP, Mahmood P. Torsion of spermatocele: a newly described entity with 2 case reports. J Urol 1985;133:683-4.

200. Takimoto K, Okamoto K, Wakabayashi Y, Okada Y. Torsion of spermatocele: a rare manifestation. Urol Int 2002;69:164-5.

201. Cullen TH, Voss HJ. Sperm granulomata of the testis and epididymis. Br J Urol 1966;38:202-7.

202. Friedman NB, Garske GL. Inflammatory reactions involving sperm and the seminiferous tubules; extravasation, spermatic granulomas and granulomatous orchitis. J Urol 1949;62:363-74.

203. Glassy FJ, Mostofi FK. Spermatic granulomas of the epididymis. Am J Clin Pathol 1956;26:1303-13.

204. Schmidt SS, Morris RR. Spermatic granuloma: the complication of vasectomy. Fertil Steril 1973;24:941-7.

205. Leader AJ, Axelrad SD, Frankowski R, Mumford SD. Complications of 2,711 vasectomies. J Urol 1974;111:365-9.

206. Schmidt SS. Technics and complications of elective vasectomy. The role of spermatic granuloma in spontaneous recanalization. Fertil Steril 1966;17:467-82.

207. Benjamin JA. Vasitis nodosa: a new clinical entity simulating tuberculosis of the vas deferens. J Urol 1943;49:575-82.

208. Kiser GC, Fuchs EF, Kessler S. The significance of vasitis nodosa. J Urol 1986;136:42-4.

209. Schned AR, Selikowitz SM. Epididymitis nodosa. An epididymal lesion analogous to vasitis nodosa. Arch Pathol Lab Med 1986;110:61-4.

210. Stout AP. Conditions of the epididymis simulating carcinoma. Proc New York Pathol Soc 1917:129-37.

211. Civantos F, Lubin J, Rywlin AM. Vasitis nodosa. Arch Pathol 1972;94:355-61.

212. Balogh K, Travis WD. The frequency of perineurial ductules in vasitis nodosa. Am J Clin Pathol 1984;82:710-3.

213. Goldman RL, Azzopardi JG. Benign neural invasion in vasitis nodosa. Histopathology 1982;6:309-15.

214. Kovi J, Agbata A. Letter: Benign neural invasion in vasitis nodosa. JAMA 1974;228:1519.

215. Heaton JM, MacLennan KA. Vasitis nodosa—a site of arrest of malignant germ cells. Histopathology 1986;10:981-9.

216. Putschar WG, Manion WC. Splenic-gonadal fusion. Am J Pathol 1956;32:15-33.

217. Walther MM, Trulock TS, Finnerty DP, Woodard J. Splenic gonadal fusion. Urology 1988;32:521-4.

218. Barton JH, Davis CJ Jr, Sesterhenn IA, Mostofi FK. Smooth muscle hyperplasia of the testicular adnexa clinically mimicking neoplasia: clinicopathologic study of sixteen cases. Am J Surg Pathol 1999;23:903-9.

219. Shah VI, Ro JY, Amin MB, Mullick S, Nazeer T, Ayala AG. Histologic variations in the epididymis: findings in 167 orchiectomy specimens. Am J Surg Pathol 1998;22:990-6.

220. Kuo T, Gomez LG. Monstrous epithelial cells in human epididymis and seminal vesicles. A pseudomalignant change. Am J Surg Pathol 1981;5:483-90.

221. Young RH, Scully RE. Testicular and paratesticular tumors and tumor-like lesions of ovarian common epithelial and mullerian types. A report of four cases and review of the literature. Am J Clin Pathol 1986;86:146-52.

222. Tulunay O, Gogus C, Baltaci S, Bulut S. Clear cell adenocarcinoma of the tunica vaginalis of the testis with an adjacent uterus-like tissue. Pathol Int 2004;54:641-7.

223. Bromberg WD, Kozlowski JM, Oyasu R. Prostate-type gland in the epididymis. J Urol 1991;145:1273-4.

224. Kaplan L. Granulomas due to "alparene no. 2" used in injection treatment of hernia. J Am Med Assoc 1952;151:1188-90.

225. Yoneda F, Kagawa S, Kurokawa K. Dystrophic calcifying nodule with osteoid metaplasia of the testis. Br J Urol 1979;51:413.

226. Honore LH. Fatty metaplasia in a postpubertal undescended testis: a case report. J Urol 1979;122:841-2.

227. Healey GB, McDonald DF. Talc granuloma presenting as a testicular mass. J Urol 1977;118(Pt 1): 122.

228. Pugh JI, Stringer P. Glove-powder granuloma of the testis after surgery. Br J Surg 1973;60:240-2.

229. Nistal M, Paniagua R. Congenital testicular lymphangiectasis. Virchows Arch A Pathol Anat Histol 1977;377:79-84.

230. Coyne J, al-Nakib L, Goldsmith D, O'Flynn K. Secondary oxalosis and sperm granuloma of the epididymis. J Clin Pathol 1994;47:470-1.

231. Casella R, Nudell D, Cozzolino D, Wang H, Lipshultz LI. Primary testicular amyloidosis mimicking tumor in a cryptorchid testis. Urology 2002;59:445.

232. Handelsman DJ, Yue DK, Turtle JR. Hypogonadism and massive testicular infiltration due to amyloidosis. J Urol 1983;129:610-2.

233. Talerman A. Granulomatous lesions in the vas deferens caused by injection of radiopaque contrast medium. J Urol 1972;107:818-20.

234. Cozzutto C, Stracca-Pansa V, Salano F. Renal dysplasia of the sacral region: metanephric dysplastic hamartoma of the sacral region. Virchows Arch A Pathol Anat Histopathol 1983;402:88-106.

235. Coyne JD, Dervan PA. Multinucleated stromal giant cells of testis. Histopathology 1997;31:381-3.

236. Schofield JB, Evans DJ. Multinucleate giant stromal cells in testicular atrophy following oestrogen therapy. Histopathology 1990;16:200-1.

Index*

*In a series of numbers, those in boldface indicate the main discussion of the entity.

D

E

F